Current Topics in Pathology

Continuation of Ergebnisse der Pathologie

69

Editors

C. L. Berry E. Grundmann W. H. Kirsten

Drug-Induced Pathology

Contributors

H.W. Altmann, H.-J. Barrach, H.V. Gärtner
M. Habs, H. Jick, H.G. Laberke, H.-J. Merker
D. Neubert, E. Perucca, A. Richens
T. Riemenschneider, D. Schmähl

Editor
E. Grundmann

With 94 Figures

Springer-Verlag Berlin Heidelberg New York 1980

C.L. Berry, Professor Dr., Department of Morbid Anatomy, The London Hospital Medical College, University of London, London E1 1BB, Great Britain

E. Grundmann, Professor Dr., Pathologisches Institut der Universität, Westring 17, D-4400 Münster/Westf., Germany

W.H. Kirsten, Professor Dr., Department of Pathology, The University of Chicago, 950 East 59th Street, Chicago, IL 60637, USA

ISBN-13:978-3-642-67863-9 e-ISBN-13:978-3-642-67861-5
DOI: 10.1007/978-3-642-67861-5

Library of Congress Cataloging in Publication Data. Main entry under title: Drug-induced pathology. (Current topics in pathology; 69) Bibliography: p. 1. Drugs – Toxicology. 2. Drugs – Side effects. I. Altmann, Hans-Werner, 1916- II. Grundmann, Ekkehard. III. Series. [DNLM: 1. Drug therapy – Adverse effects. 2. Kidney diseases – Chemically induced. W1 Cu821H v. 69 / QZ42 D793]. RB1.E6 vol. 69 [RA1238] 616.07s [615.9] 80-24184 ISBN-13:978-3-642-67863-9 (U.S.)

Softcover reprint of the hardcover 1st edition 1980

2122/3130 – 543210

Contents

Epidemiological Observation on Drug-Induced Illness.
H. Jick 1

The Pathophysiological Basis of Drug Toxicity. With 4 Figures
E. Perucca, A. Richens 17

Drug-Induced Liver Reactions: A Morphological Approach. With 27 Figures
H.W. Altmann 69

Drug-Associated Nephropathy. Part I: Glomerular Lesions. With 5 Figures
H.-V. Gärtner 143

Drug-Associated Nephropathy. Part II: Tubulo-Interstitial Lesions. A: Acute Interstitial Nephritis, Nephrotoxic Lesions, Analgesic Nephropathy. With 5 Figures
H.G. Laberke 183

Drug-Associated Nephropathy. Part II: Tubulo-Interstitial Lesions. B: Hypokalemic Alterations. With 4 Figures
Th. Riemenschneider 217

Drug-Induced Damage to the Embryo or Fetus. (Molecular and Multilateral Approach to Prenatal Toxicology). With 43 Figures
D. Neubert, H.-J. Barrach, H.-J. Merker 241

Drug-Induced Cancer. With 6 Figures
D. Schmähl, M. Habs 333

Subject Index 371

Indexed in ISR

List of Contributors

Altmann, Prof. Dr. H.-W.	Pathologisches Institut der Universität Würzburg, Luitpoldkrankenhaus, 8700 Würzburg, Germany
Barrach, Dr. H.-J.	Institut für Toxikologie und Embryopharmakologie, Freie Universität Berlin, Garystraße 9, 1000 Berlin 33, Germany
Gärtner, Dr. H.-V.	Pathologisches Institut der Universität Tübingen, Liebermeisterstraße 8, 7400 Tübingen, Germany
Habs, Dr. M.	Institut für Toxikologie und Chemotherapie, Deutsches Krebsforschungszentrum, Im Neuenheimer Feld 280, 6900 Heidelberg, Germany
Jick, Dr. H.	Boston University Medical Center, 400 Totten Pond Road, Waltham, Massachusetts 02154, USA
Laberke, Dr. H. G.	Pathologisches Institut der Universität Tübingen, Liebermeisterstraße 8, 7400 Tübingen, Germany
Merker, Prof. Dr. H.-J.	Institut für Toxikologie und Embryopharmakologie, Freie Universität Berlin, Garystraße 9, 1000 Berlin 33, Germany
Neubert, Prof. Dr. D.	Institut für Toxikologie und Embryopharmakologie, Freie Universität Berlin, Garystraße 9, 1000 Berlin 33, Germany
Perucca, Dr. E.	Institute of Neurology, Clinical Pharmacology Unit, The National Hospital, Queen Square, London WC 1N 3BG, Great Britain
Richens, Dr. A.	Institute of Neurology, Clinical Pharmacology Unit, The National Hospital, Queen Square, London WC 1N 3BG, Great Britain
Riemenschneider, Dr. Th.	Pathologisches Institut der Universität Tübingen, Liebermeisterstraße 8, 7400 Tübingen, Germany

Schmähl, Prof. Dr. D. Institut für Toxikologie und Chemotherapie, Deutsches Krebsforschungszentrum, Im Neuenheimer Feld 280, 6900 Heidelberg, Germany

Epidemiological Observation on Drug-Induced Illness

H. JICK

I. Drug Commonly Induces an Otherwise Rare Illness (Category 1, Table 1) . . 2
II. Drug Rarely Induces an Otherwise Common Illness (Category 2, Table 1) . . 4
III. Drug Rarely Induces an Otherwise Rare Illness (Category 3, Table 1) 4
IV. Drug Commonly Induces an Otherwise Common Illness (Category 4, Table 1) 5
V. Both Rates in Intermediate Range (Category 5, Table 1). 7

Case-Control Studies 8
I. Selection of the Cases 8
1. Definition of Illness 8
2. Accuracy of Diagnosis of Illness 8
3. Illness-Drug Relationship 8
4. Illness Relevance 9
5. Selection Bias 9
II. Selection of the Controls 10
III. Identification of the Exposure 11
IV. Influence of Confounding Factors 11
V. Analysis of the Data 12
VI. Interpretation of the Results 12
1. The Statistical Significance of the Association 12
2. The Strength of the Association 12
3. Repeatability 12
4. Biologic Plausibility 13
5. Epidemiologic Plausibility 13
VII. Limitations of the Case-Control Method 13
References 14

The increase in the use of drugs for both short-term and long-term treatment during the past decades has led to a corresponding increase in concern about their potential for inducing serious illnesses. As a result, the search for drug-induced disorders has achieved a high priority in medical research (*Allan* 1976; *Terselic* 1976).

In many cases the identification of drug induction of illnesses is straightforward and can be accomplished readily by informal clinical observation. Rapid discovery of a drug-illness relation tends to occur when the induced illness is dramatic and occurs within a very short period after a drug is taken – for example, penicillin-induced anaphylaxis and ethacrynic-acid-induced deafness. When a drug produces such reactions frequently, the problem is likely to be recognized during premarketing studies, and the drug may not be approved for routine clinical use. However, when a drug produces such an illness only rarely, the discovery of the adverse effect is more likely to occur in the post-marketing period, after widespread clinical use.

Under other circumstances, drug induction of serious illness may not be recognized through informal clinical experience. Clinical observation tends to be insufficient when the time necessary to induce the illness is long – weeks, months or years – especially when the drug induces the illness only rarely or when the illness is otherwise reasonably common (or both). In these circumstances, the use of formal methods rather than reliance on clinical observations is required.

Drug-induced illness may be manifested primarily by a physiologic or biochemical abnormality or it may lead to structural changes which can be readily observed by pathologists. Examples of the former are anaphylaxis, parkinsonism, symptomatic elevation of uric acid levels, and hyperkalemia leading to cardiac arrhythmia. Examples of the latter are aplastic anemia, hepatitis, and cancer.

The major concerns of the epidemiologist are, firstly, to discover previously unrecognized drug-induced illness and, secondly, to provide some quantitation of risk.

The problem of discovering drug-induced illness can be defined by the magnitudes of two risks – the added risk of illness experienced by users of a drug, and the baseline risk in the absence of the drug. Somewhat arbitrarily, each risk is taken to be "high" if the rate of newly occurring illness exceeds one per 200 per year, "low" if less than one per 10,000 per year and, otherwise, "intermediate". Table 1 lists various combinations of these magnitudes of risk. For the resulting categories, the need for formal research is determined not only by the likelihood that drug-illness relations will be missed during the process of informal clinical observation, but also by the nature of illnesses that in each category are particularly apt to be drug induced.

The strategy for research includes several basic approaches. The options are the following: *clinical trial* – an experimental study in which patients are randomly assigned for the duration of the study to one of the compared treatments and are followed forward in time, for some defined period, to ascertain the possible development of illnesses; *nonexperimental cohort study* – a follow-up study in which the choice of drug regimen is dictated by ordinary clinical practices rather than the interest of scientific comparison; and *case-control study* – a study in which patients with an illness of interest are compared to a series of people without the illness for the proportions who have and have not used any of the drugs of interest.

I. Drug Commonly Induces an Otherwise Rare Illness (Category 1, Table 1)

In this situation the rate of drug induction of a given illness is "high", and the base-line rate is low.

Need for Research. When a drug commonly induces an otherwise rare, serious illness, the likelihood is very high that the problem will be discovered in the premarketing phase. In the extraordinary circumstance in which premarketing observation fails to discover the adverse effect, as in the thalidomide disaster, discovery after marketing is likely to occur through informal clinical observation: after the necessary lag time since the introduction of the drug, a dramatic epidemic develops whose detection, although somewhat delayed, requires no formal study. An extraordinarily high proportion of the patients will have a positive history of exposure to the causative drug, and this distribution leads to the rapid identification of the drug-illness relation. Because

Table 1. Types of drug-illness relations

Category	Rate of illness[a]		Example	Primary mode of discovery	Research approach of choice		Illness of particular interest
	Drug induced	Base line			Drugs already marketed	Newly marketed drugs	
1	High[b]	Low[c]	Thalidomide-induced phocomelia	Clinical observation	Case referent	"Cohort"	Any rare illness
2	Low	High	–	Not discoverable	–	–	–
3	Low	Low	Chloramphenicol-induced aplastic anemia	1: Clinical observation 2: Formal research	Case referent	"Cohort"	Any rare illness
4	High	High	? Tolbutamide-induced cardiovascular mortality	Formal research	1: Clinical trial 2: Case referent 3: "Cohort"	1: Clinical trial 2: "Cohort"	Myocardial infarction and sudden deaths in high-risk populations
5	Intermediate	Intermediate	Estrogen-induced endometrial cancer	Formal research	Case referent	"Cohort"	Particular cancers

[a] Refers to acquired illness only

[b] Arbitrarily defined as > 1/200/yr for the purposes of this paper

[c] Arbitrarily defined as < 1/10,000/yr for the purposes of this paper

such drug-illness connections are so readily and quickly identified when they are fully manifested, it is unlikely that any adverse effects of this kind exist undiscovered for drugs already on the market. Of course, if the lag time is appreciable, recognition of an adverse effect is correspondingly delayed.

Although the needs for formal post-marketing research are minor in this category, virtually any rare illness is a potential candidate for drug induction.

Strategy of Research. Although it is exceptional for a drug to be marketed if it commonly induces an otherwise rare, serious illness, it is of interest to consider how the effect, when it occurs, may be discovered. When the phocomelia epidemic of the early 1960's became evident (*Kohler* et al. 1962), its cause was sought by the case-control approach: a series of cases of phocomelia was contrasted to healthy babies for the frequency of various prenatal experiences. In the case series a far greater proportion of mothers had taken thalidomide early in pregnancy as compared to the mothers of normal babies. Thus, it was inferred that the risk of phocomelia was very much higher in the offspring of thalidomide-using mothers than in the others. In general, the potential drug causation of an unexplained epidemic of illness is most efficiently evaluated by the case-referent approach.

The existence of Category 1 side effects of newly marketed drugs is ruled out by premarketing studies. In the extraordinary case in which they have not, untoward reactions will come to attention rapidly upon the development of the epidemic. Consequently, no special follow-up effort is indicated for Category 1 drug illnesses.

II. Drug Rarely Induces an Otherwise Common Illness (Category 2, Table 1)

When an illness is rarely induced by a drug and is common in its absence, the proportion of cases due to the drug is very small; neither general clinical experience nor formal research will identify the drug-illness relation. For example, if the incidence of an illness were one per 100 per year in the absence of drug treatment and the drug itself induced the illness in one per 50,000 per year, the risk among the users would be increased only to 1.002%. Weak relations of this kind simply will have to remain undiscovered.

III. Drug Rarely Induces an Otherwise Rare Illness (Category 3, Table 1)

There are many known examples in this category. Among the more familiar ones are the connection between chloramphenicol and aplastic anemia (*Wallerstein* et al. 1969), oral contraceptives and benign liver tumors (*Contostavlos* 1973), practolol and sclerosing peritonitis (*Brown* et al. 1974), lincomycin and pseudomembranous colitis (*Scott* et al. 1973), and diethylstilbestrol and vaginal cancer (*Herbst* et al. 1971).

Need for Research. Drug-illness relations in this category almost always escape notice in the premarketing phase since a vast experience is needed before cases of the rare illness occur. On the other hand, once experience has accrued after marketing, informal discovery of the problem is likely, particularly when a drug accounts for a large proportion of the rare illness. However, even when a relation is recognized by chance, the discovery is always delayed. Reduction of this delay is the major objective of formal research.

As previously noted, virtually any rare illness may be suspected of having been drug induced.

Strategy for Research. An example of a formally discovered relation in Category 3 is the connection between maternal use of diethylstilbestrol and vaginal cancer in the offspring (*Herbst* et al. 1971). A series of eight cases of this exceedingly rare condition was accrued and contrasted to a series of 32 normal girls. Detailed histories for a number of etiologic factors were taken in each series. Of the eight patients with cancer, seven had a history of intrauterine exposure to diethylstilbestrol in constrast to none in the reference series.

For the discovery of drug-illness relations in this category, the case-control approach is particularly feasible in the study of drugs already on the market because an appreciable number of cases of the rare illness have to accumulate. Since any given case-control study focuses on a single illness only, separate series for each of the rare illnesses of concern need to be assembled to explore the role of drug exposure fully.

For newly marketed drugs, some kind of monitoring scheme is needed to uncover adverse effects early. The most efficient means of monitoring newly marketed drugs for rare, serious toxicity might be to establish a central registry of a large number of the earliest patients who receive the drug and to follow up these patients at periodic intervals for the development of serious, unusual illness. Users of new drugs could be inexpensively and rapidly identified if notification of use (by the prescribing physician or by the pharmacist who filled the prescription) to a central registry was mandatory and automatic. Periodic follow-up observation of users with mailed questionnaires that inquire about the development of serious illness should identify most drug-illness connections within the first few cases, particularly if the illness is otherwise rare and dramatic.

IV. Drug Commonly Induces an Otherwise Common Illness (Category 4, Table 1)

An example of the high risk associated with a drug when the risk of an illness in the absence of the drug is also high is the putative effect of tolbutamide in increasing coronary mortality (University Group Diabetes Program 1970).

Need for Research. Adverse effects in this category are unlikely to be discovered informally. In the first place, a discernible epidemic would not tend to arise – for example, if the drug is taken by 10% of the population, and if it doubles the rate of the illness, the drug still accounts for only about 10% of the cases. Furthermore, the experience of any single physician would generally be insufficient to discern, say, a doubling of the rate of the illness among users of the drug or, alternatively, a doubling of the usage rate of this drug among patients with the illness. Finally, even if the drug effect were suspected informally, confounding would remain a likely explanation in the absence of formal analysis of the experience.

Since drug-illness relations in this category would tend to escape detection by routine clinical observation, the particular illnesses that may be caused by a drug deserve special attention. Aside from epidemics of certain infectious diseases, annual attack rates of at least one in 200 are associated with essentially no serious illnesses but acute manifestations of cardiovascular disease – most notably, acute myocardial infarction and sudden coronary deaths – in certain high-risk populations. Thus, research needs on the illnesses of concern tend to be quite limited in this category.

Considerable information on the influence of some drugs on the course of coronary heart disease is already available. Numerous clinical trials involving over a dozen important drugs have been carried out (University Group Diabetes Program 1970; Coronary Drug Project Research Group 1973; Veterans Administration Cooperative Study Group on Antihypertensive Agents 1967; *Grant* et al. 1966; *Green* et al. 1975; *Elwood* et al. 1974; *Wilhelmsson* et al. 1974). Beyond this experience, a large body of relevant data has been accumulated by the Boston Collaborative Drug Surveillance Program [BCDSP] (*Jick* et al. 1973): the histories of drug use in some 2,000 patients with acute nonfatal myocardial infarction have been contrasted with histories of other patients (BCDSP 1974; *Miettinen* et al. 1976; *Jick* and *Miettinen* 1976; *Rosenberg* et al. 1976). No definite indications of drug cause have emerged. The data, however, are insufficient to exclude drug associations of the order of magnitude of, say, twofold, except for reasonably commonly used drugs. Moreover, in terms of the control of confounding factors, it is not feasible to explore the potential etiologic role of drugs used to treat predisposing illnesses or to treat coronary heart disease itself.

Strategy for Research. As an example of formal research in Category 4, one can examine the origin of the hypothesis that tolbutamide is conducive to fatal coronary heart disease (University Group Diabetes Program 1970). A clinical trial had been mounted with the primary aim of assessing the relative efficacies of alternative treatments for adult-onset diabetes. Among the complications potentially prevented by the drugs were myocardial infarction and sudden death. Quite unexpectedly, these complications occurred more commonly in the tolbutamide-treated group than in the placebo-using reference series. The difference was "statistically significant", and confounding was dealt with through randomization of treatment allocation, augmented by the control of certain factors in the analyses. Despite the experimental nature of the design, there has been substantial controversy about the validity of the comparison and, therefore, about the inference itself (*Schor* 1971; *Feinstein* 1971).

Experimental evaluation of the relation of coronary heart disease to drugs at large, although it is the most valid approach because treatments are randomized, requires separate randomized series for all the drugs of concern. Experimental evaluation of a newly marketed drug and drugs of special interest can be accomplished, though it should be noted that long-term clinical trials frequently cost millions of dollars (*Wallerstein* et al. 1969; *Contostavlos* 1973). For the evaluation of the multitude of drugs already in clinical use, the experimental approach is obviously infeasible.

A nonexperimental cohort study is amenable to simultaneous evaluation of a multitude of drugs. As compared to the case-control approach, the cohort approach requires the enrollment of much larger numbers of subjects and the follow-up study of those subjects for the recording of drug use and subsequent occurrence of the illness. Thus, follow-up studies tend to be relatively costly and time consuming, particularly if conducted prospectively (Royal College of General Practitioners 1974).

The case-control approach permits evaluation of the role, in a single study, of many drugs as the cause of a particular illness. The cost of such studies, when done individually, is frequently no more than a few thousand dollars and rarely more than tens of thousands of dollars. Though very efficient and permitting the enrollment of large numbers of cases, this approach has the potential for bias from several sources, particularly in the areas of subject selection and information gathering. When these problems are insurmountable, the case-control approach is not applicable.

V. Both Rates in the Intermediate Range (Category 5, Table 1)

In this circumstance, the added risk associated with a drug is neither "high" nor "low", and the base-line risk of the illness is also in the intermediate range. An example is the apparent connection between the use of exogenous estrogens and the risk of endometrial cancer (*Smith* et al. 1975).

Need for Research. Adverse drug effects in this category are unlikely to be discovered informally, since the proportion of incident cases of the illness due to the drug is usually only a small fraction of the total cases, and no discernible epidemic occurs. Thus, even the exceedingly strong association between estrogens and endometrial cancer went undetected for over 20 years until formal case-referent studies directed to the evaluation of this specific relation were carried out.

As for illnesses of concern in Category 5, the incidence rates of the spectrum of serious illnesses that are potential candidates for drug induction reveal that all cancers, except for the rarest forms, qualify. Only a few additional illnesses meet these criteria. Among them are gallbladder disease, cataract, and peptic ulcer. Substantial series of cases of these three diseases, as well as others in Category 5, have been accrued by the (BCDSP 1973, 1974; *Levy* 1974).

Strategy for Research. An example of formally discovered relations in Category 5 is the association between oral contraceptives and gallbladder disease (BCDSP 1973). A series of 212 premenopausal women who had undergone gallbladder operations were collected by the BCDSP during a hospital survey. They were compared to 842 women hospitalized for other conditions presumed to be unrelated to oral contraceptive use. Analysis of the data yielded the estimate that users of oral contraceptives were twice as likely as nonusers to undergo gallbladder operations.

For the discovery of drug-illness relations of this kind, the case-control approach, once again, has a substantial feasibility advantage in the study of drugs already on the market. Follow-up studies would entail the monitoring of huge numbers of patients for many years to evaluate the many drugs currently marketed in relation to the illnesses of importance in this category.

For newly marketed drugs, registry and follow-up observation of early users are indicated for prompt identification of drug-illness relations. The interpretation of data, however, may be more complex than that involving rare diseases. The quantitation of the relation of a drug to an illness that occurs reasonably often in the absence of drug cause generally requires a carefully drawn reference or comparison group not exposed to the drug. This matter may be managed if a number of follow-up series are being monitored simultaneously – i.e., one for each of a number of newly marketed drugs. Under such conditions, each may act as a reference series for the other.

Case-Control Studies

As suggested above, the case-control approach is the approach most often required to study drug-induced illnesses. As such, it is most important that the correct technique be used in carrying out such studies.

There are six major areas of methodologic importance in a case-control study involving drugs: (1) selection of the cases, (2) selection of the controls, (3) identification of the exposure (to the drug(s) under study), (4) the influence of confounding factors, (5) the analysis of the data, and (6) the interpretation of the results. Important principles must be understood and applied to achieve maximum validity in each area.

I. Selection of the Cases

The following considerations should be kept in mind:

1. Definition of Illness

The illness under investigation should normally be clearly defined. This point is particularly important when studying illnesses such as coronary artery disease which have a multifactorial etiology and many manifestations. Cigarette smoking, for example, is strongly associated with the risk of acute myocardial infarction in young people, but shows a much less clear relationship with angina pectoris (*Miettinen* et al. 1976).

2. Accuracy of Diagnosis of Illness

The diagnosis of the illness should be as accurate as possible. In some instances, e.g., most cancers proven by biopsy, the accuracy of the diagnosis may be readily confirmed. However, when dealing with less well-defined illnesses such as subacute myelo-optic neuropathy (SMON – a drug-related neurologic disorder) (*Oakley* 1973) or those involving acute disturbance of liver function, misdiagnosis may produce substantial distortion.

3. Illness-Drug Relationship

The course of the illness under study should not influence the probability of being exposed to the drug of interest. This generally calls for admitting people who have been newly diagnosed as suffering from the disease (incident cases) with no premonitory symptoms or predisposing factors which would be an indication for or contraindication to the drug under investigation. For example, in studying the relationship between oral contraceptives and venous thromboembolism, subjects with recurrent thromboembolism should be excluded (or considered separately) since a previous episode of the disease would now contraindicate the use of the pill (though this was not so before the relationship was established).

4. Illness Relevance

The cases included should have some reasonable possibility of having been induced by the drug of concern. For example, cases of thromboembolism occurring during pregnancy or immediately postpartum should be excluded from a study of the pill and thromboembolism since such cases could not possibly be pill induced. Similarly, post-operative thromboembolism should be considered separately from "idiopathic" disease since surgery is a sufficient cause for the event, and the presence of oral contraceptive use may not play the same role in the etiology of post-operative disease. Inclusion of cases which do not relate to a reasonable hypothesis will, of course, dilute any association which may be present.

5. Selection Bias

Finally, it is important to be aware of possible selection biases among diagnosed cases. Such biases are of particular concern when the hypothesis being tested has previously been entertained. In these circumstances, a history of drug use may tend to increase suspicion of, or hospitalization for, an illness. For example, in regard to the pill and thromboembolism, any interpretation of the results of a current study should take into account the possibility that the illness may be selectively diagnosed (with subsequent hospitalization) in pill users as a result of a high index of suspicion in the physician. The extent of the bias introduced in such instances is usually difficult to estimate and the degree of influence on the results may be a matter of conjecture. As in all other areas of concern, the specific details of each particular study must be examined to determine what evidence there is for or against the influence of this bias.

A great deal of emphasis has been placed by some authors on the need to study a "representative" sample of cases (*Feinstein* 1973). This emphasis is misplaced. Indeed, if by "representative" it is meant that a random sample of all prevalent cases should be selected, this "representativeness" is likely to introduce substantial distortion. For example, in studying the relation between oral contraceptives and venous thromboembolism, a "representative" group of cases might be considered to include women with recurrent thromboembolism (*Feinstein* 1973), and those who developed the illness while pregnant or after the menopause. In fact, as indicated above, such women should expressly be excluded from the study.

Furthermore, a valid study may be carried out in a highly "selected" group of people. For example, a study of the relationship of oral contraceptives and benign liver tumors could be restricted to cases occurring in nurses. The control group would most likely have to consist of nurses as well, since this occupational group may have distinctive contraceptive habits. Furthermore, the results would, strictly, speaking, apply only to nurses. Nevertheless, the results themselves would be valid, if confounding were adequately controlled, despite the highly selected nature of the case and control series.

II. Selection of the Controls

The series of control subjects should be chosen in such a way that when a proper analysis is made, i.e., statistical adjustment is made for confounding factors, they are comparable with the cases in all relevant ways, except that they do not have the illness under study. When this is achieved, the controls are as likely to be users of the drug being studied as the cases (assuming that no association exists). To achieve comparability, subjects who are identified by a condition which is known to be associated with the drug under study should be excluded from the control series. Thus, when the control series consists of hospitalized patients, the following exclusions are mandatory:

(1) Patients *admitted* for conditions which are an indication for or contraindication to the drug of interest. For example, in studying the relationship of aspirin to a particular illness such as acute myocardial infarction, it would be necessary to exclude from the control series patients *admitted* to hospital because of chronic arthritis (who would be likely to have excessive aspirin use) and those *admitted* because of chronic peptic ulcer disease (who would be likely to have decreased aspirin use).

(2) Patients *admitted* for conditions which are caused or prevented by the drug under study. For example, in studying the relationship between oral contraceptives and breast disease, it would be necessary to exclude from the control series women *admitted* to hospital for thromboembolic disease (who would be likely to have excessive pill use) and those *admitted* for ovarian cyst (who would be likely to have decreased pill use).

The probability of being admitted to hospital for a given illness tends to depend on whether the condition requires mandatory hospitalization (e.g., acute myocardial infarction, severe trauma) or whether the condition is such that hospitalization is elective (e.g., hernia repair). The nature of the particular illness under study in terms of these two categories ideally calls for a control series which falls into the same category, since the likelihood of having had a drug prescribed may be correlated. In practice, this potential bias may not be of much importance. In a very large series of hospitalized patients, the age-sex standardized rates of regular drug use were closely similar in patients with mandatory admissions in comparison with those with elective admissions (*Smith* and *Jick* 1977).

The decision as to the source of the control series is generally influenced by practical considerations. Where a case series is derived from a large defined group (such as a group health plan), the control series may easily and efficiently be drawn from that group (*Klatsky* et al. 1974). When such a defined population is not available, hospital controls are generally most convenient to study. When hospital controls are used, they should be drawn from a variety of diagnostic groups so as to minimize the impact of inadvertently including an admitting illness which (unknown to the investigator) is associated either positively or negatively with the drug under study. Exposure rates for each of the control illnesses should be calculated. If the different categories are, in fact, unassociated with the exposure, the exposure rates, appropriately standardized, should be similar. "Community controls", despite their popularity, generally confer little advantage and may have considerable disadvantage in case-control studies on drug-induced illness since it is frequently difficult to obtain information from cases and controls in a comparable manner. Other factors influencing comparability may be present and, therefore, when community controls are used, they should be chosen so as to optimize the probability that they will be comparable to cases in terms of the likelihood of being hospitalized, the likelihood of being a drug user, and the likelihood of encompassing the range of confounding factors.

III. Identification of the Exposure

In studies concerned with the role of drugs in the etiology of illness, the proper ascertainment of exposure is, of course, critical. The following principles should be applied for optimum validity:

(1) The method of obtaining information on exposure must be very closely similar in cases and controls. Identical interview, abstraction, or questionnaire procedures are of prime importance. Ideally, the individual who obtains and records the information should be unaware of the hypothesis being tested and unaware of which subjects are cases and which are controls.

(2) The exposure of interest must be well defined and relevant to a reasonable hypothesis. In particular, careful consideration must be given to the length of exposure and to the time relationships between the exposure and the outcome event. Other factors related to exposure, such as dose, may be important as well.

(3) Where possible, information on drugs not suspected of being associated with the illness under investigation should be obtained. Such data enable cases and controls to be compared with regard to the level of use of drugs in general.

(4) The data source must be of identical completeness in cases and controls. This is of particular importance when medical documents are used to ascertain exposure. Information obtained from a special source (such as a hospital admission) in cases should be excluded if such information is not available for the control series (and vice versa).

(5) The information on exposure should be reasonably complete and accurate. This principle, once again, is most relevant when medical records are used as a source of information on exposure. When there is considerable doubt about the quality of records, a study should probably not be mounted.

IV. Influence of Confounding Factors

A factor or variable is said to confound a relationship when that factor is associated with both the exposure of interest (in this case, a drug) and with the illness being studied (*Miettinen* 1974). Confounding factors may be dealt with by appropriate matching of cases and controls or by statistical analyses which take confounding into account. Age and sex generally correlate both with drug use and with illness, and it should be routine, except under special circumstances, to control for these variables. Calendar year and geographic area should also routinely be controlled for. Careful examination of the data for confounding by other factors is also necessary.

V. Analysis of the Data

The correct analysis of the data collected in a case-control study is essential to the proper interpretation of the results. This matter has been extensively reviewed by *Miettinen* (1976) and will not be discussed further here.

VI. Interpretation of the Results

Proper interpretation of the results of a case-control study involves careful consideration of the validity of the design and analysis in the various areas already discussed. The question of the extent to which bias or imprecise information may have influenced the results must be faced squarely. Obviously, the more uncertainties there are, the less confidence there can be in interpreting the results.

There are a number of other considerations which contribute in an important way to a final interpretation of the results. These are:

1. The Statistical Significance of the Association

Obviously, the lower the "p value", the less likely it is that the results may have been due to chance. This point is of special importance when a study involves the simultaneous evaluation of many different drugs in the etiology of an illness or illnesses. Such studies involve multiple comparisons and thus it is to be expected that some will reach traditional levels of statistical significance by chance. Even if only one comparison is made, it should be realized that a low p value may be due to chance, just as it may be following the most perfectly designed experiment.

2. The Strength of the Association

All else being equal, the stronger the association (i.e., the higher the relative risk) the less likely it is to be due to "confounding" or selection biases. If the data reveal a biological gradient (a dose-response curve), so much the better.

3. Repeatability

Generally, the results of a single case-control study (or any other type of study for that matter) should not be used to draw causal inferences. Repetition of the findings in a number of studies carried out in different populations adds confidence to the interpretation (*Kohler* et al. 1962).

4. Biologic Plausibility

When other types of study (e.g., investigations of blood biochemistry or of tissue histology) provide results which tend to support those of an epidemiologic study, firmer conclusions can be drawn.

5. Epidemiologic Plausibility

Does a causal explanation for a proposed association make sense in the light of other data concerning, for example, the trend in the incidence of the disease with time, or differences in incidence with sex, age, social, ethnic and geographic group?

VII. Limitations of the Case-Control Method

There are a number of circumstances in which the case-control approach cannot be applied without encountering biases (or confounding) which preclude a reasonably certain interpretation of the results. The essential requirement for validity – namely, that cases and controls must have had an equal chance of being exposed to the drug of interest prior to the onset of the event which brought them into the study – identifies those problems which are not amenable to study by the case-control approach.

Circumstances where the drug may be indicated for treatment of the early manifestations of the illness or a predisposing factor. For example, it would probably not be feasible to study a postulated causal relationship between the recent use of cathartics and the development of colon cancer. In such a study it would be expected that the cases would be more likely to be users of such drugs than the controls unless the control series consisted of patients with illnesses associated with constipation. In the latter circumstance there would be little assurance that the severity of constipation and, therefore, the likelihood of being a user of cathartics would be similar.

Circumstances where use of the drug is contraindicated by early manifestations of the illness. For example, it seems doubtful that any reliable study could *now* be carried out on the relationship between oral contraceptives and acute myocardial infarction in women with predisposing illness. This is because the pill has been considered to be contraindicated in those with hypertension, diabetes, etc., since the publication of the papers by *Mann* and *Inman* (1975) and *Mann* et al. (1975). In theory, such a study might be done if it were possible to identify a control series which was "equally" at high risk. In practice, this would be a hazardous undertaking since the measures of the degree of pre-existing "risk" for an illness such as myocardial infarction are crude.

The largest epidemiologic study designed to evaluate both acute and long-term drug toxicity is the BCDSP. As of January 1, 1978, information had been obtained on about 50,000 medical inpatients and about 13,000 surgical inpatients hospitalized in seven countries. In general, the data from this study indicate, firstly, that drug usage in Western countries is extremely high, particularly in the United States and, secondly, that given the massive use of drugs, the incidence of serious drug-induced illness is quite low.

According to the latest data from this study, the rate of drug-induced deaths in hospitalized medical patients is about 0.9 per 1,000. Most of the patients who died from drug toxicity were seriously ill prior to receiving the causal drug(s). Life-threatening adverse drug effects have been noted in about 3% of patients, but since each patient received about eight drugs, the rate per course of drug treatment is about 0.4%.

Since serious adverse drug reactions are relatively infrequent, their nature and frequency are somewhat difficult to ascertain unless one has a massive reservoir of experience available. The use of national computer banks is required to provide reasonably accurate estimates.

References

Allan FN (ed) (1976) Assessing drug reactions: adverse and beneficial, philosophy and technology of drug assessment. Vol 7. Interdisciplinary Communication Associates, Washington DC

Boston Collaborative Drug Surveillance Program (1973) Oral contraceptives and venous thromboembolic disease, surgically confirmed gallbladder disease, and breast tumours. Lancet 1: 1399–1404

Boston Collaborative Drug Surveillance Program (1974) Surgically confirmed gallbladder disease, venous thromboembolism and breast tumors in relation to postmenopausal estrogen therapy. N Engl J Med 290: 15–19

Boston Collaborative Drug Surveillance Program (1974) Regular aspirin intake and acute myocardial infarction. Br Med J 1: 440–443

Brown P, Baddeley H, Read AE, Davies JD, McGarry J (1974) Sclerosing peritonitis, an unusual reaction to a β-adrenergic-blocking drug (practolol). Lancet 2: 1477–1481

Contostavlos DL (1973) Benign hepatomas and oral contraceptives. Lancet 2: 1200

Coronary Drug Project Research Group (1973) The coronary drug project: findings leading to discontinuation of the 2.5-mg/day estrogen group. JAMA 226: 652–657

Elwood PC, Cochrane AL, Burr ML, Sweetnam PM, Williams G, Welsby E, Hughes SJ, Renton R (1974) A randomized controlled trial of acetyl salicylic acid in the secondary prevention of mortality from myocardial infarction. Br Med J 1: 436–440

Feinstein AR (1971) Clinical biostatistics. VIII. An analytic appraisal of the University Group Diabetes Program (UGDP) study. Clin Pharmacol Ther 12: 167–191

Feinstein AR (1973) Clinical biostatistics: The epidemiologic trohoc, the ablative risk ratio, and retrospective research. Clin Pharmacol Ther 14: 291–307

Grant RHE, Keelan P, Kernohan RJ, Leonard JC, Nancekievill L, Sinclair K (1966) Multicenter trial of propranolol in angina pectoris. Am J Cardiol 18: 361–365

Green KG, Chamberlain DA, Fulton RM et al. (1975) Improvement in prognosis of myocardial infarction by long-term beta-adrenoreceptor blockade using practolol: a multicentre international study. Br Med J 3: 735–740

Herbst AL, Ulfelder H, Poskanzer DC (1971) Adenocarcinoma of the vagina: association of maternal stilbestrol therapy with tumor appearance in young women. N Engl J Med 284: 878–881

Jick H, Miettinen OS (1976) Regular aspirin use and myocardial infarction. Br Med J 1: 1057

Jick H, Miettinen OS, Neff RK, Shapiro S, Heinonen OP, Slone D (1973) Coffee and myocardial infarction. N Engl J Med 289: 63–67

Klatsky AL, Friedman GD, Siegelaub AB (1974) Alcohol consumption before myocardial infarction: Results from the Kaiser-Permanente Epidemiologic Study of Myocardial Infarction. Ann Intern Med 81: 294–301

Kohler HG, Fisher AM, Dunn PM (1962) Thalidomide and congenital abnormalities. Lancet 1: 326

Levy M (1974) Aspirin use in patients with major upper gastrointestinal bleeding and peptic-ulcer disease: a report from the Boston Collaborative Drug Surveillance Program. N Engl J Med 290: 1158–1162

Mann JI, Inman WH (1975) Oral contraceptives and death from myocardial infarction. Br Med J 2: 245–248

Mann JI, Vessey MP, Thorogood M, Doll R (1975) Myocardial infarction in young women with special reference to oral contraceptive practice. Br Med J 2: 241–245

Miettinen OS (1974) Confounding and effect modification. Am J Epidemiol 100: 350–353

Miettinen OS (1976) Estimability and estimation in case referent studies. Am J Epidemiol 103: 226–235

Miettinen OS, Neff RK, Jick H (1976) Cigarette-smoking and nonfatal myocardial infarction: Rate ratio in relation to age, sex, and predisposing conditions. Am J Epidemiol 103: 30–36

Oakley GP Jr (1973) The neurotoxicity of the halogenated hydroxyquinolines. JAMA 225: 395–397

Rosenberg L, Armstrong B, Jick H (1976) Myocardial infarction and estrogen therapy in post-menopausal women. N Engl J Med 294: 1256–1259

The Royal College of General Practitioners (1974) Oral Contraceptives and Health: An interim report from the Oral Contraception Study of the Royal College of General Practitioners. Pittman Publishing Corporation, New York

Schor S (1971) The University Group Diabetes Program: a statistician looks at the mortality results. JAMA 217: 1671–1675

Scott AJ, Nicholson GI, Kerr AR (1973) Lincomycin as a cause of pseudomembranous colitis. Lancet 2: 1232–1234

Smith DC, Prentice R, Thompson DJ, Hermann WL (1975) Association of exogenous estrogen and endometrial carcinoma. N Engl J Med 293: 1164–1167

Smith PG, Jick H (1977) Regular drug use and cancer. J Natl Cancer Inst 59: 1387–1391

Terselic RA (1976) Achieving safer, more effective, and less costly utilization of therapeutic drugs. Office of Technology Assessment, United States Congress, August

The University Group Diabetes Program (1970) A study of the effects of hypoglycemic agents on vascular complications in patients with adult-onset diabetes. I. Design methods and baseline results. Diabetes 19: Suppl 2, 747–830

Veterans Administration Cooperative Study Group on Antihypertensive Agents (1967) Effects of treatment on morbidity in hypertension: results in patients with diastolic blood pressure averaging 115 through 129 mmHg. JAMA 202: 1028–1034

Wallerstein RO, Condit PK, Kasper CK, Brown JW, Morrison FR (1969) Statewide study of chloramphenicol therapy and fatal aplastic anemia. JAMA 208: 2045–2050

Wilhelmsson C, Vedin JA, Wilhelmsen L, Tibblin G, Werko L (1974) Reduction of sudden deaths after myocardial infarction by treatment with alprenolol. Lancet 2: 1157–1160

The Pathophysiological Basis of Drug Toxicity

E. PERUCCA and A. RICHENS

A. Introduction 18
B. Pathogenesis of Type A Adverse Reactions 19
I. Factors inherent in the Properties of the Drug and in its Mode of Administration 20
1. The Dose and the Therapeutic Ratio 20
2. The Route of Administration 21
3. The Duration of Treatment 22
4. The Pharmaceutical Preparation 22
5. The Effects of Multiple Drug Therapy 23
II. Factors Inherent in the Patient's Responsiveness 23
1. Interindividual Differences in Pharmacokinetics 24
a) Absorption 24
b) Distribution 25
α) Plasma Protein Binding 25
β) Tissue Binding 26
γ) Active Transport 27
c) Biotransformation 28
α) Genetic Factors 28
β) Age 30
γ) Disease 30
δ) Dose-Dependent Metabolism 32
ϵ) Enzyme-Induction 33
ζ) Enzyme-Inhibition 34
η) Bioactivation 37
d) Renal Excretion 39
2. Interindividual Differences in End-Organ Responsiveness 40
a) Genetic Factors 41
b) Constitutional Factors 42
c) Pathological Factors 43
d) Supersensitivity and Tolerance 44
e) Pharmacodynamic Drug Interactions 46
C. Pathogenesis of Type B Adverse Reactions 47
I. Qualitative Abnormalities of the Pharmaceutical Preparation 47
II. Qualitative Abnormalities of the Patient's Responsiveness 48
1. Genetically Determined Abnormalities 48
a) Glucose-6-Phosphate-Dehydrogenase Deficiency 48
b) Glutathione-Reductase Deficiency 49
c) Drug-Sensitive Haemoglobins 49
d) Suxamethonium Hypersensitivity 50
e) Malignant Hyperthermia 50
f) Jaundice and Thromboembolic Associated With Oral Contraceptives . . 51
g) Rheumatoid Arthritis and Toxic Drug Reactions 51
h) Porphyria 51

2. Drug Allergy 51
a) The Drug as an Allergen 52
α) The Effect of the Molecular Size 52
β) Sensitization and Allergy 53
γ) Specific Sensitization and Cross-Allergy 53
b) Factors inherent in the Patient 54
α) Genetic Factors 54
β) Atopy 54
γ) Pathological Factors 55
c) Pathogenetic Mechanisms of Drug Allergy 55
α) Type I (Immediate) Reactions 55
β) Type II (Cytotoxic) Reactions 57
γ) Type III (Immune-Complex) Reactions 58
δ) Type IV (Cell–Mediated) Reactions 59
D. Conclusion 60
References 60

A. Introduction

Since the thalidomide disaster in the winter of 1961, the medical profession and the public have become particularly sensitive to the problem of adverse drug reactions. A more scientific approach to the study and prevention of drug toxicity has been taken, including stricter regulations for toxicological studies in animals and carefully conducted clinical trials before new drugs are released for general use. Adverse drug reactions are closely monitored so that the time lapse between the introduction of a drug into therapeutic practice and the recognition of its toxic effects has decreased dramatically (Table 1).

Almost without exception, every pharmacological agent is potentially "toxic", provided the dose administered is large enough or a susceptible individual is found. The list of adverse drug reactions is so long, and their manifestations so polymorphic, that a fully satisfactory classification is impossible to find. Classifications based on the morphological aspects of the lesions can be useful to describe drug-induced pathological changes in selected organs but, apart from being unsuitable for general purposes, usually provide little information on the mechanism of the reaction and the factors

Table 1. Latent period between introduction of a drug in therapeutic practice and discovery of important adverse effects

Drug	Date introduced	Adverse effect	Date discovered
Phenacetin	1887	Nephropathy	1953
Aminopyrine	1889	Agranulocytosis	1933
Aspirin	1899	Gastric hemorrhage	1938
Cinchophen	1908	Jaundice	1923
Phenytoin	1938	Rickets, osteomalacia	1967
Thalidomide	1957	Teratogenesis	1961
Practolol	1970	Oculo-muco-cutaneous syndrome	1974

Table 2

Type A adverse drug reactions		
Definition	Comment	Examples
Undesired effects which are closely related to the pharmacological action of the drug. They represent an exaggerated but otherwise normal pharmacological response.	Usually predictable. Dose-dependent. High frequency. Low mortality.	Dryness of mouth by anticholinergic drugs. Cardiac dysrhythmias by digitalis. Myelosuppression by antineoplastic drugs.
Type B adverse drug reactions		
Definition	Comment	Examples
Undesired effects which are unrelated to the known pharmacological action of the drug. They usually occur in a small proportion of susceptible individuals.	Unpredictable. Not always dose-dependent. Low incidence. Sometimes very severe.	Agranulocytosis by chloramphenicol Skin rashes by phenytoin. Anaphylaxis by penicillin.

involved in its management and prevention. Drug interactions are often considered separately, yet they appear to be a major source of toxic reactions both in terms of frequency and severity. In this chapter, an attempt has been made to classify adverse drug reactions on the basis of the pathophysiological mechanism involved. Although this classification provides the most rational approach, it must be realised that in many cases the mechanism is either incompletely understood or complex and multifactorial in origin. It is possible, however, to identify two fundamental types of adverse drug reactions:

1. Those which arise from the normal pharmacological action(s) of a drug, and
2. Those which represent a totally unusual and unexpected response.

According to *Rawlins* and *Thompson* (1977), these adverse drug reactions will be referred to in the present chapter as Type A and Type B reactions respectively (Table 2).

B. Pathogenesis of Type A Adverse Reactions

As summarized in Table 2, Type A reactions can be defined as undesired effects which arise from an exaggerated but otherwise normal pharmacological action of the drug. Their main characteristics are predictability, dose-dependency and occurrence in a relatively high proportion of subjects treated with the drug. Their actual incidence and severity varies for individual drugs depending on a combination of factors, partly related to the properties of the drug itself and partly to interindividual differences in drug response. These factors will be examined below in greater detail.

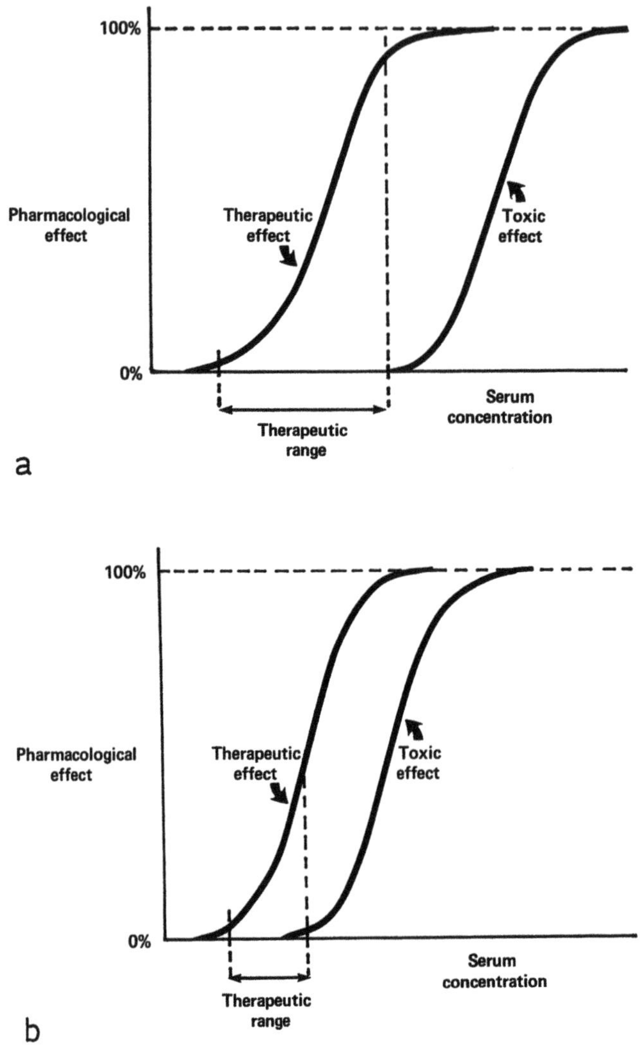

Fig. 1a, b. A simplified scheme which illustrates the dose-response relationship for drugs characterised by a high (**a**) and low (**b**) therapeutic ratio. In **a**, the concentration of the drug required to produce 90% of the full therapeutic response is insufficient to produce toxic effects. In **b**, the concentration necessary to produce the same degree of therapeutic effect also produces marked toxicity. Serum concentration is plotted on a log-scale

I. Factors Inherent in the Properties of the Drug and in its Mode of Administration

1. The Dose and the Therapeutic Ratio

These are the single most important factors which determine the manifestation of Type A adverse drug reactions. For a given drug the therapeutic ratio provides an estimate of the probability that toxic effects manifest themselves at the doses commonly used in therapeutic practice: the higher the therapeutic ratio, the safer the drug to use. Figure 1 illustrates this concept by showing the dose-response relationship for drugs characterized by a high and a low therapeutic ratio respectively. In practice, the situation is more complex than depicted in Figure 1 in that not only the severity but also the incidence of adverse effects tends to increase with increasing drug dosage. A second factor that complicates the dose-response relationship is the possibility of the drug having multiple pharmacological actions. In the latter case various types of adverse effects can be seen either at different dose levels or in different groups of patients. Carbamazepine, for example, has antineuralgic, antiepileptic and antidiuretic properties. The latter effect was originally thought to be a Type B reaction but subsequent studies showed it to be consistent, predictable and dose-dependent (*Perucca* et al. 1978). In patients with diabetes insipidus the antidiuresis is beneficial and therapeutic, but in epileptic patients it can be responsible for the development of water intoxication. This is a common occurrence with Type A adverse reactions: the same effect may prove adverse or beneficial depending on the clinical situation.

2. The Route of Administration

As the concentration of the drug is highest at the site of administration (at least until absorption or inactivation has taken place) it is not surprising that adverse reactions occurring locally are frequently observed. In some cases the reaction is a consequence of an incorrect route or mode of administration. Thus, extensive tissue necrosis may follow local extravasation during intravenous injection of highly toxic compounds, e.g. cytotoxic drugs, and irritant solvents, e.g. strongly alkaline solutions. Sterile abscesses complicate intramuscular therapy with paraldehyde so frequently that this route of administration should be used only when alternative forms of therapy are not available. Even when drugs are administered correctly, local adverse reactions are sometimes inevitable. Some degree of gastrointestinal bleeding, for example, is observed in virtually 100% of individuals ingesting therapeutic doses of aspirin (*Wood* et al. 1962), an effect that is largely related to local mucosal damage at the absorption site. Other examples of adverse reactions at the site of absorption include the alteration of the intestinal flora by broad-spectrum antibiotics, and the development of hoarseness and monilial infection in the mouth and upper airways of patients using steroid aerosols, including beclomethasone (*Lovell* and *Preuss* 1977).

Systemic adverse reactions may also be largely influenced by the route of administration. Fatalities have resulted occasionally from accidental intra-arterial injection of pharmaceutical preparations intended for intravenous use. For many drugs the dosage varies considerably depending on the route of administration. The average intravenous dose of propranolol, for example, is 10 to 40 times lower than the average oral dose and failure to recognise this principle would have disastrous effects. Misadventures have followed the intravenous administration of a preparation of adrenaline (1 : 100) designed for aerosol use (*Innes* and *Nickerson* 1975). When drugs are administered intravenously the time of infusion is often critical, adverse reactions being more frequent and more severe after rapid injection. Not well recognized is the possibility that drugs used externally might be absorbed and produce severe systemic effects. Renal failure has resulted from the absorption of copper sulphate (*Holtzman* et al. 1966) and boric acid (*Baliah* et al. 1969) from skin dressings.

3. The Duration of Treatment

It is not possible to establish a general rule which relates adverse drug reactions to duration of treatment. In many cases toxic effects manifest themselves only after a latent period has elapsed since initiation of treatment. Most frequently this latency is due exclusively to the time required for the drug to reach a steady-state concentration in body tissues (approximately 5 half-lives). Failure to take this period into account may result in gross underestimation of potentially serious toxic reactions. In the case of phenytoin, for example, it may take at least 10–15 days for the serum concentration to plateau at steady-state after starting therapy. In a similar way, the effects of digitoxin overdosage may not become apparent until one month since the last dose increment. The influence of disease must also be considered: in patients with decreased glomerular filtration rate, for example, the time required to reach steady-state serum concentrations of drugs which are excreted unchanged in urine (e.g. gentamicin, digoxin, penicillin) may be 20 times longer than in patients with normal renal function.

In some instances the latency between onset of treatment and appearance of adverse effects is much longer than expected on the basis of pharmacokinetic considerations. In these cases, more complex mechanisms are operating. For example, symptoms of folic acid and vitamin D deficiency usually become clinically manifest only several years after starting chronic therapy with antiepileptic drugs. The pathophysiological mechanism involved is likely to be induction of the hepatic microsomal enzymes which inactivate folic acid and vitamin D, and it is reasonable to assume that a prolonged period is required for the body stores of these vitamins to become depleted. Another example of adverse reaction of late onset is the respiratory disease associated with practolol therapy. Although the clinical manifestations of the disease may not be apparent until 20 months after stopping drug therapy, they often are quite severe and rapidly evolutive (*Marshall* et al. 1977).

Not infrequently, adverse drug effects show an inverse relationship with duration of treatment, i.e. they tend to decrease as the latter is prolonged. Drowsiness and fatigue, for example, are common during the initial phases of treatment with barbiturates, benzodiazepines and antihistamines but may gradually subside after a few weeks of administration. Subjects addicted to morphine or barbiturates may tolerate doses which would be lethal to individuals not previously exposed to these drugs. This phenomenon is known as tolerance and will be discussed in greater detail on page 44–46.

4. The Pharmaceutical Preparation

Between March and June, 1966, an outbreak of phenytoin intoxication was described in Australia shortly arter the excipient in phenytoin capsules had been changed from hydrated calcium sulphate to lactose (*Eadie* et al. 1968). A probable explanation for this phenomenon is that calcium sulphate reduced the absorption of phenytoin by causing flocculation of the drug particles within the gastrointestinal tract. In Scandinavia, different pharmaceutical preparations of phenytoin are available which contain either the acid or the sodium salt. The most commonly used preparation (an amorphous preparation of phenytoin acid) has less than 50% bioavailability and cases of severe intoxication have occurred when patients stabilized on this product were changed over to other preparations, subsequently found to have much higher bioavailability (*Lund* 1974). Similar differences in oral bioavailability of potential clinical significance have been reported for various pharmaceutical formulations of digoxin (*Shaw* et al. 1972; *Linderbaum* et al. 1971; *Manninen* et al. 1971; *Beveridge* et al. 1975), tolbutamide (*Varley* 1968), chloramphenicol (*Glazko* et al. 1968), quinidine (*Frigo* et al. 1977), chlormethiazole (*Fischler* et al. 1973) and phenacetin (*Prescott* et al. 1976).

It is important to stress the fact that not only the extent but also the rate of absorption may vary from one pharmaceutical preparation to another. Peak serum drug levels are higher, and systemic adverse effects more frequent, with drugs which are rapidly absorbed. One of the purposes of sustained-release preparations is to minimise the occurrence of adverse reactions shortly after intake of rapidly absorbed drugs.

An interesting example of the importance of the drug formulation in the pathogenesis of adverse reactions is provided by erythromycin. Although active hepatitis has followed on several occasions the administration of erythromycin estolate, it has not been reported after administration of the base (*Robinson* 1962). Erythromycin estolate is a combination of erythromycin propionate with the detergent lauryl sulphate, the latter being added in order to enhance the gastrointestinal absorption of the base. The suggestion has recently been made that lauryl sulphate may also enhance the penetration of erythromycin into the hepatocyte, and thus markedly potentiate its hepatotoxic properties (*Dujovne* 1978).

5. The Effects of Multiple Drug Therapy

Drug interactions are a well known source of adverse drug effects, and will be discussed in greater detail in some of the sections below.

II. Factors Inherent in the Patient's Responsiveness

As a general rule, when a standard dose of a drug is administered to a group of subjects, only in some is a fully adequate therapeutic effect produced. Many subjects are undertreated while in others the response is excessive and toxic reactions become manifest. An estimate of the degree of variability in drug response is provided by the dose range necessary to produce an optimal therapeutic effect in different subjects. In the case of guanethidine the oral antihypertensive dose may range from 10 to 1000 mg daily, a hundred-fold variation (*McMartin* and *Simpson* 1971). A similar variability is observed with warfarin, some patients requiring for optimal anticoagulant control a dose that would be virtually lethal to others. Although the risks of adverse effects are minimized by starting therapy on a small dose and increasing it gradually, toxic reactions in the most sensitive individuals are at times inevitable especially when the therapeutic ratio of the drug is narrow and when a rapid response is required. There are two main sources of variability in drug response: individual differences in drug handling (pharmacokinetic sources of variability) and individual differences in target-organ responsiveness (pharmacodynamic sources of variability).

1. Interindividual Differences in Pharmacokinetics

Interindividual differences can be observed in absorption, distribution, biotransformation and excretion. Although each of these will be considered separately, it is from a combination of these variables that inter-subject differences in drug response are produced.

a) Absorption

The rate and extent of absorption of individual drugs from the gastrointestinal tract is determined by a combination of factors such as the physico-chemical properties of the substance, the pharmaceutical preparation, the rate of gastric emptying, the intestinal motility, the integrity of the gastrointestinal mucosa, the mucosal blood flow and drug interactions in the alimentary canal. These factors may vary considerably not only between individuals but also in the same subject under different conditions including dietary habits, exercise, psychological stimuli and disease. Inter-subject differences in the rate of gastric emptying, for example, are responsible for the 80-fold variability of plasma paracetamol concentrations one hour after intake of a single dose by fasting hospital patients (*Prescott* 1974). Concurrent intake of food sometimes results in lower rate of absorption although in some cases a drastic reduction of the extent of absorption may also be seen, as for pivampicillin (*Fernandez* et al. 1973), isoniazid (*Melander* et al. 1977a) and tetracycline (*Kirby* et al. 1961). Less well known is the possibility of food enhancing drug bioavailability, as in the case of propranolol, metoprolol (*Melander* et al. 1977a) hydralazine (*Melander* et al. 1977b), canrenone (from spironolactone) (*Melander* et al. 1977c), nitrofurantoin (*Rosenberg* and *Bates* 1976) and hydrochlorothiazide (*Beermann* and *Groschinsky-Grind* 1978). Unless the time of administration is standardized in respect of meal times, the enhancement of bioavailability produced by food results in higher steady-state concentration of the drug in plasma and tissues, and toxic reactions may occur.

Ionic compounds are predominantly absorbed in their non-ionized lipid-soluble form. Therefore weakly acidic drugs such as salicylates and phenobarbitone are better absorbed at the low pH values found in the stomach whereas basic drugs such as quinidine and procainamide are preferentially absorbed in the intestine. Strong bases, however, remain almost completely ionized even at the highest physiological values of intestinal pH and their absorption is poor and erratic (e.g. guanethidine). Modifications of the luminal pH may have a profound influence on the absorption of these drugs but the effect is often unpredictable. For example, the absorption of aspirin is surprisingly enhanced in patients with gastric achlorhydria possibly because aspirin dissolves more readily in the gastric contents of these patients (*Pottage* et al. 1974).

Diseases of the gastrointestinal tract are generally associated with impaired drug absorption. The bioavailability of paracetamol (*Heading* et al. 1973) and L-dopa (*Bianchine* et al. 1971), for example, is reduced in patients with delayed gastric emptying. In patients with coeliac disease, however, the bioavailability of digoxin (*Heizer* et al. 1971) and practolol (*Parson* and *Kaye* 1974) is reduced but the bioavailability of propranolol is enhanced (*Parson* and *Kaye* 1974).

Drug interactions in the gastrointestinal tract are usually but not always associated with reduced absorption. There are a number of mechanisms by which alterations in drug absorption may occur, the formation of insoluble complexes being perhaps the most common (*Nimmo* et al. 1973; *Kunin* and *Finland* 1961). Formation of insoluble complexes is the mode by which PAS granules, for example, markedly reduce the bioavailability of rifampicin; interestingly the excipients contained in the granules and not PAS itself are responsible for this effect (*Boman* et al. 1975). These interactions generally result in a reduction of the pharmacological activity but toxic effects may readily develop when the interfering agent is withdrawn and the bioavailability of the affected drug is consequently enhanced. More rarely interactions result directly in increased drug absorption. Propantheline, for example, has been shown to increase by approximately one third the steady-state serum concentration of digoxin (*Manninen* et al. 1973). The mechanism of the interaction is probably related to the reduction of gastrointestinal motility by propantheline thus allowing digoxin to remain longer at the absorption sites. Metoclopramide, which increases gastrointestinal motility, decreased by a similar extent the serum concentration of digoxin in the same study.

b) Distribution

α) Plasma-Protein Binding

Many drugs are highly bound to plasma proteins. Since only the unbound fraction is available to produce its pharmacological effects at the site of action, it is clear that changes in the degree of plasma-protein binding can be an important source of variability in drug response. A potentiation of Type A adverse reactions would be expected in patients showing the lowest degree of plasma-protein binding. In practice, however, the situation is more complex because the increased free drug is available not only to produce biological effects but also to be distributed to tissue storage sites and to be eliminated. For these reasons changes in the binding of drugs to plasma proteins are important only for drugs having a low volume of distribution, i.e. when the amount of drug in plasma is sufficiently large as compared to the amount in tissues. Another factor which may contribute to increased incidence of adverse reactions to certain drugs in patients with reduced plasma-protein binding is the time course of unbound drug in blood during a dosing interval at steady-state. Although the average plasma concentration of unbound drug in patients with reduced binding may be similar to that in patients with normal binding, the peak concentration is generally higher in the former group (*Levy* 1976). If the pharmacological action of the drug takes place within the blood stream or the blood vessels (or highly perfused tissues), the maximum intensity of drug effect can be considerably enhanced. The importance of this principle is illustrated by the observation that the maximum hypotensive response to diazoxide (*Pearson* and *Breckenridge* 1976) after single dose administration is significantly higher in patients with reduced protein binding than in patients with normal binding. For few other drugs has evidence of clinically important effects related to changes in plasma-protein binding been presented. *Booker* and *Darcey* (1973) found that in epileptic patients the occurrence of toxic signs was very much better correlated with the unbound concentration of phenytoin than with the total concentration of the drug in plasma.

These results are indirectly supported by a report of the Boston Collaborative Drug Surveillance Program (BCDSP) (1973a). Adverse reactions to phenytoin were obersed in 11.4% of 88 hospital patients with an admission albumin level lower than 3.0 gm% but only in 3.8% of 234 patients with a normal serum albumin, despite a similar average phenytoin dose in the two groups. The authors advanced the hypothesis that decreased binding of phenytoin to serum albumin was responsible for their findings, and a negative correlation between plasma albumin level and unbound fraction of phenytoin has been confirmed in a subsequent study (*Porter* and *Layzer* 1975). Unfortunately the serum phenytoin concentration was not measured in the patients surveyed by the BCDSP and it cannot be excluded that the higher susceptibility to adverse reactions in patients with hypoalbuminemia were in fact related to concurrent liver disease and reduced rate of phenytoin metabolism. The problem is of considerable interest because a number of physiological (*Fredholm* et al. 1975; *Hayes* et al. 1975), pathological (*Blaschke* et al. 1975; *Reidenberg* et al. 1971) and pharmacological (*Reidenberg* et al. 1971) factors are known to increase the free fraction of phenytoin in plasma.

An inverse relationship between the concentration of albumin in serum and adverse reactions has also been described with diazepam (*Greenblatt* and *Koch-Weser* 1974). In more than 1200 patients monitored adverse reactions ranged from 2.9% in patients with normal serum albumin (⩾ 3.0 gm%) to 9.3% in those with hypoalbuminemia. An increased incidence of adverse reactions in patients with hypoalbuminemia has also been reported with prednisone, possibly due to increased unbound concentration of the active metabolite prednisolone (*Lewis* et al. 1971).

Patients with impaired renal function show a particular susceptibility to adverse drug reactions. Although reduced renal clearance of unchanged drug and/or toxic metabolites is often the principal cause for this finding, changes in plasma-protein binding may play a significant role. Indeed the degree of binding of many drugs has been found to be markedly reduced in uraemic patients (*Vallner* 1977; *Reidenberg* 1977b).

One drug may displace another drug from its protein binding sites and thus increase its unbound fraction in plasma. An almost endless list of such interactions have been described but only a few are likely to have clinical significance. The best known example is the displacement of warfarin by phenylbutazone (*Aggeler* et al. 1967), nalidixic acid, ethacrinic acid, diazoxide (*Sellers* and *Koch-Weser* 1970b) and trichloroacetic acid; the main metabolite of chloral-hydrate in man (*Sellers* and *Koch-Weser* 1970a). As warfarin is 99% protein bound and has low volume of distribution and low therapeutic ratio, its displacement from plasma-protein binding sites may result in marked potentiation of the anticoagulant effect with potentially serious clinical consequences.

β) Tissue Binding

A striking correlation between age and the half-life of diazepam has recently been described in adult normal subjects (*Klotz* et al. 1975). The half-life increased linearly from 20 h at 20 years of age to 90 h at 80 years. Surprisingly, the plasma clearance of the drug showed no significant age dependence and was not reduced in the elderly subjects; the marked prolongation of the half-life in the aged, therefore, was exclusively related to a progressive increase of the volume of distribution with increasing age. Since neither the plasma protein binding (97.4 ± 1.2%) nor the blood-plasma concentration ratio (0.58 ± 16) showed any correlation with age, it was concluded that the increase in distribution volume in the elderly was due to increased tissue binding of the drug. This study illustrates the possible pitfalls of interpreting half-life data when clearance values are not available. Despite the marked prolongation of the serum half-life, the constancy of the clearance indicates that the elimination of diazepam in the elderly is not impaired. Therefore the drug will not accumulate in the aged more than it does in the young and dose readjustments for different age groups may not be necessary. In the elderly, however, the time required to reach a steady-state concentration in serum and tissues will be considerably longer. An important question which remains to be answered is whether the increased tissue-binding will result in higher concentration at the receptor site and consequently enhanced pharmacological response. An increased sensitivity of elderly patients to the CNS adverse effects of benzodiazepines has been reported (Boston Collaborative Surveillance Program 1973b; *Castleden* et al. 1977) and it is tempting to speculate that it is at least in part due to changes in tissue distribution.

For a recent detailed review on the influence of various pathophysiological factors on the tissue binding of diazepam and many other drugs the reader is referred to *Klotz* (1976).

γ) Active Transport

The distribution of certain drugs within discrete regions of the body is sometimes determined by active processes. Some drugs cannot readily diffuse across the blood-brain barrier but are transported through by relatively selective transport mechanisms. For example, organic acids such as penicillin and salicylic acid are transported from the cerebrospinal fluid (CSF) to plasma by an energy-requiring pump localized in the choroid plexuses. Probenecid competes for the carrier mechanism and its administration can markedly prolong the elimination of these drugs from the CSF.

The integrity of the blood-brain barrier is altered in a number of pathological conditions, e.g. meningitis, resulting in substantial penetration into the central nervous system (CNS) of drugs that would not normally have access to it. The clinical consequences may be occasionally beneficial, e.g. enhanced penetration of an antibiotic into a septic focus, but CNS toxicity can also result.

An active transport mechanism is responsible for the uptake of various drugs from the extracellular space into the nerve terminals. The antihypertensive effect of guanethidine is dependent on the drug accumulating in relatively high concentration within the sympathetic nerve endings. This is achieved through active transport by the same pump as is responsible for the uptake of noradrenaline. Tricyclic antidepressants and phenothiazines, among other drugs, block the pump and consequently antagonise the antihypertensive action of guanethidine (*Mitchell* et al. 1970). If a tricyclic antidepressant is administered to a patient with severe hypertension controlled on guanethidine the blood pressure will rise within a few days to very high values, with potentially disastrous clinical consequences.

c) Biotransformation

Many drugs are highly lipid soluble and cannot undergo renal excretion to any important extent. Therefore they would accumulate in the body to dangerous levels if they were not transformed into more polar water soluble metabolites that can be readily excreted in urine. Biotransformation reactions require enzymatic catalysis and usually involve two steps: 1. introduction into the drug molecule of groups such as -OH, $-CO_2$ and $-NH_2$, rendering the molecule suitable for 2. conjugation with an endogenous substrate such as glucuronic acid, acetic acid, glycine, glutamine and ion sulphate. The first step is accomplished by oxidation, reduction or hydrolysis (phase I reactions) and usually results in the formation of inactive or less active metabolites, although in some cases enhancement of the pharmacological activity may occur. Phase II reactions yield what is referred to as a conjugated metabolite which is usually water soluble and readily excreted from the body. The enzymes responsible for drug metabolism are located mainly in the smooth endoplasmic reticulum (microsomes) of the hepatic cell, although a variable degree of enzymatic activity can be detected in the microsomes and the cytosol of other tissues, including the human placenta and neoplastic cells, and in infectious agents such as bacteria and protozoa. The rate at which drugs are metabolized in the body varies considerably from one subject to another. Since for most drugs metabolism is the principal determinant of the extent and duration of drug action, it is not surprising that individual differences in rate of metabolism play an important role in the pathogenesis of Type A adverse reactions. Subjects who metabolise the drug slowly tend to accumulate it in tissues and to show an exaggerated pharmacological response. This may not be true, however, for compounds which are partly or wholly converted into active metabolites (see page 37). A detailed analysis of the factors that are known to influence the rate of drug metabolism (Table 3) is beyond the purpose of this article. Their importance as a potential source of adverse drug reactions is illustrated by a few representative examples discussed below.

α) Genetic Factors

The influence of genetic factors on drug disposition is well recognized, the most notable example being the acetylator phenotype. The ability to acetylate isoniazid is inherited as a recessive autosomal trait, individuals being classified as slow or fast acetylators respectively on the basis of the rate at which they acetylate the drug. The proportion of slow acetylators varies in different populations, ranging from 82% in Egyptians and 60% in Caucasians to 15% in Chinese and 1–5% in Eskimos. Slow acetylators develop higher serum isoniazid concentrations when given ordinary doses of the drug and as a consequence show a much higher incidence of dose-related adverse effects such as peripheral neuropathy (20% as opposed to 3% in rapid acetylators) (*Devadatta* et al. 1960). Interestingly, the incidence of isoniazid-induced hepatitis is higher in fast acetylators, probably due to higher rate of formation of an hepatotoxic acetyl-hydrazide derivative in the latter group (*Lunde* et al. 1977; *Mitchell* and *Potter* 1975, for reviews).

Table 3. Factors affecting the rate of drug metabolism in man

Factor	Example
Genetic influence	Bi-modal distribution of isoniazid elimination.
Age	Reduced rate of antipyrine elimination in the elderly.
Pregnancy	Increased rate of phenytoin metabolism during pregnancy.
Liver blood flow	Increased hepatic clearance of lignocaine with increasing liver blood flow.
Protein binding	Enhanced metabolism of phenytoin in patients with reduced plasma protein-binding.
Disease (especially hepatic)	Reduced elimination of paracetamol in liver necrosis. Increased hepatic metabolism of antipyrine in renal failure.
Saturable metabolism	Dose-dependent kinetics of phenytoin (Fig. 3). Dose-dependent bioavailability of hydralazine.
Enzyme-induction	Increased warfarin elimination during phenobarbitone treatment. Reduction of the oral availability of alprenolol (induction of first-pass metabolism) by pentobarbitone.
Enzyme inhibition	Phenytoin intoxication during isoniazid treatment.

Procainamide, phenelzine, dapsone, hydralazine, the amino-metabolite of nitrazepam and certain sulphonamides are also acetylated by the same enzymatic system which metabolizes isoniazid. As expected the incidence of adverse effects to these drugs is generally higher in slow than in fast acetylators (for a recent review *Lunde* et al. 1977). Thus administration of hydralazine in doses above 200 mg/day to slow acetylators results in excessive serum concentrations of the drug and increases the probability of developing antinuclear factor autoantibodies and the systemic lupus syndrome (*Perry* 1973). *Strandberg* et al. (1976) studied 31 cases of hydralazine-induced SLE: 29 of these were slow acetylators and 25 were women. Interestingly most of their patients were treated with less than 200 mg/day. This may indicate that slow acetylators are more vulnerable to drug-induced SLE regardless of the dose or serum level of the drug. In this respect it is of considerable interest that spontaneous (e.g. non drug-induced) SLE is much more commonly associated with the slow than with the fast acetylator phenotype (*Larsson* et al. 1977). An increased incidence of a lupus-like syndrome in slow acetylators has also been described during procainamide treatment, but other workers have reported opposite findings (*Karlsson* 1978). These conflicting results may be explained by the observation that the main metabolite of procainamide retains most of the pharmacological activity of the parent drug and could therefore mediate the autoimmune reaction in fast acetylators.

β) Age

The rate of metabolism of certain drugs is reduced in both the newborn and the elderly, and failure to recognise this important principle has led to many therapeutic disasters. For example, administration of chloramphenicol in high dosages to premature neonates with low glucuronizing ability and reduced renal function has been related to the 'grey baby' syndrome observed in this age group (*Weiss* et al. 1960). Chloramphenicol half-lives of 24–28 h have been demonstrated in these newborns as compared to values of 1.5–5 h normally found in children and adults (*Sereni* and *Principi* 1968). The apparent half-life of diazepam is 75 ± 35 h in premature newborns, 31 ± 2 h in full-term newborns, 17 ± 3 h in children and 25 ± 12 h in adults (*Morselli* 1977). No doubt, the prolonged elimination of diazepam in premature newborns is at least in part responsible for their slow recovery from the toxic effects (low Apgar score, respiratory and neurological depression) of transplacentally transferred drug.

The particular vulnerability of elderly patients to adverse drug reactions is also likely to be partly related to reduced ability to metabolise certain drugs in this age group. For example, although chlormethiazole is frequently used as an hypnotic drug in elderly patients, it is not generally appreciated that in these patients serum chlormethiazole levels produced by ordinary oral doses are more than five times higher than in younger subjects (*Nation* et al. 1977). Chlormethiazole undergoes extensive hepatic first-pass metabolism, i.e. a considerable fraction of an orally administered dose is metabolized in the liver before reaching the systemic circulation: in the elderly the metabolizing capacity of this organ is reduced and a much larger fraction of the dose escapes first-pass elimination. Other drugs whose rate of metabolism has been shown to be reduced in the aged include antipyrine (*O'Malley* et al. 1971), paracetamol (*Triggs* et al. 1975), phenytoin (*Houghton* et al. 1975) and propranolol (*Castleden* et al. 1975).

γ) Disease

In view of the crucial role of the liver in drug disposition, the rate of drug metabolism could be expected to be impaired in patients with hepatic disease. The reasons for this are at least twofold: 1. hepatocellular disease can result in reduced drug-metabolizing enzyme activity and 2. disruption of the normal vascular architecture of the organ may decrease the availability of the drug at the metabolic sites. A number of studies have confirmed that drug metabolism is impaired in patients with various types of liver disease. In a careful investigation in which only age-matched and drug-free subjects were used the half-life of diazepam was found to be 106 ± 15 h in patients with cirrhosis compared with 46 ± 14 h in controls, and 75 ± 28 h in patients with acute viral hepatitis compared with 33 ± 9 h in controls (*Klotz* et al 1975). *Prescott* and colleagues (1971) determined the plasma paracetamol half-life in patients admitted to hospital after a paracetamol overdose, and found values to be twice as long in patients with hepatic necrosis than in those without (7.6 ± 0.8 versus 2.9 ± 0.3 h). Interestingly, in patients developing progressive liver damage the half-life of paracetamol increased with time: for example, in a patient who went into hepatic coma the half-life rose from 16 to 60 h over a period of a few days. *Wilkinson* and *Schenker* (1975) reviewed the literature on the subject and found evidence of impaired metabolism in liver disease for the following drugs: acetanilide, amylobarbitone, antipyrine, carbenicillin, chloramphenicol, clindamycin, diazepam, hexobarbitone, isoniazid, lignocaine, pethidine, meprobamate, paracetamol, pentobarbitone, phenobarbitone, phenylbutazone, prednisone, rifampicin, theophylline and tolbutamide.

More recent studies have focused their attention on the effects of liver disease on the disposition of drugs subject to extensive first-pass metabolism. The half-life of these drugs is determined by the rate of liver blood flow rather than by the metabolizing capacity of the organ. Unless gross alterations in hepatic blood supply occur, the disposition of these drugs after parenteral administration is little affected by hepatic disease: when the same drugs are given orally, however, the fraction of the dose which escapes first-pass elimination is considerably increased. Thus, the oral bioavailability of propranolol (*Branch* et al. 1976) and labetalol (*Homeida* et al. 1978) is twice as large in patients with cirrhosis than in normal subjects resulting, at least for labetalol, in exaggerated response in the former group (*Homeida* et al. 1978). In the case of chlormethiazole the oral availability in cirrhotic patients is ten times higher than in normal subjects and this may have a determinant role in the fatal outcome of certain cases of chlormethiazole overdose (*Pentikäinen* et al. 1978). In addition to reduced drug metabolism other factors may be responsible for the increased susceptibility to adverse drug reactions in patients with hepatic disease (Fig. 2). The complex pharmacokinetic implications of liver disease have been recently reviewed by *Blaschko* (1977).

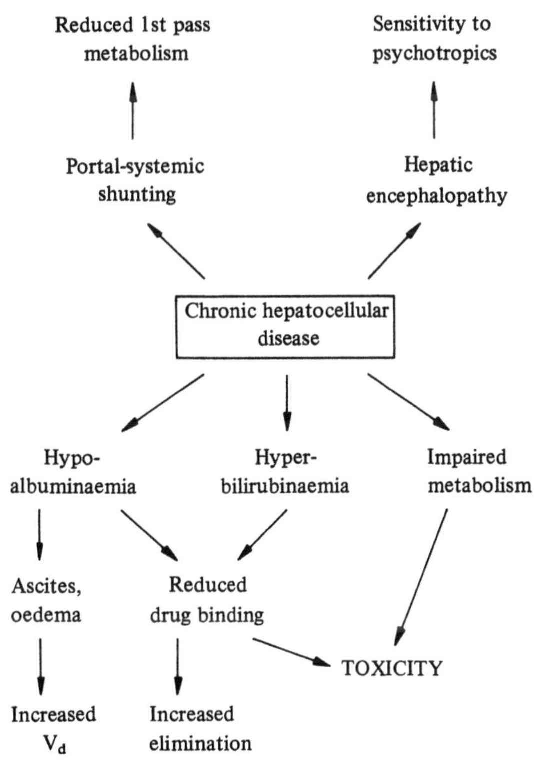

Fig. 2. Factors involved in adverse drug reactions in liver disease

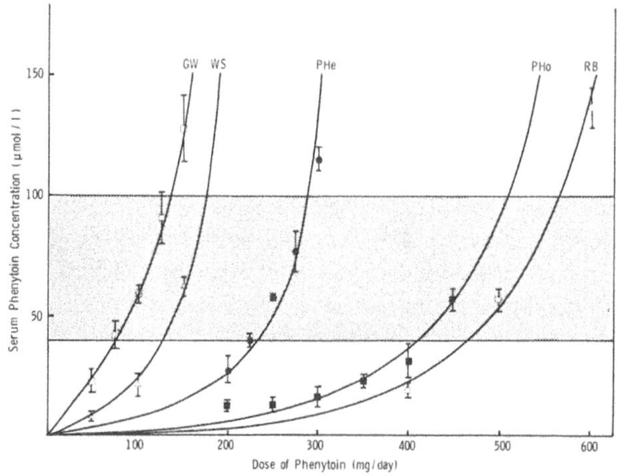

Fig. 3. Relationship between daily dose of phenytoin and resulting serum concentration in five patients on several different doses of the drug. Horizontal lines represent the limits of the therapeutic range.
Note the marked inter-subject variability in the dose at which saturation is approached (see text). (Reproduced with permission from *Dunlop* and *Richens* 1975)

δ) Dose-Dependent Metabolism

Phenytoin is hydroxylated in the liver by an enzyme-system which becomes saturated at serum concentration values commonly encountered in therapeutic practice. When saturation is approached the relationship between serum level and dose becomes increasingly steep, small increments in dose resulting in a disproportionate increase of the serum concentration at steady state (Fig. 3). Unless the dose is carefully adjusted, toxic effects may easily develop. The disastrous consequences of failing to take into account the saturable nature of phenytoin metabolism are illustrated by a case described by one of us (*Richens* et al. 1976). A 39 year old epileptic patient was admitted to a Neurological Unit in June 1974 because his seizures were poorly controlled. The serum phenytoin level was 12 μmol/l on a daily dose of 300 mg. As this was well below the therapeutic range of 40–100 μmol/l the phenytoin dose was doubled to 600 mg on the assumption, presumably, that the serum phenytoin is linearly related to dose. The patient initially improved and was discharged. When he came to our observation in November 1975 he gave a several months history of diplopia which had failed to respond to orthoptic treatment. He was restricted to a wheelchair because of severe ataxia, his speech was slurred and he showed coarse nystagmus on lateral gaze. A diagnosis of phenytoin intoxication was made on clinical grounds, and it was subsequently confirmed by a serum phenytoin level of 160 μmol/l, well into the toxic range. The drug was stopped for four days and re-started on a reduced dosage, resulting in a dramatic improvement of all symptoms and clinical signs. A computer predicted dose-serum level relationship in this patient, based on the initial value at a dosage of 300 mg/day and taking into account the saturable metabolism of the drug, clearly showed that a dose regime of 600 mg/day was expected to be toxic.

Phenytoin has a narrow therapeutic ratio and the occurrence of saturation kinetics at different doses in different subjects makes it a difficult drug to use. When the upper limit of the therapeutic range is approached, small changes in metabolic activity, e.g. due to drug interactions, can result in marked variations of the serum concentration at steady state and can be responsible for sudden development of toxicity in patients who previously had done well on the same dose.

Salicylic acid and dicoumarol (*O'Reilly* et al. 1964) have been shown also to exhibit dose-dependent kinetics when administered in therapeutic doses.

Saturation of first-pass metabolism has been demonstrated for various drugs, e.g. hydralazine (*Talseth* 1977). The oral availability of these drugs increases with increasing dosage and this may result in exaggerated pharmacological response following relatively small dose increments.

ε) Enzyme-Induction

It is now well recognized that many pharmacological agents, dietary constituents, insecticides, pesticides and industrial contaminants can stimulate the activity of the drug-metabolizing enzymes of the human liver microsomes (Table 4). The degree of stimulation is dependent on a combination of factors such as the type of inducing agent, its dosage, the route and the duration of administration, the influence of genetic factors, age and effects of concurrent disease. There are a number of ways in which stimulation of drug metabolism may result in undesired clinical effects. The most common of these is failure to produce an adequate pharmacological response when ordinary doses of a drug are given to patients receiving enzyme-inducing agents. A typical example is the stimulation of the metabolism of the oral contraceptive in women taking phenobarbitone, resulting in high incidence of breakthrough bleeding and increased risk of pregnancy (*Hempel* and *Klinger* 1976). Because of induction of warfarin metabolism, much higher doses of the anticoagulant are required to maintain a satisfactory prothrombin time during treatment with phenobarbitone and other inducing agents. If the inducing agent is withdrawn, the activity of the drug-metabolizing enzymes gradually decreases and unless the warfarin dose is reduced accordingly, potentially fatal hemorrhage may occur.

Normal body constituents such as fatty acids, steroid hormones, folic acid and vitamin D are metabolized in the liver by the same enzymatic system involved in drug

Table 4. Compounds which are known to induce the hepatic microsomal enzymes in man

Aminopyrine	Glutethimide
Antipyrine	Medroxyprogesterone
Barbiturates	Methaqualone + diphenhydramine
Carbamazepine	Pheneturide
Chlorinated hydrocarbons	Phenytoin
Dichloralphenazone	Polycyclic hydrocarbons (e.g. benzpyrene)
Ethanol	Rifampicin

Table 5. Drug-induced diseases considered to be related to induced metabolism of normal body constituents by antiepileptic drugs

Disease	Comment	Mechanism
Rickets and osteomalacia	More frequent in patients receiving no dietary supplements of vitamin D, or with reduced exposure to sunlight.	? Increased conversion of cholecalciferol to inactive metabolites.
Folic acid deficiency	Megaloblastic anaemia observed in some cases.	? Enhanced inactivation of folic acid. ? Increased utilization for cytochromic biosynthesis.
Disturbances of sex hormone metabolism	High incidence of impotence, loss of libido and reduced fertility in drug-treated epileptic patients.	? Enhanced biodegradation of androgen steroids.

metabolism. Induction of the biotransformation of these compounds is probably responsible for certain aspects of the chronic toxicity of antiepileptic drugs (Table 5) (*Perucca* 1978).

In some cases enzyme-induction results in enhancement of the pharmacological effect, due to increased rate of formation of active metabolites. This possibility is discussed at page 37.

ζ) Enzyme-Inhibition

As a general rule inhibition of drug metabolism results in prolonged and exaggerated pharmacological response and is, therefore, a typical source of Type A adverse reactions. In the clinical situation enzyme-inhibition is potentially more dangerous than enzyme-induction because it tends to occur more rapidly, generally within a few days as compared to a few weeks for enzyme-induction. A large number of drug interactions resulting in inhibition of metabolism have been reported and a selection of some of the most important in therapeutic practice is listed in Table 6. Although most of these interactions occur quite consistently their clinical manifestations are not necessarily apparent in all subjects. The same interaction may be responsible for severe adverse reactions in some cases, while in others it may pass competely unrecognized unless the serum concentration of the drugs have been carefully monitored. Such a variability in individual response is determined by a number of factors: the therapeutic ratio of the affected drug, its concentration in serum before addition of the interfering drug, the serum concentration of the inhibiting agent, the patient's age and the effects of concurrent disease. Elderly and acutely ill patients are generally more vulnerable to the adverse effects of drug interactions. Genetic influences are also important. Isonia-

Table 6. Some important examples of inhibition of drug metabolism in man

Interfering drug	Affected drug
Benzerazide	L-dopa
Allopurinol	6-mercapto-purine
Chloramphenicol Phenylbutazone	Tolbutamide
Isoniazid Sulthiame	Phenytoin
MAO-inhibitors	Tyramine etc. (see text)
Dextropropoxyphene	Carbamazepine

zid, for example, is known to inhibit phenytoin metabolism both in vitro and in vivo (*Kutt* 1972). Epidemics of phenytoin intoxication have been described in epileptic patients after administration of isoniazid for prophylaxis against tuberculosis (*Murray* 1962) but, interestingly, only slow acetylators appear to be affected (*Kutt* et al. 1970). Presumably, only slow acetylators accumulate in the hepatic microsomes a concentration of isoniazid high enough to inhibit phenytoin hydroxylation. Other drugs are known to produce phenytoin intoxication by inhibiting its metabolism and these include: chloramphenicol, dicoumarol, disulfiram, pheneturide, phenyramidol and sulthiame (for reviews *Kutt* 1972 and *Richens* 1977). The interaction with sulthiame is particularly important. *Houghton* and *Richens* (1974) determined the serum phenytoin concentration in 137 consecutive patients admitted to the Chalfont Centre for Epilepsy and found toxic levels ($\geqslant 100\ \mu$ mol/l) in as many as 40% of the patients receiving the combination sulthiame-phenytoin, as compared to only 13% of the patients receiving phenytoin but not sulthiame. These findings could not be accounted for by a difference in the phenytoin dose which was on average identical in the two groups. When the distribution of serum phenytoin levels was compared in patients receiving 300 mg/day phenytoin, values were found to be 75% higher in patients receiving sulthiame in combination (Fig. 4) but fell to normal levels in those intoxicated patients in whom sulthiame was withdrawn. A latent period of 10–20 days generally elapses between starting sulthiame treatment and the resulting rise in serum phenytoin concentration, which is suggestive of a non-competitive type of enzyme-inhibition.

Although in most cases drug metabolism interactions take place in the hepatic microsomes, there are important exceptions such as the inhibition of the monoamine oxidase (MAO) enzyme system. MAO is located in the mitochondria of a wide variety of tissues, particularly the liver and the gastrointestinal tract. The system is involved in the deamination of several biologically important amines such as dopamine, tyramine, 5-hydroxytryptamine and, to a lesser extent, adrenaline and noradrenaline. Although most of the MAO inhibitors used in clinical practice are rapidly metabolized, the in-

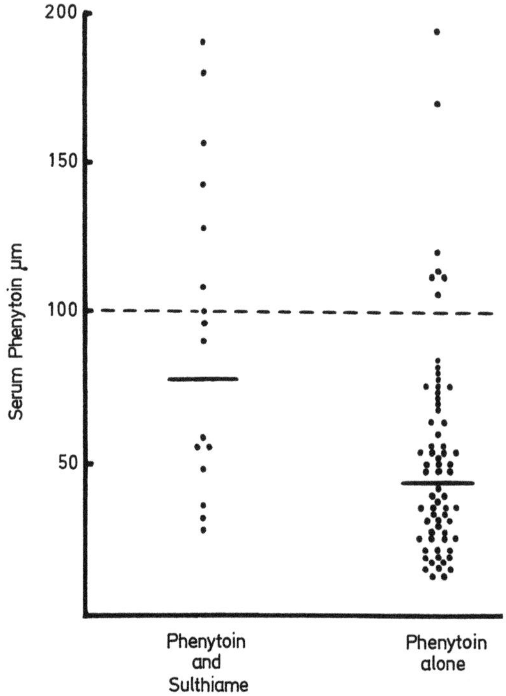

Fig. 4. Distribution of serum phenytoin levels in patients receiving 300 mg/day phenytoin, with or without the addition of sulthiame. The upper limit of the therapeutic range is marked with a dashed line. Horizontal bars represent the mean values, based on logarithmically transformed data. (Reproduced with permission from *Houghton* and *Richens* 1974)

hibition they produce is irreversible and therefore persists for a considerable time after the disappearance of these drugs from the body. Administration of MAO substrates to patients treated with MAO inhibitors can result in a disproportionate potentiation of the hypertensive effects of these substrates, with potentially fatal clinical consequences. Tyramine, in particular, is contained in relatively large amounts in various dietary products (e.g. cheese, Chianti wine, chicken liver, pickled herring). In normal subjects, after intake of these foods the amine is almost completely metabolized by the MAO in the gut and in the liver and it cannot reach the systemic circulation to any significant extent. In patients receiving MAO inhibitors the fraction of tyramine which is metabolized is markedly reduced and the drug can reach the nerve terminals in concentrations high enough to cause severe hypertensive reactions. These have been noted after ingestion of as little as 20 g of a certain Cheddar cheese (*Horwitz* et al. 1964). Many other sympathomimetic drugs such as amphetamines, ephedrine and tyramine act indirectly by releasing noradrenaline from the nerve terminals. In the presence of MAO inhibitors the amount of released transmitter is much larger than normal and the pharmacological effect of these drugs, whether they are MAO substrates or not, is correspondingly dangerously enhanced. Severe reactions have also been reported in patients receiving MAO inhibitors in combination with phenothiazines, tricyclic antidepressants, pethidine, thiazide diuretics, α-methyl-dopa, reserpine, insulin and sulphonylureas (*Sjöqvist* 1968). The clinical manifestations of these reactions are polymorphic, hypertension and central nervous system excitation being common but inconstant features, and probably reflect the wide variety of mechanisms involved (*Sjöqvist* 1968).

The number of fatalities due to MAO inhibitor interactions has fortunately decreased since more effective and safer agents have been introduced in the treatment of depressive disorders. It is not well recognized, however, that drugs still widely used in other conditions may have MAO inhibitory activity. The antineoplastic agent procarbazine is a typical example (*De Vita* et al. 1975). An example of the difficulty in recognizing even important drug interactions is provided by a clinico-pathologic-conference published in a prestigious medical journal (1970). A case of fulminant bone marrow aplasia was discussed in a patient who received allopurinol in addition to azathioprine. The clinicians, the pathologist and the journal editors all failed to recognise a supposedly 'well known' interaction. Allopurinol is a powerful inhibitor of 6-mercaptopurine metabolism. As azathioprine is converted to 6-mercaptopurine, the dosage of either drug should be drastically reduced (to about one fourth) in presence of allopurinol (*Elion* et al. 1963). This was not done in the patient discussed at the conference, and most likely caused her death.

η) Bioactivation

Numerous drugs are transformed in the body to active metabolites, and an increased rate of metabolism would be expected to potentiate their pharmacological effects. It must be remembered, however, that clinical effects are dependent not only on the intrinsic activity but also on the rate of elimination of the metabolite compared with that of the parent drug. Many metabolites are remarkably toxic when tested in vitro but their overall contribution to drug effects in vivo is often negligible because of fast elimination (or inactivation) and consequent lack of accumulation. Table 7 lists some

Table 7. Some important examples of drugs which are converted to active metabolites in man

Drug	Metabolites
Allopurinol	Oxypurinol
Amitriptyline	Nortriptyline
Carbamazepine	Carbamazepine 10, 11-epoxide
Cyclophosphamide	Aldophosphamide (and others)
Diazepam	N-Desmethyldiazepam
5-Fluoro-uracil	5-fluoro-deoxyuridine-monophosphate (and others)
Lignocaine	Monoethylglycinexylydide (and others)
Pethidine	Norpethidine
Phenacetin	Paracetamol
Phenylbutazone	Oxyphenbutazone
Potassium clorazepate	N-Desmethyldiazepam
Primidone	Phenobarbitone
Procainamide	N-acetyl-procainamide
Rifampicin	Desacetylrifampicin
Spironolactone	Canrenone

important compounds which undergo transformation to clinically relevant metabolites in man. In some cases, e.g. cyclophosphamide, the attainment of a therapeutic response rests almost entirely on the formation of the active metabolite(s). In other cases, e.g. paracetamol, the clinical importance of the metabolite(s) is exclusively due to intrinsic toxic properties that are not apparently shared by the parent drug. As a general rule, the toxicity of many of the drugs listed in Table 7 would be expected to be enhanced by administration of enzyme-inducing agent but this possibility has not been adequately investigated in clinical studies. Potentiation of the central nervous system toxicity of pethidine has recently been reported in patients treated with phenobarbitone and attributed to its more toxic N-demethylated metabolite norpethidine (*Stambaugh* et al. 1977). The toxicity of paracetamol is also enhanced by concurrent treatment with phenobarbitone (*Wright* and *Prescott* 1973). Paracetamol is a remarkably safe drug when administered in therapeutic doses. However, following the accidental or suicidal ingestion of large doses (10–20 g) it can produce massive hepatic necrosis and, more rarely, renal cortical necrosis. Characteristically, there is a latent period of 24–36 h between the ingestion of paracetamol and the first demonstrable signs of liver or kidney damage. There is convincing evidence from animal and human studies that the injury is related to the formation of an arylating metabolite which binds covalently to vital cell macromolecules (*Mitchell* and *Potter* 1975). Indeed, a positive correlation between the degree of covalent binding in vivo and the severity of hepatic necrosis has been demonstrated in the mouse (*Jollow* et al. 1973). Pre-treatment of animals with 3-methylcholanthrene, which increases several-fold the activity of the drug metabolizing enzymes in the liver but not in the kidney, potentiates the hepatotoxicity but not the nephrotoxicity of the drug. In man, treatment with enzyme-inducing agents also stimulates paracetamol metabolism (*Perucca* and *Richens* 1979) and enhances its hepatotoxicity (*Wright* and *Prescott* 1973). By contrast the hepatic and renal toxicity can be reduced by pre-treating animals with cobalt-chloride and piperonylbutoxide, which inhibit microsomal enzyme activity in both organs (*Mitchell* et al. 1977; *Mitchell* and *Potter* 1975). There is evidence that reduced glutathione can prevent the drug-induced injury in the hepatic cell by forming an active complex with the toxic metabolite. Administration of paracetamol causes a dose-dependent depletion of hepatic glutathione and its hepatotoxicity can be enhanced by diethylmaleate, which depletes glutathione stores (*Mitchell* et al. 1973) and reduced by cysteine, a glutathione precursor (*Mitchell* et al. 1974). The latter observation led to the successful use of another glutathione precursor, cysteamine, in the prevention of hepatic necrosis after paracetamol overdose (*Prescott* et al. 1974). Although the precise nature of the toxic metabolite is still unknown, it is considered to be a precursor of the cysteine and mercapturic acid conjugates which are found in urine after therapeutic and toxic doses (*Davis* et al. 1976). Following therapeutic doses the drug is predominantly converted to paracetamol glucuronide and paracetamol sulphate (*Perucca* and *Richens* 1979), only 20% of the metabolites recovered in urine being accounted for by cysteine and mercapturic acid conjugates (*Davis* et al. 1976). In these conditions only minute amounts of the toxic intermediate are probably formed which are rapidly inactivated by conjugation with reduced glutathione. Following overdose, however, conjugation with glucuronic acid and sulphate becomes saturated and a much larger fraction of the dose (up to 50% of urinary metabolites) is converted to cysteine and mercapturic acid conjugates (*Davis* et al. 1976). In these conditions the rate of formation of the toxic precursor(s) exceeds the availability of reduced glutathione and cell necrosis occurs. Indeed, a positive correlation between the amount of cysteine and mercapturic acid conjugates in urine (expressed as a fraction of total metabolites recovered) and the severity of liver damage has been described in patients admitted to hospital after a paracetamol overdose (*Davis* et al. 1976).

A mechanism similar to that discussed for paracetamol is probably responsible for the dose-dependent hepatotoxicity and nephrotoxicity of frusemide (*Mitchell* et al. 1977; *Mitchell* and *Potter* 1975). The metabolite responsible for the frusemide-induced necrosis has been recently identified almost certainly as a furan oxide derivative (*Mitchell* et al. 1976). This finding reinforces current evidence that chemically unstable epoxide derivatives mediate the toxicity of a wide variety of drugs, insecticides, pesticides, industrial contaminants and naturally occurring toxins. The discovery of the role of epoxides in bioactivation and carcinogenesis is a fascinating chapter in the history of pharmacology and toxicology, and the reader is referred elsewhere for recent reviews on the subject (*Garner* 1976; *Testa* and *Jenner* 1978).

d) Renal Excretion

A number of drugs are excreted predominantly unchanged in urine and their elimination may be impaired when renal function is reduced, e.g. in elderly patients and in kidney disease. Unless the dose and/or dosing interval are reduced accordingly the drug accumulates excessively and toxic reactions occur. The elimination half-life of certain drugs is prolonged more than 20 times in patients with severe kidney disease (Table 8) and it may take several days for the serum concentration to reach a steady-state level after each increment in dose. As a consequence, adverse effects, e.g. the ototoxicity of aminoglycoside antibiotics, can develop insidiously and may not be recognized until

Table 8. Half-life (hours) of some drugs eliminated largely by urinary excretion in patients with normal and impaired renal function

	Normal	Anuria
Ampicillin	0.9	7
Carbenicillin	1.2	12
Cephazolin	2	35
Digoxin	37	110
Erythromycin	1.4	5
Gentamicin	2.3	100
Isoniazid (fast acetylators)	1.4	2.3
Isoniazid (slow acetylators)	3.5	6.9
Kanamycin	2	70
Lincomycin	5	12
Procainamide	3.3	100
Tetracycline	9	69
Tobramycin	2	139
Vancomycin	6	231

irreversible damage has occurred. Appropriate schemes for determining the dose regime required at different glomerular filtration rates are available, although they are of little help in patients with fluctuating renal function. In many cases effective and safe drug therapy depends on the measurement of the serum drug concentration, but the latter is not always readily available.

The misconception that drugs largely eliminated by hepatic metabolism can be safely used in patients with impaired renal function has produced therapeutic disasters. Apart from the fact that hepatic drug metabolism (*Reidenberg* 1977a) and tissue distribution (*Reidenberg* 1977b) can be markedly abnormal in uraemic patients, the effects of accumulation of metabolite(s) must also be considered. Muscle weakness and tenderness associated with increased serum creatinine kinase activity have been described in five uraemic patients receiving 1–2 g of clofibrate daily (*Pierides* et al. 1975). These effects were considered to be due to excessive accumulation of the active metabolite chlorophenoxybutyric acid and were presumably potentiated by a markedly reduced protein binding of the same metabolite in plasma. It was concluded that uraemia should be regarded as a contraindication to the use of clofibrate. The toxicity of pethidine is also probably enhanced in patients with reduced renal function. Severe irritability, twitching and seizures have been described in uraemic patients treated with pethidine and considered to be related to the excitatory effects of the toxic metabolite norpethidine. The ratio of norpethidine to pethidine in the plasma of these patients was approximately ten times higher than in subjects with normal renal function, whereas the plasma concentration of the parent drug was within the normal range (*Szeto* et al. 1977). Adverse reactions probably caused by accumulation of active metabolites in patients with impaired renal function have also been reported with nitrofurantoin (*Maxwell* and *Meyer* 1978) and allopurinol (*Elion* et al. 1968).

In contrast with kidney disease there is limited evidence that changes in the degree of urinary excretion can be responsible for adverse drug reactions in patients with normal renal function. A case of quinidine toxicity has been attributed to increased tubular resorption of the drug in urine alkalinized by concurrent administration of antacids (*Zinn* 1970). A similar mechanism has been proposed to explain another case of quinidine intoxication in a patient with renal tubular acidosis receiving 'normal doses' of the drug (*Gerhardt* et al. 1969). On the contrary, acidic drugs are mainly ionized at alkaline values of urinary pH and their rate of excretion is enhanced in these conditions. Forced alkaline diuresis can be used to hasten the elimination of phenobarbitone and salicylate after ingestion of an overdose of these drugs.

Certain compounds are secreted into the renal tubule by an active process and competition for the transport mechanism may impair their elimination. This effect is used therapeutically when probenecid is associated with penicillin in order to prolong the half-life of the antibiotic but in other cases it may give rise to adverse reactions, e.g. the block of the tubular secretion of urate by frusemide, ethacrinic acid and thiazide diuretics.

2. Interindividual Differences in End-Organ Responsiveness

As a general rule the concentration of a drug in serum correlates with the concentration at the site of action in the tissues very much better than with the administered dose.

Individual differences in response arising from pharmacokinetic sources of variability can be minimized by tailoring the dose in order to achieve the desired serum level. It is a dangerous myth, however, to assume that all patients will show an identical response to the same serum level. Some patients may be clinically intoxicated despite the concentration of the drug being well below the lower limit of the 'therapeutic' range whereas others may tolerate unusually high levels without any untoward effects. Although differences in drug distribution between serum and tissues may account for part of these findings, it must be accepted that individual variation in end-organ responsiveness (pharmacodynamic variation) is an important determinant of drug response. Because of the difficulties involved in quantitating pharmacological response and drug concentration at the site of action, inter-subject differences in pharmacodynamics have been much less extensively investigated than their pharmacokinetic counterpart. Some important factors involved in the regulation of tissue sensitivity to drugs will be discussed below.

a) Genetic Factors

By reasons of accessibility, the best known and most extensively studied model of pharmacodynamic variability in man is the taste sensitivity for a drug. The lowest molar concentration at which a number of pharmacological agents can be tasted (taste threshold) varies considerably from one subject to another, and allows classification of human populations into two main groups, the sensitive and the non-sensitive drug tasters. Interestingly, the taste sensitivity to a given drug is correlated with the taste sensitivity to a variety of chemically unrelated compounds (*Fischer* and *Griffin* 1963); subjects who show a low taste threshold to quinine, for example, also tend to show a low taste threshold to phenothiazine drugs. Although the factors involved in the modulation of taste sensitivity are still incompletely known, there is clear evidence of a genetic control, at least for thiourea derivatives (*Vesell* 1975) and, to a lesser extent, for quinine (*Knopp* et al. 1966). The interest of these studies stems from the evidence that the taste sensitivity for a drug in humans may show a positive correlation with its systemic toxicity in animals (*Fischer* and *Griffin* 1963). It has been suggested that a similar correlation might also be found in man. In a double blind trial, *Knopp* et al. (1966) described a significant relationship between taste threshold to quinine and the development of systemic side-effects to a phenothiazine drug. Twenty-five female schizophrenic patients were screened for taste sensitivity to quinine before being started on a fixed treatment schedule with prochlorperazine. Patients sensitive to the taste of quinine developed extrapyramidal signs at an average cumulative dose of prochlorperazine significantly lower than that required to produce the same effects in non-sensitive tasters (97 versus 225 mg respectively). Although no attempt was made to ascertain possible differences in drug disposition between the two groups, these and other findings by the same authors (*Fischer* et al. 1965) were interpreted as indicative of a relationship between drug responses at different sites of action. These data require further investigation, especially in view of other lines of evidence (*Knopp* et al. 1966; *Kyrianthoupoulos* et al. 1962) that the susceptibility to the phenothiazine-induced Parkinsonian syndrome in patients with psychiatric disorders is partially under genetic control.

Another example of genetically determined abnormality in end-organ responsiveness is an hereditary condition known as warfarin-resistance (*O'Reilly* 1970). Two large kindreds affecting 25 individuals have been described so far. Although these subjects show normal absorption, distribution and elimination kinetics of warfarin, they require huge warfarin doses (up to 46 standard deviations above the mean normal daily dose) for a satisfactory anticoagulant response to be achieved. The sensitivity to the antagonist action of vitamin K on the warfarin-induced hypoprothrombinemia is strikingly increased in the same individuals. The mechanism underlying this abnormal response is considered to be a genetic mutation of the vitamin K-warfarin receptor transmitted as a single dominant effect on an autosomal chromosome (*Manninen* et al. 1971).

A third example of genetically controlled differences in drug response is the increase in intraocular pressure to locally applied steroids. In a randomly selected population (80 subjects) the pressure changes during chronic application of 0.1% dexamethasone-21-phosphate to the right eye showed a trimodal distribution (*Armaly* 1968). In 66% of the subjects the intraocular pressure increased by 5 mm Hg or less, in 29% the increase was between 6 and 15 mm Hg, while in the remaining 5% elevations between 18 and 22 mm Hg were observed. Family studies showed that the response can be adequately explained by a two-allele model with three genotypes P^LP^L, P^LP^H and P^HP^H being responsible for the low, intermediate and high degree of pressure increments respectively. There is evidence that the pressure response to topical steroids is correlated with certain types of glaucoma. Indeed the incidence of genotypes P^LP^H and P^LP^H is very much higher in patients with open-angle hypertensive glaucoma and low tension glaucoma than in the general population (*Armaly* 1968). In the latter study, the pressure response to topical steroids was determined in the uninvolved eye of patients with unilateral post-traumatic glaucoma.

b) Constitutional Factors

Age appears to be an important factor associated with altered tissue sensitivity to drugs. There is increasing evidence that the higher susceptibility of elderly patients to adverse drug reactions cannot solely be explained on the basis of pharmacokinetic differences such as impaired elimination or decreased plasma-protein binding. *Bender* (1964) has advocated the development in the elderly of an increased drug sensitivity at the receptor site. The adverse reactions to barbiturates so frequently observed in geriatric patients are likely to be due to this mechanism (*O'Malley* et al. 1976). The susceptibility of the same patients to hemorrhagic complications during therapy with oral anticoagulants (*Lamy* 1974) is also likely to be due to increased tissue sensitivity to warfarin in the aged. In a recent study the anticoagulant response to a loading warfarin dose was found to be significantly greater in six elderly subjects than in six younger controls, despite the use of a much smaller dose in the former group (0.57 versus 0.96 mg/kg on average). No appreciable differences in warfarin kinetics (plasma half-life, apparent volume of distribution, total body clearance, plasma-protein binding or plasma concentration of the active metabolite, warfarin-alcohol) could be demonstrated between the two groups. The inhibition of vitamin K-dependent synthesis of clotting factors at a given plasma concentration of warfarin was significantly greater in the elderly than in the young, further suggesting an increased receptor-site sensitivity to the anticoagulant drug. A similar mechanism is also likely to mediate the increased sensitivity to nitrazepam in old age (*Castleden* et al. 1977).

c) Pathological Factors

Adverse drug reactions most frequently arise when the pharmacological action is potentiated by the effects of concurring disease. A typical example of this phenomenon is provided by the enhancement of digitalis toxicity (cardiac dysrhythmias in particular) in the presence of potassium depletion. This is easy to overlook because relatively large decreases in intracellular potassium can occur in spite of normokalemia. Another example of potentiation of drug toxicity by pathological conditions is provided by the action of various antiinflammatory drugs on gastric secretion. A minor degree of gastrointestinal bleeding is observed in a large proportion of subjects treated with salicylates, indomethacin, phenylbutazone and systemic corticosteroids. In most subjects this is unlikely to cause major clinical problems, but in patients with quiescent gastro-duodenal

Table 9. Some important examples of pharmacodynamic sources of adverse drug reactions in diseased states

Disease	Drug	Risk or effect
Hepatic precoma	Morphine	Encephalopathy
Hepatic cirrhosis	Oral anticoagulants	Hemorrhage
Peptic ulcer	Aspirin Phenylbutazone Indomethacin	Gastrointesinal hemorrhage
Gout	Thiazide diuretics	Acute attack
Diabetes mellitus	Thiazide diuretics Frusemide Corticosteroids	Hyperglycaemia
Heart failure	β-adrenergic blocking drugs	Aggravation of chronic heart failure; precipitation of acute heart failure
Asthma	β-adrenergic blocking drugs	Acute asthmatic attack, status asthmaticus
Open-angle glaucoma	Corticosteroids	Increased intraocular pressure
Narrow-angle glaucoma	Anticholinergic drugs	Increased intraocular pressure
Herpetic eruptions	Corticosteroids	Deterioration of the infection

ulcers prolonged administration of the same drug is likely to activate the disease. Other important adverse drug reactions related to selected diseases are reported in Table 9. In most cases toxicity is secondary to the effects of the drug being additive to those of the underlying disease. In some instances, however, there is clear evidence of a disease-induced alteration in drug sensitivity at the receptor site. An example is the enhancement of the CNS depressant action of morphine in patients with hepatic precoma (*Laidlaw* et al. 1961), and the development of tolerance and supersensitivity to various drugs in patients with certain neurological disorders (see below). The subject of alteration of tissue-sensitivity to drugs in disease has been reviewed by *Lowenthal* (1974).

d) Supersensitivity and Tolerance

In many biological systems the sensitivity of the target cell to a given agonist is subject to dynamic modulation, being increased in conditions associated with reduced receptor stimulation and, conversely, decreased in the opposite situation. An increase in response is usually referred to as supersensitivity and a decrease as hyposensitivity (or tolerance, although the latter term is generally used in a wider sense). Although similar sensitivity changes have been observed in various tissues, including lymphocytes and insulin-dependent cells (*Raff* 1976), the best known example of supersensitivity is the exaggerated response of an effector organ to a submaximal concentration of its normal transmitter which occurs after its nerve supply has been severed (*Fleming* et al. 1973). Increased sensitivity to acetylcholine, for example, has been demonstrated in smooth muscle, secretory glands and striated muscle after degeneration of the cholinergic efferents; in the case of striated muscle, the enhanced response can be explained as the result of an increased number of acetylcholine receptors (*Fleming* et al. 1973). In the development of supersensitivity to catecholamines after post-ganglionic degeneration of the sympathetic nerve supply two separate mechanisms are operating: 1. a change in the characteristics of the adrenergic receptors at post-synaptic sites and 2. impaired uptake of the transmitter by pre-synaptic nerve terminals resulting in slower inactivation and prolonged response. Only the former mechanism, however, is responsible for the supersensitivity which develops after pre-ganglionic denervation (decentralization) (*Fleming* et al. 1973). Interestingly, decentralization supersensitivity is characterized by an increased response of the target cell not only to sympathominetic drugs but also to acetylcholine, barium, potassium, serotonin and other agents. Although most studies in this field have been performed in animal models, it is now clear that super- and hyposensitivity are clinical conditions that can develop as a result of diseases, drug treatment, and drug abuse. A typical example of denervation supersensitivity is observed in subjects with Shy-Drager syndrome, a neurological disorder associated with extensive degeneration of the pre- and post-ganglionic autonomic fibres. The dose of intravenous noradrenaline required to produce a 30% rise in systolic blood pressure is six times lower in these patients than in normal control subjects, almost certainly due to the development of denervation supersensitivity at the adrenergic receptor sites in the arteriolar smooth muscle (*Wilcox* and *Aminoff* 1976). Because of the strikingly enhanced pressor response, administration of standard doses of directly acting sympathomimetic agents may prove disastrous in patients affected by the syndrome.

The clinical manifestations of Parkinson's disease are considered to be the consequence of extensive degeneration of the dopaminergic nigro-striatal pathways (*Bernheimer* et al. 1973). There is increasing evidence that as nigro-striatal neurones degenerate the receptors on the post-synaptic membrane innervated by the degenerating fibres become supersensitive to dopamine (*Anden* 1970). In the early stages of the disease this condition is clinically beneficial because the supersensitive response compensates for the lower amount of transmitter released by the few remaining intact neurones (*Moore* and *Thornburg* 1975). In later stages, however, dopamine supersensitivity in the striatum can be responsible for the development of one of the most common and troublesome adverse effects of anti-parkinsonian therapy, the L-dopa-induced dyskinesias (*Weiner* and *Bergen* 1977). These dyskinesias are characterized by abnormal involuntary movements of limbs, hands, trunk and lingual-facial-buccal musculature. In animal models apparently similar dyskinesias can be reproduced by dopaminergic stimulation, particularly in the striatum (*Klawans* et al. 1975), and can be altered and enhanced by experimental manipulations resulting in dopamine supersensitivity in the same nucleus (*Klawans* et al. 1975; *Ungerstedt* et al. 1975; *Moore* and *Thornburg* 1975). In man, L-dopa induced dyskinesias are by far more common in patients with Parkinson's disease than in those with apparently intact nigro-striatal pathways (*Chase* et al. 1973). It has been noted by several authors that there is a correlation between the prevalence and severity of the dyskinesias and the duration of Parkinson's disease (*Weiner* and *Bergen* 1977). Presumably, the longer the duration of the disease, the more extensive the nigro-striatal degeneration and the greater the degree of dopamine supersensitivity in the striatal neurones. This interpretation is further supported by the observation that in individual patients the dyskinesias generally start on the side first affected by the disease (*Weiner* and *Bergen* 1977). Although administration of dopaminergic blocking agents effectively controls the abnormal movements (*Postma* 1972), this form of treatment is not recommended because of the resulting deterioration in Parkinsonian symptoms. Interestingly, a syndrome closely resembling L-dopa induced dyskinesias develops in a relatively high proportion of patients chronically treated with phenothiazine drugs, especially after a reduction in neuroleptic dosage (Editorial 1978). The pathogenesis of this condition, known as tardive dyskinesia to indicate its usually late onset, has also been interpreted on the basis of neuroleptic-induced dopamine supersensitivity in the basal ganglia (*Klawans* 1973). In contrast to supersensitivity, the development of tolerance at the receptor site would be expected to be associated with a reduced prevalence of Type A adverse effects. This, however, may not always be true. For example, the development of hyposensitivity to catecholamines at post-synaptic sites may explain the reduction in the CNS stimulant effects of amphetamine drugs during chronic administration and the need to increase progressively the dose in order to maintain a sustained response during abuse. There is evidence, however, that hyposensitivity may also develop at the level of pre-synaptic autoreceptors located on the membrane of adrenergic neurones, especially in the striatal and mesolimbic systems (*Schwartz* et al. 1978). This would result in enhancement of the stimulant action of these drugs and it is probably implicated in the pathogenesis of dyskinetic movements and paranoid psychoses during chronic amphetamine abuse (*Schwartz* et al. 1978). An additional factor to be considered is the persistance of the state of modified response for some time after withdrawing the abused drug. The development of dependence and the appearance of withdrawal symptoms can be explained often on the basis of modified post-synaptic sensitivity not adequately compensated by pre-synaptic sensitivity. The recent discovery of enkephalin receptors on catecholaminergic nerve endings in the CNS may greatly contribute to an improved understanding of the mechanisms involved in the manifestations of the narcotic abstinence syndrome. *Schwartz* and associates (1978) have proposed that tolerance and dependence to opi ate drugs develop as a consequence of post-synaptic supersensitivity secondary to pre-synaptic inhibition of transmitter (including catecholamines) release in different area of the brain.

e) Pharmacodynamic Drug Interactions

Clinically important drug interactions are frequently seen after administration of agents which act at the same sites or influence the same physiological system. Interactions among drugs which act primarily on the autonomic nervous system are well known and include blockade of the β-agonist effects of adrenaline by propranolol, or of the α-agonist effects of noradrenaline by phenoxybenzamine. Less well recognized is the possibility that similar interactions occur with drugs which produce secondary pharmacological effects on the same system. Phenothiazine drugs and tricyclic antidepressants, for example, possess significant α-adrenergic blocking properties and may enhance the activity of other α-blockers used in combination.

Many antibiotics, including streptomycin, neomycin, kanamycin, gentamicin, colistin, lincomycin, bacitracin, clindomycin and tetracyclines have a weak curare-like action at the neuromuscular junction. Although in most subjects this effect will pass unnoticed, in patients undergoing general anaesthesia the action of tubocurarine, gallamine and succinylcholine is markedly potentiated, and prolonged apnea may result (*Dundee* and *McCaughey* 1976). The same mechanism is responsible for the worsening of muscle weakness after administration of these antibiotics to patients with myasthenia gravis.

Because of the ease in measuring drug response, a large number of pharmacodynamic interactions involving cardiovascular drugs have been described. Some important examples include the enhancement of quinidine cardiac toxicity by phenothiazines and tricyclic antidepressants, the reversal of the antihypertensive effects of clonidine by desipramine and the potentiation of digitalis toxicity by drugs affecting the electrolyte balance. Clinically important interactions at the receptor site between psychotropic drugs include the reciprocal ptentiation of the CNS depressant effects of alcohol, benzodiazepines and barbiturates, the deterioration in psychotic symptoms induced by L-dopa in schizophrenic patients treated with neuroleptics, and the precipitation of the withdrawal syndrome by naloxone in subjects addicted to opiates. In most cases these interactions are highly predictable on the basis of the known pharmacological properties of the individual compounds. Therefore the prevention of adverse effects must rely on the clinician's knowledge of the basic mechanisms of drug action.

C. Pathogenesis of Type B Adverse Reactions

Type B adverse reactions are defined in this context as any type of undesired response which cannot be explained on the basis of the known pharmacological properties of the drug. A critical evaluation of these reaction can be exceedingly difficult for a number of reasons. Type B adverse reactions are often bizarre, and they tend to occur in a small minority of treated subjects. The mechanisms involved are largely unknown mainly because, unlike Type A effects, these reactions cannot be easily reproduced in animal models. Moreover the relationship between drug administration and adverse response is one of association, and the causative role of the pharmacological agent cannot always be established with certainty.

In most cases the pathogenesis of Type B adverse reactions can be attributed to the presence of a qualitative abnormality in drug response in susceptible patients. There are fewer cases, however, in which the qualitative abnormality can be found to be in the physico-chemical properties of the pharmaceutical preparation.

I. Qualitative Abnormalities of the Pharmaceutical Preparation

Severe adverse reactions are occasionally produced by toxic contaminants present in the pharmaceutical preparation. During September and October 1937 at least 76 subjects died in the United States poisoned by di-ethylene-glycol used as a solvent for sulphanilamide (*Geiling* and *Cannon* 1938). The nephrotoxic properties of certain formulations of phenacetin are likely to be potentiated by small amounts of p-chloro-acetanilide present as impurity (*Harvald* et al. 1950). Fatal renal tubular necrosis has been reported after parenteral administration of pharmaceutical preparations containing excessive amounts of merthiolate as preservative (*Axton* 1972). Allergic reactions to 'inert' compounds widely used as excipients in the pharmaceutical industry have been frequently reported and can be occasionally severe (*Rogers* and *Barrett* 1974). A recent report from Israel illustrates the possibility that allergic reactions to excipients may occur even with prednisone preparations (*Rubinger* et al. 1978).

In 1963, *Ehrlich* and associates described a clinical picture characterized by nausea, vomiting, polyuria, polydipsia, glycosuria, acidosis, proteinuria and aminoaciduria in children treated with outdated tetracyclines (*Ehrlich* and *Stein* 1963; *Frimpter* et al. 1963). A similar syndrome has been described in adults (*Gross* 1963). The clinical manifestations closely resemble the Fanconi syndrome and they are rapidly reversible following discontinuation of the degraded antibiotic. A facial lesion typical of systemic lupus erythematosus and photosensitivity have also been observed after ingestion of partially decomposed tetracycline: the degradation products responsible for the toxic reactions have not been identified with certainty, although anhydrotetracycline and epiandrotetracycline are likely candidates (*Sulkowski* and *Haserick* 1964).

II. Qualitative Abnormalities of the Patient's Responsiveness

1. Genetically Determined Abnormalities

a) Glucose-6-Phosphate-Dehydrogenase Deficiency

Glucose-6-phosphate-dehydrogenase (G-6-PD) deficiency is the most common of the hereditary enzymatic abnormalities in man (more than 100 million affected individuals throughout the world). The disorder is transmitted as an X-linked incomplete dominant trait; more than 80 varieties have been described, each variant being characterized by a specific abnormality in the aminoacid sequence of the enzymatic protein (*Motulski* et al. 1971). The majority of patients affected by the disease are asymptomatic, although some degree of haemolysis may occur either spontaneously or during infection. Haemolytic crises, however, almost invariably follow the administration in the same patients of various pharmacological agents, especially certain analgesics (e.g. aspirin, phenacetin), antimalarials (e.g. primaquine, quinine), sulphonamides, vitamin K, chloramphenicol, quinidine, nitrofurantoin and PAS. The basic defect in G-6-PD deficiency is a pathological increase in corpuscolar fragility under the effect of drugs or their metabolites. Older red cells are more vulnerable to haemolysis than newly formed erythrocytes. The severity of the reaction is determined mainly by the dose of the offending drug and by the degree of enzymatic deficiency. In the mild deficiency of the Negro variant, for example, haemolysis is limited to a small proportion of red cells and the resulting moderate anaemia subsides rapidly once more resistant younger erythrocytes have replaced older elements in the circulation. In subjects with the more severe Mediterranean type of the disease, however, a much larger proportion of red cells are vulnerable to haemolysis and administration of even small doses of drugs in these patients can precipitate a dramatic clinical picture characterized by fever, chills, vomiting, abdominal pain, haemoglobinuria and in some cases even death. The spectrum of substances that can induce haemolysis is also wider in patients with the Mediterranean type of G-6-PD deficiency and includes fava beans and chloramphenicol. Within groups of patients affected by the same variant of G-6-PD deficiency, the severity of the enzymatic defect is largely determined by the individual genotype. In fact, while all erythrocytes of hemizygote males and homozygote females are abnormal, heterozygote females possess two separate populations of red cells, one normal and one G-6-PD deficient. The ratio between the two populations may vary considerably, only those subjects with a sufficiently high proportion of deficient erythrocytes being liable to clinically important haemolysis (World Health Organisation 1973).

The mechanism responsible for the drug-induced haemolytic reaction is only incompletely understood. It is known that the integrity of the erythrocytes depends on the availability of reduced glutathione (GSH), which is necessary to maintain important functional groups of haemoglobin and other cellular proteins in a reduced state. The concentration of GSH is regulated by the enzyme glutathione-reductase which requires NADPH as coenzyme. In presence of G-6-PD deficiency NADPH is formed at a lower rate and the concentration of GSH in the red cell is correspondingly reduced. In these conditions oxidizing agents interact with critical groups of cellular macromolecules resulting in methaemoglobin formation, protein denaturation, structural damage and consequent haemolysis (*Weed* and *Reed* 1966). There is evidence that in many cases the oxidizing agent is a reactive metabolite derivative formed within the erythrocyte rather than the drug itself (*Fraser* et al. 1971). An explanation for the increased vulnerability of older cells is provided by the observation that G-6-PD activity progressively declines with the age of the erythrocyte. Such a decline is clearly related to the inability of the mature erythrocyte to synthetise G-6-PD and therefore compensate for the physiological enzyme-degradation during the aging process.

b) Glutathione-Reductase Deficiency

Glutathione-reductase deficiency is a relatively rare hereditary disorder transmitted as an autosomal dominant trait. Affected individuals show a variable degree of hepatosplenomegaly, thrombocytopenia, leucopenia and, in some cases, associated neurological abnormalities. The life-span of the erythrocytes is only marginally reduced in the absence of a drug challenge, but can be drastically reduced by administration of certain antimalarials, analgesics and sulphonamides and other drugs. The susceptibility to haemolytic reactions is similar to that observed in patients with intermediate degree of G-6--PD deficiency, and the pathogenesis is probably analogous.

c) Drug-Sensitive Haemoglobins

In 1962 *Frick* and coworkers described a case of severe haemolysis in a 2 year old patient treated with sulphadimethoxine in the course of a febrile illness of unknown origin (*Frick* et al. 1962). A careful medical history revealed that the same patient and her father had suffered similar episodes previously when they received courses of sulphonamide therapy. Father, daughter and fifteeen other relatives were found to have an abnormal haemoglobin (Hb_{Zurich}) with an electrophoretic mobility intermediate between that of haemoglobins A and S. The determination of the aminoacid sequence of the globin demonstrated the presence of a substitution in position 63 of the β-chain, a critical abnormality because it is at this point that the haem group is attached to the β-chain. The disorder is transmitted as an autosomal dominant and affected subjects are generally asymptomatic despite a moderate degree of haemolysis. Severe haemolytic crises, however, may follow the intake of sulphonamides or chinoline derivatives (primaquine). The crises are characterized by anaemia, reticulocytosis, marked anisocytosis with schistocytosis and associated large Heinz bodies in all erythrocytes.

A second type of drug sensitive haemoglobin is observed in a variant of α-thalassemia known as HbH disease. In adult subjects affected by this condition the majority of the haemoglobin present in the erythrocytes is composed of four β-chains. The condition is transmitted as a recessive autosomal trait and it clinically resembles β-thalassemia minor, although the manifestations are sometimes more severe. The incidence of HbH disease is particularly high in the Far East but occasional cases have been described also in European populations. In Hb disease haemolytic crises are precipitated by the same oxidant drugs described under G-6-PD deficiency.

d) Suxamethonium Hypersensitivity

Shortly after suxamethonium was introduced for the induction of general anaesthesia in 1952, it became clear that there are occasional patients who are extraordinarily sensitive to the muscle-relaxant action of the drug. Prolonged apnoea and death have been reported on several occasions. Affected individuals show a strikingly decreased serum activity of the enzyme pseudocholinesterase which is responsible for the bioinactivation of the drug (*Forbat* et al. 1953). As a result, the rate of enzymatic hydrolysis of the drug is drastically reduced and the duration of effect is prolonged from the usual 2 minutes to more than 2 hours. Apart from some patients in whom the decreased serum pseudocholinesterase activity is related to renal or hepatic disease, the enzymatic defect is observed in otherwise healthy individuals. These subjects show an inherited structural abnormality of the enzymatic protein characterized by a markedly reduced affinity for suxamethonium and other substrates (*Kalow* and *Staron* 1957). In a strict sense the adverse response arises from the prolongation of the normal pharmacological action of the drug and should therefore be classified as a Type A reaction. However, the rarity of its occurrence (1 out of 2500 individuals) and the extreme severity of the clinical manifestations are more reminiscent of a Type B reaction.

e) Malignant Hyperthermia

Malignant hyperthermia is a rare clinical condition characterized by a dramatic rise of body temperature during general anesthesia. About 200 cases have been described to date with a mortality rate of 70–80%. The condition is estimated to occur in approximately 1 out of 20,000 cases of general anaesthesia; young subject are more commonly affected than elderly patients (*Kalow* 1972). Consistent clinical features are tachycardia, hyperventilation, hypoxia, acidosis, hyperkalaemia and hypocalcemia, usually associated with muscular rigidity. In the most severe cases the temperature may rise rapidly to 42°C and the muscular rigidity may progress without interruption into rigor mortis. Malignant hyperthermia has been observed during anaesthesia with nitrous oxide, methoxyflurane, halothane, ether, cyclopropane, and it is probably more common in presence of suxamethonium or tubocurarine. The mechanism involved is only incompletely understood but it is likely to be related to a drug-induced blockade of the intracellular transport of calcium in the muscles of these subjects (*Kalow* 1972). A genetic basis has been known since *Denborough* and colleagues (1962) described ten cases of fatal hyperthermia in 38 members of the same family who underwent general anaesthesia for various surgical procedures. Subsequent studies have confirmed that the susceptibility to the condition is inherited as an autosomal dominant trait with variable expressivity and incomplete penetrance (*Kalow* 1972). An elevated serum creatine phosphokinase activity has been reported in the majority of susceptible individuals (*Kelstrup* et al. 1974), and an association with certain muscular disorders has also been described (*Harriman* et al. 1973).

f) Jaundice and Thromboembolism Associated With Oral Contraceptives

A strikingly increased incidence of cholestatic jaundice in premenopausal women on oral contraceptives has been described in certain families and in selected ethnic groups (*Orellana-Alcalde* and *Dominquez* 1966; *Eisalo* et al. 1965; *Rawlins* and *Thompson* 1977), suggesting a genetically controlled susceptibility to this adverse response. An hereditary factor is also possibly involved in the development of thromboembolic disease associated with oral contraceptives. This hypothesis is supported by the observation that young women of blood group 0 show a significantly lower incidence of thromboembolic disorders while on oral contraceptives than women of blood groups A and AB (*Jick* et al. 1969).

g) Rheumatoid Arthritis and Toxic Drug Reactions

In patients with rheumatoid arthritis a positive association has been described between adverse drug reactions and certain types of HLA alloantigens. Patients possessing HLA-B27 antigens show an increased incidence of adverse reactions to levamisole (*Veys* et al. 1978) whereas toxic complications to sodium aurothiom and penicillamine therapy are more frequently associated with DRW2 and DRW3 antigens (*Panayi* et al. 1978). Possibly, some of the adverse reactions to these drugs are mediated by immunological mechanisms controlled by the genetic loci involved in the expression of the HLA-phenotype.

h) Prophyria

In patients affected by acute intermittent porphyria severe attacks are known to be precipitated by administration of various pharmacological agents such as barbiturates, phenytoin, glutethimide, griseofulvin, oral contraceptives, sulphonamides and tolbutamide. Many of these compounds stimulate the activity of various enzymatic systems in the human liver, and it has been suggested that the porphyrogenic action of these drugs is related to induction of δ-aminolaevulinic acid-synthetase, the rate-limiting enzyme in porphyrin biosynthesis. However, it is now clear that the pathogenesis of drug-induced acute porphyria is much more complex, being probably intimately related to the negative feed-back regulation of the haem-pathway. The biochemical alterations of porphyrin metabolism under the effect of porphyrogenic drugs have been reviewed by *De Matteis* (1975) and *Maxwell* and *Meyer* (1978).

2. Drug Allergy

The term 'allergy' was first introduced in 1906 by *von Pirquet* to describe a state of specifically altered reactivity to a particular chemically-defined exogenous compound. Today the term is generally used to describe any type of adverse reaction to a foreign substance which is mediated by an immune response. Allergic drug reactions are characterized by the following features:

(i) There is a latent period between the initial exposure to the drug (allergen) and the establishment of the allergic state;

(ii) The reaction is usually reversible after withdrawing the drug, and it re-appears immediately on re-administration;

(iii) The clinical manifestations are unrelated to the pharmacological properties of the drug and generally resemble some form of immunological response, e.g. acute anaphylactic shock, acute laryngeal edema, urticaria;

(iv) The reaction shows no linear relationship to dose and may be precipitated by even minute amounts of the drug.

As allergy is dependent upon the interaction of the drug (or a drug derivative) with host antibodies or sensitized lymphocytes, it is possible to classify the factors involved in the development of the allergic state into two main groups:

1. Those related to the properties of the drug and to its mode of administration, and

2. Those related to the immunological state of the subject.

a) The Drug as an Allergen

α) The Effect of the Molecular Size

The molecular size is the most critical factor in determining the potential ability of a drug to act as an allergen. With a few exceptions (dextrans, peptides, vaccines) drugs are small molecules and therefore cannot by themselves stimulate an immunological response, a principle which apparently contrasts with the relatively high incidence of allergic reactions to compounds of low molecular weight such as penicillin, aspirin and the sulphonamides. In some cases there is evidence that the allergic reaction is mediated by macromolecular contaminants contained in the pharmaceutical preparation; macromolecular derivatives, for example, contaminate most available preparations of semisynthetic penicillins (*Knudsen* et al. 1970) and are partly responsible for the much higher incidence of allergic reactions to these antibiotics than to natural penicillins (*Assem* 1977a). In most cases, however, it is the drug itself that stimulates the immune response, often after conjugation with an endogenous macromolecule, usually a protein, and consequent formation of a complete antigen in which the drug acts as hapten, or antigenic determinant. Only drugs possessing reactive groups able to bind covalently endogenous proteins can act as haptens; the reversible binding which frequently occurs between drugs and plasma proteins is generally inadequate to stimulate an immune response (*Levine* 1966). Various compounds which act as allergens in vivo show covalent binding with proteins in vitro, whereas others do not appear to share such a property. In the latter case it is probably a breakdown product or a reactive metabolite to serve as an hapten. The best known example is provided by penicillin allergy, which is mediated by various breakdown products of the drug, particularly penicilloyl group derivatives, which are formed exogenously and endogenously and may act as haptens (*Levine* 1965). In some cases haptens are produced by exposing the drug to light. This results in chemically reactive groups being introduced into the molecule through the energy transmitted by the absorbed light. The generation of allergens by light is termed photosensitization and mediates the clinical manifestations (mainly skin rashes) of photoallergy (*Harber* and *Baer* 1972).

In sensitized individuals the unconjugated hapten is usually able to combine with its specific antibody and this may modify the clinical manifestations of allergy, although the latter are still mainly dependent on the formation of macromolecular complexes.

β) Sensitization and Allergy

Sensitization, i.e. the establishment of a specific immunological response, is not necessarily synonymous with allergy. For example, antibodies against the penicilloyl determinant can be demonstrated in the majority of adult subjects and yet only very few of these are actually allergic to penicillin (*Levine* et al. 1966). In some cases drug-induced antibodies may paradoxically have a protective action against the development of an allergic reaction to the same drug: Ig G and Ig M antibodies (blocking antibodies), for example, can attenuate and even prevent the clinical manifestations of reagin-mediated anaphylaxis, by combining with the antigen before it reaches the reaginic antibody in tissues (*Levine* 1965). As a general rule, the ability of an allergen to produce a clinically important reaction is directly correlated with the number and the duration of previous exposures (*Parker* 1975). The mode of administration is also important, allergic reactions being more frequent and more severe following intravenous administration. The latter observation can be sometimes explained by the presence in the pharmaceutical preparation of macromolecular contaminants which have direct antigenic properties or may act as substrates to which haptens subsequently bind. These macromolecules, usually proteins, have generally no important role after oral administration because they undergo degradation in the gastrointestinal tract. This does not rule out the possibility of severe reactions, e.g. acute anaphylactic shock, occurring after the oral or even after the topical route of administration (*Parker* 1975).

γ) Specific Sensitization and Cross-Allergy

Allergic reactions sometimes occur without any latent period in patients with no history of previous exposure to the drug. There are a number of observations to be made on this point. First, it is often impossible to exclude with absolute certainty previous drug intake as many patients and doctors alike are remarkably unaware of the drug composition of many proprietary preparations, especially over-the-counter medicines. Second, previous exposure may have occurred through dietary products containing sufficient amounts of drug to elicit sensitization, a possibility which is not remote for penicillin (*Levine* 1966) and other antimicrobial products. A third possibility is that sensitization had been produced by previous exposure to another drug. Although antibodies are usually hapten-specific, a certain degree of cross-reactivity with molecules showing structural similarity is a frequent occurrence. This phenomenon explains the cross allergy to drugs belonging to the same chemical class, e.g. nitrofurantoin and furazolidone, or sulphonamides and sulphonylureas. A particular type of cross-allergy is observed between drugs which are transformed to a common metabolite; in many of these cases it is the latter which acts as hapten.

b) Factors Inherent in the Patient

Allergic reactions are observed in only a minority of subjects treated with the same drug. Such a variability in response is determined by a number of factors, some of which are summarized below.

α) Genetic Factors

A genetically determined variability in immunological response can be clearly demonstrated in various animal species (*McDevitt* and *Bodmer* 1972) and it is likely to be an important factor in determining the susceptibility to allergic drug reactions in man. The association between adverse reactions mediated by immunological mechanisms and genetic markers such as the HL-A serotype in patients with rheumatoid arthritis has been mentioned above. A significant association has also been demonstrated between certain HL-A alloantigens and reagin-mediated allergy in patients tested by prick-in skin tests, the degree of response to a given allergen being clearly related to a particular haplotype (*Marsh* et al. 1973a, b). The most convincing evidence of a genetically controlled allergic response in man is provided by studies conducted in patients with atopic disease (see below). The risk of allergy has been estimated to be 3–5 times greater in the children of allergic parents than in the offspring of parents showing no history of allergic disease (*Cohen* 1974). It is likely that genetic influences affect several steps of the immune response; recognition of the antigen, activation of T and B lymphocytes, antibody production, tissue binding of the antibody, nature and amount of mediators released and tissue sensitivity to them (*Cohen* 1974; *Aas* 1978). For an extensive review of the genetic aspects of allergy see *Cohen* (1974).

β) Atopy

Atopy (from the Greek α-τοποσ – out of place) can be defined as a condition characterized by increased susceptibility to synthetise Ig E antibodies after exposure to allergens normally present in the external environment, e.g. pollen or house dust. Atopic subjects (10% of the population in most areas) show a high prevalence of allergic disease such as eczema, Ig E mediated rhinitis (hay-fever) and asthma. It is generally accepted that atopic patients are particularly susceptible to develop allergic reactions to various drugs, particularly penicillin (*Assem* 1977a; *Levine* 1966), but this view has been questioned (*Stember* and *Levine* 1973).

It is a relatively frequent occurrence for patients with previous history of allergic reactions to show an increased incidence of allergy to a variety of chemically unrelated compounds. We have observed a patient with drug induced systemic lupus erythematosus who turned out on different occasions to be allergic to phenytoin, ethosuximide, sodium valproate, carbamazepine, aspirin, cephalosporins, penicillin and erythromycin. The allergic manifestations ranged from skin rashes to severe agranulocytosis and, with some drugs, re-activation of the lupoid syndrome.

γ) Pathological Factors

The allergic response is altered in various diseases affecting the immune system such as immunodeficiency syndromes, Hodgkin's disease and the leukaemias. An increased incidence of allergic drug reactions to some antibiotics in particular has been reported in patients with glandular fever and other infectious diseases. It has been suggested that antigenic compounds of the infectious agent enhance the immune response by acting as adjuvants (*Munoz* 1964).

c) Pathogenetic Mechanisms of Drug Allergy

The clinical manifestations of allergic drug reactions are primarily determined by the mechanism involved in their pathogenesis. The most satisfactory classification of the allergic responses has been proposed by *Gell* and *Coombes* (1968), and includes four main types (Table 10). It is important to emphasise that a given drug may produce allergic reactions of different types, which may occur in the affected subject either simultaneously or in successive stages.

α) Type I (Immediate) Reactions

The typical reaction of the immediate type is anaphylaxis, either in its generalized (acute anaphylactic shock) or localized forms. The latter include allergic rhinitis, asthma, acute laryngeal oedema, atopic eczema, cutaneous erythemas, urticaria and certain types of gastrointestinal syndromes which follow acute drug administration. *Prausnitz* and *Kustner* in 1921 were first to demonstrate that the immediate type of allergy can be transferred from one subject to another by a serum component. It is now clear that the transferable factor is the Ig E (reagin) antibody. The pathogenesis of anaphylaxis can be summarized as follows (*Ishizaka* 1978):

(i) The drug in its antigenic form interacts with T-lymphocytes (T-helper cells). Following this interaction the T-helper cells stimulate the proliferation of hapten-specific B-lymphocytes into plasma cells.

(ii) Plasma cells initiate the synthesis and secretion of specific Ig E antibodies. Precursors of Ig E forming cells are different from those of Ig G and Ig M forming cells. Ig E antibodies are homocytotropic, i.e. they attach to the cellular membrane of basophils and mast-cells. As many as 40,000 Ig E molecules per cell have been enumerated in human basophils, whereas their concentration in serum is extremely low ($<$ 200 ng/ml).

Table 10. A classification of allergic drug reactions in man

Type	Terminology	Antibody	Example	Comment
I	Anaphylactic, reagin-mediated, immediate type.	Primarily Ig E	Acute anaphylactic shock Laryngeal oedema Urticaria	Reaction mediated by release of histamine from basophils and mast-cells.
II	Cytotoxic	Ig G or Ig M	Various haemolytic anaemias and certain leucopenias.	Reaction mediated by the antigen-antibody reaction at the cellular surface. Several variants known (see text). Complement may be involved.
III	Antigen-antibody complex	Ig G	Serum sickness	Reaction mediated by tissue deposition of antigen-antibody complexes. Complement may be involved
IV	Delayed, cell-mediated, tuberculin type	Sensitized lymphocytes	Contact dermatitis	Reaction mediated by local migration of lymphocytes. No serum antibody demonstrable.

(iii) Upon re-challenge, the drug rapidly and specifically binds to cellular Ig E in tissues. The cross-linking of two molecules of Ig E on the surface of the human mast cell by the allergen triggers a succession of events culminating in the release of histamine and other mediators (SRS-A, etc.) which, in turn, mediate the clinical and pathological aspects of anaphylaxis.

The clinical manifestations of the reaction depend on the predominant site(s) at which the antigen-antibody interaction occurs and on local factors such as location of smooth muscle and distribution, sensitivity to, and rate of degradation of the chemical mediators. As the latter are released only when the allergen is capable of forming a bridge between two Ig E molecules (*Ishizaka* 1978), the presence is required on the molecule of the allergen of at least two antigenic determinants; the most common occurrence is that of two haptens covalently bound to proteins. There are a number of mechanisms by which anaphylaxis may be prevented (*Assem* 1977b):

(i) excess of antigen. This is observed when antigen molecules compete for the antibody and bridge formation is prevented;

(ii) monovalent haptenic binding. This is observed when free (unconjugated) haptens or hapten-protein complexes possessing a single hapten determinant bind the Ig E antibody. The phenomenon may occur after administration of very small doses of the drug, and it can be reproduced prophylactically to induce hyposensitization;

(iii) presence of blocking antibodies in serum. These antibodies (Ig G and Ig M) bind the antigen and prevent its access to the reagin antibodies. This is a common but not the sole mechanism by which hyposensitization occurs.

Table 11. Drugs most frequently associated with acute systemic anaphylaxis

Antisera
Aspirin
Bromosulphthalein
Cephalosporins
Demethylchlortetracycline
Dextrans
Fluorescein
Heparin
Iodinated contrast media
Local anaesthetics
Nitrofurantoin
Penicillins
Sodium dehydrocholate
Thiamine
Streptomycin
Vaccines
Various polypeptide hormones

The complexity of the reactions and interactions described above explains the unpredictability of most Ig E mediated allergic manifestations, and illustrate some possible causes for the occasional failure of skin test to reveal allergy to a specific compound. In this respect it is important to remember that drug-induced clinical manifestations indistinguishable from anaphylaxis may occur without the intervention of any demonstrable immune response. The latter reactions are generally referred to as anaphylactoid reactions and include life-threatening conditions such as aspirin-induced asthma and certain acute reactions to radio-opaque dyes and other drugs which act directly as histamine releasers: codeine, morphine, heroin, pethidine, some dextrans, d-tubocurarine, polymyxin antibiotics and thiamine. Many of these compounds may produce both anaphylactoid and true anaphylactic reactions (Table 11).

β) Type II (Cytotoxic) Reactions

In Type II reactions the initial events leading to sensitization are identical to those described above except that serum antibodies, Ig G and/or Ig M are involved. The clinical manifestations of cytotoxic allergy are mediated by the formation of antigen-antibody complexes on the cellular surface: this results in structural alterations of the cell membrane which are followed by lysis or phagocytosis. Although cytotoxic reactions occur in various tissues, by reasons of accessibility the most extensively investigated are those involving the cellular elements of the blood. Many haemolytic accidents following transfusion of incompatible blood, for example, are clearly produced by Ig G or Ig M antibodies directed against the donor's red cells. In the case of drug-induced cytotoxic reactions, however, the pathogenesis of the immune response is more complex. At least two separate mechanisms have been identified:

1. Immune type. In the immune type of allergy the antibody is directed against the drug (or a drug derivative) acting as hapten. In some cases the antigen-antibody complexes are formed in serum and subsequently attach to the cell surface, resulting in phagocytosis or lysis. Complement may or may not be involved. Typical examples include haemolytic reactions to stibophen, quinine, quinidine, sulphonamides, sulphonylureas, chlorpromazine and rifampicin (*Horler* 1977). The indirect Coombs test is positive in presence of the drug.

In the second variety of immune-type reactions the antigen-antibody complex forms directly on the cell membrane, to which the hapten had previously attached. In the case of haemolysis this variant can be distinguished by a positive direct antiglobulin reaction of the γ-type when drug treated erythrocytes are exposed to the serum of a sensitized patient. Drugs which produce this type of reaction include penicillin and the cephalosporins (*Horler* 1977).

2. Auto-immune type. In the auto-immune cytotoxic reaction the antibody is directed against a native antigen, e.g. the rhesus factor, located on the cellular surface. The role of the drug probably involves conjugation with a proteinaceous component of the cell membrane which results in a conformational change of the protein molecule. The latter is no longer recognized as "self" by the immune system and stimulates auto-antibody production. In the case of drug-induced auto-immune haemolytic anaemia (ten times more common than the immune type) the reaction is indistinguishable from idiopathic auto-immune anaemia and the presence of the drug is not required for the demonstration of the antibody. A typical auto-immune reaction produced by α-methyldopa may include not only haemolytic anaemia, but also hepatitis, myocarditis (*Mullick* and *McAllister* 1977) and the development of LE cells and of autoantibodies against a variety of tissue antigens.

In many cases of cytotoxic reactions, especially of the auto-immune type, the role of the drug may only be critical in initiating the immune response. Tissue necrosis is frequently associated with release of chemical mediators and exposure of new antigenic determinants which can themselves mediate a self-perpetuating disease, sometimes of the cell-mediated immune type.

γ) Type III (Immune-Complex) Reactions

A typical example of Type III allergy is provided by the serum sickness syndrome. In the pathogenesis of this syndrome, antigen-antibody complexes formed in presence of slight antigen excess are deposited in various organs of the sensitized subject. The antibodies involved belong to the Ig G or, more rarely, to the Ig M class. Deposition of the immune complexes in tissues is followed by complement activation, migration of polymorphonuclear leucocytes, release of lysosomal enzymes and local inflammation. Vasculitis is the most common lesion, but granuloma formation with giant-cell infiltration may also occur (*Spector* and *Heesom* 1969). The clinical manifestations generally include some forms of systemic reactions such as fever, arthralgia and lymphadenopathy occasionally associated with anaphylactic features (e.g. urticaria, asthma and acute laryngeal oedema). The local manifestations are determined by the predominant site(s) of complex deposition and may include skin rashes, pneumonitis (extrinsic allergic alveolitis), myocarditis, glomerulonephritis, mono- and polyneuritis, meningo-encephalitis and polyarteritis nodosa. The nature of the reaction can be identified by the presence of precipitating antibodies in serum and by the appearance of a late onset Arthus-type skin reaction on skin testing. The drugs most frequently involved in the pathogenesis of the serum-sickness syndrome include: vaccines, penicillin (particularly the long-acting procaine derivative), streptomycin, aspirin, cholecystographic dyes, phenytoin, PAS, sulphonamides and thiouracils. Characteristically there is a latency of at least one week between the initial exposure to the drug and the manifestations of the syndrome. The period reflects the time required to synthesise sufficient amounts of antibodies for the reaction to occur.

δ) Type IV (Cell-Mediated) Reactions

Type IV reactions include various drug-induced diseases associated with the so-called delayed type of hypersensitivity. In the latter type of allergy the reaction is mediated by sensitized T-lymphocytes without the demonstrable intervention of serum antibodies. The best known example is provided by contact dermatitis. Allergic contact dermatitis results from the binding of an hapten with an epidermal protein resulting in the formation of a complete antigen. Although an immediate (Ig E-mediated) reaction may also occur, at least in some cases, the most common lesion in sensitized subjects is characterized by a delayed onset. The pathological features consist of mononuclear cell infiltrates, while the clinical manifestations are those typical of an eczematous reaction with redness, intra-epidermal oedema (spongiosis), weeping, scaling and thickening of the skin (*Solomon* and *Esterly* 1974). The lesions are localized to the area(s) exposed to the allergen and can be reproduced for diagnostic purposes by application of the suspected compound to an area of normal skin (patch test). Lymphocyte-transformation tests may also be useful in detecting the aetiological agent. Some of the most common contact allergens include mercaptobenzothiazole, potassium bichromate, paraphenylethylendiamine, nickel sulphate and turpentine oil (*Baer* et al. 1973). Drugs are also frequently involved, particularly amongst subjects susceptible to professional exposure. There is evidence that cell mediated-allergy may be implicated in immunological disease in organs other than the skin but the precise mechanisms involved in each case are only incompletely understood. It is known that many manifestations are mediated by a variety of soluble, non-antibody, proteinaceous substances which are released from lymphocytes, monocytes, macrophages and other cells involved in the cell-mediated reaction. The reader is referred elsewhere for a recent review on this subject (*Bendtzen* 1978).

D. Conclusion

An attempt has been made to illustrate some important mechanisms involved in the pathogenesis of adverse drug reactions in man. It is hoped that an improved understanding of these mechanisms will help to stimulate a more rational approach to the use of drug therapy.

References

Aas K (1978) What makes an allergen an allergen. Allergy 33: 3–14

Aggeler PM, O'Reilly RA, Leong L (1967) Potentiation of anticoagulant effect of warfarin by phenylbutazone. New Engl J Med 276: 496–501

Alvan G (1978) Interindividual differences in the disposition of drugs metabolized in the body. Clinical Pharmacokinetics 3: 155–175

Anden NE (1970) Pharmacological and anatomical implications of induced abnormal movements with L-dopa. In: Barbeau A, McDowell F (eds) L-dopa and parkinsonism. FA Davis, Philadelphia, pp 132–143

Armaly MF (1968) Genetic factors related to glaucoma. Ann NY Acad Sci 151: 861–875

Assem E-SK (1977a) Drug allergy. In: Davies DM (ed) Textbook of adverse drug reactions. Oxford University Press, Oxford, pp 380–896

Assem E-SK (1977b) Tests for detecting drug allergy. In: Davies DM (ed) Textbook of adverse drug reactions. Oxford University Press, Oxford, pp 397–410

Axton JHM (1972) Six cases of poisoning after a parenteral organic mercurial compound (Merthiolate). Postgrad med J 48: 417–421

Baer RL, Ramsey DL, Biondi Ella (1973) The most common contact allergens. Arch Dermat 108: 74–78

Baliah T, MacLeish H, Drummond KN (1969) Acute boric acid poisoning. Canad Med Ass J 101: 166–168

Beermann B, Groschinsky-Grind M (1978) Gastrointestinal absorption of hydrochlorothiazide enhanced by concomitant intake of food. Eur J clin Pharmac 13: 125–128

Bender AD (1964) Pharmacologic aspects of aging: a survey of the effect of increasing age on drug activity in adults. J Am Geriatr Soc 12: 114–134

Bendtzen K (1978) Biological properties of lymphokines. Allergy 33: 105–119

Bennett WM, Singer I, Coggins CJ (1974) A guide to drug therapy in renal failure. J Am Med Ass 230: 1544–1553

Bernheimer H, Birkmayer W, Hornykiewicz O, Jellinger K, Seitelberger F (1973) Brain dopamine and the syndromes of Parkinson and Huntington: clinical, morphological and neurochemical correlations. J Neurol Sci 20: 415–455

Beveridge T, Kalberer E, Nüesch E, Schmidt R (1975) Bioavailability studies with digoxin-Sandoz and Lanoxin. Eur J clin Pharmac 8: 371–376

Bianchine JR, Rivera-Calimlim L, Morgan JP, Dujovne CA, Lasagna L (1971) Metabolism and absorption of L-3,4-dihydroxyphenylalanine in patients with Parkinson's disease. Ann NY Acad Sci 179: 126–139

Blaschke TF (1977) Protein binding and kinetics of drugs in liver diseases. Clinical Pharmacokinetics 2: 32–44

Blaschke TF, Meffin PJ, Melinon KL, Rowland M (1975) Influence of acute viral hepatitis on phenytoin kinetics and protein binding. Clin Pharmac Ther 17: 685–691

Boman G, Lundgren P, Stjernström G (1975) Mechanism of the inhibitory effect of PAS granules on the absorption of rifampicin: adsorption on rifampicin by an excipient, bentonite. Eur J clin Pharmac 8: 293–299

Booker HE, Darcey B (1973) Serum concentrations of free diphenylhydantoin and their relationship to clinical intoxication. Epilepsia (Amst) 14: 177–184

Boston Collaborative Drug Surveillance Program (1973a) Diphenylhydantoin side effects and serum albumin levels. Clin Pharmac Ther 14: 529–532

Boston Collaborative Surveillance Program (1973b) Clinical depression of the central nervous system due to diazepam and chlordiazepoxide in relation to cigarette smoking and age. New Engl J Med 288: 277–280

Branch RA, Kornhauser DM, Shand DG, Wilkinson GR, Wood AJJ (1976) Biological determinants of propranolol disposition in normal subjects and patients with cirrhosis. Br J clin Pharmac 3: 243

Castleden CM, Kaye CM, Parsons RL (1975) The effect of age on plasma levels of propranolol and practolol in man. Br J clin Pharmac 2: 303–306

Castleden CM, George CF, Marcer D, Hallett C (1977) Increased sensitivity to nitrazepam in old age. Br Med J 1: 10–12

Cheigh JS (1977) Drug administration in renal failure. Am J Med 62: 555–563

Chase TN, Holden EM, Brody JA (1973) Levodopa-induced dyskinesias. Arch Neurol 29: 328–330

Clinicopathologic conference (1970) Hypertension and the lupus syndrome. Amer J Med 49: 519–523

Cohen C (1974) Genetic aspects of allergy. Med Clinics North Amerca 58: 25–42

Coombs RRA, Gell PGH (1968) Classification of allergic reactions responsible for clinical hypersensitivity and disease. In: Gell PGH, Coombs RRA (eds) Clinical aspects of immunology, 2nd edition. Blackwell, Oxford, p 575

Davis M, Simmons CJ, Harrison NG, Williams R (1976) Paracetamol overdose in man: relationship between pattern of urinary metabolites and severity of liver damage. Quarterly J Med 45: 181–191

De Matteis F (1975) The effect of drugs on 5-aminolaevulinate synthetase and other enzymes in the pathway of liver haem biosynthesis. In: Parke DV (ed) Enzyme induction. Plenum Press, London, pp 185–205

Denborough MA, Forster JFA, Lovell RRH, Maplestone PA, Villiers JD (1962) Anaesthetic deaths in a family. Br J Anaesth 34: 395–396

Devadatta S, Gangadharam PRJ, Andrews RH, Fox W, Ramakrishnan CV, Selhon JB, Veru S (1960) Peripheral neuritis due to isoniazid. WHO Bull 23: 587–598

De Vita VT, Hahn MA, Oliverio VT (1965) Monoamine oxidase inhibition by a new carcinostatic agent, N-isopropyl-A-(2-methyl-hydrazino)-p-toluamide (MIH). Proc Soc Exp Biol Med 120: 561–565

Dujovne CA (1978) Hepatotoxic and cellular uptake interactions among surface active components of erythromycin preparations. Biochem Pharmac 27: 1925–1930

Dundee JW, McCaughey W (1976) Drugs in anaesthetic practice. In: Avery G (ed) Drug treatment. Adis Press, Sydney, pp 214–251

Eadie MJ, Sutherland JM, Tyrer JH (1968) 'Dilantin' overdosage. Med J Aust 2: 515

Editorial (1978) Treatment of tardive dyskinesia. Drug Therapeutics Bull 16: 55–56

Ehrlich LJ, Stein HS (1963) Abnormal urinary findings following administration of achromycin V. Pediatrics 31: 697–698

Eisalo A, Jarvinen PA, Luukkainen T (1965) Liver-function tests during intake of contraceptive tablets in premenopausal women. Br Med J 1: 1416–1417

Elion GB, Callaghan S, Nathan H, Bieber S, Rundles RW, Hitchings GH (1963) Potentiation by inhibition of drug degradation: 6-substituted purines and xanthine oxidase. Biochem Pharmac 12: 85–93

Elion GB, Yü T-F, Gutman AS, Hitchings GH (1968) Renal clearance of oxipurinol, the chief metabolite of allopurinol. Am J Med 45: 69–77

Fernandez CA, Menezes JP, Ximenes J (1973) The effect of food on the absorption of pivampicillin and a comparison with the absorption of ampicillin potassium. J Int Med Res 1: 530–533

Fischer R, Griffin F (1963) Quinine dimorphism: a cardinal determinant of taste sensitivity. Nature 200: 343–347

Fischer R, Griffin F, Archer RC, Zimmeister SC, Jastram PS (1965) Weber ratio in gustatory chemoreception: an indicator of systemic (drug) reactivity. Nature 207: 1049–1053

Fischler M, Frisch EP, Örtengren B (1973) Plasma concentrations after oral administration of different pharmaceutical preparations of chlomethiazole. Acta Pharm Su 10: 483–492

Fleming WW, McPhillips JJ, Westfall DP (1973) Postfunctional supersensitivity and subsensitivity of excitable tissues to drugs. Ergebn Physiol 68: 55–119

Forbat A, Lehmann H, Silk E (1953) Prolonged apnoea following injection of succinylcholine. Lancet 265: 1067–1068

Fraser OM, Tilton BE, Vesell ES (1971) Effects of some metabolites of hemolytic drugs on young and old, normal and G-6-PD deficient human erythrocytes. Ann NY Acad Sci 179: 644–653

Fredholm BB, Rane A, Persson B (1975) Diphenylhydantoin binding to proteins in plasma and its dependence on free fatty acid and bilirubin concentration in dogs and newborn infants. Pediatr Res 9: 26–30

Frick PG, Hitzig WH, Betke K (1962) Hemoglobin Zurich. I. A new hemoglobin anomaly associated with acute hemolytic episodes with inclusion bodies after sulphonamide therapy. Blood 20: 261–271

Frigo GM, Perucca E, Teggia DM, Gatti G, Mussini A, Salerno J (1977) Comparison of qunidine plasma concentration curves following oral administration of some short and long-lasting preparations. Br J clin Pharmac 4: 449–454

Frimpter GW, Timpanelli AE, Eisenmenger WJ, Stein HS, Ehrlich LJ (1963) Reversible 'Fanconi syndrome' caused by degraded tetracycline. J Am Med Ass 184: 111–113

Garner RC (1976) The role of epoxides in bioactivation and carcinogenesis. In: Bridges JW, Chasseaud LP (eds) Progress in drug metabolism, vol 1. John Wiley and Sons, London, pp 77–128

Geiling EMK, Cannon PR (1938) Pathogenic effects of elixir or sulphanilamide (diethylene glycol) poisoning. J Am Med Ass 111: 919–926

Gerhardt RE, Knouss RF, Thyrum PT, Luchi RJ, MOrris JJ (1969) Quinidine excretion in aciduria and alkaluria. Am Int Med 71: 927–933

Glazko AJ, Kinkel AW, Alegnani WC, Helmes EL (1968) An evaluation of the absorption characteristics of different chloramphenicol preparations in normal human subjects. Clin Pharmac Ther 9: 472–483

Greenblatt DJ, Koch-Weser J (1974) Clinical toxicity of chlordiazepoxide and diazepam in relation to serum albumin concentration: A report from the Boston Collaborative Drug Surveillance Program. Eur J clin Pharmac 7: 259–262

Gross JM (1963) Fanconi syndrome (adult type) developing secondary to ingestion of outdated tetracycline. Ann Int Med 58: 523–528

Harber LC, Baer RL (1972) Pathogenic mechanisms of drug-induced photosensitivity. J Invest Derm 58: 327–342

Harriman DG, Summer DW, Ellis FR (1973) Malignant hyperpyrexia myopathy. Quart J Med 42: 639–664

Harvald B, Valdorf-Hansen F, Nielsen A (1960) Effect on the kidney of drugs containing phenacetine. Lancet I: 303–305

Hayes MJ, Langman MJS, Short AH (1975) Changes in drug metabolism with increasing age: II Phenytoin clearance and protein binding. Br J clin Pharmac 2: 73–79

Heading RC, Nimmo J, Prescott LF, Toothill P (1973) The dependence of paracetamol absorption on the rate of gastric emptying. Br J Pharmac 47: 415–421

Heizer WD, Smith TW, Goldfinger SE (1971) Absorption of digoxin in patients with malabsorption syndromes. New Engl J Med 285: 257–259

Hempel E, Klinger W (1976) Drug stimulated biotransformation of hormonal steroid contraceptives: clinical implications. Drugs 12: 442–448

Holtzman NA, Elliott DA, Heller RH (1966) Copper intoxication. New Engl J Med 275: 347–352

Homeida M, Jackson, L, Roberts CJC (1978) Decreased first-pass metabolism of labetalol in chronic liver disease. Br Med J 2: 1048–1050

Horler AR (1977) Blood disorders. In: Davies DM (ed) Textbook of adverse drug reactions. Oxford University Press, Oxford, pp 354–364

Horwitz D, Lovenberg W, Engelman K, Sjoerdsma A (1964) Monoamine-oxidase inhibitors, tyramine, and cheese. J Am Med Ass 188: 1108–1110

Hurwitz L (1969) Predisposing factors to adverse reactions to drugs. Br Med J 1: 536–540

Houghton GW, Richens A (1974) Phenytoin intoxication induced by sulthiame in epileptic patients. J Neurol Neurosurg Psychiatr 37: 275–281

Houghton GW, Richens A, Leighton M (1975) Effect of age, height, weight and sex on serum phenytoin concentration in epileptic patients. Br J clin Pharmac 2: 251–256

Innes IR, Nickerson M (1975) Norepinephrine, epinephrine, and the sympathomimetic amines. In: Goodman LS, Gilman A (eds) The pharmacological basis of therapeutics. McMillan Publishing Company, New York, pp 477–513

Ishizaka K (1978) Mechanism of reaginic hypersensitivity and immunotherapy. Lung 155: 3–22

Jick H, Slone D, Westerholm B, Inman WHW, Vessey MP, Shapiro S, Lewis GP, Worcester J (1969) Venous thromboembolic disease and ABO blood type. A cooperative study. Lancet I: 539–542

Jollow DJ, Mitchell JR, Potter WZ, Davis DC, Gillette JR, Brodie BB (1973) Acetaminophen-induced hepatic necrosis. II Role of covalent binding *in vivo*. J Pharmac exp Ther 187: 195–202

Kalow W (1972) Succinylcholine and malignant hyperthermia. Fed Proc 31: 1270–1275

Kalow W, Staron N (1957) On distribution and inheritance of atypical forms of human serum cholinesterase, as indicated by dibucaine numbers. Can d J Biochem 35: 1305–132-

Karlsson E (1978) Clinical pharmacokinetics of procainamide. Clinical pharmacokinetics 3: 97–107

Kelstrup J, Reske-Nielsen E, Haase J, Jørni J (1974) Malignant hyperthermia in a family: a clinical and serological investigation of 139 members. Acta Anaesth Scand 18: 58–64

Kirby WM, Roberts CE, Burdick RE (1961) Comparison of two new tetracyclines with tetracycline and demethylchlortetracycline. Antimicrob Agents Chemother 1: 286–292

Klawans HL (1973) The pharmacology of extrapyramidal movement disorders. In: Cohen MM (ed) Monographs in neural sciences, 2. Karger, Basel, pp 1–136

Klawans HL, Crossett P, Dana N (1975) Effect of chronic amphetamines exposure on sterotyped behavior: implications for pathogenesis of L-dopa-induced dyskinesias. In: Calne DB, Chase TN, Barbeau A (eds) Advances in neurology 9. Raven Press, New York, pp 105–112

Knopp W, Fischer R, Beck J, Teitelbaum A (1966) Clinical implications of the relation between taste sensitivity and the appearance of extrapyramidal side effects. Dis Nerv Syst 27: 729–735

Klotz U (1976) Pathophysiological and disease-induced charges in drug distribution volume: pharmacokinetic implications. Clin Pharmacokinetics 1: 204–218

Klotz U, Avant GR, Hoyumpa A, Schenker S, Wilkinson GR (1975) The effects of age and liver disease on the disposition and elimination of diazepam in adult man. J clin Invest 55: 347–359

Knudsen ET, Dewdney JM, Trafford JAP (1970) Reduction in incidence of ampicillin rash by purified ampicillin. Br Med J 1: 469–471

Kunin CM, Finland M (1961) Clinical pharmacology of the tetracycline antibiotics. Clin Pharmac Ther 2: 51–69

Kutt H (1972) Diphenylhydantoin. Interactions with other drugs in man. In: Woodbury DM, Penry JK, Schmidt RP (eds) Antiepileptic drugs. Raven Press, New York, pp 169–180

Kutt H, Brennan R, Dehejia H, Verebely K (1970) Diphenylhydantoin intoxication. A complication of isoniazid therapy. Am Resp Dis 101: 377–384

Laidlaw J, Read AE, Sherlock S (1961) Morphine tolerance in hepatic cirrhosis. Gastroenterology 40: 389–396

Lamy PP (1974) Geriatric drug therapy. Clin Med 81: 52–57

Larsson R, Karlsson E, Molin L (1977) Spontaneous systemic lupus erythematosus and acetylator phenotype. Acta Med Scand 201: 223–226

Levine BB (1965) Immunochemical mechanisms involved in penicillin hypersensitivity in experimental animals and in human beings. Fed Proc 24: 45–50

Levine BB (1966) Immunochemical mechanisms of penicillin allergy. A haptemic model system for the study of allergic diseases of man. New Engl J Med 275: 1115–1125

Levine BB, Redmond AP, Fellner MJ, Voss HE, Levytska V (1966) Penicillin allergy and the heterogenous immune response of man to benzylpenicillin. J clin Invest 45: 1895–1906

Levy G (1976) Effect of plasma protein-binding of drugs on duration and intensity of pharmacologic activity. J Pharm Sci 65: 1264–1265

Lewis GP, Jusko WJ, Burke CW, Graves L (1971) Prednisone side effects and serum protein levels. Lancet II: 778–781

Lindenbaum J, Mellow MH, Blackstone MO, Butler VP (1971) Variations in biological availability of digoxin from four preparations. New Engl J Med 285: 1344–1347

Lovell RG, Preuss L (1977) Bronchial asthma: which drugs to use and why. Modern Medicine 21: 34–41

Lowenthal DT (1974) Tissue sensitivity to drugs in disease states. New Engl J Med 58: 1111–1119

Lund L (1974) Clinical significance of generic inequivalence of three different pharmaceutical preparations of phenytoin. Eur J clin Pharmac 7: 119–124

Lunde PKM (1971) Plasma protein binding of diphenylhydantoin in man. Acta Pharmacol 29: 152–155 (Supp 3)

Lunde PKM, Frislid K, Hansteen V (1977) Disease and acetylation polymorphism. Clinical Pharmacokinetics 2: 182–197

Manninen V, Apajalahti A, Melin J, Karesoja M (1973) Altered absorption of digoxin in patients given propantheline and metoclopramide. Lancet I: 398–400

Manninen V, Melin J, Härtel G (1971) Serum digoxin concentration during treatment with different preparations. Lancet II: 934–935

Marsh DG, Bias WB, Hsu SH, Goodfriend L (1973a) Association of the H2-A7 cross reacting group with a specific reaginic antibody response in allergic man. Science 179: 691–693

Marsh DG, Bias WB, Hsu SH, Goodfriend L (1973b) Association between major histocompatibility (H2-A) antigens and specific reaginic antibody responses in allergic man. In: Goodfriend L, Sehon AH, Orange RP (eds) Mechanisms in allergy: Reagin-mediated hypersensitivity. New York, p 113

Marshall AJ, Eltringham WK, Barritt DW, Davies JD, Griffiths DA, Jackson LK, Laszlo G. Read AE (1977) Respiratory disease associated with practolol therapy. Lancet II: 1254–1257

Maxwell JD, Meyer U (1978) Pharmacogenetics in the field of heme metabolism: drug sensitivity in hereditary hepatic porphyria. In: De Matteis F, Aldridge WN (eds) Heme and hemoproteins. Springer, Berlin Heidelberg New York (Handbook of experimental pharmacology 44, pp 239–254)

McDevitt HO, Bodmer WF (1972) Histocompatibility antigens, immune responsiveness and susceptibility to disease. Amer J Med 52: 1–8

McMartin C, Simpson P (1971) The absorption and metabolism of guanethidine in hypertensive patients requiring different doses of the drug. Clin Pharmac Ther 12: 73–77

Melander A, Danielson K, Hanson A, Jansson L, Rerup C, Schersten B, Thulin T, Wahlen E (1976) Reduction of isoniazid bioavailability in normal men by concomitant intake of food. Acta Med Scand 200: 93–97

Melander A, Danielson K, Schersten B, Wåhlin E (1977a) Enhancement of the bioavailability of propranolol and metoprolol by food. Clin Pharmac Ther 22: 108–112

Melander A, Danielson K, Hanson A, Rudell B, Schersten B, Thulin T, Wåhlin E (1977b) Enhancement of hydralazine bioavailability by food. Clin Pharmac Ther 22: 104–107

Melander A, Danielson K, Schersten B, Thulin T, Wåhlin E (1977c) Enhancement by food of canrenone bioavailability from spironolactone. Clin Pharmac Ther 22: 100–103

Mitchell JR, Cavanaugh JH, Arias L, Oates JA (1970) Guanethidine and related agents. Antagonism by drugs which inhibit the norepinephrine pump in man. J Clin Invest 49: 1596–1604

Mitchell JR, Jollow DJ, Potter WZ, Gillette JR, Brodie BB (1973) Acetaminophen-induced hepatic necrosis. IV Protective role of glutathione. J Pharmac exp Ther 187: 211–217

Mitchell JR, McMurtry RJ, Statham CN, Nelson SD (1977) Molecular basis for drug-induced nephropathies. Am J Med 62: 518–525

Mitchell JR, Nelson WL, Potter WZ, Sasame HA, Jollow DJ (1976) Metabolic activation of furosemide to a chemically reactive, hepatotoxic metabolite. J Pharmac exp Ther 199: 41–52

Mitchell JR, Potter WZ (1975) Drug metabolism in the production of liver injury. Med Clinics North America 59: 877–885

Mitchell JR, Thorgeirsson SS, Potter WZ, Jollow DJ, Keiser H (1974) Acetaminophen-induced hepatic injury: protective role of glutathione in man and rationale for therapy. Clin Pharmac Ther 16: 676–684

Moore KE, Thornburg JE (1975) Drug-induced dopaminergic supersensitivy. In: Calne DB, Chase TN, Barbeau A (eds) Advances in neurology 9. Raven Press, New York, pp 93–104

Morselli PL (1977) Psychotropic drugs. In: Morselli PL (ed) Drug disposition during development. Spectrum Pub, New York, pp 431–474

Motulski AG, Yoshida A, Stamatoyannopoulos G (1971) Variants of glucose-6-phosphate dehydrogenase. Ann NY Acad Sci 179: 636–644

Mullick FC, McCallister HA (1977) Myocarditis associated with methyldopa therapy. J Am Med Ass 237: 1699–1701

Munoz J (1964) Effect of bacteria and bacterial products on antibody response. Adv Immunol 4: 397–440

Murray FJ (1962) Outbreak of unexpected reactions among epileptics taking isoniazid. Am Rev Resp Dis 86: 729–732

Myrianthoupoulos NC, Kurland AA, Kurland LT (1962) Hereditary predisposition in drug-induced parkinsonism. Archs Neurol (Chic) 6: 5–9

Nation RL, Vine J, Triggs EJ, Learoyd B (1977) Plasma level of chlormethiazole and two metabolites after oral administration to young and aged human subjects. Eur J clin Pharmac 12: 137–145

Neuvonen PJ, Elfving SM, Elonen E (1978) Reduction of absorption of digoxin, phenytoin and aspirin by activated charcoal in man. Eur J clin Pharmac 13: 213–218

Neuvonen PJ, Gothoni G, Hackman R, Bjorksten K (1970) Interference of iron with the absorption of tetracyclines in man. Br Med J 4: 532–534

Nimmo J, Heading RC, Toothill P, Prescott LF (1973) Pharmacological modification of gastric emptying: effects of propantheline and metodopramide on paracetamol absorption. Br Med J 1: 587–589

O'Malley K, Crooks J, Duke E, Stevenson IH (1971) Effect of age and sex on human drug metabolism. Br Med J 3: 607–609

O'Malley K, Judge TG, Crooks J (1976) Geriatric clinical pharmacology and therapeutics. In: Avery G (ed) Drug treatment. Adis Press, Sydney, pp 123–142

O'Reilly RA (1970) The second reported kindred with hereditary resistance to oral anticoagulant drugs. New Engl J Med 282: 1448–1451

O'Reilly RA, Aggeler PM, Leong LS (1964) Studies on the coumarin anticoagulant drugs: a comparison of the pharmacodynamics of dicoumarol and warfarin in man. Thromb Diath Haemorrh 11: 1–22

Orellana-Alcalde JM, Dominquez JP (1966) Jaundice and oral contraceptive drugs. Lancet II: 1278–1280

Panayi GS, Wooley P, Batchelor JR (1978) Genetic basis of rheumatoid disease: HLA antigens, disease manifestations, and toxic reactions to drugs. Br Med J 2: 1236–1238

Parker CW (1975) Drug allergy. New Engl J Med 292: 511–514, 732–735, 957–960

Parson RL, Kaye CM (1974) Plasma propranolol and practolol in adult coeliac disease. Br J clin Pharmac 1: 348

Patterson R, Zeiss CR, Kelly JF (1976) Classification of hypersensitivity reactions. New Engl J Med 295: 277–278

Pearson RM, Breckenridge AM (1976) Renal function, protein binding and pharmacologic response to diazoxide. Br J clin Pharmac 3: 169–175

Pentikanen I, Neuvonen PJ, Tarpila S, Syvälahty E (1978) Effect of cirrhosis of the liver on the pharmacokinetics of chlormethiazole. Br Med J 2: 861–863

Perry HM Jr (1973) Late toxicity to hydralazine resembling systemic lupus erythematosus or rheumatoid arthritis. Amer J Med 54: 58–72

Perry HM, Tan EM, Carmody S, Sakamoto (1973) Relationship of acetyl transferase activity to antinuclear antibodies and toxic symptoms in hypertensive patients treated with hydralazine. J Lab Clin Med 76: 114–125

Perucca E (1978) Clinical consequences of microsomal enzyme-induction by antiepileptic drugs. Pharmacology and Therapeutics 2: 285–314

Perucca E, Garratt A, Hebdige S, Richens A (1978) Water intoxication in epileptic patients receiving carbamazepine. J Neurol Neurosurg Psych 41: 713–718

Perucca E, Richens A (1979) Paracetamol disposition in normal subjects and in patients treated with antiepileptic drugs. Brit J clin Pharacol 7: 201–206

Pierides AM, Alvarez-Ude F, Kerr DNS, Skillen AW (1975) Clofibrate-induced muscle damage in patients with chronic renal failure. Lancet II: 1279–1282

Porter RJ, Layzer RB (1975) Plasma albumin concentration and diphenylhydantoin binding in man. Arch Neurol 32: 298–303

Postma JV (1972) Haloperidol in levodopa-induced choreoathetosis. Psychiatr Neurol Neurochir 75: 69–71

Pottage A, Nimmo J, Prescott LF (1974) The absorption of aspirin and paracetamol in patients with achlorhydria. J Pharm Pharmacol 26: 144–145

Prescott LF, Wright N, Roscoe P, Brown SS (1971) Plasma paracetamol half-life and hepatic necrosis in patients with paracetamol overdosage. Lancet I: 519–522

Prescott LF (1974) Gastrointestinal absorption of drugs. Med Clinics North America 58: 907–916

Prescott LF, Newton RW, Swainson CP, Wright N, Forrest ARW, Matthew H (1974) Successful treatment of severe paracetamol overdosage with cysteamine. Lancet I: 588–592

Prescott LF, Steel RF, Ferrier WR (1976) The effects of particle size on the absorption of phenacetin in man. Clin Pharmac Ther 11: 496–504

Raff M (1976) Self regulation of membrane receptors. Nature 259: 265–266

Rawlins MD, Thompson JW (1977) Pathogenesis of adverse drug reactions. In: Davies DM (ed) Textbook of adverse drug reactions. Oxford University Press, Oxford, pp 10–31

Reidenberg MM (1977a) The biotransformation of drugs in renal failure. Am J Med 62: 482–485

Reidenberg MM (1977b) The binding of drugs to plasma proteins and the interpretation of measurements of plasma concentrations of drugs in patients with poor renal function. Am J Med 62: 466–470

Reidenberg MM, Odar-Cederlöf I, von Bahr C, Borga O, Sjöqvist F (1971) Protein binding of diphenylhydantoin and desmethylimipramine in plasma from patients with poor renal function. New Engl J Med 285: 264–267

Richens A (1977) Interactions with antiepileptic drugs. Drugs 13: 266–275

Richens A, Dunlop A, Ahmad S, Laidlaw J (1976) Monitoring serum phenytoin. Lancet I: 699–700

Robinson MM (1962) Hepatic dysfunction associated with triacetyloleandomycin and propionyl erythromycin ester lauryl sulphate. Am J Med Sci 243: 502–509

Robinson DS, Benjamin DM, McCormack JJ (1971) Interaction of warfarin and nonsystemic gastrointestinal drugs. Clin Pharmac Ther 12: 491–495

Rogers ML, Barrett CW (1974) Problems presented by components of drug vehicles. Adv Drug Reaction Bull 47: 156–159

Rosenberg HA, Bates TR (1976) The influence of food on nitrofurantoin bioavailability. Clin Pharmac Ther 20: 227–232

Rubinger D, Friedlander M, Superstine E (1978) Hypersensitivity to tablet additives in transplant recipients on prednisone. Lancet II: 689

Samter M (1974) The 'classical' diseases of allergy. Med Clinics North America 58: 233–238

Schwartz JC, Costentin J, Martres MP, Protais P, Baudry M (1978) Modulation of receptor mechanisms in the CNS: hyper- and hyposensitivity to catecholamines. Neuropharmacology 17: 665–685

Schwartz JC, Pollard H, Llorens C, Malfroy B, Gros C, Pradelles P, Dray F (1978) Endorphins and endorphin receptors in striatum: relationships with dopaminergic neurons. In: Costa E (ed) Advances in biochemical psychopharmacology, vol 18. Raven Press, New York, pp 245–264

Sellers EH, Koch-Weser J (1970a) Potentiation of warfarin-induced hypoprothrombinemia by chloral-hydrate. New Engl J Med 283: 827–831

Sellers EM, Koch-Weser J (1970b) Displacement of warfarin from human albumin by diazoxide and ethacrinic, mefenamic and nalidixic acids. Clin Pharmac Ther 11: 524–529

Sereni F, Principi N (1968) Developmental pharmacology. Ann Rev Pharmacol 8: 453–466

Shaw TRD, Howard MR, Hamer J (1972) Variations in the biological availability of digoxin. Lancet II: 303–307

Shepherd AMM, Hewick DS, Moreland TA, Stevenson IH (1977) Age as a determinant of sensitivity to warfarin. Br J clin Pharmac 4: 315–320

Sjöqvist F (1968) Toxic interactions between monoamine oxidase inhibitors (MAOI) and other drugs. In: Monoamine oxidase inhibitors, Vol 10. Pergamon Press, Oxford New York, pp 61–74

Solomon LM, Esterly NB (1974) The adult skin and its potential for allergic reactions. Med Clinics North America 58: 165–183

Spector WG, Heesom N (1969) The production of granulomata by antigen-antibody complexes. J Pathol 98: 31–39

Stambaugh JE, Wainer IW, Hemphill DM, Schwartz I (1977) A potentially toxic drug interaction between pethidine (meperidine) and phenobarbitone. Lancet I: 398–399

Stember RH, Levine B (1973) Prevalence of allergic diseases, penicillin hypersensitivity and aeroallergen hypersensitivity in various populations. Abstract 46. Am Acad Allergy 51: 100

Strandberg J, Boman G, Hassler L, Sjöqvist F (1976) Acetylator phenotype in patients with hydralazine-induced lupoid syndrome. Acta Med Scand 200: 367–371

Sulkowski SR, Haserick JR (1964) Simulated systemic lupus erythematosus from degraded tetracycline. J Am Med Ass 189: 152–154

Szeto HH, Inturrisi CE, Houde R, Saal S, Cheigh J, Reidenberg MM (1977) Accumulation of normeperidine, an active metabolite of meperidine, in patients with renal failure or cancer. Am Int Med 86: 738–741

Talseth T (1977) Kinetics of hydralazine elimination. Clin Pharmac Ther 21: 715–720

Testa B, Jenner P (1978) Novel drug metabolites produced by functionalization reactions: chemistry and toxicology. Drug Met Rev 7: 325–369

Triggs EJ, Nation RL, Long A, Ashley JJ (1975) Pharmacokinetics in the elderly. Eur J clin Pharmac 8: 55–62

Trounce JR (1975) Drugs in the elderly. Br J clin Pharmac 2: 289–291

Ungerstedt U, Ljunberg T, Hoffer B, Siggins (1975) Dopaminergic supersensitivity in the striatum. In: Calne DB, Chase TN, Barbeau A (eds) Advances in neurology. Dopaminergic mechanisms, 9. Raven Press, New York, pp 57–65

Vallner JJ (1977) Binding of drugs by albumin and plasma protein. J Pharm Sci 65: 447–465

Varley AB (1968) The generic inequivalence of drugs. J Am Med Ass 206: 1745–1748

Vesell ES (1975) Genetically determined variations in drug disposition and response in man. In: Gillette JR, Mitchell JR (eds) Concepts in biochemical pharmacology. Springer, Berlin Heidelberg New York, pp 169–212

Veys EM, Mielants H, Verbruggen G (1978) Levamisole-induced adverse reactions to HLA B27-positive rheumatoid arthritis. Lancet I: 148

Weed RI, Reed CF (1966) Membrane alterations leading to red cell destruction. Amer J Med 41: 681–698

Weiner WJ, Bergen D (1977) Prevention and management of the side effects of Levodopa. In: Klawans HL (ed) Clinical neuropharmacology, vol 2. Raven Press, New York, pp 1–23

Weiss CF, Glazko AJ, Westein JK (1960) Chloramphenicol in the newborn infant: a physiologic explanation of its toxicity when given in excessive doses. New Engl J Med 262: 787–794

Wilcox CS, Aminoff MJ (1976) Blood pressure responses to noradrenaline and dopamine infusions in Parkinson's disease and the Shy-Drager syndrome. Br J clin Pharmac 3: 207–214

Wilkinson GR, Schenker S (1975) Drug disposition and liver disease. Drug Metab Reviews 4: 139–175

Wood PHN, Smith HEA, Dixon ASJ (1962) Salicylates and gastrointestinal bleeding. Acetylsalicylate acid and aspirin derivatives. Br Med J 1: 669–674

World Health Organization (1973) Pharmacogenetics. Wld Health Org techn Ref Ser 524

Wright N, Prescott LF (1973) Potentiation by previous drug therapy of hepatotoxicity following paracetamol overdosage. Scott Med J 18: 56–58

Zinn MB (1970) Quinidine intoxication from alkali ingestion. Texas Medicine 66: 64–66

Drug-Induced Liver Reactions: A Morphological Approach

H.-W. ALTMANN*

I. Introductory Remarks 69
II. Adaptative Phenomena 71
1. Agranuloreticular Hypertrophy (Hypertrophy of the Smooth Endoplasmic Reticulum) 71
2. Secondary Regressive Changes 73
III. Acute Liver Injury 76
1. Types and Mechanisms 76
2. Morphological Findings 85
a) Cytotoxic Lesions 85
b) Cholestatic Lesions 91
c) Granulomatous Reactions 102
IV. Chronic Liver Injury 104
V. Hepatovascular Lesions 109
VI. Tumor Induction 115
References 121

I. Introductory Remarks

Since general attention focused on manifestations of drug-induced liver injuries in the late 1950s, a wealth of original papers and a considerable number of *reviews* have been published on the different aspects of this subject (e.g. 11, 36, 37, 38, 42, 103, 120, 136, 140, 210, 216, 217, 224, 226, 249, 311, 319, 327, 342, 357–359, 393, 401, 408, 416, 417, 427, 476, 497–501, 503), among which the recently published comprehensive monograph of *Zimmerman* (503) should be emphasized. Associated clinical and biochemical phenomena were elucidated and the spectrum of morphological patterns was described. Therefore the injuring potential of drugs is well known and generally accepted, but many questions remain open with regard to even the acute manifestations of liver damage. They refer (a) to problems of pathogenesis – disturbance of cell metabolism or immunologic reactions, and if so, of which kind; (b) to the nomenclature: hepatitis, hepatosis, or hepatopathy; and (c), closely linked to this, the analysis of morphological patterns, i.e., whether liver damage can be differentiated from viral hepatitis in the event of predominating cellular necroses. Moreover, in the field of chronic progressive liver disease even the actual impact and relevance of drug-induced injuries is being discussed, whereas their pathogenetic significance for certain circulatory disorders as well as for tumor induction has already been reliably assessed through experience accumulated over recent years.

* Dedicated to Prof F. BÜCHNER on occasion of his 85th birthday (20.1.1980)

Whereas the morphology of acute liver diseases is fairly well known, the chronic, insidious, and slowly progressing forms of liver injury are far from being assessed with sufficient precision, and it is hardly possible to separate them with certainty from the other phenomena lumped together under the name of "chronic hepatitis." Moreover, the question whether the distinction is practicable is answered in the negative by most authors who discuss it. The definition of the term "hepatitis" being rather unsatisfactory, it appears preferable to drop it altogether in reference to drug-induced lesions, in favor of less prejudicial words like *"drug-induced injury"* or *"hepatopathy"*: These would permit the inclusion of the cholestatic lesions that are classified separately by the authors advocating "drug-induced hepatitis." However, even the elastic term of "drug-induced hepatopathy" fails to cover the great variety of phenomena and all their morphological or pathogenetic aspects, for the influence of drugs may provoke changes not to be interpreted as detrimental injuries, but rather as positive and progressive events, as expression of genuinely increased function, manifesting functionally conditioned hypertrophy or hyperplasia of cellular organelles. Here we are referring to drug-induced hypertrophy of the agranular endoplasmic reticulum (Figs. 1, 2) and to cellular hypertrophies and hyperplasias of the same origin. These not only dominate the morphological picture, but demonstrate the phenomenon of so-called enzyme induction, thus actually explaining a number of drug-induced injuries based on the long-term influence of the drug in question. Recognition and identification of these changes was initiated by the fundamental experimental investigations of *Remmer* and *Merker*

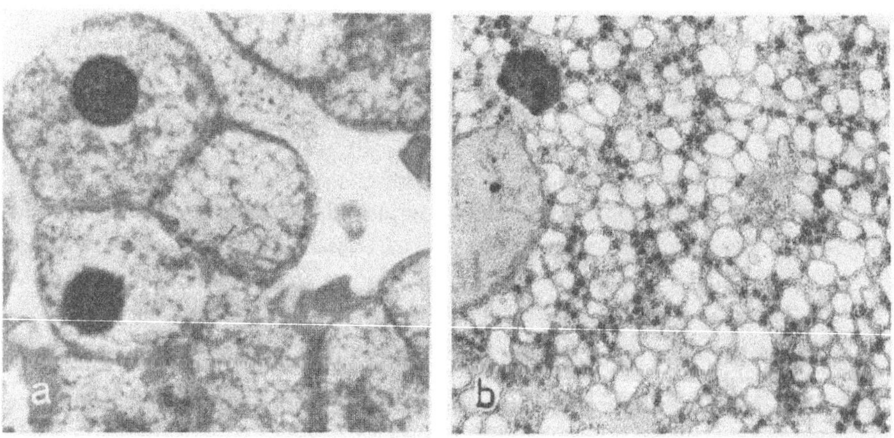

Fig. 1a,b. Drug-induced hypertrophy of the SER. **a** Finely vacuolar appearance as the light microscopic aquivalent of **b** numerous slightly dilated cisternae of the SER in the electron micrography; **a** = H & E, X 1500, **b** = X 22000

(374), who were also the first to identify and describe the correlation between hypertrophy of agranular (smooth) endoplasmic reticulum (ER) and enzyme induction.

The theory of *biotransformation* developed from these concepts is of decisive relevance for the understanding of acute as well as of chronic drug-induced liver diseases. Thus "reactions" appears preferable to "injuries" as a genetic term, even in a presentation of morphological features of drug-induced alterations. And for the same reason any discussion of these reactions should begin with a description of the drug-induced changes of the agranular ER, which even in some unequivocally regressive pathologic manifestations must be seen as the first link in a whole chain of events. In view of the limited space available, our presentation in this volume must be strictly limited to human material and primarily to discussion of light microscopic findings. In fact, the majority of publications on the subject and the diagnosis which the pathologist is asked to pronounce are based on histology. The discussion of the classic drug-induced injuries to liver cells will be supplemented by discussion of drug-induced circulatory disorders and neoplasms.

II. Adaptative Phenomena

1. Agranuloreticular Hypertrophy
(Hypertrophy of the Smooth Endoplasmic Reticulum)

When given over a longer time, a great number of pharmaceutical drugs that are metabolized in the liver will effect *induction* or enhancement of the enzymes involved in their decomposition, transformation, and conjugation (e.g., 79, 205, 371–375, 435), thus substantially influencing the response of the organism to these compounds. Insofar as these ferments are linked to the agranular ER, their increase is associated with a *hypertrophy* of this *smooth membranous system* particularly abundant in lobulocentral cells (159, 198, 259, 346). In stronger reactions, a vesicular appearance of the considerably proliferated structures defined as "type II of SE" (325) is observed both in animals and in humans (Fig. 1b). Deposites of glycogen are often found between the vesicles, while granular endoplasmic membranes and mitochondria are dislocated from their central position. A pronounced *agranuloreticular hypertrophy,* as observed in man after prolonged administration of barbiturates and especially of psychodrugs like Diazepam (195–198, 325) (Fig. 2d), of analgesics (associated regularly with lipofuscinosis) (Fig. 3), of antiepileptic drugs (Fig. 2a), but also of oral contra-ceptives (when given in the higher doses that were used until recently (150, 195, 340) (Fig. 14a), and of anabolic steroids (198), will even alter the microscopic picture (1, 2, 3, 14a).

A finely reticular appearance of the highly eosinophilic cytoplasm (435) combined with a thickening of the outher cellular membranes reflect the drug-induced hypertrophy of agranular ER. As a rule, this change of cytoplasmic structure can be readily distinguished from the particular hypertrophy observed in excess accumulations of HB_S antigens within elongated cisterns of agranular ER. Therefore, resort to orcein or aldehyde-fuchsin staining is rarely indicated, although its positive results in HB_S-bearing cells might facilitate the diagnosis in doubtful cases. Consequently, it appears rather infortunate to bring together both patterns (drug-induced agranuloreticular hypertrophy and that of viral origin) under the common name of *"ground-glass" hepatocytes* (e.g., 301, 451) – a term entirely inappropriate in describing the fine vesicular pattern that is always observed in the drug-induced form (Figs. 1a, 2). One may consider another distinctive feature to be the strictly centrolobular localization of ferment-induced hypertrophy, which affects all cells on the same level in the same way (Fig. 2a), whereas HB_S-bearing cells are always characterized by isolated or focal inci-

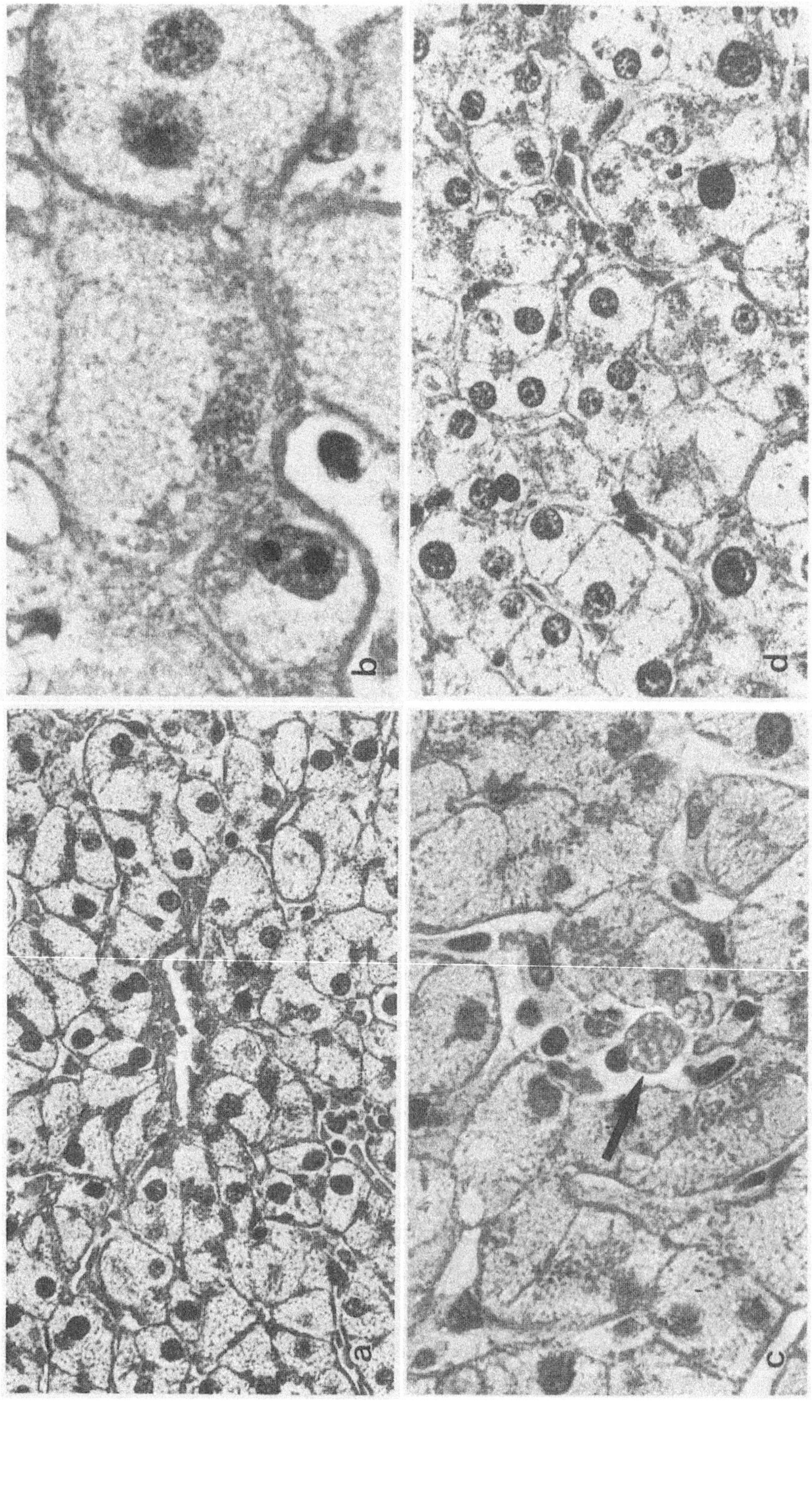

Fig. 2a–d

dence among normal-looking hepatocytes. Ferment-induced changes may show a remarkable peripheral spread, even touching the lobular borders in extreme cases, but they will always be strongest in the center of the lobules.

Hypertrophy of agranular ER, mediated by hyperplasia of its membrane systems, must necessarily increase the size of the affected cells and, consequently, lead to an enlargement of the lobule itself, clearly reflected in its increased radius. General hypertrophy of the whole liver is the obvious result, although less spectacular in man than in the rat. Moreover, in animals there is some evidence for a *numerical hyperplasia of liver cells,* induced and conditioned by an enhancement of the drug-metabolizing capacities, but in man there is no proof for such an event at present. The manner in which this ER hypertrophy takes place has not yet been elucidated. A certain inhibition of breakdown can be taken for granted and an increased formation is also probable.

That the hypertrophy of the smooth ER (SER) reverses as soon as the pressure from the respective substrate stops was learnt from animal experiments (43, 435) as well as from follow-up observations in man (11), but again, how this happens is still unclear. An increased rate of physiologic degradation seems to be a sufficient explanation. Such an event can hardly be expected to become visible in the microscopic picture. Electron microscopic morphometry (43) might be a suitable instrument for observation, provided it could catch the exact moment when the reversion occurs.

2. Secondary Regressive Changes

Our knowledge about regressive changes in hypertrophic membrane systems of the human liver is rather poor. *Concentric lamellar bodies,* consisting of concentrically arranged agranular membranes like the so-called *glatte Nebenkerne*, so well known from animal experiments with thioacetamide, DDT, or nitrosamines (see 22, 435), and which are interpreted as regressive changes, are hardly ever found in human material, not even in a most feeble form. In this context only some isolated, circumscribed plasma areas of fine vesicular, homogeneous structure which could be assessed in gradual transition to more or less homogeneous droplets (11) might be mentioned. No evidence was found, however, for an increase of agranular membrane systems without a concomitant increase of functional activity, in the sense of the hypothesis of hypoac-hypertrophic ER (183), unless marked structural changes in the SER were to be seen.

←

Fig. 2a–d. Drug-induced agranuloreticular hypertrophy. **a** Affecting all centrolobular cells; carbamazepine. Ladewig, × 480. **b** Finely vacuolar appearance of the cytoplasm and thickening of the outer cell membranes, the basophilic material being displaced to the pericanalicular pole; diphenylhydantoin. H & E, × 1200. **c** Single necrotic cell (arrow) surrounded by some mononuclear cells; psychopharmacological agents. H & E, × 950. **d** Increase of binuclear and macronuclear hepatocytes in the course of prolonged intake of psychopharmacological agents. H & E, × 600

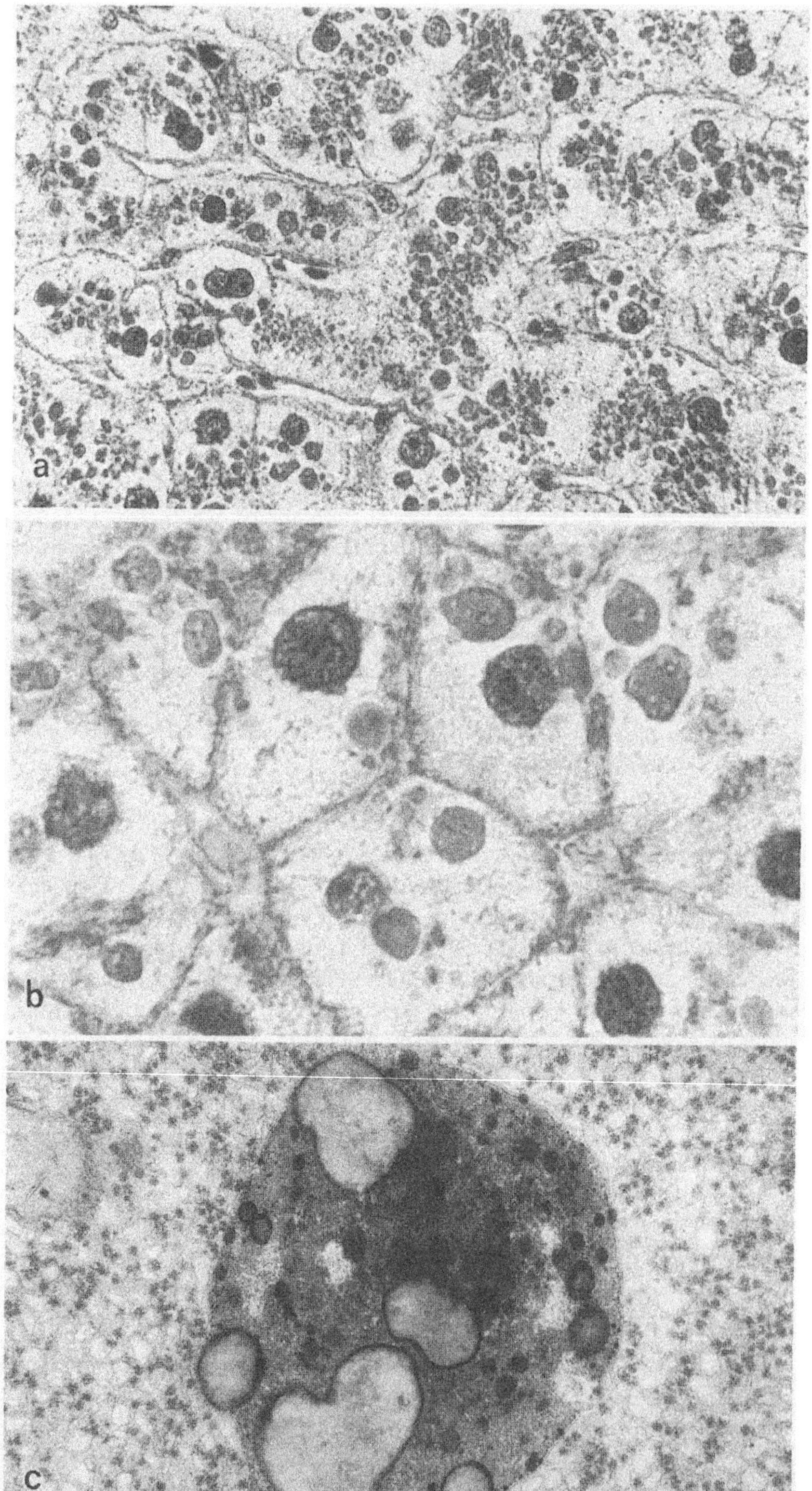

Fig. 3a–c

An interpretation of such transformed plasma areas as stages of degradation of agranular ER may be justified by the occurrence of numerous small *homogeneous droplets* under certain conditions developing in the course of agranuloreticular hypertrophy; these droplets are gradually transformed to *pigment granules of the lipofuscin type,* thus being responsible for the conspicuous *lipofuscinosis* that is frequently observed after analgesics in hypertrophic – not atrophic! – hepatocytes (Fig. 3) (1, 11, 34, 226, 227, 427, 441). The conditions for turning a simple agranuloreticular hypertrophy into the variant complicated by pigment granules seem to be created exclusively by certain drugs, namely phenacetin, acetosalicylic acid, and aminophenazone. Phenacetin has been used to provoke such pigmentation in various animal species (34, 441). The procedure seems to involve a biochemical pathway leading [possibly via free radicals (364)] from peroxidation of unsaturated lipids in the membrane system to almost or completely insoluble polymeric residues, persisting within lysosomes. These pigment pre-stages, which are less colored, are then gradually transformed into luminous pigment granules of smaller size, and with a lower amount of the formerly abundant protein. The size of these granules, the intensity of their coloration, and the peripheral spread of the pigmentation can serve as parameters for the severity and duration of phenacetin abuse. The bigger the granules, the heavier the abuse; the stronger their colors, the longer the period of administration. Therefore pigmentation spreading as far as the periphery of the lobulus signals massive drug abuse over a long time.

If drug administration is stopped, pigmentation persists much longer than the causative agranuloreticular hypertrophy itself. As far as we know today, this kind of pigmentation is induced only by the above-mentioned drugs, not by hypertrophic changes as such. Consequently, *lipid peroxidation* seems only to be mediated by certain metabolites of these drugs (139, 293) – some oxidative effects were demonstrated for phenacetin (462) , and the degradation of the membrane system seems to be visualized microscopically only if it is actually "deviated" by these drugs. Possibly, lipid peroxidation is also apt to provoke precocious membrane alterations leading to an increased rate of membrane formation.

Thus, pigmentation as such must be taken as a signal of drug-induced injury to hepatocytes, or at least to certain hepatocellular organelles. Even in plain agranuloreticular hypertrophy, the required increase in metabolic activities will sometimes exceed the limits of cellular adaptation capacity. The compensated burden turns into a decompensated overload. At any rate, scattered single *cell necroses* are sometimes found (11, 225) (Fig. 2c), especially in pigment-associated agranuloreticular hypertrophy, as are occasional small intralobular accumulations of resorptive macrophages or at least some swollen Kupffer cells containing lipofuscin as a sign of its having phagocytosed pigment-bearing hepatocytes.

From such cases there is a gradual transition to others that exhibit liver cell injury only after a long period of medication, i.e., after the induction of the SER has reached such an extent that enough reactive metabolites are produced to damage liver cells. Clinically the above-mentioned necroses of single liver cells are accompanied by slight-

Fig. 3a–c. Drug-induced lipofuscinosis (with hypertrophy of SER); phenacetin abuse; many coarse pigment deposits; finely vacuolar cytoplasm. **a** Ladewig, × 600; **b** Ladewig, × 1500; **c** × 20000 ly elevated transaminase levels. In this way not only cell degradation but also regenerative cell proliferation is enhanced. Mitoses are rare, but in cases of prolonged drug abuse we never fail to observe marked *differences in nuclear volumes* (Fig. 2d) and increase of binucleate cells within the potentially pigment-bearing inner zones of the lobules (11). The reason may be found in the comparative scarcity of actual cell necroses, which is able to stimulate regenerative cell proliferation but not to such a degree that the karyokinetic process is regularly completed. Instead of a perfect mitosis resulting in two daughter cells, typical for regenerating liver epithelia after severe cell loss or partial hepatectomy, there is incomplete karyokinesis resulting in multi- or meganucleated single cells (Fig. 2d). That implies an intensification of the basically identical process which normally occurs during the course of adult life and leads to the well-known rise of meganuclei in advanced age. Thus "nuclear unrest" in drug-induced agranuloreticular hypertrophy may illustrate a certain increase of cell renewal and, logically, of *hepatocyte turnover.* The process might be interpreted as a premature "ageing" of the liver, according to the age-related trend toward meganuclearity, especially in the central parts of the lobules.

III. Acute Liver Injury

1. Types and Mechanisms

The *medical drugs* liable to cause more or less acute clinical symptoms are usually divided into two groups: compounds provoking regularly dose-related and reproducible liver lesions, and compounds causing these lesions only occasionally and without any identifiable reason. Consequently, authors refer to directly or indirectly hepatotoxic agents (e.g., 4, 42, 103, 106), to predictable or unpredictable lesions (e.g., 342, 405, 408, 415–418), and to "intrinsic hepatotoxicity" or host-dependent "idiosyncratic liver lesions" (497–501, 503; see 475). We prefer to use the terms *obligatory and facultative hepatotoxicity.* Regardless of terminology, a borderline zone of fluid transition exists between the two groups; the number of facultatively affected persons may appear rather great, or perhaps a slight affection of the liver is an almost regular finding, whereas only the culmination in more severe injuries appears uncommon and hardly predictable.

In the same way the majority of *acute hepatic injuries* can be divided into two basically separable groups that do, however, have fluid borders: The first is characterized by the alteration of intermediate hepatocellular metabolism involving varying dangers to the life of the affected cells. The other involves only the excretory hepatic function. This type comprises all cases whose morphology is dominated by intralobular cholestasis with visible bile plugs and which are generally classified as *"cholestatic reactions."* In German publications these cases are often defined as *"cholestatic hepatosis (hepatopathy)."* The first group comprises all forms dominated by regressive epithelial changes of fatty or hydropic nature, or even involving more or less extensive necrosis. Whereas fatty changes are nearly always identified and classified as such, the necrotic forms have commonly been defined as "drug (-induced) hepatitis" – a term that is now employed for lighter forms with only isolated cell necroses as well as for the rare acute liver failure of the same etiology, which is called "fulminating drug

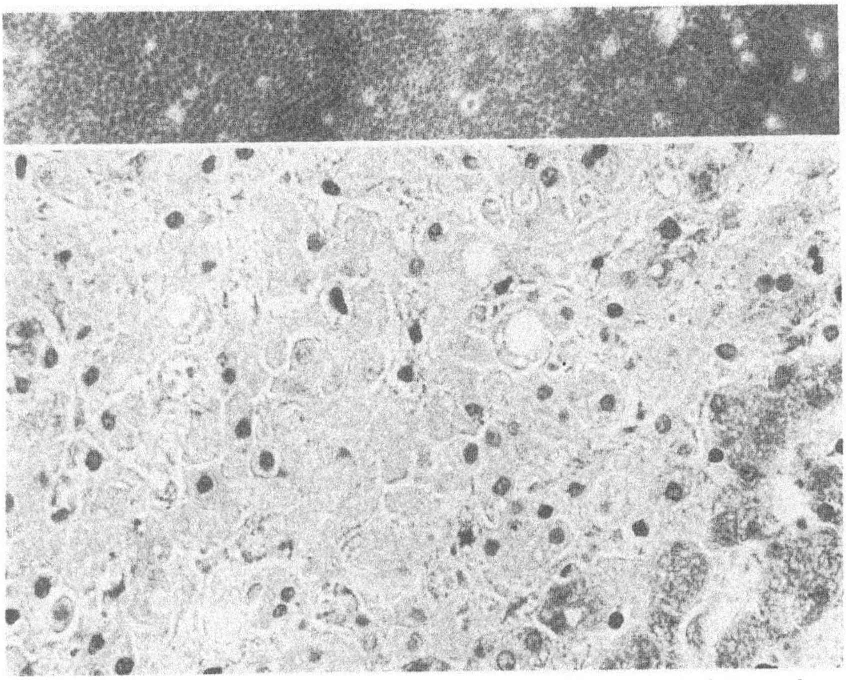

Fig. 4a, b. Acute centrolobular necrosis; cytostatics. **a** Macroscopic. **b** Loss of cytoplasmic basophilia, pyknosis of nuclei. Cresyl violet, X 375

hepatitis." This usage is based on several factors. The clinical picture, for instance, is hardly distinguishable, even in its variability, from that of genuine virus-induced hepatitis, and the morphological differentiation may be just as difficult. But in opposition to general opinion (e.g., 408), we feel that this similarity applies only to the aforesaid "fulminate" forms of hepatitis, i.e., to acute liver dystrophy, and not to the more common lighter injuries. The term *"cytotoxic liver injury" (Cytotoxic hepatosis, cytotoxic hepatopathy)* seems to fit this type of drug-induced liver damage more appropriately than does "toxic hepatitis" (meaning an inflammatory lesion), although morphological distinction will sometimes be difficult or impossible. With greater precision we may speak of "cytotoxic necrotizing hepatopathy," of "cytotoxic hepatopathy with single or grouped necroses," and, possibly, of "cytotoxic liver dystrophy." This terminology is further supported by the general term *"toxic hepatopathy,"* which is suitable – in contrast to "hepatitis" – for covering other plainly regressive changes, e.g., changes of a fatty character and cholestatic lesions.

Therefore, under the general heading of drug-induced toxic hepatopathy (hepatosis) we shall distinguish between a principally cytotoxic (e.g., Figs. 4, 5, 7, 10) and a cholestatic reaction (e.g., Figs. 11–13, 16). The two basic forms are, however, not strictly separated; we know *mixed forms* where both reactions are equally conspicuous and where cholestasis must not be interpreted as an independent manifestation, but rather as part of the general cytotoxic injury (Figs. 6a, 12a). This combined forms, considered by many authors as the most common of drug-induced reactions (e.g., 103), is sometimes classified separately as "cholestasis with hepatitis." On the other hand it is well known that while certain substances provoke chiefly cytotoxic reactions, other provoke almost exclusively cholestatic manifestations, but that one and the same drug may also evoke a cytotoxic response in one patient, a cholestatic one in another, or even mixed forms. However, such observations are not meant to qualify the principal concept of differentiating these two types of reaction.

In addition, we feel that a third form has to be added, namely the *granulomatous reaction,* though it is rarely found. It is characterized by intra- and extralobular, often epithelioid granulomas and periportal infiltration of more or less eosinophilic granulocytes (Figs. 17–19); cytotoxic or cholestatic phenomena may also be present. These special cases are dealt with separately and may be left aside in our survey of the acute reactions in general.

Compounds of *obligatory hepato(cyto)toxicity* are hardly, if ever, represented among the modern therapeutic drugs. The relatively well-known liver poisons like carbon tetrachloride, chloroform, or amanitine relate to our present problem only insofar as they may demonstrate the spectrum of morphological changes induced by fully analyzed pathogenic mechanisms. Tannic acid, too, can be cited in this context; after some use in the therapy of skin burns, it had to be eliminated on account of its obligatory hepatotoxicity (e.g., 58). Morphologically, the nature of all these injuries is cytotoxic, with occasional admixture of a slight cholestatic component resulting from the severe impairment of hepatocellular metabolism.

However, if we also include dosage problems, obligatory hepatotoxicity is encountered in a much larger number of drugs, among them such familiar and often prescribed substances as acetosalicylic acid and acetaminophen. Aspirin, for instance, of which a single excess dose will provoke markedly toxic fatty changes (459), is liable to induce liver necroses of varying intensity when given at high doses over a long time, as in rheumatism therapy (189, 317, 334, 383, 412, 489, 502, 505). The nature of the immediate cytotoxic mechanism was investigated and demonstrated in animal experiments and in vitro cell cultures (456). Occasional evidence of mild portal inflammation (141, 383, 489) illustrates the potential association of the latter with primary epitheliotoxic lesions, exemplifying their reactive nature. Paracetamol (acetaminophen), a phenacetin derivative quite harmless in the usual low dosage, will provoke considerable liver injuries as soon as a certain threshold level in passed; this has been observed in attempted poisoning or suicide as well as in animal experiments (46, 98, 289–292). Their manifestations vary from toxic fatty changes through single cell necroses and focal centrolobular necroses to fully developed liver dystrophy (23, 71, 101, 130, 157, 194, 248, 322, 362, 363, 450, 485). The decisive factor seems to be the formation of a *metabolite* which induces irreversible covalent linkage to cellular macromolecules (90, 139, 140, 203, 343), possibly acting via lipid peroxidation (65). Since this metabolite may be trapped by SH groups preventing its attack on cellular macromolecules (90, 139, 140, 203, 240, 292, 343), the glutathione level of cells is of decisive influence upon the toxic threshold: cellular injuries will not occur unless the glutathione level drops to below 30% of normal values (292). Since the metabolite is produced within the agranular ER, pretreatment with phenobarbital will enhance the toxicity of paracetamol, whereas reduced activity of P_{450} will lead to reduced cellular injury (289, 293, 492). Therefore, much depends on the actual status of the affected tissue and of the *drug-metabolizing system;* that prolonged administration of smaller doses (4 g being by no means a negligible quantity!) may eventually provoke chronic liver injury and portal infiltration (44) is easily understood.

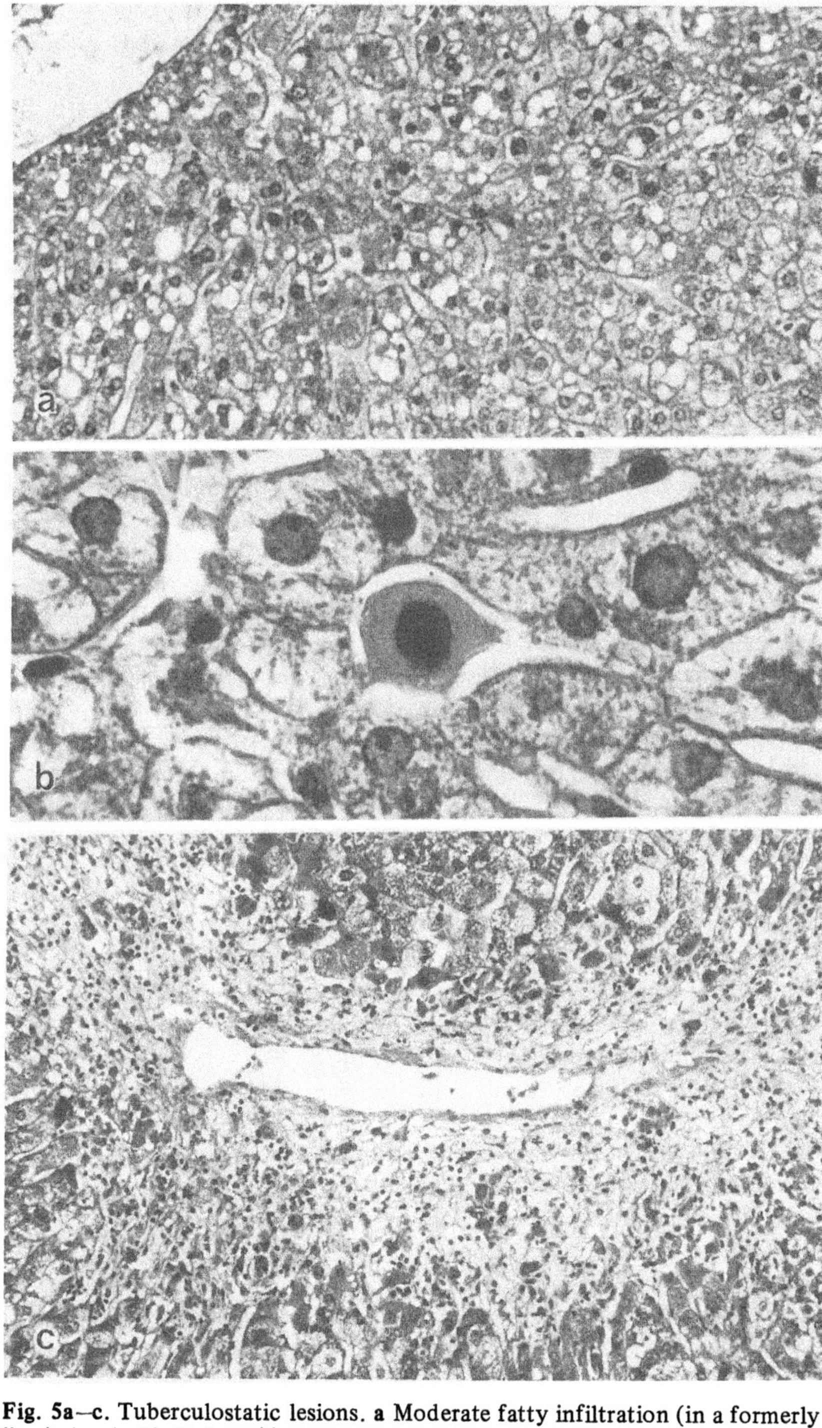

Fig. 5a–c. Tuberculostatic lesions. **a** Moderate fatty infiltration (in a formerly fat-free liver), isoniazid. H & E, × 240. **b** Single cell necrosis; isoniazid. H & E, × 960. **c** Centrolobular cell loss; isoniazid + rifampicin. Tri-PAS, × 150

Obligatory hepatotoxicity must also be attributed, we feel, to those cytostatic drugs that are liable to affect the liver, such as mercaptopurine (70, 117, 135, 501, 503), mitomycin (295), mithramycin (368), and methotrexate, when given in the treatment of malignant lymphoma or psoriasis (11, 86, 182, 328, 405, 501, 503) as a single agent or in combination with other, possibly enhancing cytostatics in the so-called de Vita schedule (311, 389, 473) (Fig. 4). Accordingly, animal experiments have illustrated dose-dependent acute and chronic injuries (24). Tetracyclines (see 76, 403) are equally liable to induce liver injuries if given in excess doses or if renal insufficiency, preventing speedy excretion, results in abnormal concentration of these agents in the blood. Inhibiting the cellular protein synthesis, tetracyclines cause a deficiency in carrier proteins and eventually impede triglyceride release (see 435); the result is a highly characteristic diffuse accumulation of fine fat droplets which resembles the so-called "fatty liver of pregnancy" and is regularly associated with some scattered hepatocytic necroses.

None of the liver reactions to the drugs of this group differ principally from the reaction to classic hepatotoxines. They always manifest morphologically as toxic hepatopathy (hepatosis), i.e., as toxic hepatopathy of the cytotoxic type. In contrast, there seem to be no drugs of *obligatory cholestatic* effect, notwithstanding the fact that certain steroids will regularly affect certain predisposed patients – but only these –, provoking cholestasis by direct attack on the biliary excretion apparatus. Thus, the terms "obligatory" and "facultative" only describe the regularity of the liver injuries, not the particular mechanisms involved.

The group of drugs with *facultative hepatotoxicity* provoking cytotoxic, cholestatic, or granulomatous reactions, is much larger. A first observation (jaundice after Atophan) was published as early as 1923 (491); today, the number of drugs in this category exceeds 200. The most common of them have been repeatedly listed and tabulated (e.g., 42, 103, 503); however, the dangerous property of one and the same substance varies considerably: It can increase with the course of treatment or with the repetition of a single dose, as in halothane narcosis (186, 187) (Fig. 6), but it can equally diminish under such conditions.

Toxic effects of some drugs have been documented in only a few isolated cases (Fig. 5a); the complications of some others are common enough to be assessed in percentages: monotherapy with isoniazid produces cytotoxic liver injuries in 1% of cases (320, 433, 501), while combined therapy with rifampicin and isoniazid does so in 10% (Fig. 5b, c). Cholestatic reactions to chlorpromazine were reported in 0.5%–5% of cases (216, 217, 249, 357, 498) (Fig. 16). Some drugs were found to induce a minor subclinical impairment of liver functions rather frequently, but also unexpected more severe changes in some rare cases. Methyldopa (293, lit.) may be taken as an example, for many patients receiving this drug show minor liver injuries manifesting in a slight rise of transaminase levels (121, 138, 262, 385, 461, 484). In the field of facultative cholestatic reactions, estrogen therapy was found to induce some delay of bile excretion in most women (e.g., 321), but genuine cholestatic reactions (Fig. 11) were morphologically verified in only a very small number of patients. With regard to chlorpromazine, the above-mentioned cholestatic reactions in up to 5% of jaundice cases must be seen in context, with mild functional disorders occurring in no less than 50% of cases. It is not the disturbance of the excretory function as such, but its abnormal and excessive increase that should be interpreted as an unpredictable "surprise." The relevance of dosage is illustrated once more by the fact that these reactions are becoming less frequent since the reduction of estrogen components in modern contraceptives.

In all of these cases the nature of the drug is less influential on the causation of liver injuries than the *personal and individual susceptibility* of the patient. When unexpected reactions occur we might even characterize the condition as an *allergic reaction* in the broadest sense of this term (11), or as an *idiosyncrasy* (497–501, 503; see 475, 479), obviously without immediately implying that this peculiarity has an immunologic basis.

As regards the *mechanism of action* of these drugs of facultative hepatotoxicity, two groups can be distinguished. One is dominated by *hypersensitivity reactions,* the other by the effect of *toxic metabolites* of either unusual nature or unusual quantity (see 139, 140, 288, 289, 343). The borderline separating them is drawn differently by different authors; recent experiences favor a shift of weight toward the second group, i.e., the abnormal primary metabolic reactions. Even the effects of halothane (Fig. 6), much discussed and previously at most supposed to induce some sort of hyperergic damage, was recently explained, not least in consequence of experimental findings, in terms of an induction of hepatotoxic metabolites under the specific conditions of hypoxia and ferment induction (32, 83).

Such harmful *reactive metabolites,* commonly not present at all or only in small quantities, may either directly attack the cellular macromolecules, producing an immediate cytotoxic effect, or evoke, as haptens linked to cellular macromolecules, a cytotoxic immune response resulting in indirect damage to the cell. With regard to primarily metabolic reactions of drugs of facultative hepatotoxicity, we might speak of *direct* of *indirect* cytotoxic injuries (see 106), bearing in mind that the meaning of these adjectives differs from common usage in our context: they are not synonymous to obligatory and facultative hepatotoxicity, nor are they used according to the interpretation of *Zimmerman,* who wants to characterize the nature of cytotoxic attacks by calling a generalized damage "direct," and using "indirect" to describe the interruption of only one vital metabolic pathway.

In contrast, the unusual, typical feature of the second category of reactions is not the presence of a certain metabolite, but the onset of an immunologic response mediated either by the drug itself or by its physiologic metabolites.

The categories are differentiated not only by pathogenetic criteria, but also according to their clinical and morphological manifestations. Clinically, the second group alone is associated with the usual *phenomena of hypersensitivity,* which in the first group are either never found or only in a modified and reduced manner (see 489–501, 503). Morphologically, metabolic cytotoxic lesions are dominated by the reactions known from the classic liver poisons and commonly termed "toxic liver injuries" (e.g., Figs. 4, 5): a variety of regressive epithelial changes and centrolobular necroses. In the second category local mesenchymal reactions of unexpected strength, sometimes extending to granuloma (Figs. 17–19), and marked portal infiltrations often with strong eosinophilia (Fig. 15) are signs of a hyperergic component which, however, must not be held responsible for the accompanying uniform cellular necroses.

Obviously, in some cases no satisfactory diagnostic decision between the two groups will be obtainable, even by synoptic evaluation of all morphological and clinical

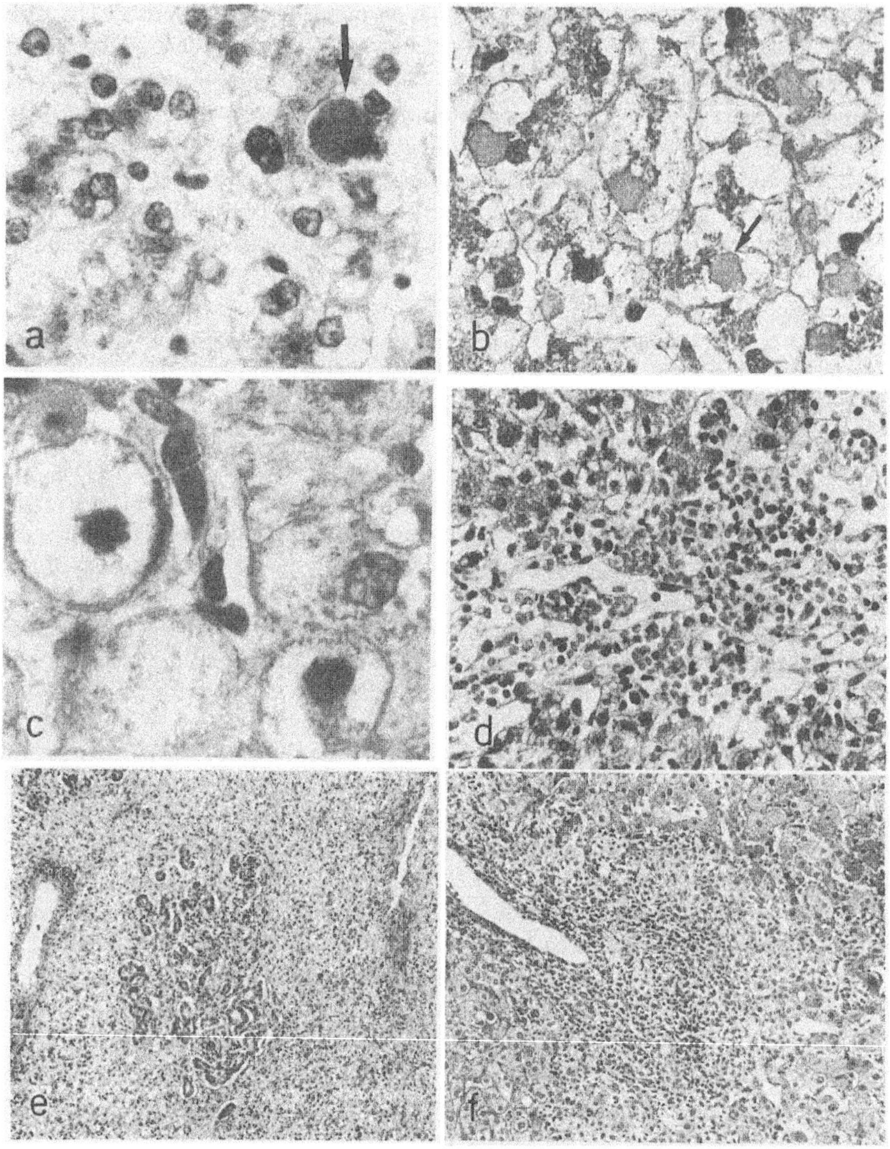

Fig. 6a–f. Patterns of halothane-induced liver lesions. **a** Fatty infiltration with bile plug (arrow). H & E, × 960. **b** Hydropic changes with sharply demarcated drop-like inclusions. Masson, × 460. **c** Single cell necrosis and two mitotic figures with clumped chromosomes (second narcosis). Ladewig, × 1500. **d** Centrolobular loss of hepatocytes (second narcosis). Ladewig, × 375. **e** Subacute liver dystrophy (third narcosis). H & E, × 95. **f** Granulomatous reaction in the portal areas (second narcosis). H & E, × 150

findings. Combined or mixed reactions are conceivable since cytotoxic *and* antigenic effects of one and the same metabolite are not necessarily exclusive nor incompatible. In this connection both reactions may contribute to the development of the morphological injury, or the immunologic phenomena are no more than an additional process, not damaging the liver but sometimes dominating the clinical picture. Nor is a certain drug always certain to exert its facultative hepatotoxicity in the same fashion (see 139), as illustrated by the very different reactions that have been observed in response to one drug (Figs. 6, 8). Halothane-induced reactions may provide an example (Fig. 6): Some are dominated by cytotoxic epithelial lesions like hydropic or fatty changes, others by allergic responses with portal eosinophilia (Figs. 6f, 18a), and yet others by acute or subacute, and possibly fatal, liver dystrophy (e.g., 420).

In primary *metabolic facultative liver injuries,* a decisive role is often assigned to *genetic particularities,* as exemplified in cholestasis after contraceptives (3, 88). There is a familial disposition (88, 436) al well as individual and statistical correlations with the so-called pregnancy jaundice of the last trimester (3, 41, 107, 161, 281, 318, 321, 321, 397, 418), during which estrogen values rise to an exceptional level. Further arguments are taken from the geographic variation of incidence rates, which are 1:10000 in the United States, but 1:4000 in Scandinavian countries and in Chile (324, see 103, 281, 318). Anthropological investigations in Chile proved the genetic disposition of certain Indian tribes (Araucanians) to be responsible for increased risk of pregnancy jaundice as measured by the incidence of the pruritus of pregnancy (327). However, the biochemical or structural properties dependent on this genetic factor are as unknown as the mechanism of steroid cholestasis to which they are supposed to predispose.

With regard to some other drugs, the genetic factor provoking or promoting a certain drug-induced injury is better known (207, 246, 249, 468–470). In their reaction to the tuberculostatic isoniazid, patients capable of rapid transformation of this compound (*"fast acetylators"*) by virtue of an autosomal dominant factor (207, 268) will show other incidence risks than patients whose lower acetyltransferase activity results in a considerable retardation of the same process (*"slow acetylators"*). The crucial substance seems to be an acetylated metabolite (acetylhydrazine) that is also capable of inducing experimental liver necrosis and that can be neutralized by prolonged acetylation. Logically, sometimes the fast acetylators with their high rate of metabolites (39, 238, 288, 294) and sometimes the slow acetylators with their delayed degradation (238, 303) may be subject to increased risk and therefore show a higher percentage of structural or functional liver injuries. The slow acetylators are also at a disadvantage during diphenylhydantoin therapy for epilepsia, because a toxic metabolite persists over too long a period (320). In other cases genetic factors may open, via an alteration of hepatocellular ferments, some new and unphysiologic pathways of metabolism, evoking new and unusual metabolites (249, 420) which, in turn, cause direct or indirect damage to the cells.

Great importance is to be attributed to the *activity of the drug-metabolizing enzymes* and therefore to the amount of functionally active agranular ER. Ferment induction by previous or simultaneous administration of other drugs may lead, via unusually enhanced metabolites, to an injury that would hardly ever or never occur otherwise (139, 288, 290, 343, 361, 503). This may explain why drug-induced liver damage some-times appears only after the drug in question has been administered for a longer period, leading to an easily recognizable hypertrophy of the agranular endoplasmic reticulum. In such cases genetic factors may be involved too, as suggested by the fact that the rate of induction is related to species- and person-specific differences (62, 89, 323). An appropriate example is found in combined tuberculostatic therapy (Fig. 5b, c) with rifampicin and isoniazid, wherein liver injuries are more frequent and more severe (18, 238, 244, 288, 289, 320, 344, 346, 347) than in monotherapy with either isoniazid or even rifampicin (29, 409, 446). Rifampicin, being an enzyme inductor (283, 320, 343, 346, 375), leads to a higher concentration of directly cytotoxic metabolite of isoniazid acetylhydrazine. Similar effects of enzymatic induction of actual hepatotoxicity were also demonstrated in iproniazid, a monoamine oxidase inhibitor prescribed as an antidepressant (293, 343). Even halothane will, under similar conditions and under simultaneous reduction of oxygen pressure, evoke reduced metabolites capable of regular induction of centrolobular liver necrosis (Fig. 6d–e) even in experimental animals (32, 54, 62, 83, 93, 378, 426, 436, 482).

The second category of idiosyncratic liver injury caused by facultative liver toxins is characterized by an *uncommon immunologic response* to the drug itself or to its normal or abnormal metabolites. When a metabolite bound to the cellular macromolecules evokes cellular damage only under such a condition, i.e., as a result of a peculiar reactivity of the immune system, the findings have to be classified in this category. Whether and when this special case will occur hardly appears predicable so far, certainly not on the basis of morphological findings. So this category is up to now mainly represented by cases manifesting clinical and morphological symptoms of hyperergic reactions. These are – in contrast to widespread opinion – quite rare in the field of cytotoxic reactions. In addition, they are less commonly associated with cholestatic lesions than they were thought to be and are also of lesser importance. Sufficient proof for hyperergic reaction was collected, however, from reactions to halothane in cases undergoing repeated anesthesia (186, 187, 304, 440) whose corresponding clinical manifestations and morphological findings demonstrated eosinophilic infiltration and a trend toward granuloma development (Figs. 6f, 17). Similar pictures were observed in cases of reexposition to oxyphenisatin-containing laxatives (Fig. 15a). Nevertheless, we cannot definitely exclude the possibly important influence of unusual metabolites produced by genetic or acquired alterations of the normal pathways of degradation. Last but not least, it is hard to decide whether allergic or hyperergic reactions are provoked by just those substances that are responsible for the simultaneous *cytotoxic damage*. Repeated penicillin medication, for instance, is known to cause allergic or hyperergic reactions rather frequently, but genuine liver injuries are surprisingly rare, both clinically and morphologically (149, 466, 501, 503) (Fig. 17). So if drug-related hypersensitivity reactions are associated more often with hepatic lesions, we may be sure that the drug in question is also directly affecting the hepatocytes (501, 503). For some of the frequently hypersensitivity-provoking drugs, evidence of resulting milder liver injuries could actually be demonstrated in isolated perfused livers as well as in cell cultures (e.g., 109, 211, 212, 501, 503, 504). Therefore, allergic–hyperergic injury is hardly conceivable unless the drug in question or one of its metabolites reacts directly with, or even alters the hepatocytes.

The morphological picture of liver injury induced by drugs of facultative hepatotoxicity is much too varied (Figs. 6, 8) to be explained by uniform mechanism. Except for the occasional abundance of eosinophils (Figs. 8, 13, 15) and the sometimes coinciding, sometimes isolated occurrence of granulomatous reactions (Figs. 17–19), morphological findings failed to yield conclusive evidence for cellular or humoral immune reactions being involved in the causation of explicit hepatocellular changes whose nature can be characterized as either cytotoxic or cholestatic.

2. Morphological Findings

a) Cytotoxic Lesions

Cytotoxic alterations of liver tissue are found with drugs of facultative as well as of obligatory hepatotoxicity. *Fatty changes* are frequent, though rather unspecific (Fig. 7). Among them, the fatty changes following glycocorticoid therapy are exceptional, because they can hardly be classified as cytotoxic in the true sense of the word. They show storage of larger lipid droplets and are free from single cell necroses, but there may be occasional small tubercles indicative or recidivating and disseminating tuberculosis.

All other drug-induced fatty changes should always be interpreted as symptoms of a direct cytotoxic mechanism attacking the cellular metabolism. Obviously no immunologic mechanism is at play. Such changes are seen after cytostatics (11, 86, 389) (Fig. 7c), in which case they are usually associated with single cell necrosis and, occasionally, with cytotoxic cholestasis. They are also found after (a) tuberculostatic drugs (Fig. 5a), expressing only minor damage; (b) high doses of aspirin (459); (c) paracetamol (322); (d) phenylbutazon (114), and (e) anesthesia with halothane (222, 223, 228, 349, 420) (Fig. 6a) as one of several possible reactions to this drug. Similar results may be observed after prolonged medication with antidepressants or antiarrhythmics like ajmaline (Fig. 8a) or parajmalintartrate, again as one of several possible reactions. In these cases we see selective centrolobular fatty changes with medium-sized droplets and varying peripheral spread. This pattern, differing characteristically from alcohol-induced fatty changes, should always alert the observer to the possibility of drug-related causation (Figs. 7, 8a). Tetracyclines will, as a rule, provoke characteristical poly-vacuolar changes (see 76, 348, 403) with the afore-mentioned striking resemblance to the so-called fatty liver of pregnancy.

Another regressive lesion is the so-called *"cellular hydrops"* (Fig. 9), likewise designated as hydropic (e.g., 115, 427) or toxic swelling of cells (223, 224, 226) or as cell-ballooning (e.g., 412). All of these terms are rather poorly defined, covering a great diversity of ultrastructural changes even if we exclude the so-called "feathery degeneration" (Fig. 11c) provoked by the effect of retained or accumulated bile acids. This special form of feathery hydrops is, in fact, very rare among the drug-induced changes, being found only in focal manifestation during prolonged cholestasis. All other cases thus classified can be traced back to a combination of two separate basic reactions: one is the abnormal *storage of glycogen* due to inhibition of glycogen degradation (11, 226) and with the resulting typical picture of plant-like cells (Fig. 9c); the other consists of a considerable *dilatation of the ER cisterns*, resembling, to some extent, the pattern found in chronic alcoholism, although it develops more rapidly, and equally associated with a decrease of the granular compartments of ER, that is, with a reduction of "cytoplasmic basophilia." Microscopic pictures of this dilatation (Figs. 6b, 9a, b) are much more irregular and rather varied, often being associated with nuclear changes like condensation of chromatin or, reversely, reparative nuclear swelling with bigger nucleoli. The two types are not always distinctly separable because the second is apt to show intercisternal glycogen accumulation at the same time. The second form is certainly more common, often being linked with cell destruction or cell loss. It can be found, for instance, after ajmaline (Figs. 8c, 9b) or halothane (Fig. 6b). Occasionally some cytoplasmic inclusions of a more or less homogeneous nature are to be seen (see 223; Fig. 6b), which may be interpreted as the result of an acute intracisternal protein retention. Changes of this kind indicate a direct toxic influence and should alert the observer to the possibility of drug-induced injuries.

Necroses, when found, are as a rule of the coagulation type, manifesting as either single cell (Figs. 5b, 6c, 9c, 10, 11b, 12a, 15b, 18b, c) or focal necroses (Fig. 4), the latter having a clear preference for the centrolobular area and being sharply demarcated (see Figs. 5c, 6d). This fact can be correlated with either particularly active drug metabolism in this area (202, 203, 291, 343) or with insufficient oxygen supply, and must be interpreted in either case, even under halothane influence (349, 420, 475, 487, 503), in terms of a direct cytotoxic lesion. Extensive necrosis as a sign of acute liver failure is rare, at least in our region. Consequently, reports that such cases account for 25%–30% of the total number of fatal liver insufficiencies (e.g., 58, 349, 457, 501, 503) seem rather exaggerated. They were described, for instance, after methyldopa (e.g., 178, 261, 370, 411, 455, 463), tuberculostatics (21, 39, 260), excess doses of paracetamol (23, 71, 101, 322, 485), and halothane (see 187, 223, 228, 349, 420). As a rule, morphological differentiation from acute liver dystrophy in "fulminating viral hepatitis" is hardly possible. The actual pathogenesis of this extreme reaction to drugs given in normal doses is still unknown and the idea of an extreme production of hepatotoxic metabolites, not yet proven. A protacted course of the disease leads to a subacute liver dystrophy; survivors later show the typical picture of postdystrophic (postnecrotic) cirrhosis.

Fig. 7a–c. Drug-induced fatty infiltration. **a** "Multivacuolar"; psychopharmacological agents. H & E, X 375. **b** Centrolobular fatty infiltration combined with intra-cellular bile deposits (arrowheads); diphenylhydrazine. H & E, X 600. **c** Centrolobular fatty infiltration with single cell necrosis (arrowhead); cytostatics (de Vita). H & E, X 240

Fig. 8a–d. Liver lesions, induced by ajmaline. **a** Univacuolar fatty infiltration. H & E, X 125. **b** Intracanalicular cholestasis (after the first intake). H & E, X 960. **c** Scattered hydropic cells. Ladewig, X 240. **d** Eosinophilic portal infiltration with fibrosis. Congo red, X 375

Fig. 9a–c. Drug-induced "hydropic" changes. **a** Equivalent of dilatation of the hyperplastic cisternae of SER; many different agents, mostly psychotropic. H & E, X 600. **b** Some hydropic cells (dilatation of SER cisternae), accompanied by a generalized swelling of mitochondria and one necrosis (arrowhead); ajmaline. H & E, X 600. **c** Glycogen accumulation with single cell necrosis; contraceptives. H & E, X 960

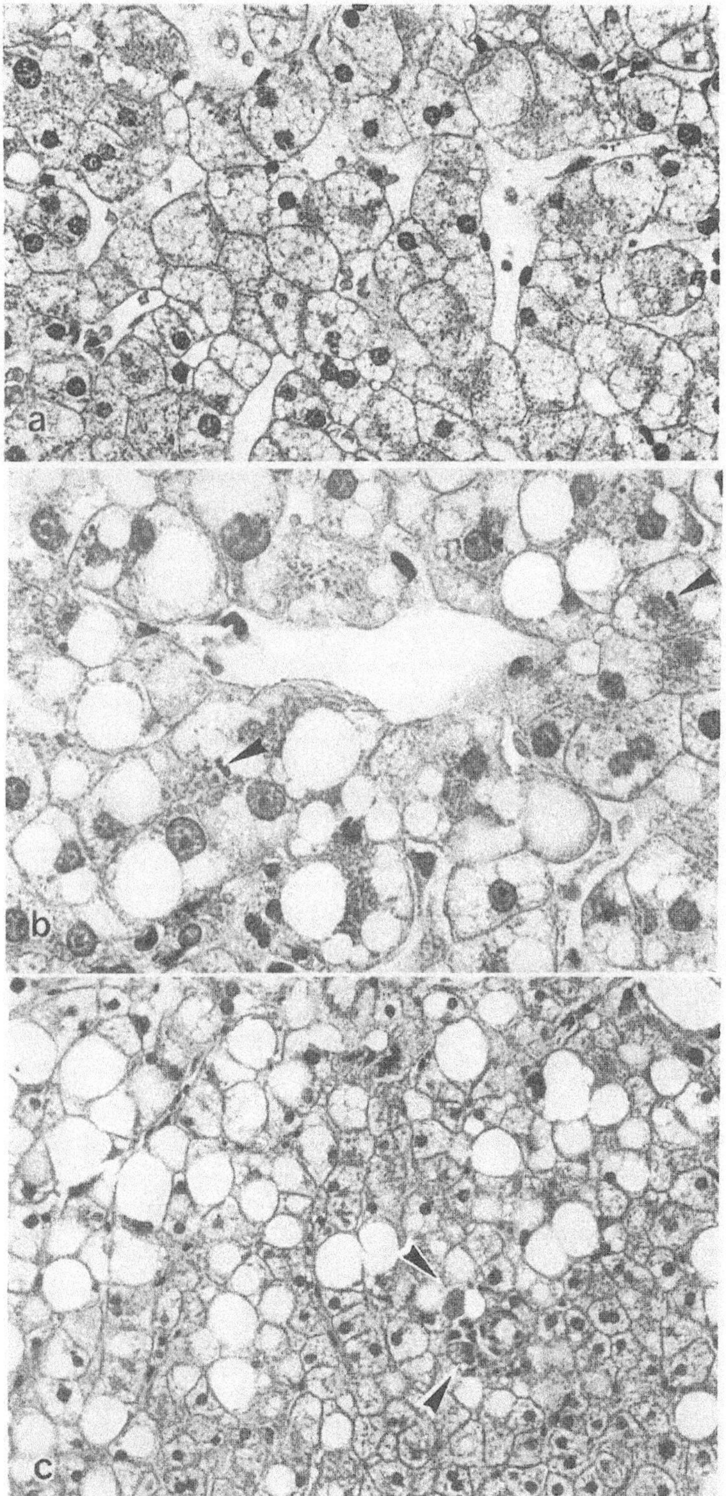

Fig. 7a–c

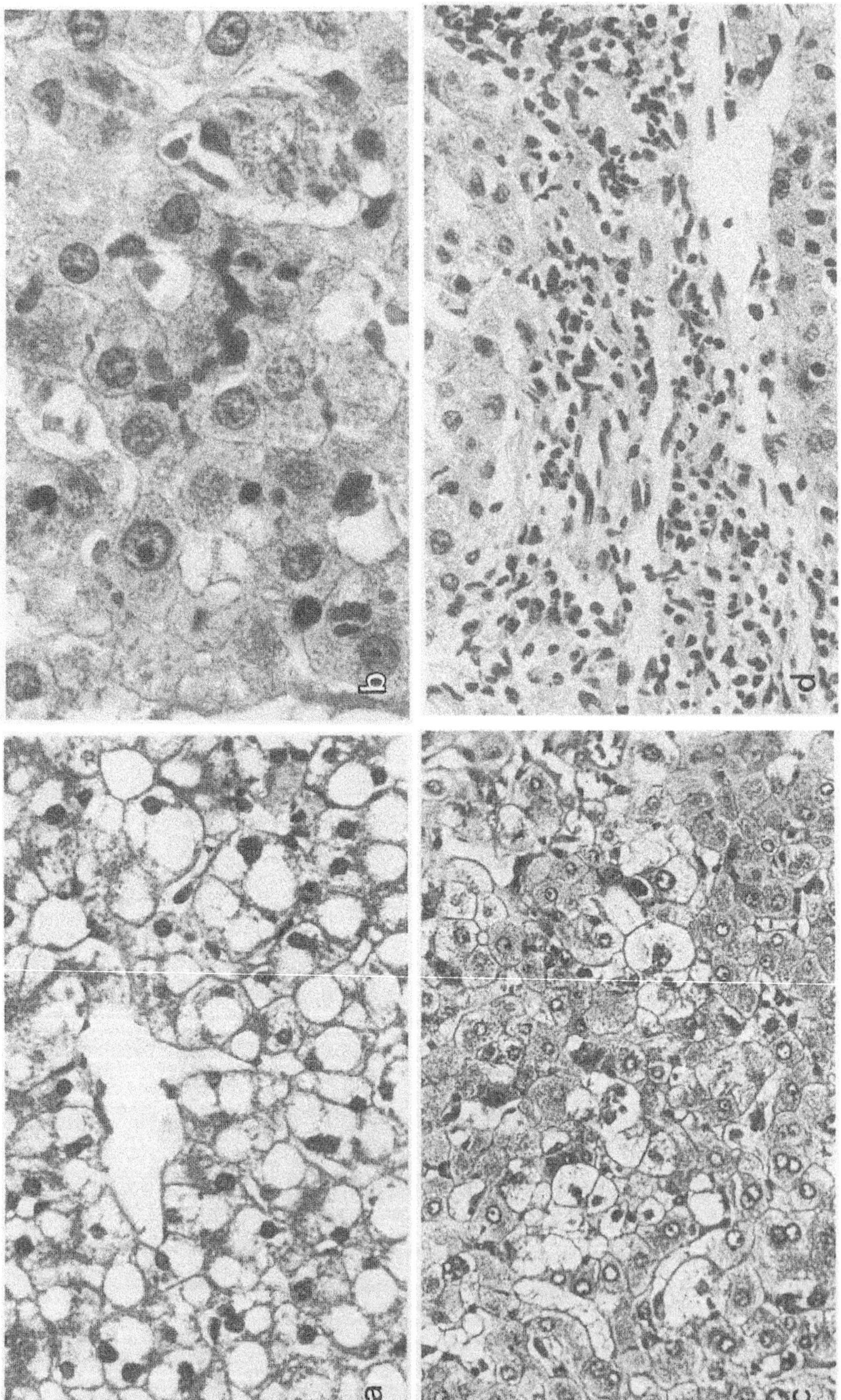

Fig. 8a—d

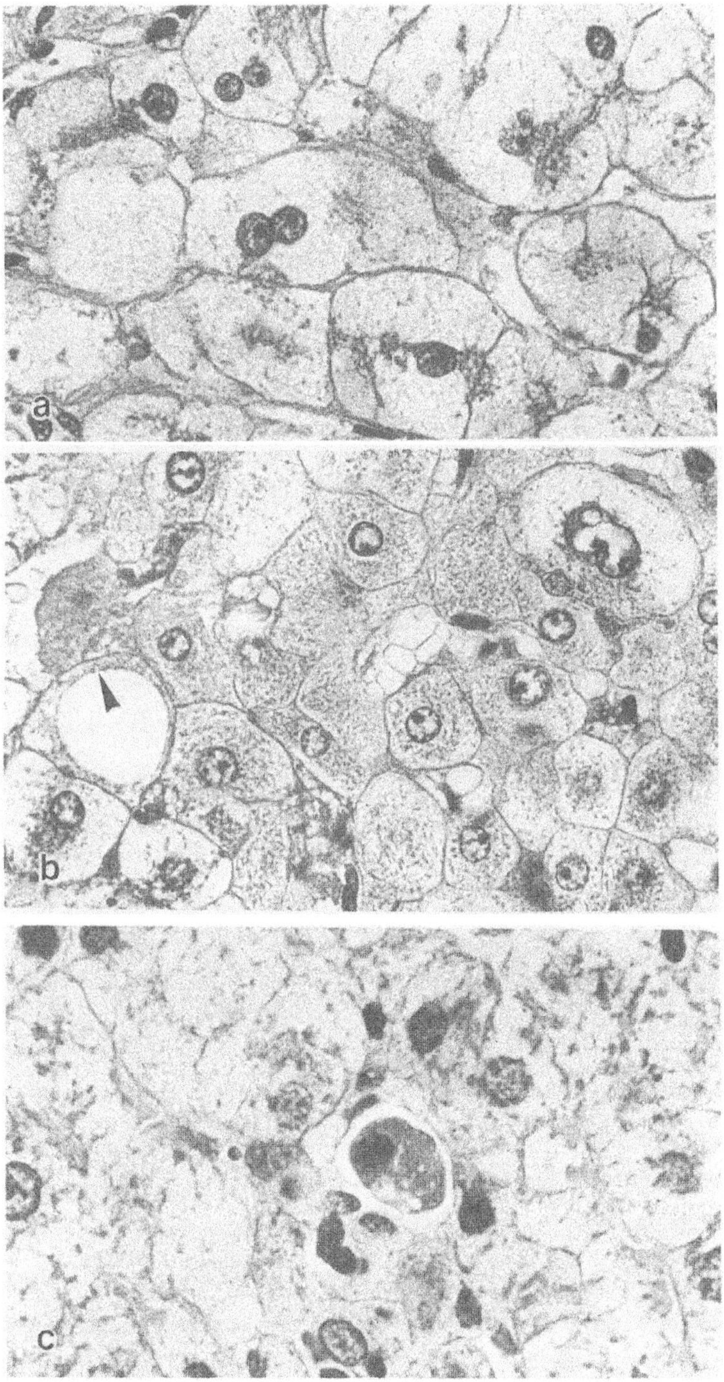

Fig. 9a–c

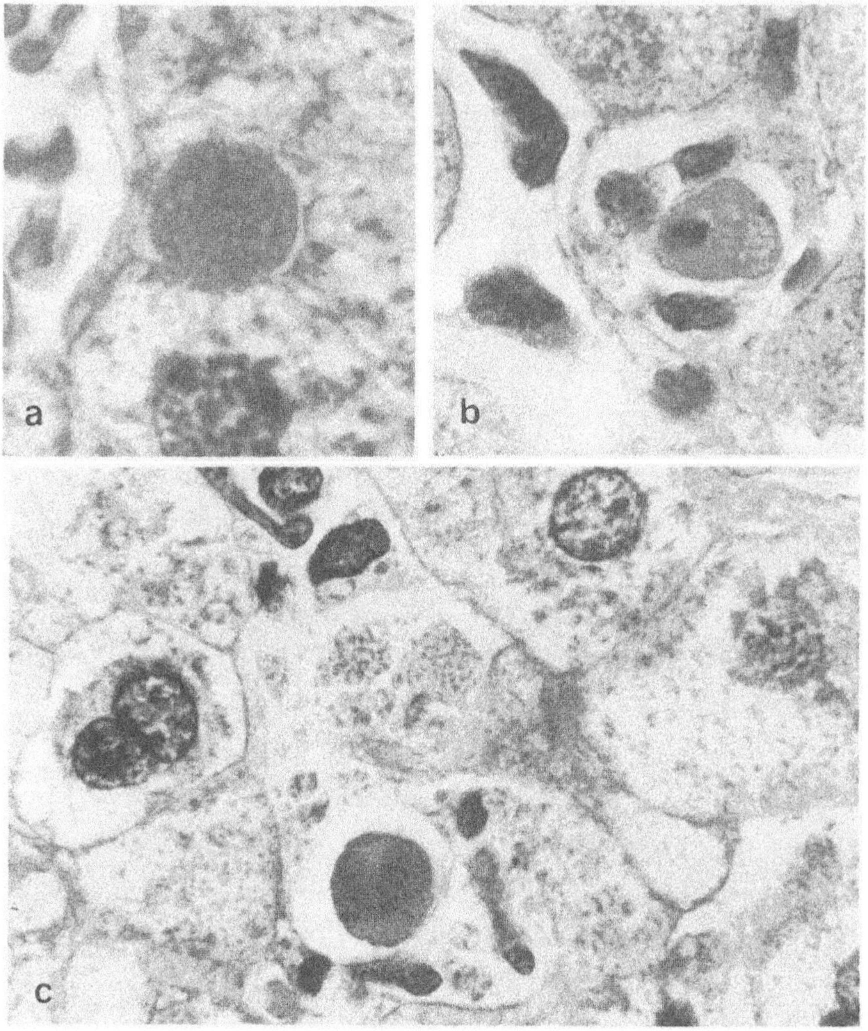

Fig. 10a–c. Single cell necrosis. **a** Rounded and condensed necrotic cell, without any adjacent mononuclear cell; phenytoin. H & E, × 2400. **b** Necrotic cell surrounded by small mononuclear cells; in the adjacent sinusoid, activated Kupffer cells; antiepileptics. H & E, × 1500. **c** A necrotic cell and a resorptive macrophagic nodulus with ceroid pigment; oxyphenisatin, reexposition. H & E, × 1500

Necrotic hepatocytes sometimes but not always immediately surrounded by mononuclear cells (Fig. 10b) are removed by macrophages, often transforming the phagocytized debris into ceroid pigment (Fig. 10c) and also, especially in focal necroses, storing some hemosiderin after simultaneously phagocytozing erythrocytes. If the process of cell necrosis continues, ceroid pigment becomes visible in the portal macrophages. Infiltration of mononuclear leukocytes into the portal fields may or may not be present. In cases with clinical hyperergic reactions, eosinophilic granulocytes are prominent (Figs. 8a, 15, 18). When multiple necroses have developed, a number of regenerative mitoses may be found in the parenchymal tissue (Figs. 6c, 15b, 17a), some of them exhibiting anomalies of the karyokinetic process, such as small or misfunctioning spindles with anaphase disturbances, clumping or aberrations of chromosomes, or suppression of cell division. Under prolonged administration of an adverse drug, the regenerative capacity of the liver will be even more severely impaired and largely suppressed. Instead of the foregoing centrolobular necroses and parenchyma loss (Figs. 5c, 6d), a small *fibrous focus* is now to be seen, which, on the other hand, may arise from converging single cell necroses too. Because the development of single or focal cell necroses sometimes, quite in contrast to the less harmful, bland cholestasis, lacks any conspicuous clinical symptoms, being realized only by a control of the transaminases, even greater areas of hepatocellular loss can appear in a quite imperceptible manner.

In other cases sudden drug-induced cell necroses are accompanied by a clinical picture closely mimicking that of viral hepatitis. It is therefore most important to *differentiate drug-induced liver injuries* from viral hepatitis by means of distinctive morphological criteria. The attempt is rarely made, although it often does not present any great difficulties, especially if a case, quite apart from the associated regressive changes, shows only isolated, poorly reacting cell necroses without remarkable portal infiltration. Those were the findings that *Popper* and his co-workers (358) have called "unspecific drug hepatitis." There are often cases, of course (called "hepatitis-like," if we want to insist on further differentiation from the aforementioned type of reaction), where differentiation is less readily made or even impossible, at least if the changes are induced by facultative liver toxins. However, differentiation is certainly more often practicable than it is thought to be (408), except in cases of acute liver dystrophy with massive necrosis. The common signs of a drug-induced injury or at least a toxic lesion are: preference for centrolobular areas (406, 487, 503), localized and minor reactions of Kupffer cells and macrophages, and, as distinctive negative items, the missing diffuse Kupffer cell reactions and the absence or paucity of portal infiltration. Differential diagnosis may become difficult, however, if, during prolonged drug-induced injuries, inflammatory cells tend eventually to accumulate in the portal triads (Fig. 20), widening the range of alternatives from the rather readily distinguishable acute to the ill-defined chronic active viral hepatitis. In cases of hepatic injuries associated with acute hyperergic reactions, viral hepatitis may be excluded on account of numerous eosinophils in portal fields and sinusoids. Confusion with shock sequelae appears possible when extended centrolobular necroses are present; a differential diagnostic lead can be found in the fact that necrotizing circulatory disturbances, unlike toxic lesions, will always result in an extensive loss of glycogen as a first result.

b) Cholestatic Lesions

In all cases of toxic liver injuries previously mentioned, findings of bile plugs may reflect that bile excretion is also affected (Fig. 6a). In this case, we speak of a *"combined cytotoxic–cholestatic drug injury"* or, if we want to apply the term of hepatitis to all necrotizing liver lesions, of "drug-induced hepatitis with cholestasis." However, cholestasis will always be less conspicuous morphologically than the severe cellular damage in these cases.

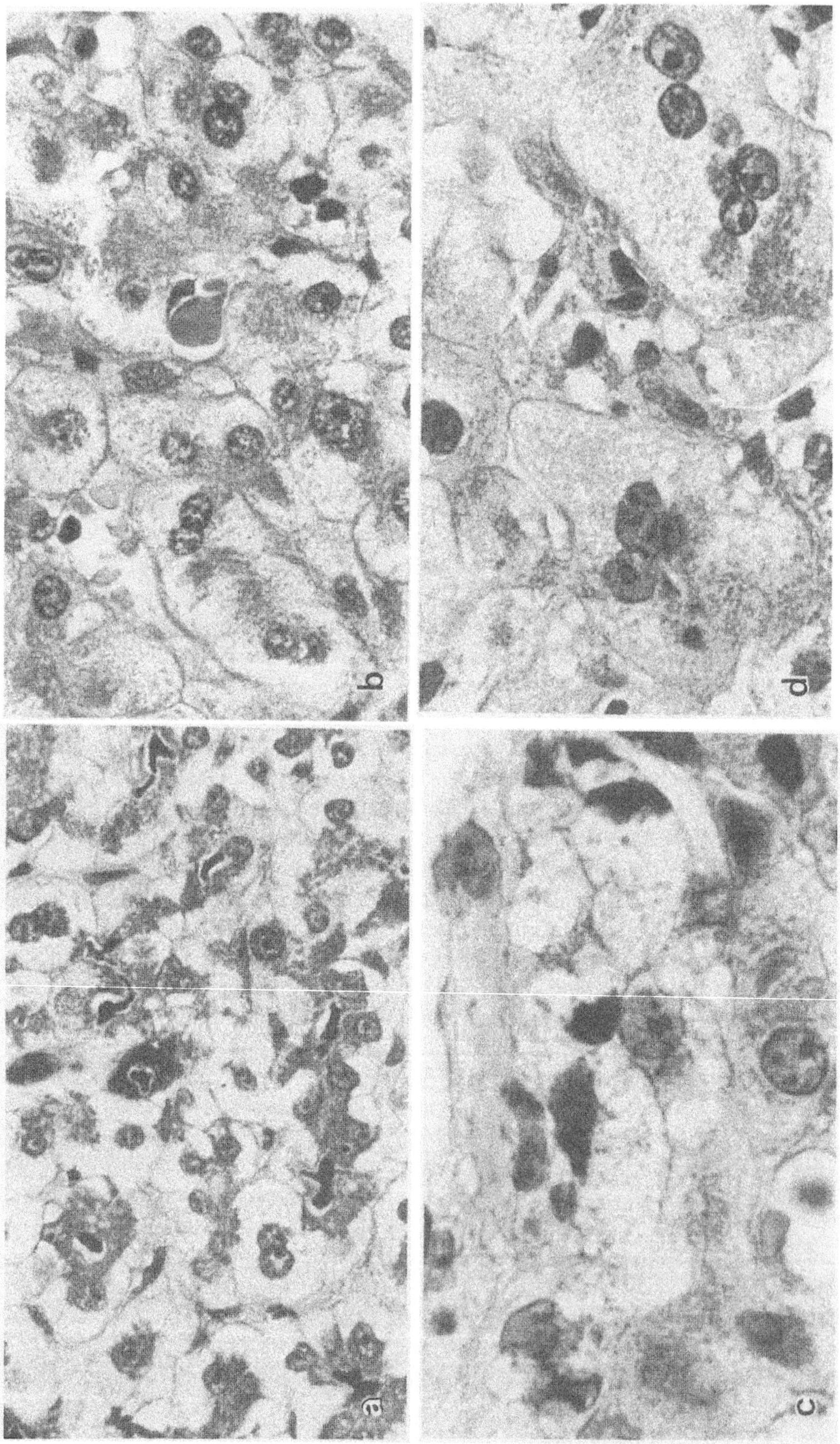

Fig. 11a–d

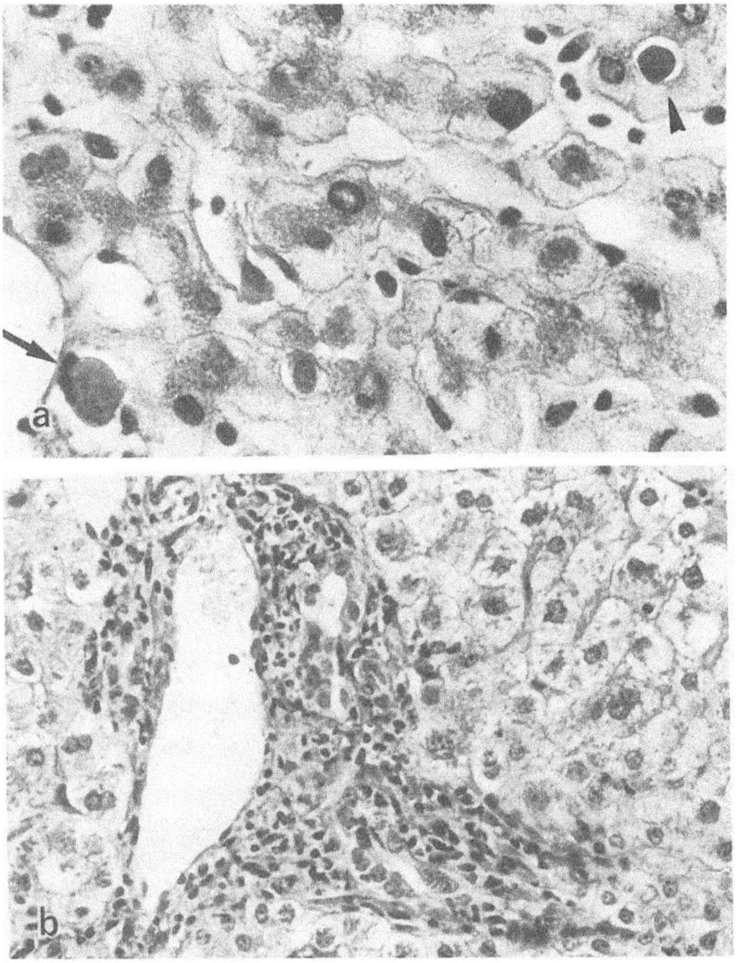

Fig. 12a, b. Drug-induced cholestatic reaction. **a** Bile cast in dilated canaliculi (arrowhead) and single cell necrosis (arrow), slight cellular "hydrops"; imipramine. H & E, × 960. **b** Accompanying portal infiltration with numerous granulocytes; thyrostatic. H & E, × 300

In contrast, cholestasis dominates the picture of *properly cholestatic drug injuries* (Figs. 8b, 11, 12, 16) which, being associated with jaundice, are readily detected and therefore have been known for a long time. Since they only affect one function of the liver, cholestatic lesions are less severe and less consequential. The jaundice in such cases is always the result of intralobular (postmicrosomal) excretory dysfunction with increasing blood levels of bilirubin, bile acids, and alkaline phosphatase, and often with generalized pruritus. The *morphological picture* is dominated by intercellular *bile plugs*

←

Fig. 11a–d. Cholestasis and related lesions after contraceptives. **a** Bile plugs in dilated canaliculi with condensation of the basophilic material around the canaliculi. H & E, × 375. **b** Scattered single cell necrosis. H & E, × 770. **c** Feathery degeneration of centrolobular hepatocytes during prolonged cholestasis. H & E, × 1500. **d** Multinucleated giant cells (result or cell confluence) beside Kupffer cells with bile casts. H & E, × 950

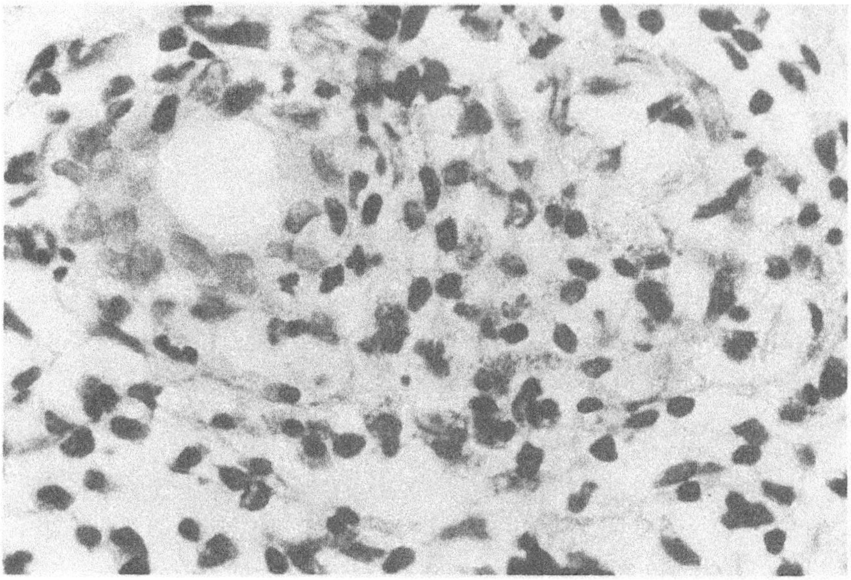

Fig. 13. Eosinophilic infiltration in the edematous portal area, mainly around the ductuli. Methyltestosterone. Congo red, X 1500

(Figs. 8b, 11a, 12a, 15a, 16) within the central part of the lobules, while intracellular bile deposits, in contrast to alcoholic cholestasis, are almost or completely absent. Dilatation of biliary canaliculi is observed even in noncholestatic areas and is therefore a primary and perhaps the initial phenomenon (see 351), associated ultrastructurally with a loss of microvilli (e.g., 195, 351, 358, 360, 399, 402). The basophilic material is collected around the canaliculi, readily visualized by appropriate staining methods (Fig. 11a), and the so-called extoplasma is clearly broadened in some cases. Centrolobular hepatocytes show various alterations: they are often swollen and somewhat hydropic even in those areas where only dilatation of canaliculi and not cholestasis is to be seen (Figs. 11a, b, 12, 16). This "clearing up" is probably due to retention of bile acids. Single cell necroses (Figs. 11b, 12b, 15b) may be rare or abundant. In later phases of prolonged cholestasis, confluent giant cells (Fig. 11c) can be observed as well as, occasionally, small but typical foci of feathery degeneration (Fig. 11c). *Portal infiltration,* if present, sometimes contains abundant eosinophils accumulated near minor bile ducts (Figs. 13, 15), thus presenting the picture of "eosinophilic pericholangitis" or even "eosinophilic cholangitis (190, 250, 342, 503) that was observed recently, e.g., after reexposition to oxyphenisatin laxatives (169, 170, 255, 257) (Fig. 15c).

The existence or the lack of portal infiltrations of this kinds offers one of the essential morphological criteria for *subclassifying* drug-induced cholestasis (see 103, 106, 216, 217, 342, 357, 400, 401, 405, 414, 416, 417, 418, 501, 503): A first group, represented by cholestasis after contraceptives or C-17-alkylated anabolic steroids (Fig. 11), is commonly thought to be characterized only or predominantly by the presence of bile thrombi, while single cell necroses are scarce and portal infiltrations, missing.

In contrast, the second group, comprising all other manifestations or drug-induced cholestasis (chlorpromazine-induced jaundice being its prototype) (Figs 8b, d, 12, 16), is said to be characterized by more abundant cellular necrosis and by evidence of inflammatory portal infiltration which may occur during early phases only and disappear subsequently in spite of persisting jaundice (358, 401, 405, 408). Terminological alternatives are "uncomplicated cholestasis" versus "unspecific drug hepatitis with cholestasis" or "drug-induced cholestatic hepatitis" (342, 358, 408); *"steroid icterus* or nonsensitive icterus" versus *"hypersensitivity icterus"* (106, 414–418); and *"bland or canalicular cholestasis"* versus *"cholangiolitic or hepatocanalicular cholestasis"* (278, 501, 503). Obviously, the proposed terms imply certain clinical observations and pathogenetic concepts. Steroid cholestases are interpreted as an effect of direct alterations to the bile-excreting system, the others as result of hyperergic immunologic reactions.

Whether this strict differentiation is feasible or correct in every case is hard to decide, nor can the line between the two groups – if accepted at all – always be drawn in the proposed fashion. Anyway, we have occasionally seen examplary eosinophilic infiltrations in some cases of steroid-induced cholestases (Fig. 13), after contraceptives as well as after anabolics (11; see 242, 400); equally, we have seen bland cholestases in the initial phases of classic drug-induced jaundice. For these reasons, and also because cellular necroses are never completely absent in steroid-induced jaundice nor in cholestasis during pregnancy, we prefer to interpret both reactions, as far as cholestasis is concerned, as variants of one and the same disturbance, affecting the terminal pathway of hepatocellular excretion. At any rate, the portal infiltrations are phenomena only accompanying, but never causing the jaundice. Perhaps they are provoked by drained metabolites or other products of the altered hepatocellular metabolism.

The jaundice following *contraceptives* (e.g., 3, 84, 104, 107, 242, 281, 313, 318, 321, 324, 339, 417, 452, 501, 503) (Fig. 11) is now thought to be correlated to a direct hepatocellular effect of te estrogens administered. Consequently it is observed both after therapeutic doses of estrogen alone and in patients treated with estrogens for carcinoma of the prostate, while it fails to occur after the minipill, which contains progesterone derivatives only (339, 342). The jaundice appears to be dose dependent, showing increased incidence in proportion to higher estrogen doses (106, 339); it has recently occurred less frequently, in accordance with the lower hormone doses of modern contraceptives. Subclinical excretory disorders were demonstrated with more sophisticated methods, in every hormone-treated patients in two studies (318, 321) as well as in experimental animals. Therefore some authors want to include the so-called pill cholestasis among the predictable biochemical reactions (399, 405), but this is hardly recommendable since only the aggravation of such subclinical deviations is of importance – and this is never predictable unless it is preceded by jaundice of pregnancy or recurrent benign cholestasis (45).

Mutatis mutandis, the above also applies to jaundice induced by *anabolic steroids* as we have known it for 30 years (480). Here, too, reduction of bromsulphalein excretion and of maximum bile excretion was reported in humans (e.g., 110, 326, 395), as well as reduction of bile flux in certain animal species (96, 245).

However, the actual *mechanism of icterogenesis* is still as unknown as the precise point at which steroids affect the liver cells. It has only been ascertained with certainty

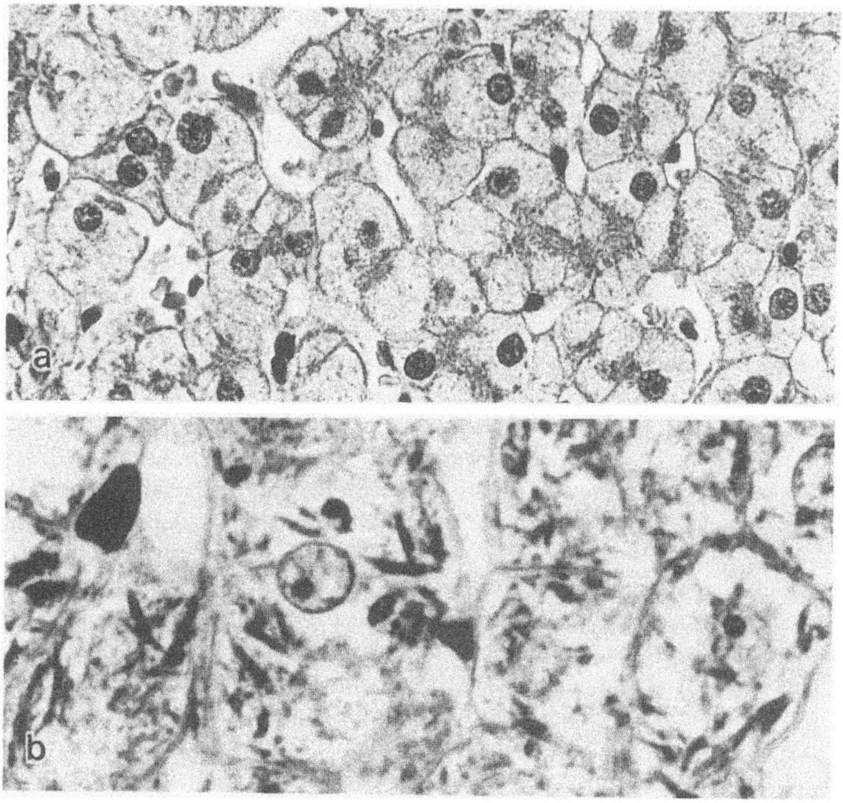

Fig. 14a, b. Harmless contraceptive-induced liver reactions. **a** Hypertrophy of SER (with some enlarged nuclei) after 5 years use. H & E, × 960. **b** Giant mitochondria. Iron hematoxylin, × 1500

that the injury must concern the terminal part of the hepatocellular excretory pathway. Many points were made supporting a leading role of actomyosin-containing pericanalicular *microfilaments* (see Fig. 16b), whose responsibility for intracanalicular bile transport was demonstrated using cytochalasin (350–353). Quite recently *Phillips* and co-workers, in an experimental assay (351) with anabolic steroids, were able to reveal not only canalicular ectasia and reduction of microvilli, but also loss of identifiable microfilaments. Further observations concerned alternations of membrane ATPase (94), but a number of other cellular lesions illustrating a broad spectrum of activities and attacks are also to be found. Contraceptive drugs, for instance, may provoke morphological changes in mitochondria with evidence of elongated *giant mitochondria* with crystalline inclusions (150, 263, 339–342) that are visible microscopically (Fig. 14b). But these changes are also found after the minipill (339, 341), though in small numbers, as well as in many other cases; so a correlation to cholestasis does not seem to exist.

More weight must be attributed to the almost ubiquitous evidence of some single cell necroses appearing from the very start of cholestasis and not only in its later phases. They are reflected in the elevated transaminase levels that are found in all cases (235, 249, 318, 321). Hypertrophy of the agranular endoplasmic reticulum, so often to be found during prolonged and otherwise undisturbed administration (Fig. 14a) is only rarely visualized microscopically probably, because it is still rather feeble when jaundice sets in during the first cycles of contraceptive medication. However, that some hypertrophy must be developing in submicroscopic dimensions may be inferred from the fact that the pill-induced jaundice is apt to regress in some cases despite continued medication. For the sake of completeness, some findings of elevated transaminase levels without any evidence of cholestatic syndromes should be mentioned [allegedly in 6%–18% of cases (242)]; this may again be interpreted in terms of diffuse cellular impairment which, in such cases, is morphologically expressed in the evidence of scattered cell necroses (104, 297).

Nonsteroid drugs capable of provoking jaundice or cholestatic hepatosis (see 483) are numerous and belong to very different types of chemical compounds and therapy schedules (see 42, 103, 216, 217, 342, 357, 417, 503): antirheumatics (phenylbutazone), chemotherapeutics (sulfonamides), cytostatics (6-mercaptopurine), thyrostatics (methylthiouracil, thiamazol) (Fig. 12b), uricosurics (cinchophen, prophylthiouracil), antiarrhythmics (ajmaline, parajmalintartrate) (Fig. 8b), which have gained increasing interest in recent years (30, 100, 171, 256, 336, 376), laxatives (oxyphenisatin) (e.g., 169, 257, 379, 380, 461) (Fig. 15), antimetabolites (azathioprine) (160), and last but not least, psychotropic drugs (Figs. 12a, 16), the most prominent among them being chlorpromazine (Fig. 16).

The pathogenetic pathways and *mechanisms* of these drugs are even less well explained than those of the steroids. "Hyperergic" clinical and morphological phenomena are not infrequent, but are sometimes very discrete and by no means obligatory. Therefore theories about the hyperergic origin of these injuries are not very convincing, at least not in every case and without further ado. At all events there seems to be no explanation without considering genetic factors, certain chemometabolic target effects of the causative drugs, and some basic impairment of hepatocytes (498, 499, 503).

Substantial proof for the above is at hand, even for prototypic chlorpromazine. The genetic factor is exemplified by a family in which members of three generations manifested an unusual susceptibility to that drug (415). Basic impairment is illustrated by the rather large number of patients (40%–50%) showing mild functional disorders, as in the case of these using contraceptive drugs, in contrast to the low percentage (1%–2%) of actually diseased patients (190, 357, 415, 503), even if the mild disorders tend to regress (via ferment induction) under persisting medication. The concept is confirmed by certain experimental findings of secretory inhibition (318) and of subclinical morphological cholestasis (399). Extensive but rather subtle cellular changes were also found in isolated perfused livers (180, 211, 212); and leakages of intracellular enzymes were demonstrated in liver cell cultures and interpreted as a symptom of a genuine cytotoxic effects (109, 504). Moreover, glutathione was shown to exert a neutralizing effect against chlorpromazine as well as against the doubtlessly cytotoxic paracetamol (394). On this basis, and at least for these effect on experimental animals, some authors tend to speak of "predictable impairments of bile flow" for which direct toxic injuries to membrane ATPase could be held responsible (394) – a

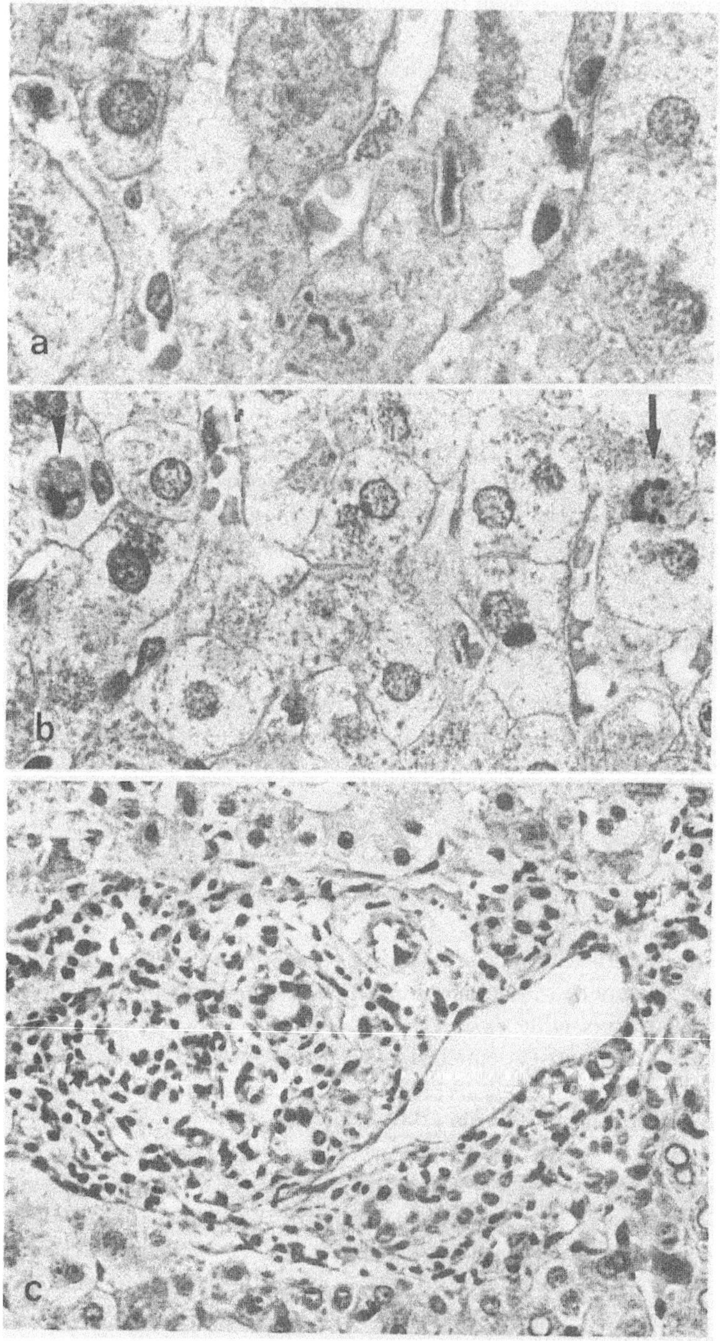

Fig. 15a–c. Cholestatic liver lesions by oxyphenisatin-containing laxatives. **a** Bile plugs in dilated canaliculi. H & E, × 960. **b** Accompanying single cell necrosis (arrowhead) and disturbed mitosis (arrow). H & E, × 770. **c** Portal infiltration, mainly with granulocytes; reexposition. H & E, × 600

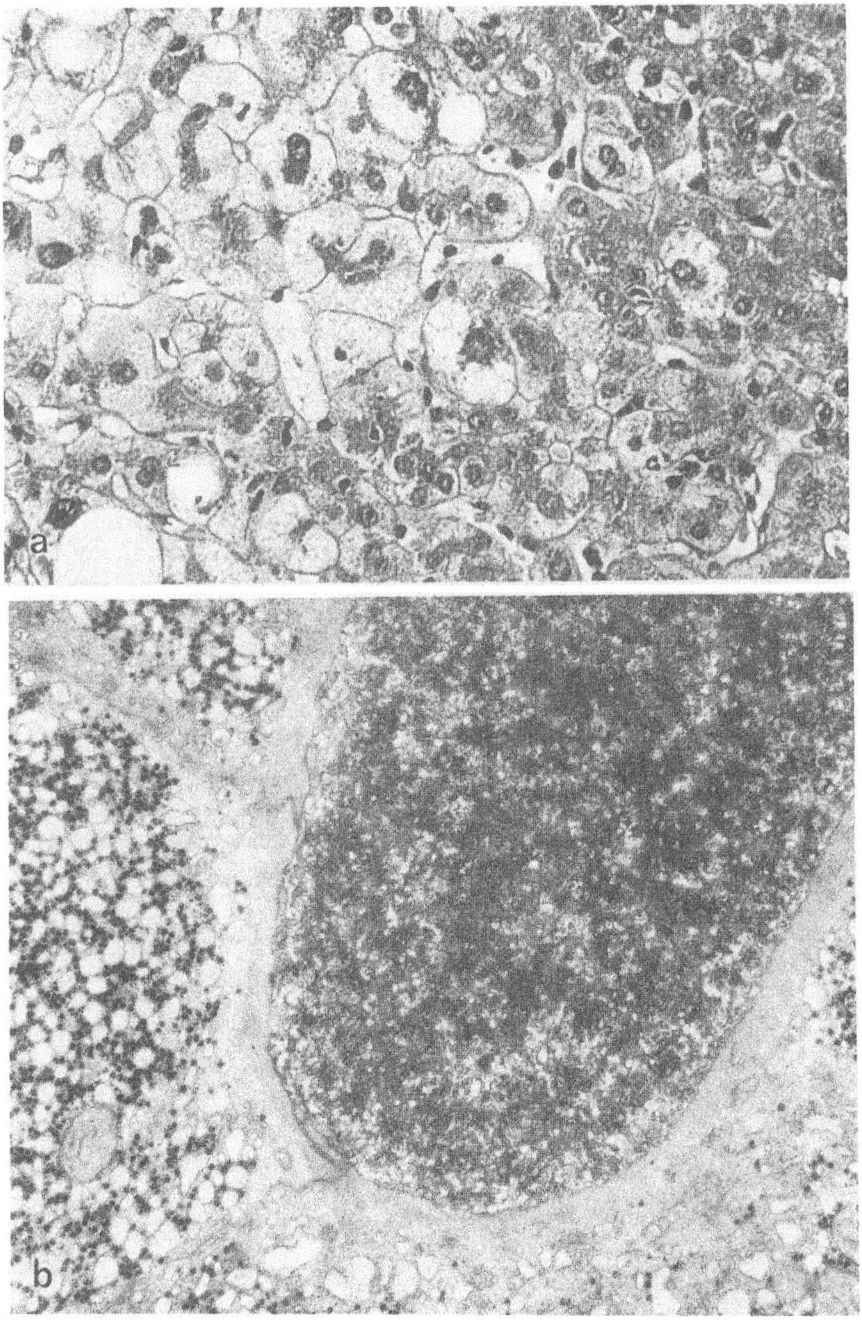

Fig. 16a, b. Chlorpromazine-induced cholestasis. **a** With hydropic changes in the mainly affected centrolobular area. H & E, X 325. **b** Bile plug in dilated canaliculus, devoid of microvilli; prominent fibrillar pericanalicular ectoplasm, dilated hyperplastic cisternäe of SER, many glycogen rosettes. X 13 800 remarkable concept insofar as the same point of attack is being discussed for contraceptive drugs (94). Perhaps the two forms of cholestasis are, actually, not so far apart as current opinion would have it. It is of special interest that a patient who developed jaundice after chlorpromazine as well as after methylestosterone (16) is known.

Diagnostic problems in drug-induced jaundice relate not so much to the exact separation from cholestatic forms of hepatitis, but rather to differentiation from obstructive jaundice. The following may be considered as indicative of intralobular cholestasis: extensive cellular changes of a hydropic nature, weak staining of bile thrombi, their presence in only the centrolobular areas – without spreading to the periphery as observed in nearly every case of extrahepatic obstruction –, and the absence of portal edema or ductal epithelial swelling. The absence of dilatation of ductal lumina is a less reliable sign. Portal infiltrations, if present, are interpreted as suggesting a cholestatic drug reaction if they show a loose arrangement of cells, no neutrophilic covering of ductules, but higher content of eosinophils (Figs. 8d, 12b, 13, 15c), the latter being qualified insofar as evidence of eosinophilic granulocytes may also be found in cholestasis and cholangitis of extrahepatic origin.

As a rule, drug-induced jaundice will *regress* clinically soon after therapy is stopped; morphologically, bile thrombi may persist for quite some time, like in other cholestases, appearing even in Kupffer cells in phagocytized form. In some cases, however, jaundice may *persist* obstinately over several weeks, as *Hanger* and *Gutman* (164) pointed out in their first description of a drug-induced cholestasis (after Salvarsan in 1940). According to our own observations, this can happen even after contraceptives (144, 281, 321, 339), but mainly after chlorpromazine and its derivatives, for which persistence of jaundice over several months was described (167, 190, 232, 305, 439) with subsequent complication by hypercholesterinemia and pseudoxanthoma (30, 181, 190, 216, 217, 250, 305, 359, 367, 415, 427, 474). The reason for this unusual behavior is still unknown; a plausible explanation can be seen in an irreversible blockade of long-living macromolecules, eventually lifted by the definitive breakdown of the latter.

In such cases the summation of single cell necroses must lead to increased production of fibers in the central as well as in the peripheral parts of the lobules; in the latter, such a *fibrosis* may be associated with scanty cellular infiltration, even with occasional temporary ductular proliferation (190). Stronger periportal fibrosis is a common feature, but the full picture of cirrhosis has so far never been reported. Apparently such a cirrhotic pattern could never resemble that of *"primary biliary cirrhosis,"* as supposed in previous publications, the latter being a late manifestation of destructive nonsuppurative cholangitis and therefore of extralobular origin, quite in contrast to the hypothetical drug-induced type. In addition, no clues are found for typical secondary destructive changes with subsequent destruction of bile ducts that may occur in

Fig. 17a–c. Hyperergic granulomatous liver reaction, induced by penicillin. **a** Scattered single-cell necrosis (arrow) and reparative mitotic figures. H & E, X 600. **b** Intralobular granuloma with epithelioid cells, eosinophils, and a central fibrin deposit. H & E, X 770. **c** Intralobular granuloma, surrounded by fibrin threads, containing a small multinucleated cell (the clear area in its center being the sphere with the centrioles). H & E, X 960

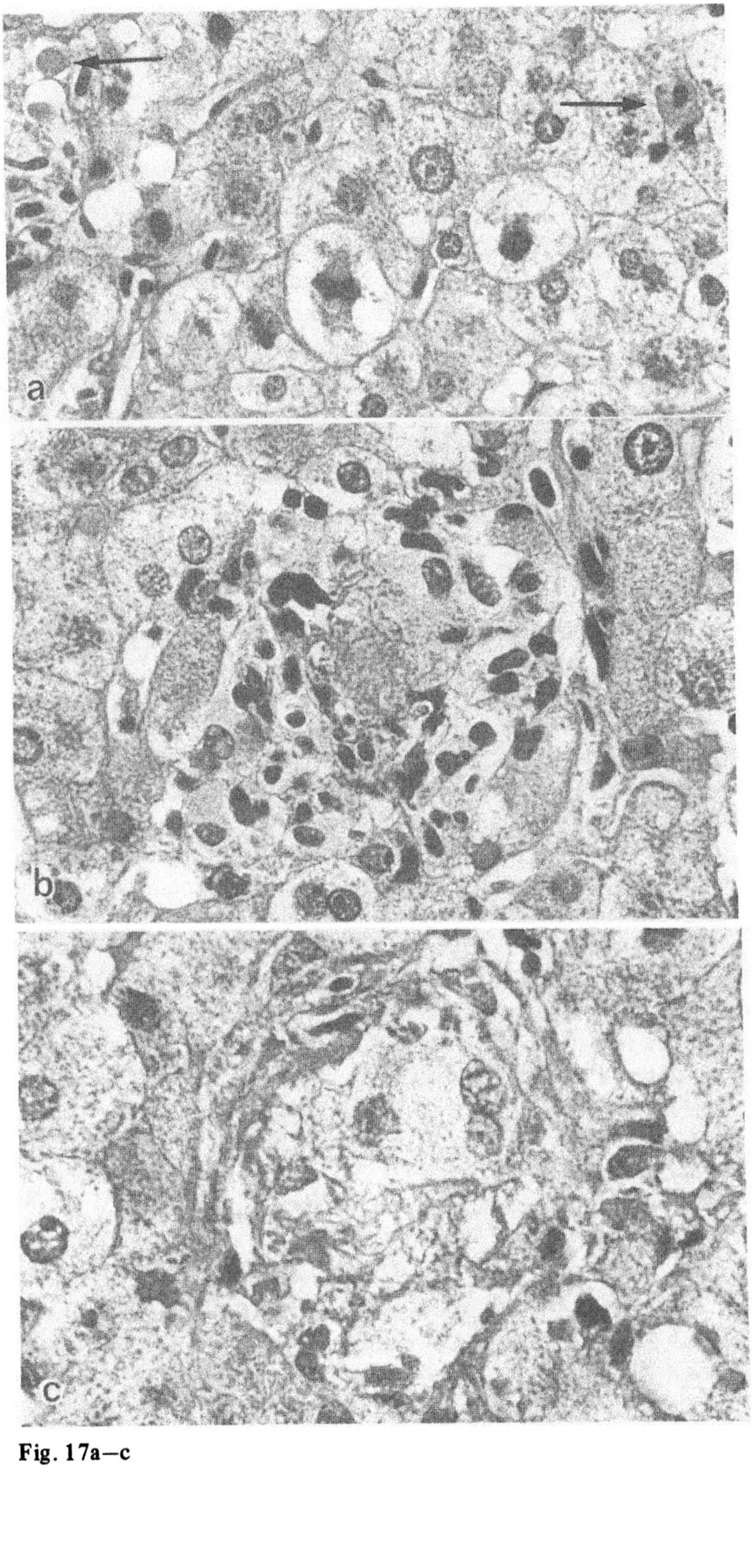

Fig. 17a–c

the course of primary intralobular cholestasis (190, 250), nor do we have any proof for a potentially drug-related causation of destructive cholangitis.

c) Granulomatous Reactions

That immunologic processes may be involved in the hepatic reaction to drugs is documented by abundant evidence of *eosinophilic leukocytes* in the portal triads in certain cases of cytotoxic as well as in cholestatic liver injuries. Occasional occurrence of *granulomas* (Lit. see 93, 274, 287) (Figs. 17–19), restricted to only a few predisposed persons, which disappear when therapy is stopped, may be interpreted in the same sense. Granulomas were first described after sulfonamides (298; 40, 60, 125, 384); they have since been reported, mainly as unusual and isolated cases, in the course of very different medications: mostly after phenylbutazone (111, 147, 191), but also after allopurinol (124, 277, 424, 442), diazepam (217), hydralazine (204), hydantoin (165), methotrexate (33), methyldopa (285), penicillin (478) (Fig. 17), quinidine (63), and halothane (105, 217, 228) (Fig. 6f).

Unfortunately, the morphological data of these reports often fail to give sufficient detail for an adequate visualization of the nature and localization of the granulomas and their associated phenomena. Apparently, the general term of "granuloma ' covers two different or, at least, distinguishable lesions with, in fact, more or less fluid transitions. The first is the noncaseous epitheloid cell granulomes with multinucleated giant cells situated mainly, if not exclusively, within the portal fields (277). They are often classified as *sarcoid-like lesions,* to be distinguished from Boeck granulomes by the absence of sclerosis and by the almost regular admixture of eosinophilic leukocytes. Single cell necroses in parenchymal areas are very scarce, if occurring at all. In many cases granulomas are developing simultaneously in different organs (40, 125, 147, 204, 298, 384, 478), thus manifesting generalized allergic reaction without hepatospecificity. Consequently, these granulomes should be interpreted as phenomena of an immunologic process, rather than as a cause of appreciable liver injury.

The second type, which could be called *"minifocal epithelioid cell reaction,"* is characterized by smaller granulomas developing preferably in the lobules, but also in the portal triads (Figs. 17–19). In the lobules, they often arise from necrotic liver cells (but also without such a focus) and then induce subsequent alteration or necrosis of adjacent hepatocytes initiated by a condensation of nuclei and cytoplasm (Fig. 18b, c). There may also be some evidence of fibrin or of an adjacent eosinophil (Fig. 17b). When situated in the portal fields, granulomas may spread into the adjacent parenchymal tissue, destroying the neighboring liver cells (Figs. 18b, 19a). Lying within the lobuli they may (Fig. 19b) show a certain resemblance to lipophagic granulomas that occur around necrotic fatty liver cells, e.g., in chronic alcoholism; they are, however,

Fig. 18a–c. Granulomatous liver lesion after second halothane narcosis. **a** Periportal epithelioid granulomata, invading the lobulus and replacing necrotic liver cells; abundant eosinophils. Congo red, X 375. **b** Margin of a portal granuloma with a necrotic hepatocyte at the front of it. H & E, X 600. **c** Intralobular granuloma, with a lot of eosinophils, surrounding a necrotic hepatocyte. H & E, X 600

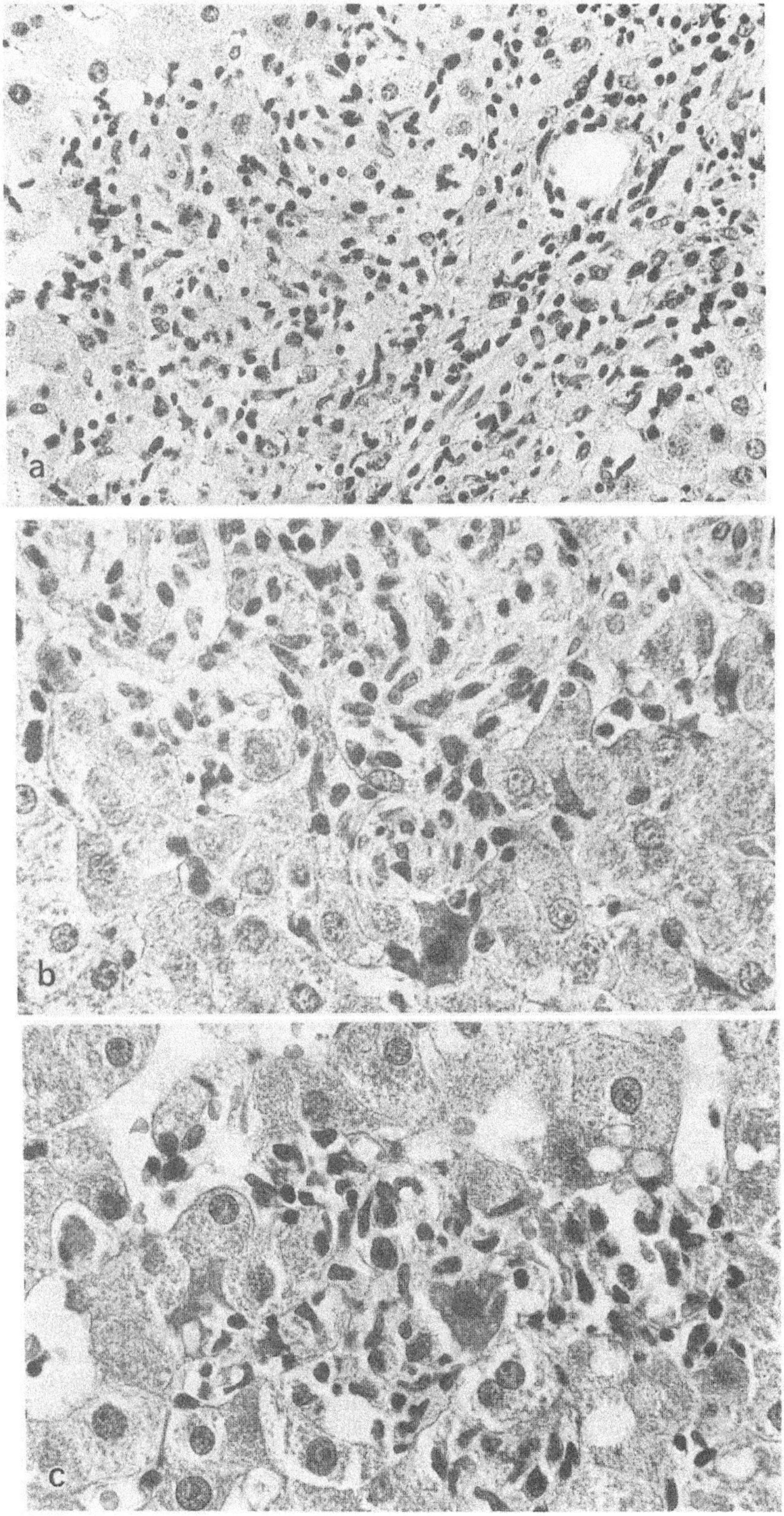

Fig. 18a–c

readily distinguished from the latter by the almost regular admixture of eosinophilic leukocytes (see 274). As a rule, they do not contain ceroid pigment – in sharp contrast to swollen Kupffer cells that are occasionally found –, nor do they show any noticeable signs of phagocytosis (465). Multinucleate cells may be found (Fig. 17c), but there are no giant cells of the Langhans type. Associated epithelial changes with or without discrete cholestasis can hardly be overlooked (Figs. 17a, 18b, c). Mitoses may be occasionally found in abundance (Fig. 17a), and are often characterized by the well-known signs of a disturbed karyokinetic process. The portal triads contain many eosinophils (Fig. 18a) and may present the picture of *eosinophilic cholangitis* (442).

As a rule other sites of the body fail to show corresponding changes (but see 442), so these granulomas seem to be hepatospecific, indicating that the liver must be the target of allergic reactions to the drugs in question. Causative factors can be sought in the metabolites produced in the course of hepatocellular biotransformation. Clinical manifestations are hyperergic phenomena as well as symptoms of liver injury. It is remarkable that they may occur soon or immediately after the second or third dose of the drug, e.g., after halothane (Fig. 18) or penicillin therapy (Fig. 17), while in other cases clinical symptoms will appear rather late after prolonged medication without any earlier complications, e.g., with allopurinol (277, 442). This delay may be due to a metabolite which needs some time or some special condition to appear in a sufficient amount.

IV. Chronic Liver Injury

Chronic drug administration can induce pathologic liver changes – this is an established fact exemplified by the above-cited cases of agranuloreticular hypertrophy, particularly if a certain regressive influence is illustrated by extreme lipofuscine deposits, single cell necrosis, or cellular polymorphism with an increase of meganuclei. Some of the just-mentioned spectacular cases of prolonged cholestasis might also be cited in this context; however, the persistance of changes after and despite the discontinuation of medication suggests that they must be separated from the reactions that are obviously bound to long-term administration of a drug. In recent years, and in particular since *Reynolds* published his results about liver lesions induced by oxyphenisatin laxatives (380–382; 81, 97, 142, 148, 169, 170, 255, 257, 379) (Fig. 20a, see Fig. 15), examples of this type of drug-induced hepatopathy have been reported in considerable numbers (see 42, 103, 262, 503). They concern, among others, methyldopa (148, 178, 385, 411, 484), chlorpromazine (392), halothane (449), ajmaline (171) (Fig. 20b), and even isoniazid (39) and aspirin (412). These reports are now usually collected under the common heading of *"chronic active hepatitis"* capable of progressing to cir-

→

Fig. 19a–c. Hyperergic granulomatous reaction; many different drugs, especially analgesics and psychopharmacological agents. **a** Portal epithelioid granulomata, invading the lobulus. H & E, × 375. **b** Intralobular epithelioid granuloma with circumscribed destruction of the sinusoid wall. Ladewig, × 960. **c** Intralobular granuloma, with destruction of the reticulin fibers. Gömöri, × 770

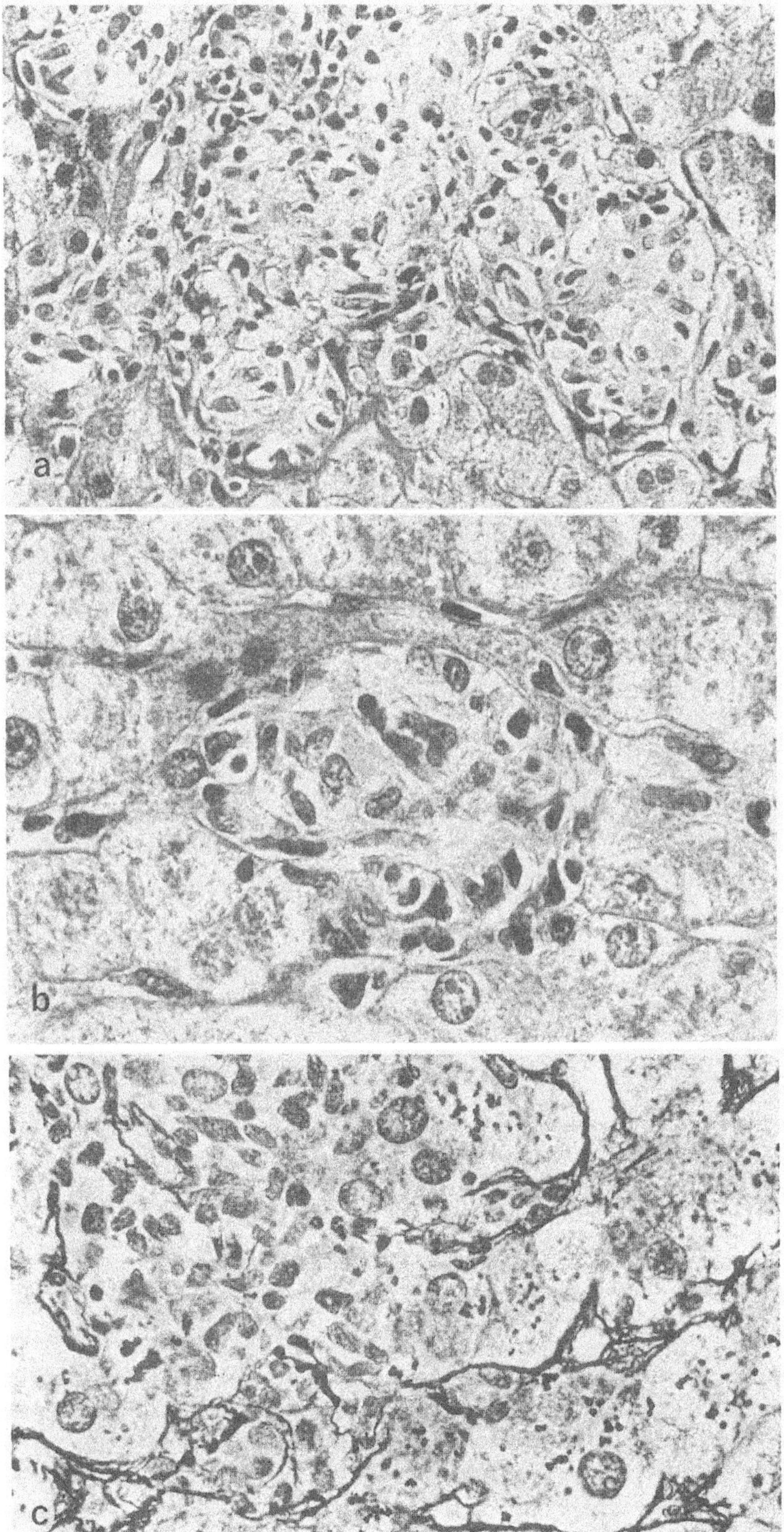

Fig. 19a–c

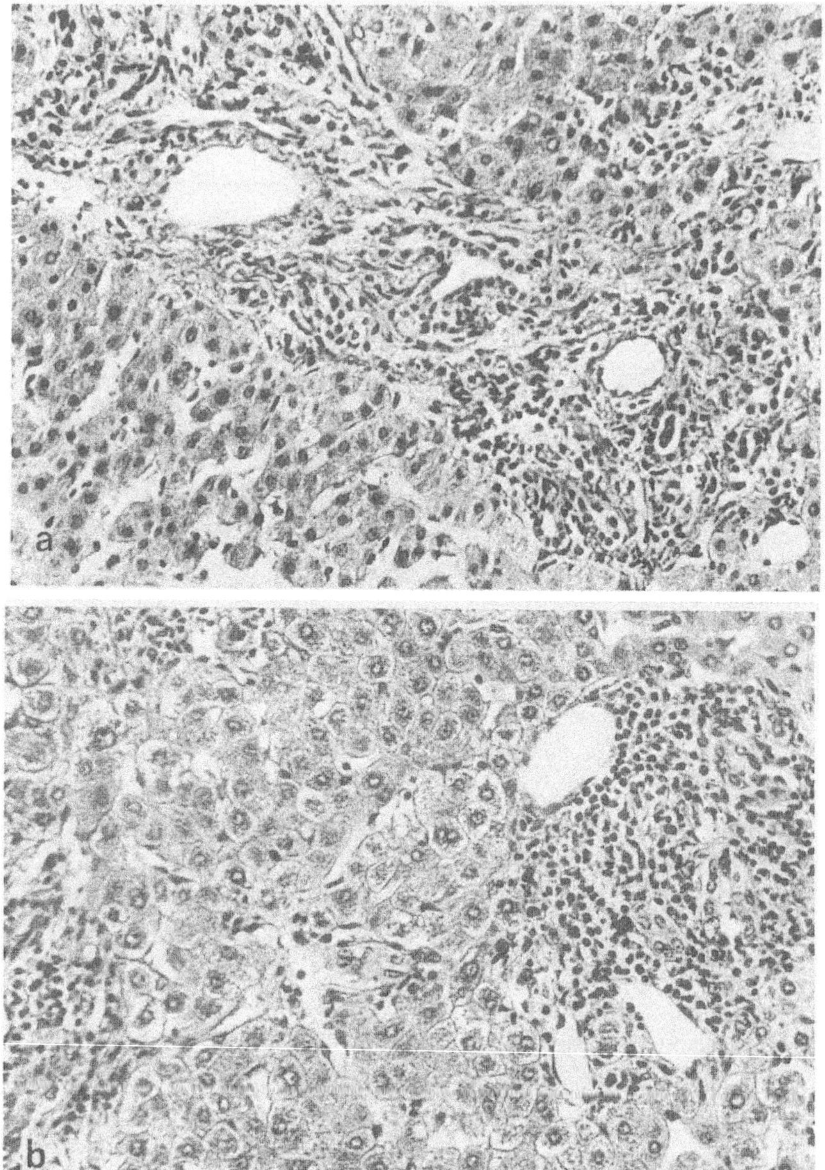

Fig. 20a, b. Drug-induced portal fibrosis and cellular infiltration; "drug-induced chronic hepatitis." **a** Oxyphenisatin; van Gieson, × 240. **b** Prajmalium bitartrate; H & E, × 240

rhosis. Several authors want to attribute considerable importance to this "drug-induced form of chronic hepatitis," which is said to resemble above all the so-called lupoid type of this disease (501). *Henning* (169, 170), for instance, thought that phenolisatin abuse (oxyphenisatin) was the causative factor of chronic hepatitis, liver cirrhosis, or liver scarring in at least 10% of all patients (in 20% of female patients) examined in several large sanatoria, a percentage that appears exaggereted when compared to the material at our disposal. Data suggesting that one-third of all liver cirrhoses of apparently nonviral origin must be traced back to chronic drug influence (81, 97, 142, 148) should also be regarded with scepticism.

The liver injuries so classified fail to show any uniformity with regard to their pathogenesis, morphogenesis, and morphological appearance; they are rather inadequately brought together under the overstretched term of "chronic hepatitis," often taken as synonymous to chronic liver injury in general, thus referring to an assumed, but actually nonexistent entity. Certainly the presence of a few free cells in a portal field should not be interpreted as a sufficient criterion for a diagnosis of "chronic hepatitis" – they are equally found in prolonged purely cytotoxic lesions such as poisoning by mushrooms or carbon tetrachloride, where they must be interpreted as resorptive or reactive side effects.

Even if we disregard the more or less stationary cases of *postdystrophic liver cirrhosis,* representing the consequence of one single but severe liver damage (e.g., Fig. 5c), we apparently have to distinguish at least two types of chronic liver injury, the *first type* resulting from *cumulation* of minor cytotoxic changes, most of them *direct cytotoxic,* that are familiar from the acute liver injuries and potentially complicated by one or several consecutive episodes of extensive necrosis. In this context neither clinical nor morphological significance is attributed to immunologic hypersensitivity reactions.

We see an appropriate example in chronic liver injuries induced by tuberculostatic drugs, which are characterized by peripheral spread of an initially lobulocentral "drop out" of necrotic liver cells (see Fig. 5c). First to be destroyed are the cells of the innermost layer; adjacent epithelia follow, while regeneration is suppressed, the vacated epithelial spaces being collapsed and later occupied by newly formed collagenous fibers. Except for genuine alcohol-specific changes, the picture closely resembles that of alcoholic centrolobular sclerosis, and in the same fashion, parenchyma loss and fibrosis may proceed toward the periphery along the borders of Rappaport's acinus, eventually resulting in cirrhotic transformation. If the process alternates with phases of more extensive cell destruction, the result may be formation of bridging necrosis (261, 432), and even of postnecrotic cirrhosis as described after isoniazid (39) or methyldopa (148, 261, 262, 411). The "chronic hepatitis" found after prolonged administration of aspirin in high doses (412) is also classified in this category, owing to its direct cytotoxic effects devoid of associated hypersensitivity reactions. The same argument relating to chronic liver injuries after paracetamol (44) was substantiated by successful experimental induction of cirrhosis by this drug (47). Both these examples illustrate that portal cell infiltrations may occur even in purely cytotoxic lesions, where they represent a reactive or resorptive response without the involvement of any immunologic process whatsoever. In our opinion, chronic liver injuries after methotrexate, a directly cytotoxic drug (24), must also be classified here; the – dose-related (312) – reaction is observed in lymphoma as well as in psoriasis patients; it eventually results in cirrhotic transformation via peripheral fibrosis (11, 74, 75, 82, 86, 122, 182, 273, 300, 308, 312, 328, 392, 405, 445, 454, 477). The peripheral localization of the substitutive fibrosis, particularly conspicuous in hepatic infiltrations during lymphoma, is explained by the immediate attack on those liver cells that are first reached and affected by the drug, possibly supported by an additional effect of degradation products from decompasing lymphoma cells (11). The fact that folic acid antagonists tend to inhibit proliferation and, logically, regeneration of liver epithelia, is certainly favorable to the development of portal substitutive fibrosis.

The *second* group comprises a number of agents that are initially tolerated without difficulty by most patients, but which may induce the clinical picture of chronic liver injury in a limited number of patients *rather slowly* and after a longer period of a symptomless "incubation." Their etiologic significance is revealed by the fact that discontinuing administration will renormalize clinical, biochemical, and morphological parameters, whereas *reexposition,* even after prolonged delay, will reevoke the picture of acute hepatic disease with *allergic–hyperergic manifestations.* Laxatives containing phenolisatins are the best-documented models of this type (42, 75, 85a, 97, 142, 148, 169, 170, 209, 255, 257, 272, 280, 338, 378–380, 460, 486), with many reports about voluntary or involuntary reexposition.

The significant feature common to all these cases is a comparatively minor, but chronic impairment initiating slow, gradual transformation of the architecture of the liver. The process may be manifested in various ways and shapes, among which epithelial lesions associated with necrosis and minor cholestasis usually predominate (85a, 280, 338, 381, 382), while portal infiltration, preferably of lymphocytes (85a), is said to be prominent in some cases (Fig. 20), while in others it is only slight (209, 272, 338). The difference could result from variations in the patient's individual susceptibility or from varying dosage, the latter possibility being supported by the fact that rather high single doses may provoke severe, extensive, occasionally fatal liver necrosis (148), and that reexposition will commonly provoke reactions stronger than those observed in simple chronic liver disease (255): there are not only abundant single cell necroses and marked cholestasis, but also an unusual accumulation of eosinophils in close relationship to the small ducts (acute eosinophilic cholangiohepatitis) (255, 257) (Fig. 15). Since oxyphenisatin is excreted with bile (129), we might think of a reaction to the intraductular presence of the drug, the more so as a delay in bile flow can be taken for granted under these circumstances.

The ensemble of changes and phenomena is best explained by a concept of drugs mediating and gradually inducing a certain mechanism affecting and injuring the liver cells which is liable to be subsequently enhanced and modified by immunologic and hyperergic reactions (501, 503). The fact that among persons with abuse of laxatives not more than a small number, apparently women only, are affected, is nothing unusual in the field of drug reactions. Salient features, however, are the *long latency* (suggesting that a thorough change in biotransformation is necessary to produce the incriminated metabolite) and the effectiveness of reexposition after a delay of unusual length (suggesting that the changes inflicted on biotransformation have become irreversible). Evidence for an involvement of autoimmune processes is neither clinically nor morphologically demonstrable.

Seen as a whole, the *morphological picture* of this category differs markedly from that of common chronic viral hepatitis, not only in cases exacerbated by reexposition, but also in the common chronic course. For there are so many morphologic peculiarities that suspicion of chronic drugs injury appears justified. Characteristic features are the predominance and variability of epithelial changes, the frequency of bile plugs, the low activity of Kupffer cells, lower number of portal infiltrations, and scarcity of peripheral destructive processes (piecemeal necroses) (Fig. 20). From the paradigmatic example of laxative-induced injuries we may conclude that other agents administered over a long time are liable to provoke similar changes, although it is not yet possible to nominate any candidate with certainty, with the possible exception of methyldopa (148, 178, 385, 411, 455, 484).

The above-discussed lesions have been known for quite some time; recent reports have focused on chronic liver lesions of a very different nature, but again suggestive of direct drug cytotoxicity. Japanese authors described *drug-induced phospholipidosis* in liver cells (177, 185, 193, 421, 422, 494) after long-term administration of a coronary dilatant (2,4-diethylaminoetoxyhexestrol = coralgil) as a result and expression of a generalized impairment of phospholipid metabolism that is reproducible in animal experiments (2, 494). The alteration is manifested by typical intralysosomal *myelin bodies* of concentric structure, observed microscopically as paracanalicular "dense bodies." Affected liver cells show hydropic swelling; prolonged administration results in an increasing number of cell necroses as well as in portal fibrosis, ductal proliferation, and cellular infiltration, although authors have not used the term hepatitis in these cases (as might have been expected). The myelin bodies seem to consist of unphysiologic phospholipids arising from drug-induced disorders of synthesis. Normal lysosomal ferments are nearly or completely unable to break down these bodies (185, 258), so that they persist and can be demonstrated for quite a long time after medication is discontinued (2, 177).

Similar lamellar bodies were observed recently after *perhexiline maleate therapy* of several months' duration (26, 27, 234, 237, 254, 269, 335, 345). This direct hepatotoxic drug used in angina pectoris therapy is of particular interest insofar as it initially leads only to fat infiltration and scattered single cell necrosis (234), but in the course of time in some patients gives rise to genuine *Mallory bodies* and to cell necroses surrounded by leukocytes (26, 27, 269, 335, 345), thus mimicking a alcoholic hepatitis, and eventually leads to cirrhosis.

V. Hepatovascular Lesions

Under the influence of certain drugs, primary morphological changes may occur in the vascular bed of the liver. We know of lesions affecting the afferent vessels, of others occurring preferably in the sinusoids themselves, and also of lesions affecting the efferent venous system.

Drug-induced disorders of the *afferent vessels* are found in the *portal veins* only, due to stenosing intimal proliferation in the big and median portal branches preceded by direct endothelial damage with subsequent edema. Vascular changes of this kind formerly classified under M. Banti, are now commonly defined as *hepatoportal sclerosis* (284). The lesion always results from direct toxicity and may be provoked, for instance, by prolonged application of arsenic in Fowler's solution as used in psoriasis therapy (230, 299, 472). Smaller intrahepatic branches of the portal artery are, however, equally liable to be occluded by similar intimal proliferations, e.g., under metho-

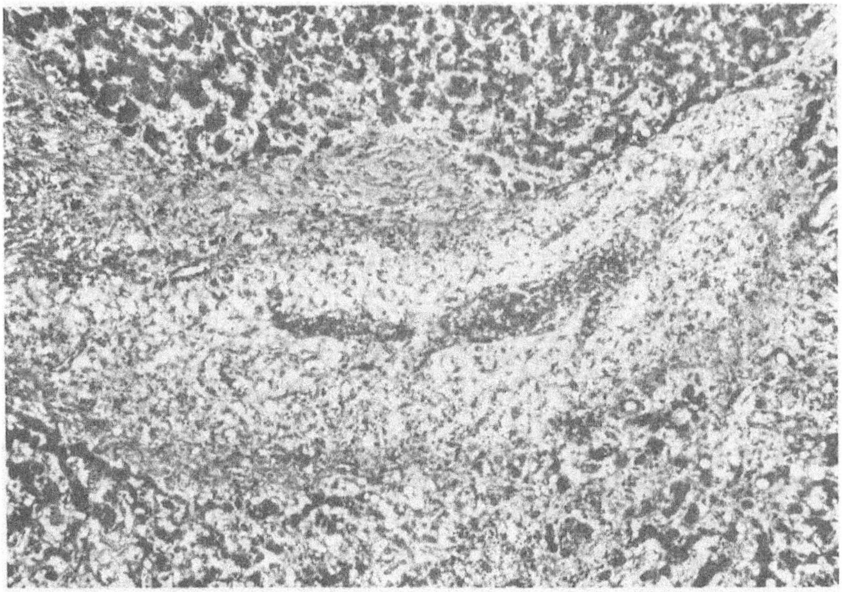

Fig. 21. "Endophlebitis" of a branch of the portal vein; methotrexate-treated lymphosarcoma. Masson, X 60

trexate therapy for lymphosarcomatous cell infiltrations (11) (Fig. 21). It is an open question as yet whether the intimal damage in these cases is chiefly caused by the cytostatic drug or by the by-products of decomposition from the attacked lymphomatous infiltrations.

The potential occurrence of drug-induced changes in *intralobular vascular pathways* was first assessed by *Gordon* and co-workers (152) who, after norethrandolone medication, found not only cholestasis, but also evidence of peliosis hepatis characterized by intralobular blood spaces of varying width. Since then, observations of *peliosis* and of its pre-stages (Fig. 22), not necessarily progressing, were reported in such numbers in connection not only with C-17-alkylated anabolic steroid (used as bone marrow stimulant) (19, 35, 66, 158, 206, 214, 236, 269, 271, 276, 306, 307, 337, 413, 447, 464, 481, 495), but also with contraceptives (107, 206, 297, 356, 437, 488) and conjugated estrogens alone (307), that there can be no doubt about the connection. Apparently the range of incriminated drugs is still growing; corresponding changes were also found after glucocorticoid monotherapy (388), chenodesoxycholic acid (252), and azathioprine (95, 423); the latter was also successfully used to induce experimental circumscribed sinus ectasias.

→

Fig. 22a–c. Patchy hyperemia and peliosis. **a** Contraceptives H & E, X 150. **b** Within a focal nodular hyperplasia (multinodular adenoma) in a 19-year-old girl after contraceptives for 2 years. H & E, X 150. **c** Within a true (mononodular) adenoma in a 30-year-old man. H & E, X 150

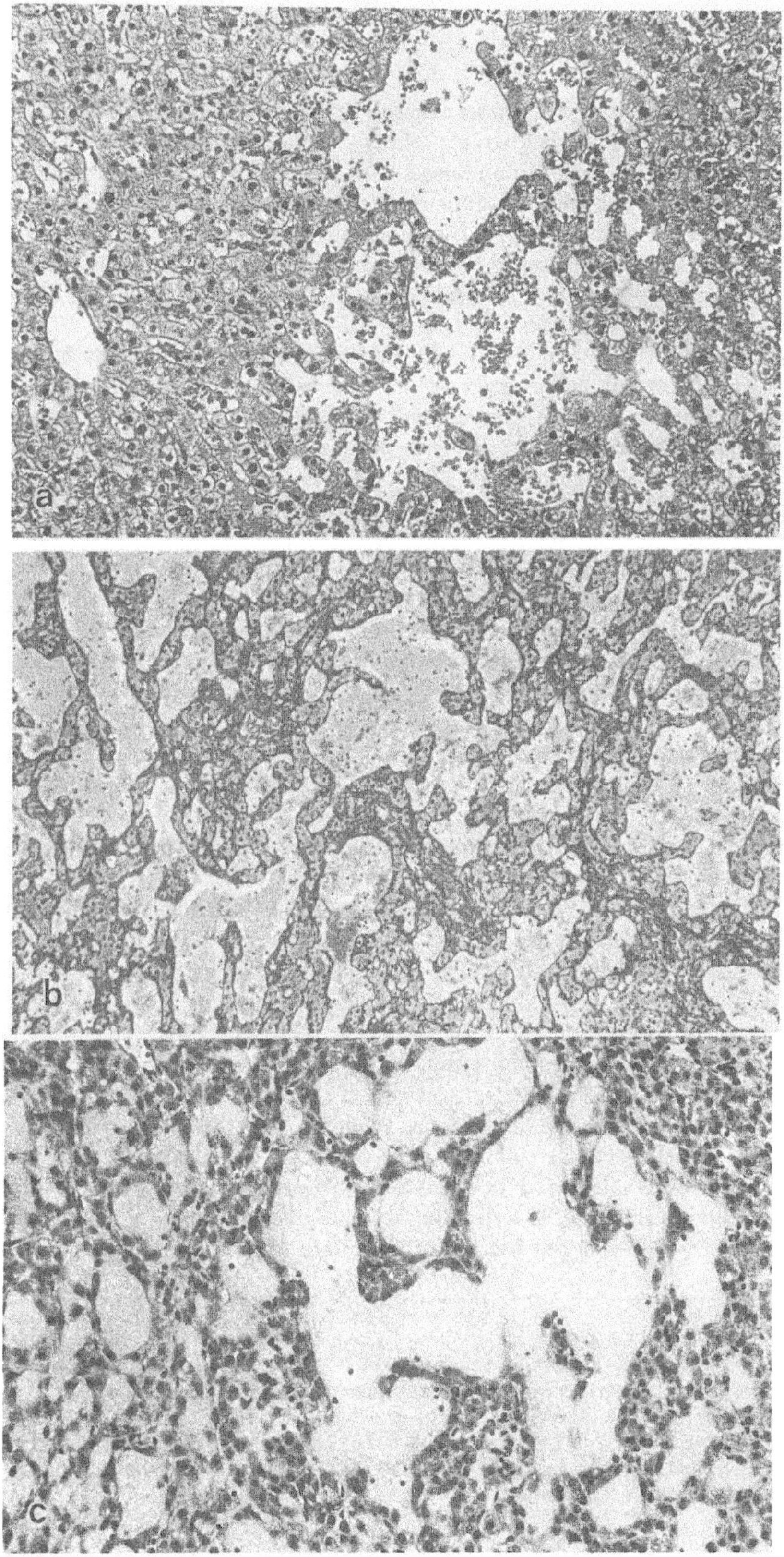

Fig. 22a–c

Such *patchy dilatation* of sinuses seems to be the initial stage of peliosis (Fig. 22a). Associated with circumscribed atrophy of hepatocytes, this may lead – with or without isolated or focal hepatocyte necroses – to excessive overextension of the parenchymal plates, to epithelial discontinuity, to rupture of sinusoidal walls, including their reticular fibers, and finally, to the formation of large, more or less rounded blood spaces bordered by the persisting but protruded outer epithelial lamellas surrounding the original focus. Only this picture should be appreciated as genuine peliosis and termed accordingly. This stage might be termed *"major form of peliosis"* (95) to distinguish it from the *"minor form"* with its less clearly outlined, patchy hyperemia, which seems, however, better designated as *"prepreliosis"* (Fig. 22a). The blood-filled spaces show first incomplete, then continuous endothelial lining, subsequently developing a fibrous bordering. They may even become thrombotic with secondary organization. The livers thus changed are larger than normal, hyperemia being correlated with a true quantitative increase of the blood volume. These foci may become the source of severe, occasionally fatal hemorrhage (e.g., 19, 306). On the other hand, prepeliotic dilatations are still completely reversible if steroid therapy is stopped in time (19, 306) – a fact proving their origin from and maintenance by steroid hormones. Therefore it was a logical inference to hold these hormones equally responsible for the patchy hyperemias in *benign steroid-induced liver tumors* (19, 35, 107, 276, 356) (Fig. 22b), but this idea is not quite conclusive insofar as hyperemia is often limited to the actual tumor area, which also shows other signs of local circulatory disorders. Moreover, a patchy hyperemia associated with the full picture of peliosis was also found in a hepatocellular adenoma occurring spontaneously in a male patient without any conspicuous endocrine levels and without any preceding medication (Fig. 22c). Finally, we have to remember that foci of peliosis may occur without any drug influence, as described in previous reports about chronic pulmonary tuberculosis.

The common cause of their development seems to be a limited disbalance between the intensity of intrasinusoidal pressure and the resistance of the surrounding tissues, which depends not only on the cells in sinusoidal walls, but also on the reticular fibers and on the epithelia proper. Increased intrasinusoidal pressure occurs in many cases, arising, for instance, as a result of (a) heavy coughing fits in chronic pulmonary tuberculosis or (b) almost exclusively arterial supply of the not adaptable low-pressure system of sinusoids in liver adenoma. A decrease of resistance, on the other hand, may be supposed to result from focal epithelial necroses occurring in macronodular liver adenomas as well as in tuberculosis. In steroid-induced focal peliosis occurring in livers of normal structure (less often or not at all in benign liver tumors), the *reduction of tissue resistance* seems to be a decisive factor too. Possibly the essential changes are located in the mesenchymal wall cells (306), since focal steroid-induced peliosis has

⟶

Fig. 23a–c. Budd-Chiari disease, induced by contraceptives. **a** "Endophlebitis hepatica obliterans" of a larger hepatic vein with almost total obliteration of the lumen. Ladewig, × 120. **b** Early hyperemia in the lobulocentral region with dilatation of sinusoids, loss of liver cells, and accumulation of erythrocytes within the former areas of liver cells. Ladewig, × 770. **c** End stage, with nearly complete loss of liver cells and at least partial destruction of the sinusoids and the reticulin fibers; on the right, a hyperplastic regenerative nodule. Masson, × 15

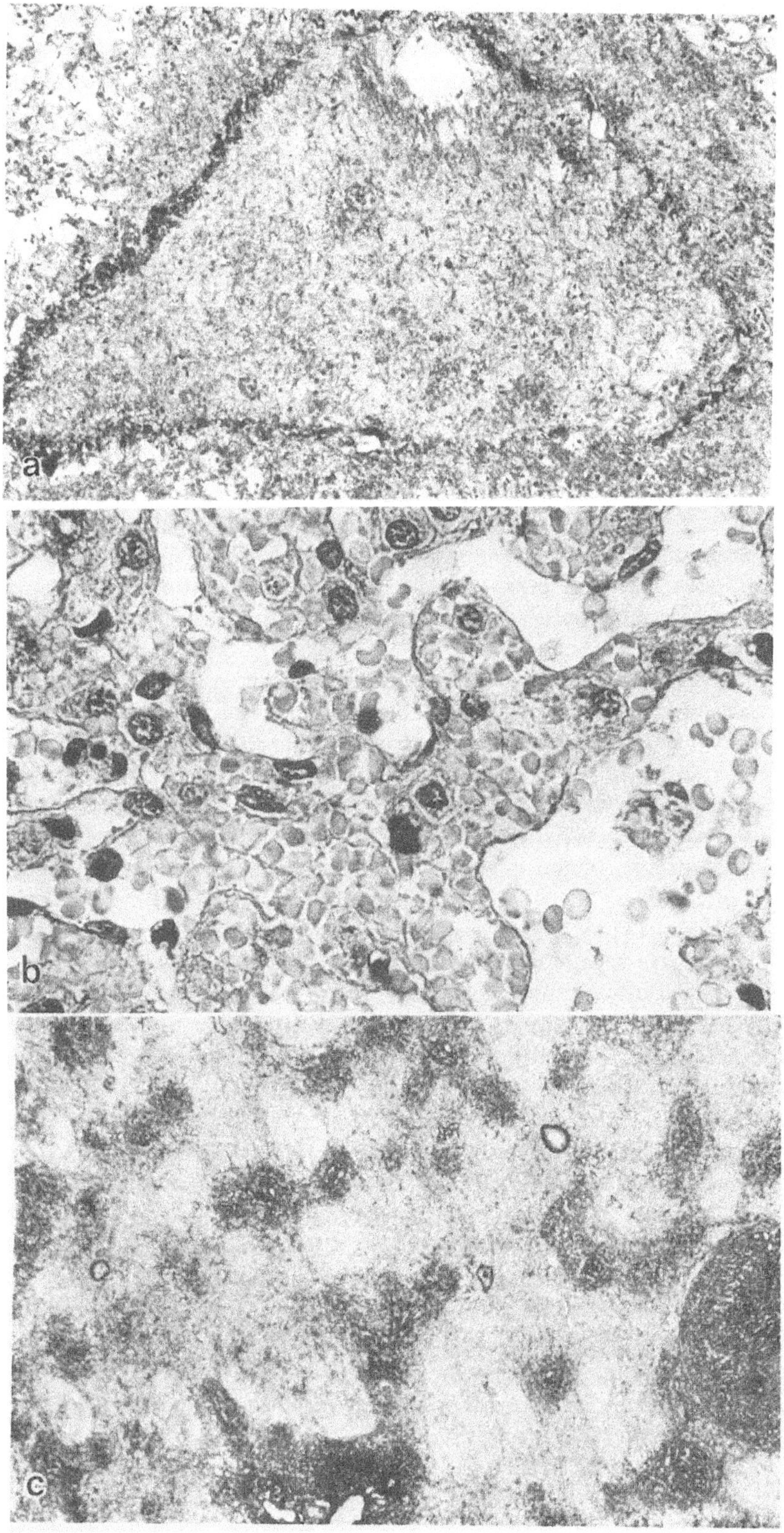

Fig. 23a–c

even been found in the spleen (66, 447). According to our own experience, an obstruction of efferent vessels by radicular endophlebitis hepatica obliterans is unlikely to play any role in the development of genuine peliosis. It seems more likely that a concomitant intimal proliferation of this type (95, 337) is due to the same damaging mechanism that affects the endothelia of efferent veins, eventually provoking sclerosing subintimal edema.

Drug-induced disorders in the *efferent venous system* may arise from the radical or truncal parts of hepatic veins. The disorder termed *radicular form of endophlebitis hepatica obliterans,* which affects the central veins and corresponds closely to the changes observed in *veno-occlusive disease* provoked by Senecio alkaloids (see 50), was found after treatment with urethane (153, 275, 499), azathioprine (95, 264), 6-mercaptopurine (70), thioquanine (156), and other cytostatic drugs (174, 423). The same type of radicular disorder may be provoked by ionizing irradiation [X-ray as well as cobalt (253, 315, 367)] and may occur in the vicinity of large deposits of Thorotrast (11). The basic lesion must be, in every case, some endothelial injury resulting in subintimal edema and subsequent stenosing or obliterating fibrosis. Centrolobular necrosis may result from the same provocation at the same time, or from endophlebitic obstruction of efferent vessels, in which case it is always accompanied by considerable sinus dilatation (see 95).

Disorders of *truncular* origin are more frequent, arising from slowly progressing, early organized thrombosis of the large hepatic veins, to be interpreted as true *Budd-Chiari disease.* Causation of such disorders by drugs has so far been observed only after prolonged ingestion of oral contraceptives (Fig. 23), a fact that explains the incresing incidence in younger women as well as the resulting shift in the sex-adjusted incidence rates (7, 17, 73, 112, 132, 145, 154, 179, 249, 313, 390, 429, 438, 471, 493). The predisposition factor is found in an increased clotting tendency of the blood provoked by the contraceptives (17, 108, 221), perhaps combined with an estrogen-related alteration of the intima (188, 189). The special topographic localization of the thrombotic process in the large hepatic veins, especially where they enter into the vena cava, must be due to purely local anatomic conditions. Properly hepatic causation – such as preceding necrosis with efflux of clotting-prone blood – cannot be demonstrated. Prolonged persistence of thrombosis is correlated with predominance of organization processes, which is responsible for the name "endophlebitis" (Fig. 22a).

Increasing congestion may lead to edematous impregnation of the walls in preceding veins down to the central radiculae, where it gives rise to obliterating intimal proliferations without previous thrombosis. These after-effects, as well as the degree of damage to sinusoidal areas, depend on the extent of venous occlusion; another decisive factor is seen in the possibility of finding new pathways of intrahepatic efflux if the efferent branches are not altogether obstructed (132). It appears remarkable that the veins draining the lobus caudatus are often unaffected (162): timely identification of this condition by way of scintigraphic examination with appropriate thrombolytic therapy may help to prevent the progress of the disease (239). Depending on the severity of the obstruction, the sinusoidal areas may present the picture of severe liver obstruction as found in cardial congestion (Fig. 23b) or they may show some gross destruction (otherwise never occurring) leading eventually to a widespread epithelial loss in large areas and to extensive destruction of vascular walls with formation of large "blood lakes" (Fig. 23c). The typical picture of hepatic peliosis, however, is absent because the hyperemia is not localized, but rather generalized and because the stagnating erythrocytes are being destroyed.

VI. Tumor Induction

Since the first directive reports of *Baum* et al. in 1972 (25), the suspicion that *oral contraceptives* are a causative factor in the development of liver tumors has been substantiated by conclusive evidence. The number of formerly rare tumors that are now occurring in younger women under the influence of ovulation inhibitors (see 5, 8, 10, 13, 52, 67–69, 114, 116, 127, 128, 133, 146, 153, 218, 231, 267, 309, 310, 331, 332, 404, 419, 437, 467), and after therapeutic administration of sex hormones is too great (133, 419). The initial confusion with regard to interpretation, classification, and nomenclature (see 10, 127, 128, 218, 267, 350, 331, 419) was resolved by defining two different kinds of benign tumors or tumorlike lesions, classified by *Edmondson* (113) as *true (uninodular) adenoma* (Fig. 24) and *focal (multi)nodular hyperplasia* (Fig. 25). However, evidence was accumulated for the neoplastic nature of both types, which was at first attributed only to true adenoma; both were found to be linked by transitional forms and now typical adenoma and typical focal nodular hyperplasia are seen as the most characteristic cornerstones of a longer, uninterrupted series of lesions (9, 10, 218, 309, 310, 419). Logically we prefer using the word adenoma for both types, defining them as either *uninodular* or *multinodular hepatocellular adenoma.*

The fundamental *morphological difference* between the two types is not found in the type of cells – which in any case deviates from the normal in terms of the increased nuclear and cellular volume and the higher content of glycogen (Figs. 24b, 25c) and often of fat. Nor does it lie in the histologica arrangement of epithelia, which may show pluricellular rows of fine or coarse trabeculae in either type. Rather it is the behavior of connective tissues which represents the chief distinguishing feature. In the uniform classic adenoma, collagenous fibers are rare in the interior and are never formed into larger fibrous layers or bundles with well-developed bile ducts. On the other hand, there is often a more or less well-defined capsule at the surface of the tumor. In contrast, multinodular neoplasia presents an almost cirrhosis-like picture with larger strands of connective tissue pervading the transformed area (Fig. 25c). These strands often show inflammatory infiltration and occasional epithelioid cell granulomas (10, 386) (Fig. 26b), frequently containing bile ducts or ductlike tubules and arteries of abnormal muscularity (Fig. 26a) and with marked intimal cushioning. In spite of the missing capsule, the tumor's borders against the normal tissue are sharply delineated by the diversity of epithelial appearance (Fig. 25c) as well as by the cellular and tissular displacement that are evident in the surrounding normal hepatic tissue as an expression of the neoplastic growth pressure. Transitional forms between the two types are characterized by a missing capsule and by the presence of focal infiltrating fibrous strata, mostly associated with ductal proliferation, within tumors of an otherwise purely adenomatous structure (see 9, 10, 13, 92, 146, 434).

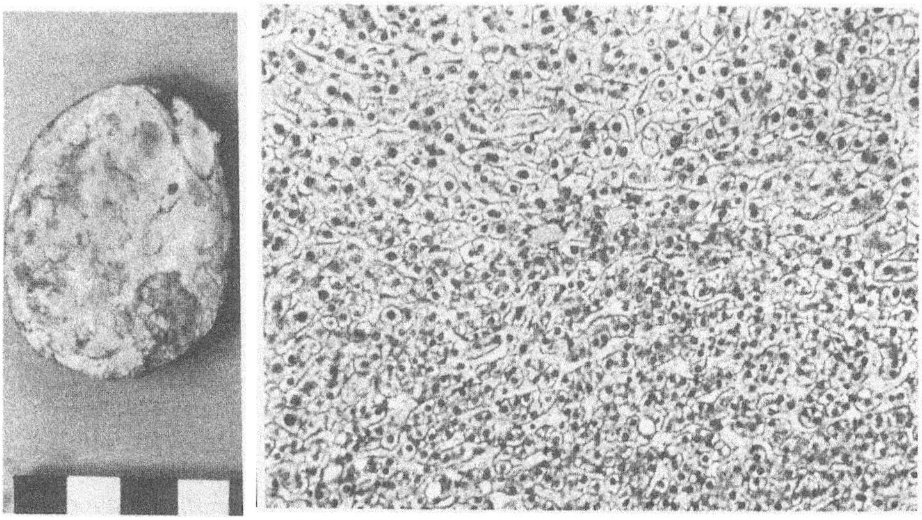

Fig. 24. Mononodular adenoma in a 34-year-old woman; 7 years contraceptives. Tri-PAS, X 150

In both types of adenoma, the neoplastic areas are even macroscopically distinctly set off from the remaining noncirrhotic liver tissue by their different, yellowish coloring. In uninodular adenoma the focus will appear more or less homogeneous, although occasionally interspersed with necrotic or hemorrhagic cavities; in multinodular neoplasia the focus looks segmented, often showing a star-shaped scar in the center of larger nodules (Fig. 25b, c). Tumor volumes vary, of course, the size being of decisive influence on clinical symptoms. Small tumors may not exceed the size of a walnut, growing very slowly, if ever, and their detection is often quite incidental. Others may grow rapidly in size, causing pressure phenomena in the upper abdomen and often manifesting themselves unexpectedly by giving rise to severe, almost fatal hemorrhage, a complication facilitated by their localization near the surface. Pedunculated tumors are a not infrequent finding, especially in the category of focal (multi)nodular neoplasms.

The macroscopic and microscopic differences between the two types certainly do not depend on the presence or absence of regressive changes which are thought to transform a previously uniform adenoma into a multinodular neoplasia with secondary segmentation by circumscribed scarring (309, 310). Even the small foci without any signs of damage may show typical segmentation which, logically, must have been present from the beginning of tumor development. In our opinion (9, 10), the essential difference depends on whether the tumor arises *unifocally* from one coherent area, *or multifocally* and more or less simultaneously from several adjacent lobules. The result will be uninodular adenoma in the first type of development, and multinodular adenoma

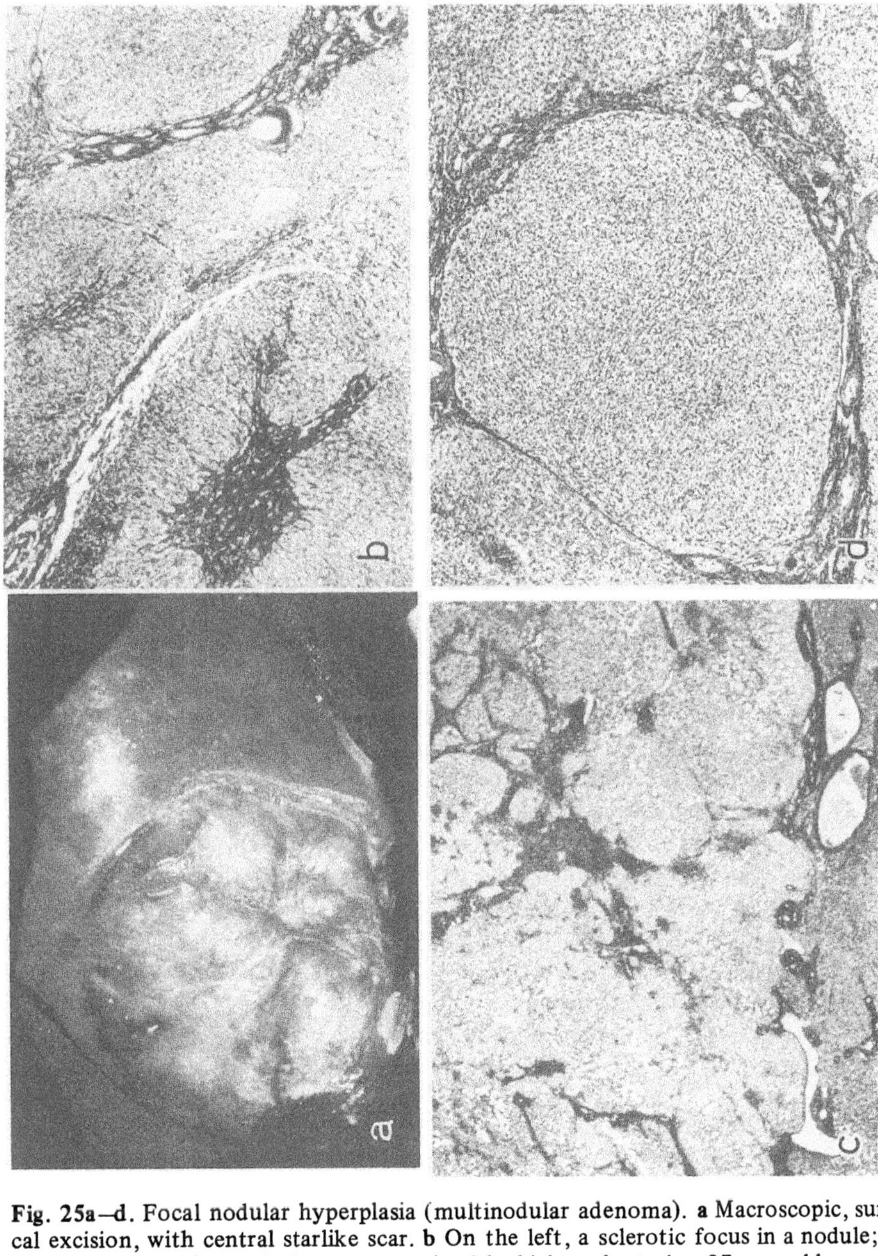

Fig. 25a–d. Focal nodular hyperplasia (multinodular adenoma). **a** Macroscopic, surgical excision, with central starlike scar. **b** On the left, a sclerotic focus in a nodule; on the right, a portal area (primary septum) with thickened arteries. 37-year-old woman. Gömöri, × 40. **c** Margin of the lesion sharply demarcated, the tumor cells being larger and clearer (high glycogen content). 19-year-old woman. 2 years on contraceptives. Ladewig, × 15. **d** One nodule, compressing the fribotic portal areas (with consequent thickening of the arteries). 37-year-old woman. Ladewig, × 60

or multifocal nodular neoplasia in the second. The fibrous septa characteristic for the latter represent included and compressed, preformed portal areas (Fig. 25b, d) with increasing fiber content, inflammatory infiltration, and true ductal structures (primary septa), or secondary, newly formed centrally located sclerotic foci (Fig. 25b) caused by circulatory disorders and containing more or less hepatocellular pseudotubules. The big central star-shaped scar (Fig. 25a), which is always missing in smaller nodules, is also seen as a secondary sclerotic focus of this kind.

Both types of adenomas are predominantly supplied by arterial vessels (see 49). Uninodular adenomas possess this kind of vascularization from the beginning; in multinodular neoplasms it is secondary to compression with subsequent destruction of certain branches of the portal vein that were originally present in the primary septa. By eliminating the portal inflow, this leads to a solely arterial supply of the parenchyma, which is considerably enhanced above the usual rate, and therefore to an increased pressure in the originally low-pressure system of the sinusoids. This must be one of the factors responsible for the frequent occurrence of patchy hyperemia and foci of *peliosis* in both types of adenoma (8, 49, 52, 80, 92, 218, 229, 437). Another factor is seen in the not infrequent occurrence of smaller necrotic foci impairing the resistance of sinusoidal border zones. The necroses may be the consequence of alterations of the arteries, which, being more perfused and simultaneously compressed by the expanding nodules, not only show muscular or intimal thickening but even genuine muscular obliteration (Fig. 26a). Steroid hormones may contribute to the changes affecting the terminal vascular pathways, but this factor should not be given too much weight, firstly, because the corresponding changes are but seldom visible in the adjacent normal hepatic tissue and secondly, because fully developed foci of peliosis may also be found in nonsteroid-induced adenomas.

At any rate, local disorders of circulation, necroses, and the mainly arterial blood supply certainly play an important role in the most important clinical complication endangering these tumor patients, that is, *hemorrhage* into the abdominal cavity, which is said to occur in some 25% of larger tumors (64, 68, 310) and may prove acutely fatal. This complication is favored by the localization of the tumor in the superficial parts of the liver, where it sometimes is separated from the organ capsule only by a small rim of normal tissue.

Etiologic connections with the administration of sex hormones are certainly obvious and fairly well corroborated experimentally, at least in male animals and with very high doses (77), but the exact mode of action is still unexplained. Effects on the nuclear DNA appear plausible since steroid hormones, which, bound to a cytoplasmic receptor, enter the nucleus (see 119), are known to act via an immediate attack on chromatin. A particular risk attached to certain estradiol derivatives (114) could not be confirmed and was probably only simulated by the different date of introduction of the respective compounds. That a particular combination of factors is necessary to launch the tumorigenic properties of antiovulants is substantiated beyond doubt by the very small number of cases that have been reported so far. In the United States, the *true tumor risk* is estimated at present at 1:80 000 (199) or 1:33 000 (490). The *relative risk* increases with the dose of steroid, with the age of the user, and with the duration of use. As a recently published WHO study has pointed out, the risk will rise

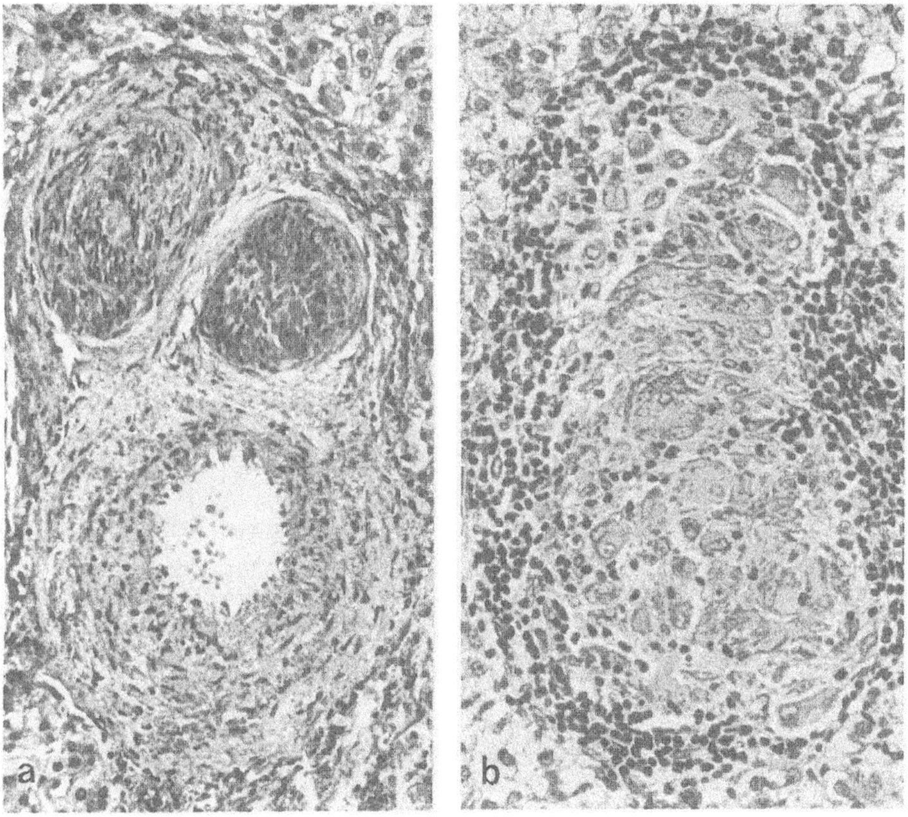

Fig. 26a, b. Additional features of focal nodular hyperplasia, induced by contraceptives. **a** Vascular changes within included portal treads: fibrosis and hyperplasia of muscle cells in the portal vein, muscular obliteration of the arteries. 28-year-old woman. Ladewig, × 240. **b** Epithelioid granuloma, with surrounding lymphocytes. 28-year-old woman. Ladewig, × 150

to 100-fold after 3–5 years and even to 500-fold after more than 7 years as compared with an application time of 1 year only. The influence of some genetic factors might be postulated (see 310), but there seems to be no correlation to those genetic factors that are held responsible for the development of cholestasis. That estrogen reduction in modern contraceptive pills is apt to at least delay the development of a tumor may be presumed; that the introduction of the minipill is an effective prevention may not be improbable.

Under present conditions, development of liver adenoma requires use of the "pill" for an average of *4 years* (310, 419), although 13% of cases were found after less than 2 years (310); even shorter periods of influence (as little as 4–6 months; e.g., 25, 68, 218, 310, 404) have been cited. This would suggest that cellular transformation can be effected in rather a short time. Occasional cases of multiple adenomas of both the uni-

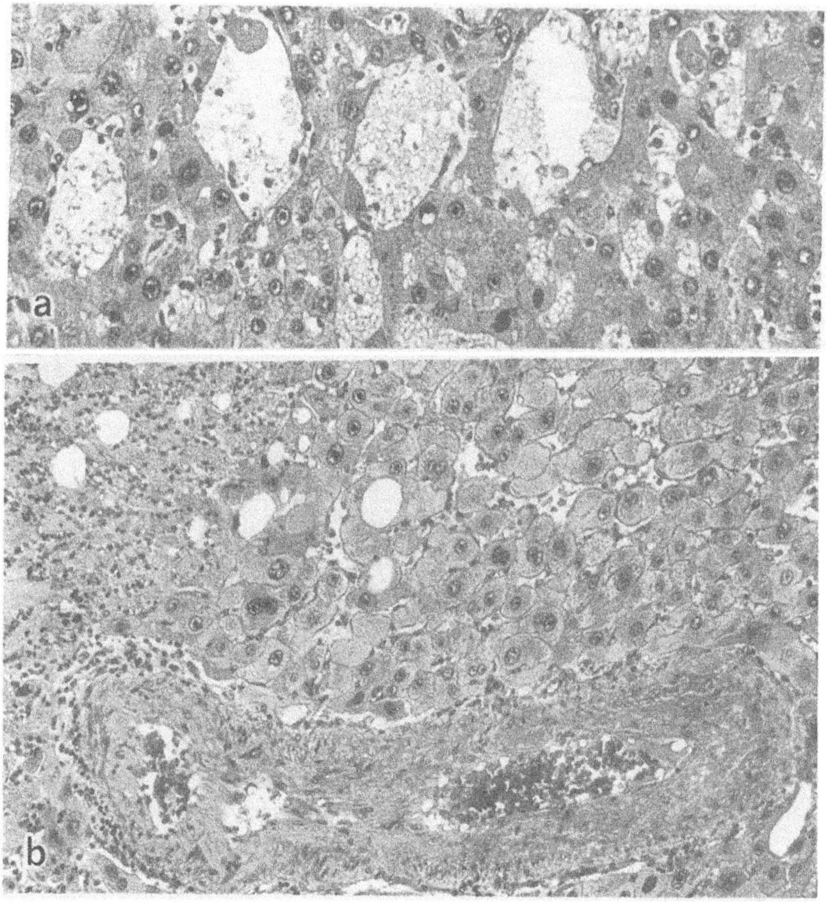

Fig. 27a, b. Hepatocellular carcinoma arising in a 38-year-old woman after 13 years on contraceptives, leading to death by abdominal hemorrhage. **a** Peliosislike foci, with cell necrosis. H & E, X 240. **b** Trabecular pattern, with small cells on the left and large ones on the right. Artery with hypertrophic media. Masson, X 150

nodular and the multinodular type are less surprising than the tendency of such tumors to stop growth or even to regress, to a certain degree, when medication is stopped (5, 14, 114, 116, 208, 266, 267, 366, 387, 434), although no details of the respective morphological process have been elucidated so far. These findings emphasize once more the inductive influence of hormones, and demonstrate at the same time that at least in such cases the complete autonomy, i.e., the independence of all organismic regulatory mechanisms, is by no means reached.

On the other hand, there cannot be any doubt, in contrast to an opinion that prevailed for a long time, that the transfer to actual malignancy, i.e., to *hepatocellular carcinoma,* is possible (92, 146, 218). However, the resulting carcinomas (Fig. 27) seem to have some pecularities – e.g., arteries with considerable muscular hypertrophy (Fig. 27b) and an immanent tendency to hemorrhages – which are related to their genesis and which separate them from the usual liver carcinomas arising in cirrhosis. It is hard to decide whether all carcinomas that were observed in younger women after antiovulants (8, 51, 52, 67, 134, 143, 163, 166, 172, 218, 243, 267, 279, 282, 331, 365, 404, 410, 448, 453, 458) or estrogen therapy (431, 448) necessarily developed via adenomas of the above description. But these reports would suggest or even prove, in combination with our previous data, that contraceptives are capable of transforming human liver tissue into real malignancy at varying speeds and via varying pre-stages or steps.

It could be expected that C-17-alkylated androgenic *anabolic steroids* would also be able to induce *adenomatous tumors*. That the reports about them, concerning uninodular adenomas (48, 55, 173, 247, 302, 316, 443, 444) as well as multinodular types (213, 443, 444), were rather late in appearing may be due to the small number of patients treated over sufficiently long periods. But it is very remarkable that real *carcinomas*, sometimes with apparent pre-stages (413), were reported with comparable frequency. Concerning their architecture and the shape of their cells, these tumors are rather well differentiated. Moreover, they show a conspicuous tendency to regress after stopping drug administration, demonstrating a certain hormone dependency (10, 35, 48, 55, 126, 151, 168, 200, 201, 276, 296, 404, 413, 496). They were found particularly in younger people receiving testosterone derivatives over several years of therapy for aplastic anemia, regardless of the specific type. At any rate, the development of hepatocellular carcinomas is by no means (55, 126, 496) bound to Fanconi anemia, characterized by its tendency toward fragmentation of chromosomes.

A plausible conclusion would be that juvenile, growing liver tissue is particularly sensitive and susceptible to these drugs. The occurrence of mixed hepatoblastoma in early infancy after antiovulant medication of the mother at the time of conception and during the first trimester of pregnancy (333) could be more than coincidental and calls for increased anamnestic vigilance in such tumor cases.

References

1. Abrahams D, Wheatley A, Rubenstein AH, Stables D (1964) Hepatocellular lipofuscin after excessive ingestion of analgetics. Lancet II: 621
2. Adachi S, Matsuzawa Y, Yokomura T, Ishikawa K, Uhara S, Yamamoto A, Nishikawa M (1972) Studies on drug-induced lipidosis (V). Changes in the lipid composition of rat liver and spleen following the administration of 4,4'-diethylaminoethoxyhexestrol. Lipids 7: 1
3. Adlercreutz H, Tenhunen R (1970) Some aspects of the interaction between natural and synthetic female sex hormones and the liver. Amer J Med 49: 630
4. Affolter H (1965) Die medikamentöse Leberschädigung. Schweiz med Wschr 95: 706
5. Aldinger K, Ben-Menachem Y, Whalen G (1977) Focal nodular hyperplasia of the liver associated with high-dosage estrogens. Arch Intern Med 113: 357
6. Alpers DH, Isselbacher KJ (1975) Fatty liver: Biochemical and clinical aspects. In: Schiff L (ed) Disease of the liver. 4th ed.I.P. Lippincott, Philadelphia, pp 815–832

7. Alpert LI (1976) Veno-occlusive disease of the liver associated with oral contraceptives: case report and review of literature. Human Path 7: 709
8. Alpert E, Fernucci J, Athanasoulis C, Malt RA, Galdabini J (1978) Primary hepatic tumor. Gastroenterology 74: 759
9. Altmann H-W (1977) Consideraciones sobre el significado y la nomenclature de los tumores hepaticos en el hombre. In: Llombart-Bosch A (ed) Patologia del cáncer de higado. Soc. Espanola de Anatomia Pathológica, pp 1–16
10. Altmann H-W (1978) Pathology of human liver tumours. In: Remmer H, Bolt H, Bannasch P, Popper H (eds) Primary liver tumors. MTP-Press Ltd, Lancaster, pp 53–71
11. Altmann H-W, Klinge O (1972) Drogen-Hepatopathie. Morphologische Reaktionen menschlichen Lebergewebes auf Pharmaka. Verh Dtsch Ges Path 56: 194
12. Altmann H-W, Pfeifer U (1979) Pathomorphologische Grundreaktionen menschlichen Leberparenchyms. In: Kühn H-A, Wernze H (eds) Klinische Hepatologie 1. Thieme, Stuttgart, p 18
13. Ameriks JA, Thompson NW, Frey ChF, Appelman HD, Walter JF (1975) Hepatic cell adenomas, spontaneous liver rupture, and oral contraceptives. Arch Surg 110: 548
14. Andersen PhH, Packer JT (1976) Hepatic adenoma. Observations after estrogen withdrawal. Arch Surg 111: 898
15. Anthony PP (1975) Hepatoma associated with androgenic steroids. Lancet I: 685
16. Arias IM, Nemark J (1957) Recent developments in the understanding of chlorpromazine jaundice. Amer J Gastroenterol 28: 371
17. Asbeck F, Joist H, Löhrs U (1972) Lebervenenthrombose und Ovulationshemmer. Ein weiterer Fall von Budd-Chiari-Syndrom nach Einnahme eines oralen Kontrazeptivum. Med Klinik 67: 82
18. Austerhoff A, Kindler U, Knop P, Knieriem H-J (1974) Lebertoxizität einer Rifampicin-Kombinationstherapie. Dtsch med Wschr 99: 1182
19. Bagheri SA, Boyer JL (1974) Peliosis hepatis associated with androgenic-anabolic steroid therapy. A severe form of hepatic injury. Ann intern Med 81: 610
20. Bailey WC, Thompson DH, Carson B, Greenberg HB (1973) Fetal hepatic necrosis in a woman receiving chemoprophylaxis with isoniazid. Amer J Gastroenterol 59: 512
21. Bailey WC, Weill H, DeRouen TA, Ziskind MM, Jackson HA, Greenberg HB (1974) The effect of isoniazid on transaminase levels. Ann Intern Med 81: 200
22. Bannasch P (1968) The cytoplasm of hepatocytes during carcinogenesis. Electron- and light-microscopical investigations of the nitrosomorpholine-intoxicated rat liver. Recent Results in Cancer Res. 19: 1. Springer, Berlin Heidelberg New York
23. Barbhoo SP, Owens D, Sherlock Sh (1972) Acute liver failure due to paracetamol. Digestion 6: 298
24. Baskerville A, Cox CS (1978) Histopathological effects of methotrexate on mouse liver. Br J exp Path 59: 32
25. Baum JK, Holtz F, Bookstein JJ, Klein EW (1973) Possible association between benign hepatomas and oral contraceptives. Lancet II: 926
26. Beaugrand M, Chousterman M, Callard P, Carnilleri JP, Petite JP, Ferrier JP (1977) Hépatites au maléate de perhexiline (Pexid) évoluant vers la cirrhose malgré l'arrêt du traitment (2 cas). Gastroent clin Biol 1: 745
27. Beaugrand M, Poupon R, Levi V-G, Callard P, Lageron A, Lecomte D, Darnis F, Ferrier J-P (1978) Lésions hépatiques dues au maléate de perhexiline. Etude dinique, biologique, histopathologique, ultrastructurale et biochimique de 7 cas. Gastroenterol clin Biol 2: 579
28. Becker FF, Lane BP (1968) Regeneration of the mammalian liver. VI. Retention of phenobarbital induced cytoplasmic alterations in dividing hepatocytes. Am J Path 52: 211

29. Beckert W (1973) Zentrilobuläre Parenchymnekrosen der Leber. Beitrag zur Kenntnis arzneimittelbedingter Leberschäden. Zbl allg Path path Anat 117:219
30. Beermann B, Ericsson JLE, Hellström K, Wengle B, Werner B (1971) Transient cholestasis during treatment with ajmaline, and chronic xanthomatous cholestasis after administration of ajmaline, methyltestosterone and ethinylestradiol. Two case reports. Acta med Scand 190: 241
31. Beeson PB, Bass DA (1977) The eosinophil. IN: Smith jr LH (ed) Major problems in internal medicine, 14. Saunders, Philadelphia London Toronto
32. Bennetts FE (1978) Halothane, hypoxia, and hepatitis. Lancet II: 673
33. Berge G, Lundquist A, Rorsman H, Ackerman M (1970) Liver biopsy in psoriasis. Brit J Derm 82: 250
34. Berneis K, Studer A (1967) Vermehrung von Lipofuscin in der Leber als Folge von Phenacetinabusus. Zentrifugation von menschlicher und tierischer Leber im Dichtegradienten. Virchows Arch 383: 75
35. Bernstein MS, Hunter RL, Yachnin S (1971) Hepatoma and peliosis hepatis developing in a patient with Fanconi's anemia. New England J Med 284: 1135
36. Berthelot P (1973) Mechanisms and prediction of drug-induced liver disease. Gut 14: 332
37. Berthelot P, Sicot C, Benhamou JP, Fauvert R (1965) Les hépatites médicamenteuses. Rev franc Étud clin biol 10: 34–39, 140
38. Bertrand L, Descomps B, Blanc F (1978) Drug induced hepatitis. Ann Gastroentérol 14: 283
39. Black M, Mitchell JR, Zimmermann JR, Ishak KG, Epler GR (1975) Isoniazid-associated hepatitis in 114 patients. Gastroenterology 69: 289
40. Bloodworth JMB (1963) Morphologic changes associated with sulfonylurea therapy. Metabolism 12: 287–301
41. Boake WC, Schade SG, Morrissey JF, Schaffner F (1965) Intrahepatic cholestatic jaundice of pregnancy followed by enovid-induced cholestatic jaundice. Ann Int Med 63: 302
42. Bode H (1978) Arzneimittelschäden der Leber. Med Welt 29: 559
43. Bolender RP, Weibel ER (1973) A morphometric study of the removal of phenobarbital-induced membranes from hepatocytes after cessation of treatment. J Cell Biol 56: 746
44. Bonkowky HL, Mudge GH, McMurtry RJ (1978) Chronic hepatic inflammation and fibrosis due to low doses of paracetamol. Lancet I: 1016
45. Bosseckert H, Krause W (1978) Benigne rezidivierende Cholestase und Schwangerschaft. Dtsch Gesundheitswe 33: 10
46. Bottinger LE, Dalen E, Hallen B (1976) Halothane-induced liver damage: an analysis of the material reported to the Swedish Adverse Drug Reaction Committee 1966–1973. Acta anaesthesiolog Scand 20: 40
47. Boyd EM, Bereczky GM (1966) Liver necrosis from paracetamol. Brit J Pharmacol 26: 606
48. Boyd PR, Mark GJ (1977) Multiple hepatic adenomas and a hepatocellular carcinoma in a man on oral methyl testosterone for eleven years. Cancer 40: 1765
49. Brander WL, Vosnides G, Ogg CS, West IE (1976) Multiple hepatocellular tumours in a patients treated with oral contraceptives. Virchows Arch, Abt A 370: 69
50. Bras G (1973) Aspects of hepatic vascular diseases. In: Gall EA, Mostofi FK (eds) The liver. Williams and Wilkins Comp, Baltimore, pp 406-430
51. Breining H, Stolpmann R, Laubenthal F, Hatzibujas J (1979) Maligner Lebertumor nach oraler Kontrazeption. Med Welt 30: 747
52. Britton WJ, Gallagher ND, Little JM (1978) Liver tumours associated with oral contraceptives. Med J Australia 65: 223
53. Brodsky I, Johnson H, Killman SÅ, Cronkite EP (1961) Fibrosis of central and hepatic veins, and perisinusoidal spaces of the liver following prolonged administration of urethane. Amer J Med 30: 976

54. Brown BR, Sipes IG (1977) Biotransformation and hepatotoxicity of halothane. Biochem Pharmacol 26: 2091
55. Bruguera M (1975) Hepatoma associated with androgenic steroids. Lancet I: 1295
56. Burger RA, Marcuse PM (1952) Peliosis hepatis. Report of a case. Amer J clin Path 22: 569
57. Byrd RB, Nelson R, Elliot RC (1972) Isoniazid toxicity. A prospective study in secondary chemoprophylaxis. J Amer Med Assoc 220: 1471
58. Caravati CM, Hooker TH (1971) Acute massive hepatic necrosis with fatal hepatic failure. Amer J Dig Dis 16: 803
59. Carcinogenicity tests on oral contraceptives. Report by the committee on safety of medicine. Her Majesty's Stationary Office, London 1974
60. Carmelita RE, Kim TS, Levine RA (1968) Granulomatous hepatitis associated with sulfadimethoxine hypersensitivity. J Amer Med Assoc 202: 985
61. Cascorbi HF, Vessell ES, Blake DA, Helrich M (1971) Halothane transformation in man. Ann New York Acad Sci 179: 214
62. Cascorbi HF, Vessell ES, Blake DA, Helrich M (1971) Genetic and environmental influence on halothane metabolism in twins. Clin Pharm Ther 12: 50
63. Chajek T, Lehrer B, Geltner D, Levij IS (1974) Quinidine-induced granulomatous hepatitis. Ann Intern Med 81: 774
64. Chan CK, Detmer DE (1977) Proper management of hepatic adenoma associated with oral contraceptives. Surg Gynec Obstet 144: 703
65. Chiu S, Bhakthan NMG (1978) Experimental acetaminophen-induced hepatic necrosis. Biochemical and electron microscopic study of cysteamine protection. Lab Invest 39: 193
66. Chopra S, Edelstein A, Koff RS, Zimelman AP, Lacson A, Neiman RS (1978) Peliosis hepatis in hematologic disease. Report of two cases. J Amer Med Assoc 240: 1153
67. Christopherson WMM, Mays ET (1976) Liver tumours and oral contraceptives. Lancet I: 1076
68. Christopherson WM, Mays ET (1977) Liver tumors and contraceptive steroids: Experiences with the first one hundred registry patients. J Natl Cancer Inst 58: 167
69. Christopherson W, Mays T, Barrows G (1977) A clinicopathologic study of steroid related liver tumours. Amer J Surg Path 1: 31
70. Clark PA, Hsia YE, Huntsman RG (1960) Toxic complications of treatment with 6-mercaptopurine. Brit med J I: 393
71. Clark R, Borirakchanyavat V, Davidson AR, Thompson RPH, Widdop B, Goulding R, Rilliams R (1973) Hepatic damage and death from overdose of Paracetamol. Lancet I: 66
72. Clinch J, Tindall V (1969) Effects of oestrogens and progesterons on liver function in the puerperium. Brit med J I: 602
73. Clubb AW, Giles C (1968) Budd-Chiari syndrome after oral contraceptives. Brit med J 1: 252
74. Coe RO, Bull FE (1968) Cirrhosis associated with methotrexate treatment of psoriasis. J Amer med Assoc 206: 1515
75. Colsky J, Greenspan EM, Warren TN (1955) Hepatic fibrosis in children with akute leukemia after therapy with folic acid antagonists. Arch Path 59: 198
76. Combes B, Whalley PJ, Adams RH (1972) Tetracycline and the liver. In: Popper H, Schaffner F (eds) Progress in liver disease, vol 4. Grune and Stratton, New York London, pp 589–596
77. Committee on the Safety of Medicine (1975) Carcinogenicity test of oral contraceptives. Her Majesty's Stationery Office, London
78. Conn HO (1974) Halothane-associated hepatitis. A disease of medical progress. In: Eliakim M, Eshchar J, Zimmerman HJ (eds) International Symposium on hepatotoxicitiy. Academic Press, New York London, pp 110–121

79. Conney AH (1968) Pharmacological implications of microsomal enzyme induction. Pharmacol Rev 19: 317
80. Contostavlos DL (1975) Benign hepatomas and oral contraceptives. Lancet II: 1200
81. Cooksley WGE, Cowen AE, Powell LW (1973) The incidence of oxyphenisatin ingestion in active chronic hepatitis: a prospective controlled study of 29 patients. Aust NZJ Med 3: 124
82. Coughlin GP, Henderson DW, Reid JH, Grant AK (1973) Cirrhosis following methotrexate administration for psoriasis. Med J Aust 2: 499
83. Cousins M, Gourlay GK, Sharp JH, Adams JF, Hall P, O'Brien P, Haynes WD (1978) Halothane hepatitis. Lancet II: 1197
84. Cullberg G, Lundström R, Stenram U (1965) Jaundice during treatment with an oral contraceptive, lyndiol. Brit med J I: 695
85. Custer RP, Freeman-Narrod M, Narrod StA (1977) Hepatotoxicity in Wistar rats following chronic methotrexate administration: A model of human reactions. J Natl Cancer Inst 58: 1011
85a. Dahinden U, Flippini L, Rondez R (1973) Hepatitis durch Laxantien. Ein Beitrag zum Oxyphenisatin-Ikterus. Schweiz med Wschr 103: 960
86. Dahl MGC, Gregory MM, Scheuer PJ (1972) Methotrexate hepatotoxicity in psoriasis. Comparison of different dose regimes. Brit med J I: 654
87. Dahl P, Schmid E (1969) Arzneimittelikterus durch Östrogene beim Mann. Z Gastroenterol 7: 183
88. Dalen E, Westerholm B (1974) Occurrence of hepatic impairment in women jaundiced by oral contraceptives and in their mothers and sisters. Acta med scand 195: 459
89. Davies DS, Thorgeirsson SS (1971) Mechanism of hepatic drug oxidation and its relationship to individual differences in rates of oxidation in man. Ann New York Acad Sci 179: 19
90. Davis DC, Potter WZ, Jollow DJ, Mitchell JR (1974) Species differences in hepatic glutathione depletion, covalent binding and hepatic necrosis after acetaminophen. Life Sciences 14: 2099
91. Davis JS, Kuafman RH (1966) Tetracycline toxicity. A clinicopathologic study with special reference to liver damage and its relationship to pregnancy. Amer J Obstet Gynec 95: 523
92. Davis M, Portmann B, Searle M, Wright R, Williams R (1975) Histological evidence of carcinoma in a hepatic tumour associated with oral contraceptives. Brit med J 4: 496
93. Davis M, Vergani D, Eddleston ALWF, Williams R (1979) Halothane hepatitis – toxicity and immunity. In: Eddleston ALWF, Weber JCP, Williams R (eds) Immune reactions in liver disease. Pitman Medical, London, pp 235–246
94. Davis RA, Kern F jr, Showalter R, Sutherland E, Sinensky M, Simon FR (1978) Alterations of hepatic Na^+, K^+-ATPase and bile flow by estrogen: effects on liver surface membrane lipid structure and function. Proc Nat Acad Sci USA 75: 4130
95. Degott C, Rueff B, Kreis H, Duboust A, Potet F, Benhamou JP (1978) Peliosis hepatis in recipients of renal transplants. Gut 19: 748
96. Despopoulos A (1970) Excretion of sulfobromophthalein by perfused rat liver as influenced by steroidal hormones. J Pharmacol Exp Ther 173: 37
97. Dietrichson O, Juhl E, Nielson JO, Oxlund JJ, CHristoffersen P (1974) The incidence of oxyphenisatin-induced liver damage in chronic non-alcoholic liver disease. A controlled investigation. The Scand J Gastroenterol 9: 473
98. Dixon MF, Nimmo J, Prescott LF (1971) Experimental paracetamol-induced hepatic necrosis: a histopathological study. J Path 103: 225
99. Dölle W (1972) Arzneimittel und Leberschäden. Dtsch med J 23: 643
100. Dölle W (1972) Leberschädigung durch Paracetamol-Vergiftung. Internist 13: 429
101. Dölle W (1962) Intrahepatische Cholestase durch Ajmalin. Med Klinik 57: 1648

102. Dölle W (1973) Suchlisten für potentiell leberschädigende Medikamente. In: Demling L (Hrsg) Klinische Gastroenterologie. Thieme, Stuttgart, pp 646–649
103. Dölle W, Martin GA (1978) Leber. In: Heintz R (Hrsg) Erkrankungen durch Arzneimittel. Diagnostik, Klinik, Pathogenese, Therapie, 2. Aufl. Thieme, Stuttgart, pp 288–329
104. Dooner HP, Hoyl C, Aliaga C, Parada J (1971) Jaundice and oral contraceptives. Acta hepato-splenol 18: 84
105. Dordal E, Glagov S, Orlando RA, Platz C (1970) Fatale halothane hepatitis with transient granulomas in the liver. New England J Med 383: 357
106. Drill VA (1963) Pharmacology of Hepatotoxicity agents. Ann NY Acad Sci 104: 858
107. Benign cholestatic jaundice of pregnancy and benign cholestatic jaundice from oral contraceptives. Amer J Obstetrics Gynecol 119: 165
108. Drill VA (1975) Oral contraceptives and thromboembolic disease. Human Path 4: 454
108a. Dujovne CA, Shoeman D, Bianchine J, Lasagna L (1972) Experimental bases for the different haptotoxicity of erythromycin preparations in man. J Lab clin Med 79: 832
109. Dujovne CA, Zimmerman HJ (1969) Cytotoxicity of phenothiazines on chang liver cells as measured by enzyme leakage. Proc Soc Exper Biol Med 131: 583
110. Dunning MF (1958) Jaundice associated with norethandrolone (Nilevar) administration. J Amer Med Assoc 167: 1242
111. Ecker JA (1965) Phenylbutazone hepatitis. Amer J Gastroenterol 43: 23
112. Ecker JA, McKittrick JE, Failing RM (1966) Thrombosis of the hepatic veins. The Budd-Chiari syndrome – a possible link between oral contraceptives and thrombosis formation. Amer J Gastroent 45: 429
113. Edmondson HA (1958) Tumors of the liver and intrahepatic bile ducts. Atlas of tumor pathology, Sect VII, 25. Armed Forces Institute of Pathology
114. Edmondson HA, Henderson B, Benton B (1976) Liver cell adenoma associated with use of oral contraceptives. New England J Med 294: 470
115. Edmondson HA, Peters RL (1967) Diagnostic problems in liver biopsies. Pathology annual 2: 213
116. Edmondson HA, Reynolds TB, Henderson B, Benton B (1977) Regression of liver cell adenomas associated with oral contraceptives. Ann Intern Med 86: 180
117. Einhorn N, Davidsohn I (1964) Hepatotoxicity of mercaptopurine. J Amer Med Assoc 188: 802
118. Eisenfeld AJ, Aten RF, Weinberger MJ (1978) Oral contraceptives – possible mediation of side effects via an estrogen receptor in liver. Biochem Pharmacol 27: 2571
119. Eisenfeld AJ, Aten R, Weinberger M, Haselbacher G, Halpern K (1976) Estrogen receptor in the mammalian liver. Science 191: 862
120. Eliakim M, Eshchar J, Zimmerman HJ (1974) International symposium on hepatotoxicity. Academic Press, New York London
121. Elkington SG, Schreiber WM, Conn HO (1969) Hepatic injury caused by L-alphamethyldopa. Circulation 40: 589
122. Epstein EH jr, Croft JD (1969) Cirrhosis following methotrexate administration for psoriasis. Arch Dermatol 100: 531
123. Erlinger S (1974) Influence of drugs on bile flow. In: Eliakim M, Eshchar J, Zimmerman HJ (eds) International symposium of hepatotoxicity. Academic Press, New York London, pp 60–66
124. Espiritu CR, Alalu J, Glueckauf LG, Lubin J (1976) Allopurinol-induced granulomatous hepatitis. Digest Dis 21: 804
125. Espiritu CR, Kim TS, Levim RA (1967) Granulomatous hepatitis associated with sulfodimethoxine hypersensitivity. J Amer Med Assoc 202: 985

126. Farrell GC, Joshua DE, Uren RF, Baird PJ, Perkins KW, Kronenberg H (1975) Androgen-induced hepatoma. Lancet I: 430
127. Fechner RE (1977) Benign heptic lesions and orally administered contraceptives: A report of seven cases and a critical analysis of the literature. Human Path 8: 255
128. Fechner RE (1977) Hepatic tumors and oral contraceptives. Path annual 12: 293
129. Ferleman G, Vogt W (1965) Entacetylierung und Resorption von phenolischen Laxantien. Naunyn Schmiedebergs Arch 250: 479
130. Forrest JAH, Roscoe P, Prescott LF, Stevenson IH (1974) Abnormal drug metabolism after barbiturate and paracetamol overdose. Brit med J 4: 499
131. Fowler PD, Woolf D, Alexander S (1975) Phenylbutazon and hepatitis. Rheum Rehab 14: 71
132. Frederick WC, Howard RG, Spatola S (1974) Spontaneous rupture of the liver in patients using contraceptive pills. Arch Surg 108: 93
133. Fuji S, Tsujioka E, Takewa M, Yukawa S, Nomoto H, Nagasaki Y, Ohsawa Y, Tanaka T (1978) A case of focal nodular hyperplasia of the liver associated with female sex hormone treatment. Acta hepatol jap 19: 41
134. Ganse W van, Caenen P (1976) Hepatocarcinoom met langdurige overleving bij een jonge vrouw (met enkele beschouwingen over de mogelijke relatie tussen primaire levertumoren en geslachtssteroiden). Tijdschrift voor gastro-enterologie 19: 263
135. Gerhartz H (1961) Hepatotoxische Nebenwirkungen unter cytostatischer Therapie. Arzneimittel-Forsch 11: 191
136. Gerok W, Sickinger K (1975) Drugs and the liver. Schattauer, Stuttgart New York
137. Gilbert EF, DaSilva AQ, Queen DM (1963) Intrahepatic cholestasis with fatal termination following norethandrolone therapy. J Amer Med Assoc 185: 538
138. Gillespie L jr, Oates JA, Grout JR, Sjoerdsma A (1962) Clinical and chemical studies with α-Methyldopa in patients with hypertension. Circulation 25: 281
139. Gilette JR (1979) The role of reactive metabolites. In: Eddleston ALWF, Weber JCP, Williams R (eds) Immune reactions in liver disease. Pitman Mecial, London
140. Gilette JR, Mitchell JR, Brodie BB (1975) Biochemical mechanisms of drug toxicity. Ann Rev Pharmacol 14: 271
141. Githin N, Dietrich B, Spektor F (1974) Salicylate hepatitis. A case report. South Afric Med J 48: 1990
142. Gjone E, Blomhoff JP, Ritland S, Husby G (1972) Laxative induced chronic liver disease. Scand J Gastroent, Suppl 16
143. Glassberg AB, Rosenbaum EH (1976) Oral contraceptives and malignant hepatoma. Lancet I: 479
144. Glober GA, Wilkerson JA (1968) Biliary cirrhosis following the administration of methyltestosterone. J Amer Med Assoc 204: 170
145. Goebell H, Dölle W (1972) Budd-Chiari-Syndrom nach Einnahme eines Ovulationshemmers. Dtsch med Wschr 97: 1701
146. Goldfarb S (1976) Sex hormones and hepatic neoplasia. Cancer Res 36: 2584
147. Goldstein G (1963) Sarcoid reaction associated with phenylbutazone hypersensitivity. Ann intern Med 59: 97
148. Goldstein GB, Lam KC, Mistilis SP (1973) Drug-induced active chronic hepatitis. Digest Dis 18: 177
149. Goldstein LK, Ishak GK (1974) Hepatic injury associated with penicillin therapy. Arch Pathol 98: 114
150. Gonzalez-Angulo A, Aznar-Ramos R, Bautista-O'Farril J, Martinez-Manautou J (1970) The fine structure of liver cells in women under steroid effect. Contraceptive therapy, normal pregnancy, and trophoblastic growth. Lab Invest 22: 498
151. Goodman MA, Laden AMJ (1977) Hepatocellular carcinoma in association with androgen therapy. Med J Australia 1: 220

152. Gordon BS, Wolf J, Krause T, Shai F (1960) Peliosis hepatis and cholestasis following administration of norethandrolone. Amer J clin Path 33: 156
153. Grabowski M, Stenram U, Bergquist A (1975) Focal nodular hyperplasia of the liver, benign hepatomas, oral contraceptives and other drugs affecting the liver. Acta Path microbiol Scand, Sect A 83: 615
154. Grayson MJ, Reilly MCT (1968) Budd-Chiari syndrome after oral contraceptives. Brit med J 1: 512
155. Gregory DG, Zaki GF, Sarcosi GA, Carey jr JB (1967) Chronic cholestasis following prolonged tolbutamide administration. Arch Pathol 84: 194
156. Griner PF, El-Baldawi A, Parkman H (1976) Veno-occlusive disease after chemotherapy for acute leukemia. Report of two cases. Ann Int Mecicine 85: 578
157. Groarke JF, Averett JM, Hirschowitz BI (1977) Acetaminophen and hepatic necrosis. The New England J Med 296: 233
158. Groos G, Arnold OH, Brittinger G (1974) Peliosis hepatis after long-term administration of oxymetholone. Lancet I: 874
159. Gumucio JJ, DeMason LJ, Miller DL, Krezoski SO, Keener M (1978) Induction of cytochrome P-450 in a selective subpopulation of hepatocytes. Amer J Physiol 234: C 102
160. Haas J, Patzold U, Stamm T (1978) Intrahepatische Cholestase, eine allergische Reaktion bei Azathioprin-Therapie. Dtsch med Wschr 103: 1576
161. Haemmerli UR (1966) Jaundice during pregnancy. With special emphasis on recurrent jaundice during pregnancy and its differential diagnosis. Springer, New York
162. Hales MR, Scatliff JA (1966) Thrombosis of the inferior vena cava and hepatic veins (Budd-Chiari-Syndrome). Ann Int Med 65: 768
163. Ham JM, Stevenson D, Liddelow AG (1978) Hepatocellular carcinoma possibly induced by oral contraceptives. Dig Dis 23: 38s
164. Hanger FM jr, Gutman AB (1940) Post-arsphenamine jaundice apparently due to obstruction of intrahepatic biliary tract. J Amer Med Assoc 115: 263
165. Harinasatu U, Zimmerman HJ (1968) Diphenylhydantoin sodium hepatitis. J Amer Med Assoc 203: 1015
166. Hatzibujas J, Ueberberg H, Stoldt R, Breitning H (1978) Elektronenmikroskopische Befunde eines malignen Hepatoms nach orlaer Kontrazeption. Z Gastroenterol 16: 616
167. Haubrich WS, Sancetta SM (1954) Spontaneous recovery from hepatobiliary disease with xanthomatosis. Gastroenterol 26: 658
168. Henderson JT, Richmond J, Sumerling MD (1973) Androgenic-anabolic steroid therapy and hepatocellular carcinoma. Lancet I: 934
169. Henning H (1978) Die Leberschädigung durch Phenolisatine. Eine klinische Studie zur hepatotoxischen Medikamentennebenwirkung. Thieme, Stuttgart
170. Henning H, Braun HHv, Look D, Lüders CJ, Vogel H-M (1973) Zur Hepatotoxizität von Laxantien. Ergebnisse von Expositionen mit Phenolisatinen. Z Gastroenterol 11: 75
171. Henning H, Vogel H-M, Ihlenfeld J, Buchegger K, Lüders CJ (1975) Leberschäden unter N-propyl-Ajmalin-Bitartrat (NPAB). Z Gastroenterol 13: 501
172. Hermann RE, David TE (1973) Spontaneous rupture of the liver caused by hepatomas. Surgery 74: 715
173. Hermandez-Nieto L, Bruguera M, Bombi JB, Comacho L, Rozman C (1977) Benign liver-cell adenoma associated with long-term administration of an androgenic-anabolic steroid (methandienone). Cancer 40: 1761
174. Hill K, Jüngst B-K (1969) Therapiebedingte lokale Endophlebitis hepatica obliterans and Hepatosklerose bei kindlicher Leukose. Acta hepato-splenol 16: 297
175. Hitzig WH, Schäfer K (1960) Lebercirrhose bei Antifolsäurebehandlung akuter Paraleukoblastenleukämien. Helvet paediatr Acta 15: 235

176. Holdsworth CD, Atkinson M, Dossett JA, Goldie W (1961) Hepatitis caused by the newer amine-oxidase-inhibiting drugs. II: 621
177. Horii Y, Takino T, Kaibara H, Sugino S, Okanoue T, Tanisawa Y, Masuda M (1974) Drug induced phospholipidosis of the liver – the fate of inclusions –. Gastroenterol japon 9:
178. Hoyumpa AM jr, Connell AM (1973) Methyldopa hepatitis. Report of three cases. Digestiv Dis 18: 213
179. Hoyumpa AM jr, Schiff E, Helfman L (1971) Budd-Chiari syndrome in women Taking oral contraceptives. Amer J Med 50: 137
180. Hruban Z, Tavoloni N, Reed JS, Boyer JL (1978) Ultrastructural changes during cholestasis induced by chlorpromazine in the isolated perfused rat liver. Virchows Arch B Cell Path 26: 189
181. Hurt P, Wegmann T (1961) Protrahierter Largactilikterus mit Übergang in primäre biliäre Cirrhose. Acta hepato-splen 8: 87
182. Hutter RVP, Shipkey FH, Tan CTC, Murphy ML, Chowdhury M (1960) Hepatic fibrosis in children with acute leukemia. A complication of therapy. Cancer 13: 288
183. Hutterer F, Klion FM, Wengraf A, Schaffner F, Popper H (1969) Hepatocellular adaptation and injury. Structural and biochemical changes following Dieldrin and methylbutter yellow. Lab Invest 20: 455
184. Iancu Th, Elian E (1976) Ultrastructural changes in aspirin hepatotoxicity. Amer J clin Path 66: 570
185. Iglesia FA de la, Feuer G, Takada A, Matsuda Y (1974) Morphologic studies on secondary phospholipidosis in human liver. Lab Invest 30: 539
186. Inman WHW, Mushin WW (1974) Jaundice after repeated exposure to halothane: an analysis of reports to the Committee on Safety of Medicine. Brit med J I:5
187. Inman WHW, Mushin WW (1978) Jaundice after repeated exposure to halothane: a further analysis of reports to the Committee on Safety of Medicine. Brit med J II: 1455
188. Irey NS, Manion WC, Taylor HB (1970) Vascular lesions in women taking oral contraceptives. Arch Path 89: 1
189. Irey NS, Norris HJ (1973) Intima vascular lesions associated with female reproductive steroids. Arch Path 96: 227
190. Ishak KG, Irey NS (1972) Hepatic injury associated with the phenothiazines. Clinicopathologic and follow-up study of 36 patients. Arch Path (Chicago) 93: 283
191. Ishak KG, Kirchner JP, Dhar JK (1977) Granulomas and cholestatic-hepatocellular injury associated with phenylbutazone. Report of two cases. Dig Disease 22: 611
192. Ishak KG, Rabin L (1975) Benign tumors of the liver. Med Clin N Am 59: 995
193. Itoh S, Tsukada Y (1973) Clinico-pathological and electron microscopical studies on a coronary dilating agent: 4-4'Diethylaminoethoxyhexestrol-induced liver injuries. Acta Hepato-Gastroent 20: 204
194. James O, Lesua M, Roberts SH, Pulman L, Douglas AP, Smith PA, Watson AJ (1975) Liver damage after paracetamol overdose: comparison of liver function test, fasting serum bile acids, and liver histology. Lancet II: 579
195. Jézéquel AM (1976) Ultrastructural changes induced by drugs. In: Taylor W (ed) The hepatobiliary system. Fundamental and pathological mechanism. Plenum Press, New York London, pp 179–200
196. Jézéquel AM, Kock M, Orlandi F (1974) A morphometric study of the endoplasmic reticulum in human hepatocytes. Correlation between morphological and biochemical data in subjects under treatment with certain drugs. Gut 15: 737
197. Jézéquel A, Orlandi F (1962) Elextron microscopy of the human liver after methandrostenolone administration. In: Martini GA (Hrsg) Aktuelle Probleme der Hepatologie. Thieme, Stuttgart, p 41

198. Jézéquel A-M, Orlandi F (1972) Fine morphology of the human liver as a tool in clinical pharmacology. In: Orlandi F, Jezequel A-M (eds) Liver and drugs. Academic Press, London New York, pp 145–192
199. Jick H, Herman R (1978) Oral-contraceptive-induced benign liver tumors – The magnitude of the problem. J Amer Med Assoc 240: 828
200. Johnson FL (1976) Androgenic-anabolic steroids and hepatocellular carcinoma. In: Okuda K, Peters RL (eds) Hepatocellular carcinoma. J. Wiley and Sons, New York London Sidney Toronto, pp 95–103
201. Johnson FL, Feagler JR, Lerner KG, Majerus PW, Siegel M, Hartmann JR, Thomas ED (1972) Association of androgenic-anabolic steroid therapy with development of hepatocellular carcinoma. Lancet 2: 1273
202. Jollow DJ, Mitchell JR, Potter WZ, Davis DC, Gillette JR, Brodie BB (1973) Acetaminophen-induced hepatic necrosis. II. Role of covalent binding in vivo. J Pharmacol exper Therap 187: 195
203. Jollow DJ, Mitchell JR, Zampaglione N, Gillette JR (1974) Bromobenzene induced liver necrosis. Protective role of glutathione and evidence for 3,4-bromobenzene oxide as the hepatotoxic metabolite. Pharmacology 11: 151
204. Jori GP, Peschle C (1973) Hydralazine disease associated with transient granulomas in the liver. Gastroenterol 64: 1163
205. Kahl GF (1971) Veränderungen der Abbaugeschwindigkeit von Arzneimitteln und ihre Bedeutung für die Pharmakotherapie. Klin Wschr 49: 384
206. Kaira TMS, Mangla JC, DePapp EW (1976) Benign hepatic tumors and oral contraceptive pills. Amer J Med 61: 871
207. Kalow WP, Inaba T (1976) Genetic factors in hepatic drug oxidation. In: Popper H, Schaffner F (eds) Progress in liver disease, vol 5. Grune and Stratton, New York San Francisco London, pp 246–258
208. Kay S (1977) Nine year follow-up of a case of benign liver cell adenoma related to oral contraceptives. Cancer 40: 1759
209. Keeley AF, Trey C, Gottlieb LS (1971) Dealose-Plus R associated jaundice: documentation of abnormal liver function and ultrastructure after challenge. Gastroenterol 60: 195
210. Keeling PWN, Thompson RPH (1979) Drug-induced liver disease. Brit med J I: 990
211. Kendler J, Anuras S, Laborida O, Zimmerman HJ (1972) Perfusion of the isolated rat liver with erythromycin estolate and other derivatives. Prov Soc Exp Biol Med 139: 1272
212. Kendler J, Bowry S, Seeff LB, Zimmerman HJ (1971) Effect of chlorpromazine on the function of the perfused isolated liver. Biochem Pharmacol 20: 2439
213. Kessler E, Bar-Meir S, Pinkus J (1976) Focal nodular hyperplasia and spontaneous hepatic rupture in aplastic anemia treated with oxymetholone. Harefuah 90: 521
214. Kintzen W, Silny J (1960) Peliosis hepatis after administration of fluoxymesterone. Canad med Assoc J 83: 860
215. Klatskin G (1969) Clinical aspects. Symposium on toxic hepatic injury. Gastroenterol 38: 789
216. Klatskin G (1974) Drug-induced hepatic injury. In: Schaffner F, Sherlock S, Leevy CM (eds) The liver and its diseases. Thieme, Stuttgart, pp 163–178
217. Klatskin G (1975) Toxic and drug induced hepatitis. In: Schiff L (ed) Diseases of the liver, 4th Ed. Lippincott, Philadelphia, pp 604–710
218. Klatskin G (1977) Hepatic tumors; possible relationship to use of oral contraceptives. Gastroenterol 73: 386
219. Klatskin G, Kimberg DV (1969) Recurrent hepatitis attributable to halothane sensitization in an anesthesist. New England J Med 280: 515
220. Klatskin G, Smith DP (1975) Halothane-induced hepatitis. In: Gerok W, Sickinger K (eds) Drugs and the liver. Schattauer, Stuttgart, pp 289–294

221. Kletter G (1973) Tödliche Thrombosen bei Frauen im gebährfähigen Alter. Münch med Wschr 115: 1017
222. Klinge O (1965) Toxische Hepatosen bei Halothan-Narkosen. Klin Wschr 43: 1042
223. Klinge O (1972) Morphologie und Ätiologie Halothan-induzierter Leberschäden. Verh Dtsch Ges Path 56: 548
224. Klinge O (1973) Cytologic and histologic aspects of toxically induced liver. Current Topics in Pathology 58: 91
225. Klinge O (1976) Agranuläres endoplasmatisches Retikulum. – Die strukturelle Grundlage der Biotransformation in der Leber. In: Wannagat L (Hrsg) Toxische Leberschäden. Medikamente und Leber. G. Thieme, Stuttgart, pp 21–33
226. Klinge O, Altmann HW (1973) Punktathistologie drogenbedingter Leberalterationen. In: Kühn HA, Markoff NG, Meyer MS (Hrsg) Aktuelle Hepatologie. 4. Lebersymposion in Vulpera 1971. G. Thieme, Stuttgart, pp 8–22
227. Klinge O, Pfeifer U (1979) Pigmentablagrungen derLeber. In: Kühn HA, Wernze H (Hrsg) Klinische Hepatologie. G. Thieme, Stuttgart, pp 1.43–1.52
228. Klion FM, Schaffner F, Popper H (1967) Hepatitis after exposure to halothane. Ann Intern Med 71: 467
229. Knapp WA, Ruebner BH (1974) Hepatomas and oral contraceptives. Lancet 16: 270
230. Knolle J, Förster E, Roessner A, Themann H, Höhn P, Meyer zum Büschenfelde K-H (1974) Die nicht-zirrhotische portale Fibrose (hepatoportale Sklerose) nach chronischer Arsenvergiftung. Klinische und pathologisch-anatomische Befunde. Dtsch med Wschr 99: 903
231. Knowles II DM, Wolff M (1976) Focal nodular hyperplasia of the liver: a clinicopathologic study and review of the literature. Human Path 7: 533
232. Kohn NN, Meyerson RM (1961) Xanthomatous biliary cirrhosis gollowing chlorpromazine jaundice. Amer J Med 31: 665
233. Kohner JA, Lucke B (1921) A study of the histologic changes produced experimentally in rabbits by arsphenamin. Arch Dermat Syphilol 3: 483
234. Kopelman O, Morgan PGM (1977) Liver camage after perhexiline maleate. I: 705
235. Krüskemper HL, Noell G (1967) Steroidstruktur und Lebertoxizität. Untersuchungen mit C_1- und C_{12}-methylierten Androstanderivaten. Acta endocrin (Kbh) 54: 73
236. Kuhböck J, Radaszkiewicz T, Walek H (1975) Peliosis hepatis, eine Kompoikation der Anabolikatherapie. Med Klin 70: 1602
237. Lageron A, Poupon R, de Saint-Maur PP, Levi VG (1977) Liver ganglioside storage after perhexiline maleate. Lancet I: 483
238. Lal S, Singhal SN, Burley DM, Crossley G (1972) Effect of rifampicin and isoniazid on liver function. Brit med J I: 148
239. Langer B, Stone RM, Colapinto RF, Meindok H, Phillips MJ, Fisher MM (1975) Clinical spectrum of the Budd-Chiari syndrome and its surgical management. Amer J Surg 129: 137
240. Laradarios D, Davis M, Portmann B, Williams R (1977) Paracetamol-induced hepatic necrosis in the mouse-relationship between convalent binding, hepatic glutathione depletion and the protective effect of mercaptopropionylglycine. Biochem Pharmacol 26: 31
241. Larsson-Cohn U (1965) Oral contraception and liver function tests. Brit med J I: 1414
242. Larsson-Cohn U, Stenram U (1967) Liver ultrastructure and function in icteric and non-icteric women using oral contraceptive agents. Acta med Scand 181: 257
243. Leclere J, Meot B, Marchal F, Mizrahi R, Collard F, Begue J-Y, Rauber G, Hartemann P (1979) Tumeur maligne primitive du foie associtée à la prise d'estroprogestatifs. Nouvelle Presse Medical 1979: 346

244. Lees AW, Allan GW, Smith J, Tyrell WF, Fallon RJ (1972) Toxicity from rifampicin plus isoniazid and rifampicin plus ethambutol therapy. Tubercle 52: 579
245. Lennon HD (1965) Effect of several anabolic steroids on sulfobromophthalein (BSP) retention in rabbits. Steroids 5: 361
246. Lenz W (1968) Pharmagogenetik. Einige genetisch bedingte ungewöhnliche Arzneireaktionen. Münch med Wschr 110: 1225
247. Lesna M, Spencer J, Walker W (1976) Liver nodules and androgens. Lancet I: 1124
248. Lesna M, Watson AJ, Douglas AP, Hamlyn AN, James OFW (1976) Evaluation of paracetamol-induced damage in liver biopsies. Acute changes and follow-up findings. Virchows Arch, Abt A 370: 333
249. Levi AJ (1967) Drug hepatitis. In: Read AE (ed) The liver. Butterworth, London, pp 165–177
250. Levine RA, Briggs GW, Lovell DM (1966) Chronic chlorpromazine cholangiolitic hepatitis. Gastroenterology 50: 665
251. Levine RA, Espiritu C, Kim TS (1967) Granulomatous hepatitis associated with sulfadimethoxine hypersensitivity. Gastroenterology 52: 1005
252. Levy VG, Bouma ME, Lageron A, Darnis F, Infante R (1978) Hepatic sinusoidal dilatation after chenodeoxycholic-acid therapy. Lancet I: 206
253. Lewin K, Millis RR (1973) Human radiation hepatitis. A morphologic study with emphasis on the late changes. Arch Path 96: 21
254. Lewis D, Wainwright HC, Kew MC, Wzi S, Isaacson C (1979) Liver damage associated with perhexiline maleate. Gut 20: 186
255. Lindner H, Du Bosque G, Dammrmann R, Klöppel G, Krause D (1975) Phenolisatin-induzierte Lebererkrankungen. Sicherung der Pathogenese durch Exposition und Langzeitbeobachtung bei 14 Patientinnen. Dtsch med Wschr 100: 2530
256. Lindner H, Weber D, Klöppel G (1976) Prajmaliumbitartrat-induzierte Leberschäden. Dtsch med Wschr 101: 1876
257. Lüders CJ, Riske WEO, Henning H, Vogel H-M (1975) Die Histomorphologie der Leber bei Schädigung mit phenolisatinhaltigen Laxantien (rezidivierende chronische Cholangiohepatitis). Virchows Arch A Path Anat Histol 365: 309
258. Lüllmann H, Lüllmann-Rauch R, Wassermann O (1975) Drug-induced phospholipidoses. CRC Crit Rev Toxicol 4: 185
259. Ma MH, Biempica L (1970) The normal human liver cell. Cytochemical and ultrastructural studies. Am J Path 62: 353
260. Maddrey WC, Boitnott JK (1973) Isoniazid hepatitis. Ann Intern Med 79: 1–12
261. Maddrey WC, Boitnott JK (1975) Severe hepatitis from methyldopa. Gastroenterology 68: 351
262. Maddrey WC, Boitnott JK (1977) Durg-induced chronic liver disease. Gastroenterology 72: 1348
263. Martinez-Manautou J, Aznar-Ramos R, Bautista-O'Farrill J, Gonzalez-Anzulo A (1970) The ultrastructure of liver cells in women under steroid therapy. II. Contraceptive therapy. Acta Endocrin 65: 207
264. Marubbio AT, Panielson B (1975) Hepatic veno-occlusive disease in a renal transplant patient receiving azathioprine. Gastroenterol 69: 302
265. Mays ET (1976) Standard nomenclature for primry hepatic tumors. A critical need. J Amer Med Assoc 236: 1469
266. Mays ET, Christopherson WM, Barrows GH (1974) Focal nodular hyperplasia of the liver. Possible relationship to oral contraceptives. Amer J clin Path 61: 735
267. Mays ET, Christopherson WM, Mahr MM, Williams HC (1976) Hepatic changes in young women ingesting contraceptive steroids. Hepatic hemorrhage and primary hepatic tumors. J Amer Med Assoc 235: 730
268. McAvoy JM, Tompkins RK, Longmire jr WP (1976) Benign hepatic tumors and their association with oral contraceptives. Arch Surg 111: 761

269. McDonald EC, Speicher CE (1978) Peliosis hepatis associated with administration of oxymetholone. J Amer Med Assoc 240: 243
270. McDonald GSA (1977) Liver damage after perhexiline maleate. Lancet I: 1056
271. McGiven AR (1970) Peliosis hepatis: case report and review of pathogenesis. J Path (Edinb) 101: 283
272. McHardy G, Balart LA (1970) Jaundice and oxyphenisatin. J Amer Med Assoc 211: 83
273. McIntosh S, Davidson DL, O'Brien RT, Pearson HA (1977) Methotrexate hepatotoxicity in children with leukemia. J Pediatrics 90: 1019
274. McMaster KR, Henninger GR (1979) Drug-induced granulomatous hepatitis. Lab Invest 40: 272
275. Meacham GC, Tillotson FW, Heinle RW (1952) Liver damage after prolonged urethane therapy. Am J clin Path 22: 22
276. Meadows AT, Naiman JL, Valdes-Dapena M (1974) Hepatoma associated with androgen therapy for aplastic anemia. J Pediatr 84: 109
277. Medline A, Cohen LB, Tobe BA, Sellers EM (1978) Liver granulomas and allopurinol. Brit med J 1: 1320
278. Melrose AG (1960) Drug-induced jaundice. Scot Med J 5: 250
279. Menzies-Gow N (1978) Hepatocellular carcinoma associated with oral contraceptives. Br J Surg 65: 316
280. Merker H-J, Henning H, Vogel H-M (1976) Beitrag zum elektronenmikroskopischen Bild des Oxyphenisatinschadens der Leber. Z Gastroenterol 14: 796
281. Metreau J-M, Dhumeaux D, Berthelot P (1972) Oral contraceptives and the liver. Digestion 7: 318
282. Meyer P, LiVolsi V, Cornog JL (1974) Hepatoblastoma associated with an oral contraceptive. Lancet II: 1387
283. Miguet JP, Mavier P, Soussy CJ, Dhumeaux D (1977) Induction of hepatic microsomal enzymes after brief administration of rifampicin in man. Gastroenterol 72: 924
284. Mikkelsen WP, Edmondson HA, Peters RL, Redeker AG, Reynolds TB (1965) Extra- and intrahepatic portal hypertension without sclerosis (hepatoportal sclerosis). Ann Surg 162: 602
285. Miller AC, Reid WM (1976) Methyldopainduced granulomatous hepatitis. J Amer Med Assoc 235: 2001
286. Miguel J, Oro J, Bensch KG, Johnson jr JE (1977) Lipofuscin: fine structural and biochemical studies. In: Pryor WA (ed) Free radicals in biology, vol 3. Academic Press, New York San Francisco London, pp 133–182
287. Mir-Madjlessi SH, Farmer RG, Hawk WA (1973) Granulomatous hepatitis. A review of 50 cases. Am J Gastroenterol 59: 122
288. Mitchell JR, Jollow DJ (1974) Biochemical basis for drug-induced hepatotoxicity. In: Eliakim M, Eshchar J, Zimmerman HJ (eds) International Symposium on Hepatotoxicity. Academic Press, New York London, pp 18–24
289. Mitchell JR, Jollow DJ (1975) Metabolic activation of drugs to toxic substances. Gastroenterol 68: 392
290. Mitchell JR, Jollow IJ, Gillette JR (1974) Relationship between metabolism of foreign compounds and liver injury. In: Eliakim M, Eshchar J, Zimmerman HJ (eds) International Symposium of Hepatotoxicity. Academic Press, New York London, pp 45–51
291. Mitchell JR, Jollow DJ, Potter WZ, Davis DC, Gillette JR, Brodie BB (1973) Acetaminophen-induced hepatic necrosis. I. Role of drug metabolism. J Pharmacol exper Ther 187: 185
292. Mitchell JR, Jollow D, Potter WZ, Gillette JR, Brodie WB (1973) Acetaminophen-induced hepatic necrosis. IV. Protective role of glutathione. J Pharmacol exper Ther 187: 211

293. Mitchell JR, Nelson SD, Thorgeirsson SS, McMurtry RJ, Dybing E (1976) Metabolic activation: biochemical basis for many drug-induced liver injuries. In: Popper H, Schaffner F (eds) Progress in liver diseases, vol 5. Grune and Stratton, New York San Francisco London, pp 259–279
294. Mitchell JR, Zimmerman HJ, Ishak KG, Thorgeirsson UP, Timbrell JA, Snodgrass WR, Nelson SD (1976) Isoniazid liver injury: Clinical spectrum, pathology, and proble pathogenesis. Ann Intern Med 84: 181
295. Moertel CG, Rectemeier RJ, Hahn RG (1968) Mitomycin C therapy in advanced gastrointestinal cancer. J Amer Med Assoc 204: 1045
296. Morkrohisky ST, Ambruso DR, Hathaway WE (1977) Fulminant hepatic neoplasia after androgen therapy. New England J Med 296: 1411
297. Mölleken K, Stahl E, Bretzke G (1979) Morphologische und klinische Leberbefunde nach Einnahme oraler Kontrazeptiva. Z ges inn Med 34: 79
298. More RH, McMillan GC, Duff GL (1946) The pathology of sulfonamide allergy in man. Amer J Path 22: 703
299. Morris JS, Schmid M, Newman S, Scheuer PJ, Sherlock S (1974) Arsenic and noncirrhotic portal hypertension. Gastroenterol 64: 86
300. Müller SA, Farrow GM, Martalock DL (1969) Cirrhosis caused by methotrexate in treatment of psoriasis. Arch Derm 100: 523
301. Mullick FG, Ishak KG (1979) Hepatic injury associated with diphenylhydantoin therapy. Lab Invest 40: 274
302. Mulvihill JJ, Ridolfi RL, Schultz FR, Borzy MS, Haughton BPT (1975) Hepatic adenoma in Fanconi anemia treated with oxymetholone. J Pediatrics 87: 122
303. Musch E, v Oldershausen H-F (1978) Klinik und Pathogenese der "INH-Hepatitis". Therapiewocke 28: 3267
304. Mushin WW, Rosen M, Jones EV (1971) Post-halothane jaundice in relation to previous administration of halothane. Brit med J III: 18
305. Myers JD, Olson RE, Lewis JH, Moran TJ (1957) Xanthomatous biliary cirrhosis following chlorpromazine, with observations indicating overproduction of cholesterol, hypoprothrombinemia and the development of portal hypertension. Trans Ass Amer Phys 70: 243
306. Nadell J, Kosell J (1977) Peliosis hepatis. Twelve cases associated with oral androgen therapy. Arch Pathol 101: 405
307. Naheim F, Copper PH, Semion AA (1973) Peliosis hepatis. Possible etiologic role of anabolic steroids. Arch Path 95: 284
308. Nesbit M, Krivit W, Heyn R, Sharp H (1976) Acute and chronic effects of methotrexate on hepatic, pulmonary and skeletal systems. Cancer 37: 1048
309. Nissen ED, Kent F, Kent DR (1975) Liver tumors and oral contraceptives. Obstet Gynecol 46: 460
310. Nissen ED, Nissen SE, Kent DR (1977) Contraceptive steroid-induced liver tumors. In: Berk JE (ed) Developments in digestive disease: Clinical relevance. Lea and Febiger, Philadelphia, pp 97–110
311. Nolan JP (1976) Liver disease associated with toxins and drugs. In: Dietschy JM (ed) Disorders of the gastrointestinal tract. Disorders of the liver. Nutritional disorders. Grune and Stratton, New York San Francisco London
312. Nyfors A (1977) Liver biopsies from psoriatics related to methotrexate therapy. 3. Findings in post-methotrexate liver biopsies from 160 psoriatrics. Acta path microbiol scand Sect A 85: 511
313. Ockner RK, Davidson CS (1967) Hepatic effects of oral contraceptives. New England J Med 276: 331
314. Oda M, Phillips MJ (1977) Bile canalicular membrane pathology in cytochalasin B-induced cholestasis. Lab Invest 37: 350
315. Ogata K, Hizawa K, Yoshida M, Kitamura T, Akazi G, Kagawa K, Fukuda F (1963) Hepatic injury following irradiation. Tokushima J exper Med 2: 240

316. Ogle SJ, Westaby D, Swale J, Randell J, Murray-Lyon IM (1976) Prevalence of liver disease among androgen takers. Digestion 14: 538
317. O'Gorman Th, Koff RS (1977) Salicylate hepatitis. Gastroenterol 72: 726
318. Oldershausen H-F von (1968) Schwangerschaftsikterus und ovulationshemmende Steroide. Dtsch med J 19: 394
319. Oldershausen H-F von (1971) Arzneimittel und Leberschäden. Therapiewoche 21: 2339
320. Oldershausen H-F von (1975) Tuberkulostatika. In: Gerok W, Sickinger K (eds) Drugs and the liver; Arzneimittel und Leber. F.K. Schattauer, Stuttgart New York, pp 301–317
321. Oldershausen H-F von, Eggstein M, Dold U, Knörr K (1965) Ikterus bei intrahepatischer Cholestase nach Gaben von antikonzeptionellen Steroiden. Dtsch med Wschr 90: 1290
322. Olsson R (1978) Increased hepatic sensitivity to paracetamol. Lancet II: 152
323. O'Malley K, Crooks J, Duke E, Stevenson IH (1971) Effect of age and sex on human drug metabolism. Brit med J 3: 607
324. Orellana-Alcalde JM, Dominguez JP (1966) Jaundice and oral contraceptive drugs. Lancet II: 1278
325. Orlandi F, Bamonti F, Dine M, Koch M, Jézéquel AM (1975) Hepatic cholesterol synthesis in man: Effect of diazepam and other drugs. Europ J clin Invest 5: 139
326. Orlandi F, Jézéquel AM (1966) On the pathogenesis of the cholestasis induced by 17 alkylated steroids: Ultrastructural and functional changes of the liver cells during the treatment. Rev Intern Hepatol 16: 331
327. Orlandi F, Jézéquel AM (1972) Liver and drugs. Academic Press, London New York
328. O'Rourke RA, Eckert GE (1964) Methotrexate-induced hepatic injury in an adult. Arch Intern Med 113: 191
329. Orrenius S, Jones DP (1978) Functions of glutathione in drug metabolism. In: Sies H, Wendel A (eds) Functions of glutathione in liver and kidney. Springer, Berlin Heidelberg New York, pp 164–175
330. O'Sullivan JP (1976) Oral contraceptives and liver tumours. Proc roy Soc Med 69: 351
331. O'Sullivan JP, Rosswick RP (1976) Oral contraceptives and malignant hepatic tumours. Lancet I: 1124
332. O'Sullivan JP, Wilding RP (1974) Liver hamartomas in patients on oral contraceptives. Brit med J 3: 7
333. Otten J, Smets R, de Jager R, Gerard A, Maurus R (1977) Hepatoblastoma in an infant after contraceptive intake during pregnancy. New England J Med 297: 222
334. Paine D (1958) Fatal hepatic necrosis associated with aminosalicylic acid. Review of literature and report of case. J Amer Med Assoc 167: 286
335. Paliard P, Vitrey D, Fournier G, Belhadjali J, Patricot L, Berger F (1978) Perhexiline maleate-induced hepatitis. Digestion 17: 419
336. Pantlen H (1976) Intrahepatische Cholestase durch Prajmaliumbitartrat. Dtsch med Wschr 101: 1855
337. Paradinas FJ, Bull TB, Westaby D, Murray-Lyon IM (1977) Hyperplasia and prolapse of hepatocytes into hepatic veins during longterm methyltestosterone therapy: possible relationship of these changes to the development of peliosis hepatis and liver tumours. Histopathology 1: 225
338. Pearson AJG, Grainger JM, Scheuer PJ, McIntyre N (1971) Jaundice due to oxyphenisatin. I: 994
339. Perez V, Goodisch S (1974) Female sex hormones and the liver. In: Schaffner F, Herlock SS, Leevy CM (eds) The liver and its diseases. G. Thieme, Stuttgart, pp 179–190
340. Perez V, Gorodisch S, Marire J de, Nicholson R, DiPaola G (1969) Oral contraceptives: Long-term use produces fine structural changes in liver mitochondria. Science 165: 805

341. Perez V, Gorodisch S, Nynaltan B van, Casavilla F (1972) Liver studies during oral contraception with low doses of megestrol acetate. Int J Fert 17: 197
342. Perez V, Schaffner F, Popper H (1972) Hepatic drug reactions. In: Popper H, Schaffner F (eds) Progress in liver disease, vol 4. Grune and Stratton, New York, London, pp 597–625
343. Pessayre D, Benhamou J-P (1978) Hépatites medicamenteuses dues ã des métabolites instables. Acta Gastro-Enterolog Belg 41: 574
344. Pessayre D, Bentata M, Degott C, Nouel O, Miguet J-P, Rueff B, Benhamou J-P (1977) Isoniazid-rifampin fulminant hepatitis. A possible consequence of the enhencement of isoniazid hepatotoxicity by enzyme induction. Gastroenterology 72: 284
345. Pessayre D, Bichara M, Feldmann G, Degott C, Potel F, Benhamou J-P (1979) Perhexiline maleate-induced cirrhosis. Gastroenterology 76: 170
346. Pessayre D, Mazel P (1976) Induction and inhibition of hepatic drug metabolizing enzymes by rifampicin. Biochem Pharmacol 25: 943
347. Pessayre D, de Saint-Louvent P, Degott C, Bernuau J, Rueff B, Benhamou J-P (1978) Iproclozide fulminant hepatitits. Possible role on enzyme induction. Gastroenterol 75: 492
348. Peters RL, Edmondson HA, Mikkelsen WP, Tatter D (1967) Tetracycline-induced fathy liver in nonpregnant patients. A report of six cases. Amer J Surg 113: 622
349. Peters RL, Edmondson HA, Reynolds TB, Meister JC, Curphey TJ (1969) Hepatic necrosis associated with halothane anestesia. Amer J Med 47: 748
350. Phillips MJ, Oda M, Funatsu K (1978) Ultrastructure of cholestasis. In: Farber E, Fisher MM (eds) Toxic injury of the liver. M. Dekkar Co Inc, New York
351. Phillips M, Oda M, Funatsu F (1979) Evidence for microfilament involvement in Norethandrolone-induced intrahepatic cholestasis. Amer J Path 93: 729
352. Phillips MJ, Oda M, Mak E, Fisher MM, Jeejeebhoy KN (1975) Microfilament dysfunction as a possible cause of intrahepatic cholestasis. Gastroenterol 69: 48
353. Phillips MJ, Oda M, Mak E, Steiner JW (1976) Fine structure of the biliary tree. In: Taylor W (ed) The hepatobiliary system. Fundamental and pathological mechanisms. Plenum Press, New York London, pp 245–263
354. Pierce EH, Chesler DL (1978) Possible association of granulomatous hepatitis with clofibrate therapy. The New England J Med 299: 314
355. Pihl E, Rais O, Zeuchner E (1968) Functional and morphological liver changes in women taking oral contraceptives. A clinical and ultrastructural study with special reference to the occurrence of cholestasis. Acta chir scand 134: 639
356. Pliskin M (1975) Peliosis hepatis. Radiology 114: 29
357. Popper H (1973) Drug-induced liver injury. In: Gall EA, Mostofi FK (eds) The liver. The Williams and Wilkins Comp, Baltimore, pp 182–198
358. Popper H, Rubin E, Gardiol D, Schaffner F, Paronetto F (1965) Drug-induced liver disease. A penalty for progress. Arch int Med 115: 128
359. Popper H, Schaffner H (1959) Drug induced hepatic injury. Ann int Med 51: 1230
360. Popper H, Schaffner F (1970) Pathophysiology of cholestasis. Hum Path 1: 1
361. Potter WZ, Davis DC, Mitchell JR, Jollow DJ, Gillette JR, Brodie BB (1973) Acetaminophen-induced hepatic necrosis. III. Cytochrome P-450-mediated covalent binding in vitro. J Pharmacol Exp Ther 187: 203
362. Prescott LF (1973) Acute hepatic necrosis from paracetamol overdosage. Internat Symp on Hepatotoxicity, Tel Aviv 25: 3
363. Prescott LF, Wright N, Roscoe P, Brown SS (1971) Plasma-paracetamol half-like and hepatic necrosis in patients with paracetamol overdosage. Lancet I: 519
364. Pryor WA (1970) Free radicals in biological systems. Scientific Amer 223/II: 70
365. Pryor AC, Cohen RJ, Goldman RL (1977) Hepatocellular carcinoma in a woman on long-term oral contraceptives. Cancer 40: 884

366. Ramseur W, Cooper R (1978) Asymptomatic liver cell adenomas. Another case of resolution after discontinuation of oral contraceptive use. J Amer Med Assoc 239- 1647
367. Read AE, Harrison CV, Sherlock Sh (1961) Chronic chlorpromazine jaundice, with particular reference to its relationship to primary biliary cirrhosis. Am J Med 31: 249
368. Ream NW, Perlia CP, Wolter J, Taylor SG (1968) Mithramycin therapy in disseminated germinal testicular cancer. J Amer Med Assoc 204: 1030
369. Reed GB, Cox jr AJ (1966) The human liver after radiation injury. A form of veno-occlusive disease. Am J Pathol 48: 597
370. Rehmann VU, Keith ThA, Gall EA (1973) Methyldopa-induced submassive hepatic necrosis. J Amer Med Assoc 224: 1390
371. Remmer H (1964) Drug-induced formation of the smooth endoplasmatic reticulum and of drug metabolizing enzymes. Proceed Europ Soc study of drug toxicity 4: 57
372. Remmer H (1970) The role of the liver in drug metabolism. Amer J Med 49: 617
373. Remmer H (1972) Induction of drug-metabolizing enzyme system in the liver. Europ J clin Pharmacol 5: 116
374. Remmer H, Merker H-J (1963) Enzyminduktion udn Vermehrung von endoplasmatischem Reticulum in der Leberzelle während der Behandlung mit Phenobarbital (Luminal). Klin Wschr 41: 276
375. Remmer H, Schoene B, Fleischmann RA (1973) Induction of unspecific microsomal hydroxylase in human liver. Drug Metabol Dis 1: 224
376. Rexroth W, Dittrich J, Spaan G, Stein U (1976) Intrahepatische Cholestase nach N-propyl-Ajmalin-bitartrat (NPAB). Inn Med 3: 496
377. Reyes H, Gonzales MC, Ribalta J, Aburto H, Matus C, Schramm G, Katz R, Medina E (1978) Prevalence of intrahepatic cholestasis of pregnancy in Chile. Ann int Med 88: 487
378. Reynolds ES, Moslen MT (1974) Liver injury following halothane anesthesia in phenobarbital-pretreated rats. Biochem Pharmacol 23: 189
379. Reynolds JDH, Wilber RD (1972) Chronic active hepatitis associated with oxyphenisatin. Amer J Gastroenterol 57: 566
380. Reynolds TB (1969) Recurring jaundice associated with ingestion of a laxative "Dialose plus". Gastroenterol 56: 418
381. Reynolds TB (1975) Laxative liver disease. In: Gerok W, Sickinger K (eds) Drugs and the liver. Arzneimittel und Leber. F.K. Schattauer, Stuttgart New York, pp 319–325
382. Reynolds TB, Peters RL, Yamada S (1971) Chronic active and lupoid hepatitis caused by a laxative, oxyphenisatin. New England J Med 285: 813
383. Rich RR, Johnson JS (1973) Salicilate hepatotoxicity in patients with juvenile rheumatoid arthritis. Arthritis Rheum 16: 1
384. Rigberg LA, Robinson MJ, Esperitu C (1976) Chlorpromamide-induced granulomas. A probable hypersensitivity in liver and bone marrow. J Amer Med Assoc 235: 409
385. Rodman JS, Deutsch DL, Gutman SI (1976) Methyldopa hepatitis. A report of six cases in the literature. Amer J Med 60: 941
386. Roschlau G (1977) Noduläre Hyperplasie der Leber bei kontrazeptiver Behandlung. Zbl allg Path 121: 517
387. Ross D, Pina J, Mirza M, Galvan A, Ponce L (1976) Regression of focal nodular hyperplasia after discontinuation of oral contraceptives. Ann Intern Med 85:
388. Ross RC, Kovacs K, Horvath E (1972) Ultrastructure of peliosis hepatis in a percutaneous biopsy. Path europ (Brüssel) 7: 273
389. Roth A, Cerlek S, Dominis M, Kolaric K (1978) Liver changes induced by cytostatic drugs in patients with non Hodgkin's lymphomas. Acta Hepato-Gastroenterol 25: 353

390. Rothwell-Jackson RL (1968) Budd-Chiari syndrome after oral contraceptives. Brit med J 1: 252
391. Ruiz-Esquide M, Ribalta J, Reyes H (1978) Prevalencia de la colestasia intrahepatica de la embarazada en los Angeles, Chile. Rev Med Chile 106: 518
392. Russell RI, Allan JG, Patrick R (1973) Active chronic hepatitis after chlorpromazine ingestion. Brit Med J I: 655
393. Sameshima Y, Mizuno T, Sasakawa M, Shiozaki Y, Tatsumi K (1976) Drug-induced hepatic injury. A review of the Japanese articles for the past 50 years. Japanese J Gastroenterol 73: 1214
394. Samuels AM, Carey MC (1978) Effects of chlorpromazine hydrochloride and its metabolites on Mg^{2+} and Na^{+}, K^{+}, ATPase activities of canalicular-enriched liver plasma membranes. Gastroenterol 74: 1183
395. Schaffner F (1965) Effect of anabolic steroids in man. In: McIntyre N, Sherlock S (eds) Therapeutic agents and the liver. Blackwell Scientific Publ, Oxford, pp 99–117
396. Schaffner F (1968) Ultrastructure of liver in intrahepatic and extrahepatic cholestasis. In: Beck K (ed) Ikterus. FK Schattauer, Stuttgart New York, pp 143–149
397. Schaffner F (1974) Halothane hepatitis. In: Ingelfinger FJ, Ebert RV, Finland M, Relman AS (eds) Controversy in internal medicine II. WB Saunders, Philadelphia London Toronto
398. Schaffner F (1976) Drug-induced chronic liverdisease. In: Gentilini P, Popper H, Teodori U (eds) Chronic hepatitis. S Karger, Basel München Paris London New York Sydney, pp. 156–159
399. Schaffner F, Kniffen JC (1963) Electron microscopy as related to hepatotoxicity. Ann New York Acad Sci 104: 847
400. Schaffner F, Popper H, Chesrow E (1959) Cholestasis produced by the administration of norethandrolone. Amer J Med 26: 249
401. Schaffner F, Raisfeld IH (1969) Drugs and the liver. A review of metabolism and adverse reactions. Arch Intern Med 15: 221
402. Schaffner F, Sasaki H (1965) Induced cholestasis. Ultrastructural studies on drug. Rev Int Hepat 15: 461
403. Schenker S, Breen KJ, Heimberg M (1976) Pathogenesis of tetracycline-induced fathy liver. In: Gerok W, Sickinger K (eds) Drugs and the liver. FK Schattauer, Stuttgart, pp 269–280
404. Scheuer A, Lehmann F-G (1977) Lebertumoren bei Therapie mit Kontrazeptiva und Anabolika. Internist 18: 208
405. Scheuer PJ (1973) Liver biopsy interpretation. 2nd ed. Williams and Wilkins Comp, Baltimore
406. Scheuer PJ (1975) Liver lesions and androgenic steroid therapy. Lancet II: 1099
407. Scheuer PJ (1975) Hepatotoxicity of methotrexate and anathioprine. In: Gerok W, Sickinger K (eds) Drugs and the liver. FK Schattauer, Stuttgart New York, pp 281–286
408. Scheuer PJ, Bianchi L (1974) Guidelines for diagnosis of therapeutic drug-induced liver injury in liver biopsies. Review of an international group. Lancet I: 854
409. Scheuer PJ, Summerfield JA, Lal S, Sherlock S (1974) Rifampicin hepatitis. A possible complication of oral contraceptive steroids. Med J Australia 1: 215
410. Schweitzer IL, Peters RL (1974) Acute submassive hepatic necrosis due to methyldopa. A case demonstrating possible initiation of chronic liver disease. Gastroenterol 66: 1203
412. Seaman WE, Ishak KG, Plotz PH (1974) Aspirin-induced hepatotoxicity in patients with systemic lupus erythematosus. Ann intern Med 80: 1
413. Shapiro P, Ikeda RM, Ruebner BH, Connors MH, Halsted CC, Abildgaard CF (1977) Multiple hepatic tumors and peliosis hepatis in Fanconi's anemia treated with androgen. Amer J Dis Child 131: 1104

414. Sherlock Sh (1965) Hepatic reactions to therapeutic agents. Ann Rev Pharmacol 5: 429
415. Sherlock Sh (1966) Prediction of hepatotoxicity due to therapeutic agents in man. Medicine (Baltimore) 45: 453
416. Sherlock S (1967) The prediction of hepatotoxicity due to therapeutic agents in man. In: Wolstenholme GEW, Porter R (eds) Drug responses in man. Little and Brown, Boston, pp 138–154
417. Sherlock S (1968) Drugs and the liver. Brit med J I: 227
418. Sherlock Sh (1975) Diseases of the liver and biliary system. 5th ed. Blackwell Scientific Publ, Oxford London Edinburgh Melbourne
419. Sherlock S (1975) Hepatic adenomas and oral contraceptives. Gut 16: 753
420. Sherlock Sh (1978) Halothane hepatitis. Lancet II: 364–365
421. Shikata T, Kanetaka T, Endo Y, Nagashima K (1972) Drug-induced generalized phospholipidosis. Acta path jap 22: 517
422. Shikata T, Oda T, Naito Ch, Kanetaka T, Suzuki H (1970) Phospholipid fatty liver: a proposal of a new concept and its electron microscopical study. Acta path jap 20: 467
423. Shulman HM, McDonald GB (1979) Hepatic venoocclusive disease following human bone marrow transplantation. Lab Invest 40: 285
424. Simmons F, Feldman B, Gerety D (1972) Granulomatous hepatitis in a patient receiving allopurinol. Gastroenterol 62: 101
425. Simon FR, Sutherland E, Accatino L, Vial J, Mills D (1977) Studies on drug induced cholestasis: Effect of ethinyl estradiol on hepatic bile acid receptors and (NA3-K+)-ATPase. Bile acid metabolism in health and disease. Paumgartner G, Stiehl A (eds). MTP Press, Lancaster/England
426. Sipes IG, Brown BR (1976) An animal model of hepatotoxicity association with halothane anestesia. Anesthesiology 45: 522
427. Smetana HF (1963) The histopathology of drug-induced liver disease. Ann NY Acad Sci 104: 821
428. Smuckler EA, Arcasoy A (1969) Structural and functional changes of the endoplasmic reticulum of hepatic parenchymal cells. Int Rev exper Path 7: 305
429. Somayaji BN, Eeles GH, Paton A, Parker RGF (1968) Budd-Chiari syndrome after oral contraceptives. Brit med J 1: 53
430. Somayaji BN, Paton A, Price JH, Harris AW, Flewell TH (1968) Noresthisterone jaundice in two sisters. Brit med J II: 281
431. Sontaniemi EA, Alvaikko MJ, Kaipainen WJ (1975) Primary liver cancer associated with long-term oestrogen therapy. Ann clin Res 7: 287
432. Spitz RD, Keren DF, Boitnott JK, Maddrey WC (1978) Bridging hepatic necrosis. Etiology and prognosis. Amer J Dig Dis 23: 1076
433. Spyridis P, Sinaniotis C, Papadea I, Oreopoulos L, Hadjiyiannis S, Papadatos C (1979) Isoniazid liver injury during chemoprophylaxis in children. Arch Dis Childhood 54: 65
434. Stauffer JR, Lapinski MW, Honold DJ, Myers JK (1975) Focal nodular hyperplasia of the liver and intrahepatic hemorrhage in young women on oral contraceptives. Ann int Med 83: 301
435. Stenger RJ (1970) Organelle pathology of the liver. The endoplasmic reticulum. Gastroenterol 58: 554
436. Stenger RJ, Johnson EA (1972) Effects of phenobarbital pretreatment on the response of rat liver to halothane administration. Proc Soc Exper Biol Med 140: 1319
437. Stenwig AE, Solgaard T (1975) Ruptural benign hepatoma associated with an oral contraceptive. Virchows Arch A 367: 337
438 Sterup K, Mosbech J (1967) Budd-Chiari syndrome after taking oral contraceptives. Brit med J 4: 660

439. Stolzer BL, Miller C, White WA, Zuckerbrod M (1950) Postarsenical obstructive jaundice complicated by xanthomatosis and diabetes mellitus. Am J Med 9: 124
440. Strunin L (1977) The liver and anesthesia. WB Saunders Comp Ltd, London Philadelphia Toronto
441. Studer A, Schärer K (1965) Langfristige Phenacetinbelastung am Hund mit Berücksichtigung der Leber- und Nierenpigmentierung. Schweiz med Wschr 95: 933
442. Swank LA, Chejfec G, Nemchausky BA (1978) Allopurinol-induced granulomatous hepatitis with cholangitis and a sarcoid-like reaction. Arch intern Med 138: 997
443. Sweeney EC, Evans DJ (1975) Liver lesions and androgenic steroid therapy. Lancet II: 1042
444. Sweeney EC, Evans DJ (1976) Hepatic lesions in patients treated with synthetic anabolic steroids. J clin Path 29: 626
445. Talerman A, Thompson RB (1966) Hepatic fibrosis in a child possibly due to prolonged methotrexate. J clin Path 19: 81
446. Taranger J, Girbal JB, Giacchero G (1970) Rifampicine et functions hépatique. A propos de 72 ponctionsbiopsies. Rev Tuberc (Paris) 34: 717
447. Taxy JB (1978) Peliosis: A morphologic curiosity becomes an iatrogenic problem. Human Path 9: 331
448. Thalassinos NC, Lymbertos C, Hadjioannou J, Gardikas C (1974) Liver-cell carcinoma after long-term oestrogen-like drugs. Lancet I: 270
449. Thomas FB (1974) Chronic aggressive hepatitis induced by halothane. Ann intern Med 81: 487
450. Thompson RPH, Clark R, Willson RA, Borirakchanyavat V, Widdop B, Goulding R, Williams R (1972) Hepatic damage from overdose of paracetamol. Gut 13: 836
451. Thomsen P, Poulsen H, Petersen P (1975) Different types of ground glass hepatocytes in human liver biopsies: morphology, occurrence and diagnostic significance. Scand J Gastroent 11: 113
452. Thulin KE, Nermark J (1966) Seven cases of jaundice in woman taking an oral contraceptive, Anovlar. Brit med J I: 584
453. Tigano F, Ferlazzo B, Barrile A (1976) Oral contraceptives and malignant hepatoma. Lancet II: 196
454. Tobias H, Auerbach R (1973) Hepatotoxicity of long-term methotrexate therapy for psoriasis. Arch intern Med 132: 391
455. Toghill PJ, Smith PG, Benton P, Brown RC, Matthews HL (1974) Methyldopa liver damage. Brit med J 3: 545
456. Tolman KG, Peterson P, Gray G, Hammar SP (1978) Hepatotoxicity of salicylates in monolayer cell cultures. Gastroenterol 74: 205
457. Trey C, Davidson CS (1970) The management of hepatic failure. In: Popper H, Schaffner F (eds) Progress in liver disease, vol 3. Grune and Stratton, New York, p 282
458. Trias R, Rius X, Autonell J, Algaba F (1978) Hepatocarcinoma and oral contraceptives. Lancet I: 821
459. Troll MM, Menten MI (1945) Salicylate poisoning: report of four cases. Amer J Dis Childr 69: 37
460. Trülzsch D, Klinge O, Zilly W, Richter E (1975) Cholestatischer Ikterus nach dem Laxans Normolaxol. Med Klin 70: 771
461. Tysell JE jr, Knauer CM (1971) Hepatitis induced by methyldopa (Aldomet). Am J Dig Dis 16: 849
462. Uehlecke H, Schnitzer F (1969) Stoffwechsel von Phenacetin und p-Phenacetin in der Niere. Naunyn-Schmiedebergs Arch 264: 319
463. Uppala AR, Steinheber FU (1977) Fulminant hepatic failure associated with methyldopa. Amer J Gastroenterol 68: 578
464. Usatin MS, Wigger HJ (1976) Peliosis hepatis in a child. Arch Path Lab Med 100: 419

465. Uzunalimoglu B, Yardley JH, Boitnott JK (1970) The liver in mild halothane hepatitis: Light and electron microscopic findings with special reference to the mononuclear cell infiltrate. Amer J Path 61: 457
466. Valdivia-Barriga V, Feldman A, Orellana J (1963) Generalized hypersensitivity with hepatitis and jaundice after the use of penicillin and streptomycin. Gastroenterol 45: 114
467. Vana J, Murphy GP, Aronoff BL, Baker HW (1977) Primary liver tumors and oral contraceptives. J Amer M Assoc 238: 2154
468. Vesell ES (1972) Individual variations in drug response. In: Orlandi F, Jezequel AM (eds) Liver and drugs. Academic Press, London New York, pp 1–40
469. Vesell ES (1974) Pharmacogenetic factors as determinants of hepatotoxicity. In: Eliakim M, Eshchar J, Zimmerman HJ (eds) International Symposium on Hepatotoxicity, Tel Aviv 1973. Academic Press, New York, pp 40–44
470. Vesell ES, Passananti GT, Greene FE, Page JG (1971) Genetic control of drug levels and of the inductions of drug metabolizing enzymes in man. Ann New York Acad Sci 179: 752
471. Vessey MP, Weatherall JAC (1968) Venous thromboembolic disease and the use of oral contraceptives. Lancet II: 94
472. Villeneuve JP, Huet PM, Joly J-G, Marleau D, Coté J, Légaré A, Lafortune M, Lavoie P, Viallet A (1976) Idiopathic portal hypertension. Amer J Med 61: 459
473. Vila VT de jr, Serpick AA, Carbone PP (1970) Combined chemotherapy in the treatment of advanced Hodgkin's disease. Ann Int Med 73: 881
474. Walker CO, Combes B (1966) Biliary cirrhosis induced by chlorpromazine. Gastroenterol 51: 631
475. Walton B (1978) Anaesthesia, surgery and immunology. Anaesthesia 33: 322
476. Wannagat L (1976) Toxische Leberschäden. Medikamente und Leber. G Thieme, Stuttgart
477. Warin AP, Landells JW , Levene GM, Baker H (1975) A prospective study of the effects of weekly oral methotrexate on liver biopsy: findings in severe psoriasis. Brit J Dermatol 93: 321
478. Waugh D (1952) Myocarditis, arteritis and focal hepatic, systemic and renal granulomas apparently due to penicillin sensitivity. Am J Path 28: 437
479. Weck AL de (1971) Drug reagtions. In: Samter M (ed) Immunological diseases, vol 1, 2nd ed. Little, Brown and Comp, Boston, p 415
480. Werner SC, Hanger FM, Kritzler RA (1950) Jaundice during methyltestosterone therapy. Amer J Med 8: 325
481. Westaby D, Ogle SJ, Paradinas FJ, Randell JB, Murray-Lyon IM (1977) Liver damage from long-term methyltestosteron. II: 261
482. Widger LA, Gandolfi AJ, van Dyke RA (1976) Hypoxia and halothane metabolism in vivo: Release of inorganic fluoride and halothane metabolite binding to cellular constituents. Anesthesiology 44: 197
483. Wildhirt E (1966) Cholestatischer Ikterus. Arg inn Med Kinderheilk 24: 80
484. Williams ER, Khan MD (1967) Liver damage in patient on Methyldopa. J Ther clin Res 1: 5
485. Williams R (1975) Paracetamol hepatotoxicity in man. In: Gerok W, Sickinger K (eds) Drugs and the liver; Arzneimittel und Leber. FK Schattauer, Stuttgart New York, pp 337–345
486. Willing RL, Hecker R (1971) Oxyphenisatin and liver damage. Med J Austr 1: 1179
487. Wills EJ, Walton B (1978) A morphologic study of unexplained hepatitis following halothane anesthesia. Amer J Pathol 91: 11
488. Winkler K, Poulsen H (1975) Liver disease with periportal sinusoidal dilatation. A possible complication to contraceptive steroids. Scand J Gastroenterol 40: 699
489. Wolfe JD, Metzger AL, Goldstein RC (1974) Aspirin hepatitis. Ann Int Med 80: 74

490. World Health Organization (1978) Steroid contraception and the risk of neoplasia. Report of a WHO scientific group. World Health Organization Technical Report Series 619. World Health Organization, Geneva
491. Worster-Drought C (1923) Atophan poisoning. Brit med J I: 148
492. Wright N, Prescott LF (173) Potentiation by previous drug therapy of hepatotoxicity following paracetamol overdosage. Scot Med J 18: 50
493. Wu Sh-M, Spurny OM, Klotz AP (1977) Budd-Chiari Syndrome after taking oral contraceptives. A case report and review of 14 reported cases. Am J Dig Dis 22: 623
494. Yamamoto A, Adachi S, Kitani T, Shinji Y, Nasu KST, Nishikawa M (1971) Drug induced lipidosis in human cases and in animal experiments. J Biochem (Tokyo) 69: 613
495. Yanoff M, Rawson AJ (1964) Peliosis hepatis. An anatomical study with demonstration of two varieties. Arch Path 77: 159
496. Ziegenfuss J, Carabasi R (1973) Androgens and hepatocellular carcinoma. Lancet I: 262
497. Zimmerman HJ (1963) Clinical and laboratory manifestations of hepatoxicity. Ann NY Acad Sci 104: 954
498. Zimmerman HJ (1968) The spectrum of hepatotoxicity. Perceptives in Biology and Medicine 12: 135
499. Zimmerman HJ (1972) Drug-induced hepatic injury. In: Samter M (ed) Hypersensitivity to drugs. Pergamon Press Inc, New York, pp 299–365
500. Zimmerman HJ (1974) Drug-induced hepatic disease. In: Eliakim M, Eshchar J, Zimmerman HJ (eds) International symposium on hepatotoxicity. Academic Press, New York London, pp 92–103
501. Zimmerman HJ (1974) Hepatic injury caused by therapeutic agents. In: Becker FF (ed) The liver. Marcel Dekker, New York, pp 225–302
502. Zimmerman HJ (1974) Aspirin-induced hepatic injury. Ann Intern Med 80: 103
503. Zimmerman HJ (1978) Hepatotoxicity. The adverse effects of drugs and other chemicals on the liver. Appleton-Century-Crofts, New York
504. Zimmerman HJ, Kendler J (1970) Relationship between structure of phenothiazines and in-vitro cytotoxicity. Prov Soc Exp Biol Med 135: 201
505. Zucker P, Daum F, Cohen MI (1975) Aspirin hepatitis. Amer J Dis Child 129: 1433

Closed, Mai 1979

Drug-Associated Nephropathy

Part I: Glomerular Lesions

H.-V. GÄRTNER

Foreword . . . 144
Introduction . . . 145
I. Glomerular Damage Resulting from a Direct Drug Action . . . 146
1. Glomerular Lesions Associated with Aminonucleoside . . . 147
a) Introduction . . . 147
b) Clinical Findings . . . 147
c) Morphological Findings . . . 147
d) Pathogenesis . . . 149
2. Glomerular Lesions Associated with Daunomycin (Daunorubicin) . . . 149
a) Introduction . . . 149
b) Clinical Findings . . . 149
c) Morphological Findings . . . 149
d) Pathogenesis . . . 150
3. Glomerular Lesions Associated with Other Cytostatic Drugs . . . 150
4. Glomerular Lesions Associated with Penicillamine . . . 151
5. Glomerular Lesions Associated with Other Drugs . . . 151
II. Indirect Effects of Drugs Upon Glomerular Structures Mediated by Immune Mechanisms . . . 152
1. Penicillamine-Associated Glomerular Lesions (Penicillamine Nephropathy) 153
a) Introduction . . . 153
b) Frequency of Renal Side-Effects . . . 154
c) Clinical Findings . . . 154
d) Morphological Findings . . . 154
e) Clinical and Morphological Correlations . . . 156
f) Course of the Disease and Prognosis . . . 157
g) Pathogenesis . . . 158
2. Glomerular Lesions Associated with Gold Preparations . . . 159
a) Introduction . . . 159
b) Frequency of Renal Side-Effects . . . 159
c) Clinical Findings . . . 159
d) Morphological Findings . . . 160
e) Clinical and Morphological Correlations . . . 161
f) Course and Prognosis of the Disease . . . 161
g) Pathogenesis . . . 161
3. Glomerular Lesions Produced by Mercury (Mercury Nephropathy) . . . 162
a) Introduction . . . 162
b) Frequency of Renal Side-Effects . . . 162
c) Clinical Findings . . . 162
d) Morphological Findings . . . 162
e) Pathogenesis . . . 163
4. Glomerular Lesions Associated with Trimethadione (Tridione) and Distraneurine Therapy . . . 164
a) Clinical Findings . . . 164
b) Morphological Findings . . . 164
c) Pathogenesis . . . 164
5. Glomerular Lesions Associated with Captopril . . . 165
a) Introduction . . . 165
b) Clinical and Morphological Findings . . . 165
c) Pathogenesis . . . 165

6. Glomerular Lesions Produced by Sulphadiazine-Silver Therapy 165
7. Glomerular Lesions Associated with Drug-Induced Systemic Lupus Erythematosus (SLE) with Secondary Renal Involvement 166
   a) Introduction 166
   b) Clinical Findings 168
   c) Morphological Findings 168
   d) Pathogenesis 169
8. Glomerular Lesions Produced by Heroin (Diacetylmorphine) 170
   a) Introduction 170
   b) Frequency of Renal Side-Effects 170
   c) Clinical Findings 170
   d) Morphological Findings 170
   e) Pathogenesis 171
9. Glomerular Lesions Associated with the Inhalation of Volatile Hydrocarbons 171
   a) Introduction 171
   b) Clinical Findings 172
   c) Morphological Findings 172
   d) Pathogenesis 172
10. Indirect Effects Via Electrolyte and Water Imbalance: Glomerular Changes Associated with Laxative and Diuretic Abuse 172

Conclusions 173
References 174

Foreword

The kidney, along with the liver, represents the most important excretory organ for drugs and their metabolites. Since the kidney has both a particularly high blood through-put, in fact some 25% of the coronary output, and because it is the major site for the elimination of many pharmaceutical preparations, this organ is particularly predisposed to drug-dependent damage. Drug-induced damage of the kidney is facilitated by a number of aspects of renal physiology including the metabolic activity of the kidney and the high concentration of drugs and their metabolites, produced by the counter current effect, in the relatively unvascularised renal medulla. In addition drugs may become particularly concentrated in tubular cells through the mediacy of active resorption and secretion processes. Furthermore, the vulnerability of the kidney to drug damage may be to some extent a product of the filtration process itself since the deposition of circulating immune complexes or the in situ immune complex formation in glomeruli may subsequently lead to a damaging of the glomerular structures. Drug-induced renal damage might also be expected in cases of renal insufficiency where the reduced elimination of a drug results in its accumulation in the kidney. Since the kidney plays a major role in water and electrolyte balance, acute or chronic alterations in the plasma ion levels or plasma volume may lead to both morphologically and clinically detectable kidney changes.

The manifestation of drug damage may be recognised in all the structural elements of the kidney. Thus, pathological changes may be observed in the glomeruli, the tubuli, in the interstitium as well as in the vessels. The pathogenetic basis of these alterations include toxic, as well as immunological and circulatory mechanisms. However, most instances of drug-induced renal damage are dose-dependent, with those rare instances of dose-independent damage appearing to be based upon various immunological pathomechanisms.

One and the same drug may induce quite different morphological damage depending upon the dose given and the length of administration. For instance the administration of a high dose of mercuric salts may result in an acute tubular necrosis, whereas long-term therapy with low doses of the same salt can lead to an immune-complex glomerulonephritis.

In general drug-induced kidney diseases are reversible if the intake of the noxious substance is ceased in time. Occasionally, however, a disease process which was initiated by a medicament becomes progressive, when, despite a cessation of drug therapy, there is no disappearance of renal symptoms, rather there appears a chronic renal insufficiency.

The theme of "drug-associated nephropathy" will be dealt with in the following review from the point of view of morphological and pathogenetic considerations. Morphological aspects of the disease process will be subdivided into glomerular and interstitial lesions. On the other hand pathogenetic factors will divide toxic and immunological mechanisms from secondary lesions caused by alterations in the electrolyte balance. In the first part of this review glomerular lesions will be discussed, with especial consideration being given to drug-induced immune-complex glomerulonephritis.

Part II deals with tubulo-interstitial renal damage. Section A of Part II considers acute interstitial nephritis, nephrotoxic damage and analgesic nephropathy as examples of primary chronic damage. Section B takes as its theme tubulo-interstitial alterations within the framework of hypokalaemic nephropathy.

Introduction

Since the kidney has such a high blood through-put rate (in fact some 25% of the coronary output) and because this organ has relative to its weight the largest endothelial cell surface, it is not unsurprising that, as a consequence of the filtration process, the glomerular structures are particularly predisposed to drug damage.

As drug-associated renal damage is not combined with any specific clinical symptoms, the establishment of a causal correlation between the two requires a close temporal relationship between the intake of the drug in question and the appearance of renal symptoms. Further evidence of a causal correlation is the reversibility of the renal symptoms following cessation of the drug intake as well as the reappearance of symptoms upon re-exposure. In general glomerular damage leads to an increase in the permeability of the glomerular basement membrane with a resulting proteinuria, this being no less the case in instances of drug-associated glomerular lesion, whatever their pathogenesis. Thus the appearance of a proteinuria, that is, a nephrotic syndrome, is the dominant clinical symptom of this disease state.

Various pathomechanisms lie at the root of drug-associated glomerulopathy. Thus glomerular lesions may be the result either of a dose-dependent (i.e., toxic) drug effect, or a dose-independent effect. Basically drug-induced glomerulopathy may be attributed to three different pathogenetic rudiments, which may possibly be induced by only one drug and which may all appear at the same time in one individual.

I. Direct (dose-dependent, toxic) influence upon glomerular structures (basement membrane, mesangium, epithelial cells)

II. Indirect (dose-independent) effects upon glomerular structures via immunological reactions. In this instance two distinct theoretical mechanisms could be considered as being involved.

1. The drug acts as a hapten or full antigen and induces antibody production which results in:
a) the formation of *circulating* antigen-antibody complexes
b) *in situ* immune complex formation.

2. The drug elicits an autoimmune mechanism by producing changes in humoral structures with the subsequent development of:
a) a systemic disease (SLE) with a secondary renal involvement produced through the deposition of immune complexes (here the autologous antigens are cell nuclei or at least nuclear components).
b) a Heymann nephritis (in this instance the autologous antigens are tubular structures).
c) anti-basement-membrane GN, i.e., a Goodpasture syndrome (the autologous antigens are basement membrane components).

III. Indirect effects generated by alterations of water and electrolyte balance (hypokalaemic nephropathy).

These mechanisms will now be discussed in more detail.

I. Glomerular Damage Resulting from a Direct Drug Action

Drugs which may be classified under this heading are known mainly from animal experiments; in fact it may have been the outcome of these experiments which has resulted in some of these drugs not being used in human medicine. The following drugs which have a direct effect upon glomerular structures will now be considered individually:

1. Aminonucleoside (observations made in animal experiments and in man).
2. Daunomycin (daunorubicin) (observations made in animal experiments)
3. Other cytostatic drugs: azathioprine (Imurek) (observations made in animal experiments), cyclophosphamide (Endoxan) (observations made in animals and man) triethylenebenzoquinine (Trenimon) (observations made in animal experiments).
4. D-penicillamine (Metalcaptase, Trolovol) (observations made in animal experiments).
5. Miscellaneous drugs: probenicid, perchlorate, tolbutamide (observations made in humans although with some questionable relationships).

1. Glomerular Lesions Associated with Aminonucleoside

a) Introduction

The aminonucleoside of puromycin (6-dimethylaminopurin-3-amino-D-ribose) is undoubtedly the most extensively examined drug known to possess a direct toxic activity upon the glomerular structures. Thus, in 1963 *Nussenzveig* and co-workers reported the appearance of a severe nephrotic syndrome in patients suffering from Chagas' disease who had been treated with the aminonucleoside, the notion underlying the therapy being that the aminonucleoside would inhibit the purine metabolism of the causative agent of Chagas' disease (*Trypanosoma cruzii*). The morphological changes observed in the kidney were described as being relatively unspecific and took the form of an increased protein storage. In only one case was there any indication of a mild thickening of the basement membrane and an increase in glomerular cell number (*Nussenzveig* et al. 1963).

Because of the considerable nephrotoxic activity of the aminonucleoside it is now only really of historical interest for human medicine. However, following the first reports of *Frenk* et al. (1955) this substance has become the classical agent for inducing and studying the nephrotic syndrome in animals (the so-called aminonucleoside nephrosis).

b) Clinical Findings

In agreement with other authors (*Wilson* et al. 1958; *Borowsky* et al. 1961; *Lannigan* et al. 1962) we can also demonstrate (*Schöll* et al. 1974) that one injection of aminonucleoside is sufficient to induce a nephrotic syndrome in Wistar rats. Furthermore, in our experiments the progress of the disease is clinically biphasic, there being a first peak of proteinuria on experimental day 7 which subsides during the next three months. Subsequently the proteinuria rises dramatically until the fifteenth month with the concomitant development of a slow progressive renal insufficiency.

c) Morphological Findings

The morphological changes which occur in the glomeruli following a single i.v. injection (100–150 mg aminonucleoside/kg body weight) or daily subcutaneous injections (5–10 days, 17 mg/kg body weight) of aminonucleoside may be divided into early and late stages which also correspond to the clinical course of the condition.

As revealed by electron microscope studies (*Vernier* et al. 1959; *Harkin* and *Recant* 1960; *Farquhar* and *Palade* 1961; *Kortge* et al. 1961; *Lannigan* et al. 1962; *Metcoff* et al. 1963; *Ryan* and *Karnovsky* 1975; *Caulfield* et al. 1976) the early morphological changes, which are correlated with the appearance of a severe proteinuria, are characterised by lesions of the epithelial cells, which are already recognisable after a few days.

These lesions represent both a fusion and loss of foot processes, a reduction in the number of filtration slits and a development of occluding junctions in the region of the residual filtration slits with displacement of the slit diaphragms (*Ryan* and *Karnovsky* 1975; *Caulfield* et al. 1976). Simultaneously there appears a swelling of the epithelial cells and an increase in the number of phagosomes and lysosomes with further evidence of elevated pinocytosis and protein resorption. On the basement membrane itself a narrowing of the lamina densa is to be observed, with a corresponding widening of the lamina rara externa (*Caulfield* et al. 1976).

Whereas the early changes of the disease seem to be reversible, the further progress of the condition involves irreversible glomerular damage combined with the reappearance of a massive proteinuria. Besides the evidence pointing to a metabolic disturbance, that is, an increase in the number of phagosomes and a decrease in lysosomes in the epithelial cells, there is an occasional detachment of the epithelial cells from the basement membrane. There is formed, therefore, a "naked" basement membrane area, i.e. a region where basement membrane is in direct contact with the Bowman's capsule, which may be responsible for the massive proteinuria. In addition there is the synthesis of new basement membrane material in the region between the basement membrane and the partially detached epithelial cells (*Caulfield* et al. 1976). It is this which finally leads to a folding and twisting of the glomerular basement membrane. Out of these irreversible late lesions develop, during the following months, alterations which have been variously termed as glomerulosclerosis (*Vernier* et al. 1959) or chronic proliferating glomerulonephritis (*Borowsky* et al. 1961). These alterations are characterised by further elevated basement membrane synthesis, mesangial cell proliferation as well as fusion and crescent formation with final scarring of the glomeruli.

In our own animal experiments (*Schöll* et al. 1974) the light microscopical findings in the late stages of aminonucleoside nephrosis (15 months after a single injection of the drug) revealed glomerular changes which could be described as representing focal/segmental hyalinisation with fatty degeneration of the endothelial cells and fusion with the Bowmans capsule. The electron microscope revealed in addition to an irregular thickening and folding of the glomerular basement membrane and the fusion of the foot processes a massive deposition of electron-dense material in the region of the focal/segmental hyalinisation.

In short the glomerular lesions which we have examined do not seem to represent the picture of a "chronic proliferative glomerulonephritis" (mesangio-proliferative glomerulonephritis with scarring), but rather resemble the focal sclerosis of a human glomerulonephritis, especially because the juxtamedullary glomeruli are affected.

In contrast to the seemingly uniform descriptions of the light and electron microscopically identifiable changes occurring in this disease are the varied and diverse reports concerning immunohistological findings. Whereas the study of *Treser* et al. (1964) indicated a negative immunohistological result, we have found a focal deposition of γ-globulin in the region of the focal/segmental hyalinisation. We could not, however, detect the presence of complement, which is in contrast to the report of *Shimizu* (1970), who found besides a deposition of γ-globulin also C_3 in the rat. We are, however, in agreement with the above-cited author that there is no characteristic or regular immunofluorescence pattern. *Lannigan* et al. (1962) have also reported the detection of γ-globulin deposits in control animals.

These results as well as the observation that the type and extent of the immunohistological findings are dependent upon the severity of the histological changes (*Okuda* et al. 1965) contra-indicate the existence of an immune-complex glomerulonephritis. Rather, they support the idea of an unspecific deposition in the sense of an absorption process in the region of the damaged glomerular structures.

d) Pathogenesis

The cause of the glomerular changes associated with aminonucleoside is currently thought to lie in a direct effect of this drug upon the metabolic process (nucleotide synthesis?) of the epithelial cells. The disruption of these metabolic steps is then thought to result in an unhinging of basement membrane production and the synthesis of defective basement membrane material. Thus it is that the severity of the glomerular changes is dependent upon both the dosage and the duration of administration of the aminonucleoside (*Shimizu* 1970). Furthermore, it has been shown that in aminonucleoside nephropathy the negative charge decreases not only in the region of the epithelial cells (*Michael* et al. 1970) but also in the area of the glomerular basement membrane (*Caulfield* and *Farquhar* 1978). The resulting increase of permeability to anionic macromolecules may be regarded, therefore, as one causative factor of the nephrotic syndrome accompanying the aminonucleoside nephropathy.

The following points all argue in favour of a toxic mechanism and against an immunological pathomechanism for the aminonucleoside-associated glomerular lesions:

1) The lack of a latent period between the i.v. injection and the appearance of the glomerular changes. The earliest glomerular alterations are already apparent only a few hours after the administration of the drug.
2) The severity of the morphological changes in the glomerular region is dependent upon the dose and duration of drug therapy.
3) The immunohistological findings in the region of the glomeruli are uncharacteristic and do not represent any of the immunohistological patterns known to be indicative of an immunopathomechanism.

2. Glomerular Lesions Associated with Daunomycin (Daunorubicin)

a) Introduction

Daunomycin, a metabolite of *Streptomyces peucetius,* belongs to the anthracycline group of antibiotics, its main clinical application being as a cytostatic agent in tumour therapy, and most notably in cases of acute leucosis. This drug exerts its effects by the formation of complexes with RNA and DNA (*di Marco* 1967), which then results in an inhibition of growth in cells exhibiting a high mitotic rate. Clinical observations have established a variety of toxic side-effects of daunomycin (*Gerhartz* 1967; *Kreiter* et al. 1968; *Obrecht* et al. 1970), particularly a potentially lethal cardiotoxicity and suppression of the bone marrow. However, renal complications in man have until now not been reported.

b) Clinical Findings

On the other hand the administration of only one injection of daunomycin (15 mg/kg body weight) to the rat results in a nephrotic syndrome (*Sternberg* 1970) and a development of an increasing renal insufficiency. Daunomycin thus presents the same activity as aminonucleoside and, like the latter, represents a model substance both for the induction and study of the nephrotic syndrome.

c) Morphological Findings

In fact the morphological changes of the glomerular basement membrane observed in daunomycin nephrosis are markedly more impressive than those seen in aminonucleoside nephrosis. The earliest morphological changes which we are capable of detecting occur after some four days (*Kronenberg* et al. 1972), and consist of both protein droplets in the glomerular epithealial cells and the fusion of the foot processes. In the later course of the disease process, from day six onwards, basement membrane changes occur which include twisting and folding of the lamina densa with, as a consequence, obliteration of the capillaries. Such alterations have not been observed until the present in aminonucleoside nephrosis.

Glomerular changes comparable with those observed in the rat following daunomycin therapy have not been reported in man. If one accepts that daunomycin exerts its activity via a toxic effect then one might suggest that the lack of glomerular changes in man is a result of the fact that in human medicine markedly lower doses of this drug are applied, doses which are insufficient to generate renal symptoms. Furthermore, it is not possible to exclude a species-specific predisposition to the development of nephrotic changes following daunomycin, as is known to be the case for aminonucleoside.

d) Pathogenesis

The pathogenesis of daunomycin nephrosis can also be explained by a metabolic disturbance. Thus daunomycin, by adversely influencing DNA and RNA metabolism, results in a disruption of protein synthesis with the subsequent production of defective basement membrane material.

On the basis of the morphological findings seen in both aminonucleoside and daunomycin nephrosis a list of morphological criteria may be presented which when taken together point to a direct toxic effect of the drug upon glomerular structures:

1) Degenerative changes of the epithelial cells.
2) Fusion and loss of foot processes with a decrease in filtration slits and with an alteration of the residual filtration slits.
3) Alteration of basement membrane structure.
4) Separation of the epithelial cells from the basement membrane.
5) *De novo* synthesis of defective basement membrane material.
6) Lack of a constant and characteristic immunohistological fluorescence pattern.
7) Lack of a latent period between the i.v. application of the drug and the appearance of morphological changes.
8) The dependence of the degree of severity of the morphological changes in the glomerular region upon the dose and duration of the drug therapy.

3. Glomerular Lesions Associated with Other Cytostatic Drugs

A direct damage to the glomerular structures by other cytostatic agents has also been reported in individual instances. Thus, in both rat and guinea pig, the long-term administration of azathioprine (Imurek) has been reported to produce an increase of the mesangial matrix and a mesangial cell proliferation (*Wehner* 1975), although no functional deficiency was apparent. Both cyclophosphamide (Endoxan) and triethylenebenzoquinine (Trenimon) have been reported to induce a proteinuria in animals and also elicit glomerular changes, notably a thickening of the glomerular basement membrane with a secondary protein storage in the tubular epithelial cells (*Tessmann* et al.

1972). These alterations proved to be reversible following the withdrawal of the therapy.

Lopes (1967) first noted the appearance of a nephrotic syndrome in man following a cyclophosphamide therapy. *Kallenbach* and *Schattenfroh* (1961) further observed tubular necrosis following the administration of cyclophosphamide, and indeed in her report, *Lopes* (1967) also pointed out the presence of tubular necrosis in addition to the previously mentioned glomerular changes. This raises the question as to whether these glomerular lesions described by *Lopes* (1967) and *Tessmann* et al. (1972) might not be the result of an autoimmune mechanism. Thus, the direct nephrotoxic action of the cytostatic drug upon the tubular epithelial cells may lead to the production of autoantigens from this tissue. There may then ensue the formation of antibodies and immune complexes which might then be secondarily deposited in the region of the glomerular basement membrane and there lead to basement membrane thickening.

4. Glomerular Lesions Associated with Penicillamine

Whilst the renal side-effects appearing during penicillamine therapy are generally of immunological origin, there may also be an additional direct action of this drug upon glomerular structures. The evidence for this second direct pathomechanism has been provided by *Batsford* et al. (1976). Thus following the oral administration of a single dose of penicillamine (300–1500 mg/kg body weight) in the rat, a proteinuria was observed in association with both glomerular changes, which included a mesangial cell proliferation and an increase of the mesangial matrix, and tubular lesions characterised by the appearance of giant mitochondria in the tubular epithelial cells. Immunofluorescence findings were, however, with the exception of one case, completely negative. *Batsford* and co-workers (1976) considered that these negative immunofluorescence findings and the fact that the severity of both the glomerular changes and the clinical symptoms were dose-dependent, could be taken as indications of a direct effect of D-penicillamine upon the kidney.

It is possible that in one and the same organism both the direct, i.e. toxic effect and the later discussed indirect, immunological effect of penicillamine may play a role in the induction of glomerular lesions.

5. Glomerular Lesions Associated with Other Drugs

Finally it should be noted that individual reports point to an association between the administration of probenicid (an uricosuric) and the appearance of a nephrotic syndrome (*Ferris* et al. 1961; *Hertz* et al. 1972). Whereas in the report of *Ferris* et al. (1961) no morphological alterations were mentioned, *Hertz* et al. (1972) observed glomerular changes which took the form of a fusion of the foot processes combined with negative immunofluorescence findings. These morphological lesions, which are not indicative of an immune-complex glomerulonephritis but rather of a minimal proliferating intercapillary GN, as well as the fact that the nephrotic syndrome immediately disappears following withdrawal of the probenicid, are suggestive of a direct mechanism of action upon the kidney.

Moreover, it should be pointed out that one case has been reported where perchlorate therapy for thyrotoxicosis led to a nephrotic syndrome which appeared to be the result of toxic glomerular damage (*Lee* et al. 1961). Very questionable, however, is the claim made by *Schnall* and *Wiener* (1958) of a relationship between tolbutamide therapy and the appearance of a nephrotic syndrome, especially as no morphological examination was performed.

II. Indirect Effects of Drugs Upon Glomerular Structures Mediated by Immune Mechanisms

In principle every drug may be capable of influencing the immune system and may elicit hypersensitivity reactions of types I–IV. The drug may itself act as an antigen or, as is the case for most drugs, function as a hapten, which upon binding to a carrier protein (hapten-protein conjugate) constitutes the full antigen, thus inducing the immune response. Of importance is the fact that antigenicity may not only reside in the intact, pharmacologically active, form of the drug but also in its metabolites. Thus in one patient several antibodies may appear with varying specificities to a single drug and its metabolites.

Neither the type I hypersensitivity reaction, in the form of a generalised or local anaphylaxis (e.g. following penicillin), nor the cell-mediated immune reaction (the type IV hypersensitivity reaction, e.g. contact dermatitis) is currently thought to play any role in the pathogenesis of drug-induced glomerular changes. Rather the most significant pathogenic mechanism leading to the immunological glomerular damage seems to be the type III hypersensitivity reaction (Arthus phenomenon, serum sickness) and occasionally type II. These two latter immune reactions involve antigen-antibody interactions and may theoretically express themselves via two different mechanisms.

1. The drug or its metabolites act either as hapten or full antigen to induce antibody production, these substances in general representing the antigenic determinants. These antibodies may lead in one instance to the formation of circulating immune complexes which may then become deposited in the glomerular structures (e.g. subepithelial, subendothelial, mesangial), leading, via the resulting inflammatory process, to the induction of glomerular damage. A typical example of this is the animal model of acute and chronic serum sickness nephritis (type III hypersensitivity reaction) (*Dixon* et al. 1961; *Germuth* and *Rodriguez* 1973). This condition is triggered by the single administration of an exogenous antigen, which in this case is the drug or its metabolite acting as a hapten or full antigen.

Besides this form of immune-complex glomerulonephritis which is elicited by the deposition of circulating antigen-antibody complexes, a second form of immune-complex glomerulonephritis has been recently described (*van Damme* et al. 1978; *Salant* et al. 1979). Here it appears that the cause of the glomerular damage may be attributable to in situ immune complex formation. That is, free circulating antibody binds to extrarenal antigens (drug or metabolite) which have been previously entrapped in the glomerular structures, resulting in the triggering of a secondary inflammatory reaction.

2. A second, autoimmune, mechanism may also be invoked as playing a role in drug-induced glomerular damage. It might be envisioned that a drug or its metabolite

could produce alterations in somatic structures such that cell and tissue structures may subsequently act as antigenic determinants in addition to any antigenic properties of the drugs per se. That is, these structures represent autoantigens which lead to the production of autoantibodies.

The most important example of a drug-associated glomerular lesion produced by the deposition of circulating autologous antigen and antibody complexes is a drug-induced SLE with secondary renal involvement. In this case drug effects lead to the production of autoantibodies directed against cell nuclei or nuclear components. An autoimmune mechanism involving a drug-induced production of tubular autoantigens is also responsible for the development of an immune-complex glomerulonephritis. The animal model of this disease is the autologous immune-complex glomerulonephritis known as Heymann nephritis (*Heymann* et al. 1959; *Edgington* et al. 1968; *Glassock* et al. 1968).

Whereas these forms of autoimmune-complex glomerulonephritis might be compared with a type III hypersensitivity reaction, the autoimmune mechanisms present in an anti-basement-membrane glomerulonephritis might be better classified as a type II hyersensitivity reaction. In this instance chemical substances, which need not necessarily be drugs, produce an alteration in the glomerular basement membrane with the subsequent development of autoantigens and the induction of (cytotoxic) glomerular basement membrane antibodies. It is the interaction of these autoantibodies with the basement membrane which then leads, via a complement-mediated immunological process, to the morphological picture of an anti-basement-membrane glomerulonephritis.

The notion of the induction of an anti-basement-membrane glomerulonephritis by anti-basement-membrane antibodies is based upon the results obtained from animal experiments (*Steblay* 1962; *Lerner* and *Dixon* 1966), which seem to be equivalent to Goodpasture's syndrome observed in humans.

1. Penicillamine-Associated Glomerular Lesions (Penicillamine Nephropathy)

a) Introduction

Penicillamine (β-β-dimethylcystein), a breakdown product of penicillin, was discovered by *Abraham* et al. in 1943. Because of its ability to chelate copper ions, penicillamine was first introduced into medicine as a therapy for Wilson's disease (*Walshe* 1956) and later as a treatment for heavy metal poisoning. Based upon additional postulated therapeutic mechanisms of D-penicillamine, the range of indications for this drug has been extended to include the treatment of cystinuria, rheumatoid arthritis, chronic active hepatitis, primary biliary cirrhosis, scleroderma and interstitial lung fibrosis. Theories and hypotheses concerning the mode of action of the drug range from a depolymerisation of macromolecules via a reduction of the disulphide linkage, to an influence on collagen formation through an inhibition of intermolecular cross-linkages by binding to the aldehyde groups of tropocollagen, to an action upon the immune system, an inhibition of DNA and RNA synthesis, and finally to antiviral properties. However, the convincing and recognised efficacy of D-penicillamine in the treatment of the above-mentioned diseases stood in contrast to its high incidence of side-effects which were originally thought to be attributable only to the L-variant of the racemate. Thus, in 30% of the patients receiving penicillamine in the usual dose range (0.6--1.8 g/day) the therapy had to be discontinued on account of severe side-effects. These side-effects, besides those of gastrointestinal symptoms, taste impairment, allergic skin reactions, neurological disorders, haematological findings (aplastic anaemia, haemolytic anaemia, agranulocytosis, thrombocytopenia) and the development of an SLE syndrome, involved, above all, renal complications presenting as a proteinuria and nephrotic syndrome.

b) Frequency of Renal Side-Effects

The appearance of renal complications, which may be viewed along with disturbances of the haemopoietic system as the most serious side-effects of penicillamine, has been noted in some 10% (*Gros* and *Zwirner* 1975; *Dische* et al. 1976) to 20% of cases (Multicentre Trial Group 1973; *Day* and *Golding* 1974; *Huskisson* 1975; *Jaffe* 1974).

c) Clinical Findings

The results of our own investigations (*Hallauer* et al. 1974; *Gärtner* et al. 1975; *Gärtner*, Habilitation Thesis, 1977; *Neild* et al. 1979) as well as those of *Bacon* et al. (1976) and *Dische* et al. (1976) are in good agreement concerning the clinical symptomatology of penicillamine nephropathy. Typically following a mean period of therapy of 9.5 months renal symptoms appear which are characterised by proteinuria. In the majority of cases the proteinuria appeared as a nephrotic syndrome with a low-grade haematuria also being often present. On the other hand blood pressure, serum creatinine, and creatinine clearance are in most cases within the normal range.

d) Morphological Findings

The morphological changes observed in our own cases (*Hallauer* et al. 1974; *Gärtner* et al. 1975; *Lüttgen* et al. 1975; *Gärtner*, Habilitation Thesis, 1977; *Neild* et al. 1979) are in general agreement with those descriptions of individual cases which have been reported to date (*Jaffe* et al. 1968; *Lachmann* 1968; *Tribe* et al. 1975; *Bacon* et al. 1976; *Dische* et al. 1976). Thus it was possible to observe glomerular changes presenting the typical picture of perimembranous glomerulonephritis (Figs. 1 and 2) first in 31 renal biopsies (*Gärtner* et al. 1975) and later in 60 biopsies from 51 patients (*Gärtner*, Habilitation Thesis, 1977). Whereas examination of our biopsy material from penicillamine cases exclusively revealed perimembranous glomerulonephritis, the work of *Sternlieb* et al. (1975) and *Gibson* et al. (1976) records the presence of two cases and one case, respectively, exhibiting mesangio-proliferative glomerulonephritis with crescents. However, immunohistological examinations by these two groups revealed no linear fluorescence pattern but rather, in the instance of *Sternlieb* et al. (1975), a picture typical of immune-complex glomerulonephritis, whilst the immunofluorescence findings of *Gibson* et al. (1976) were negative.

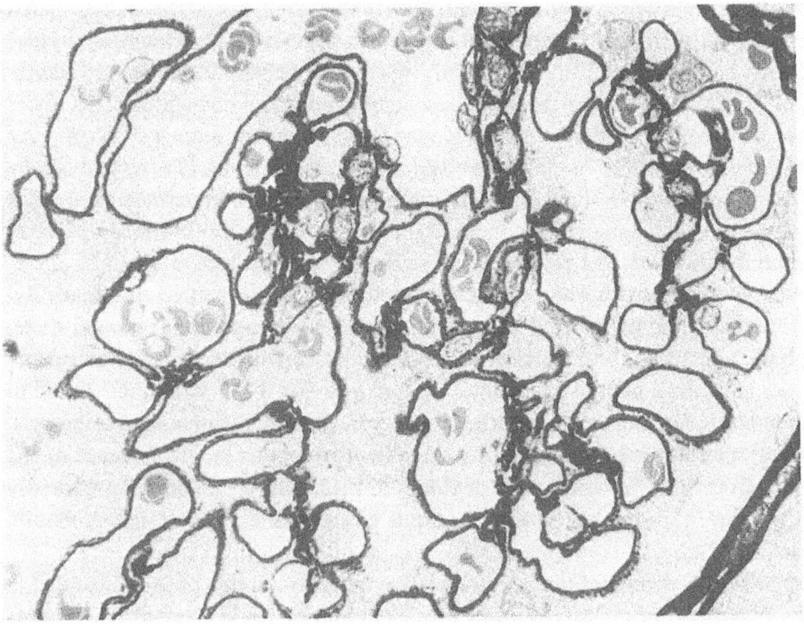

Fig. 1. Stage II of penicillamine-associated perimembranous glomerulonephritis: semithin section. Silver impregnation (Movat) X 900

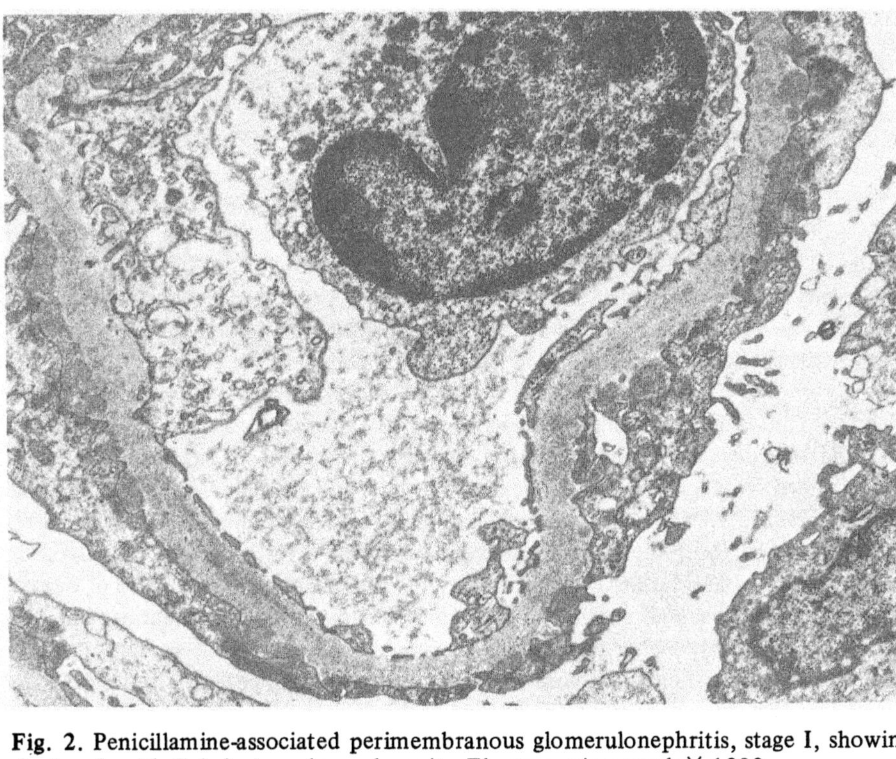

Fig. 2. Penicillamine-associated perimembranous glomerulonephritis, stage I, showing single subepithelial electron-dense deposits. Electron micrograph X 1200

In penicillamine-induced perimembranous glomerulonephritis the subepithelial deposits are markedly smaller than those observed in idiopathic perimembranous glomerulonephritis and are in addition often only deposited segmentally (*Gärtner*, Habilitation Thesis, 1977). Hence, the resulting basement membrane changes are of a lower intensity and of a segmental character. Such changes explain the findings of *Lachmann* (1968), *Henningsen* et al. (1973), *Tribe* et al. (1975), *Bacon* et al. (1976) and *Dische* et al. (1976) who reported their light microscopical observations either as an MPI or as inconspicuous, in spite of a concomitant positive immunofluorescence result and the demonstration of electron-dense deposits. In the instance of penicillamine-associated glomerulonephritis the basement membrane transformation processes develop in a manner identical to that seen in idiopathic perimembranous glomerulonephritis. This fact justifies the classification of these basement membrane changes occurring in penicillamine nephropathy into the same stages I–V as defined for idiopathic perimembranous glomerulonephritis. However, as penicillamine-associated perimembranous glomerulonephritis frequently shows only a segmental involvement of the basement membrane, the various stages of this condition follow one another markedly more quickly than in idiopathic perimembranous glomerulonephritis (*Gärtner,* Habilitation Thesis, 1977).

The diagnosis of perimembranous glomerulonephritis has also been established in our patients following an immunofluorescence examination. In agreement with the results of *Jaffe* et al. (1968), *Lachmann* (1968), *Tribe* et al. (1975) and *Dische* et al. (1976) we have also observed in practically all cases a fine granular fluorescence pattern of co-deposits of IgG and C_3, with the fluorescence intensity of the latter being in general lower than that of the IgG.

e) Clinical and Morphological Correlations

A result of our investigations was the fact that neither the duration of therapy nor the dosage of penicillamine administered had any influence upon the stage of the disease presented at the time of biopsy (*Gärtner*, Habilitation Thesis, 1977). Furthermore, our results also indicated that the degree of proteinuria observed at the time of biopsy was, like the disease stage, independent of both the duration and the dosage of penicillamine therapy (*Gärtner*, Habilitation Thesis, 1977). In fact the severity of the proteinuria was only dependent upon the degree of the glomerular basement membrane changes. Thus with increasing duration of the disease there was a tendency for the proteinuria to decrease; it had practically disappeared by stage V (Fig. 3).

Whereas the degree of the proteinuria is independent of the total penicillamine dosage (*Henningsen* et al. 1973; *Bacon* et al. 1976; *Gärtner*, Habilitation Thesis, 1977) the duration of the proteinuria does seem to be related to the quantity of the drug given (*Gärtner*, Habilitation Thesis, 1977). Thus, it was apparent that those of our patients who still presented a persistent proteinuria after one year of treatment had received a significantly higher total dosage of penicillamine during the same period than had the group of patients in whom the proteinuria had disappeared. This suggests the possibility that the quantity of the antigen-antibody complexes deposited or formed in situ might play a role in the duration of the repair process.

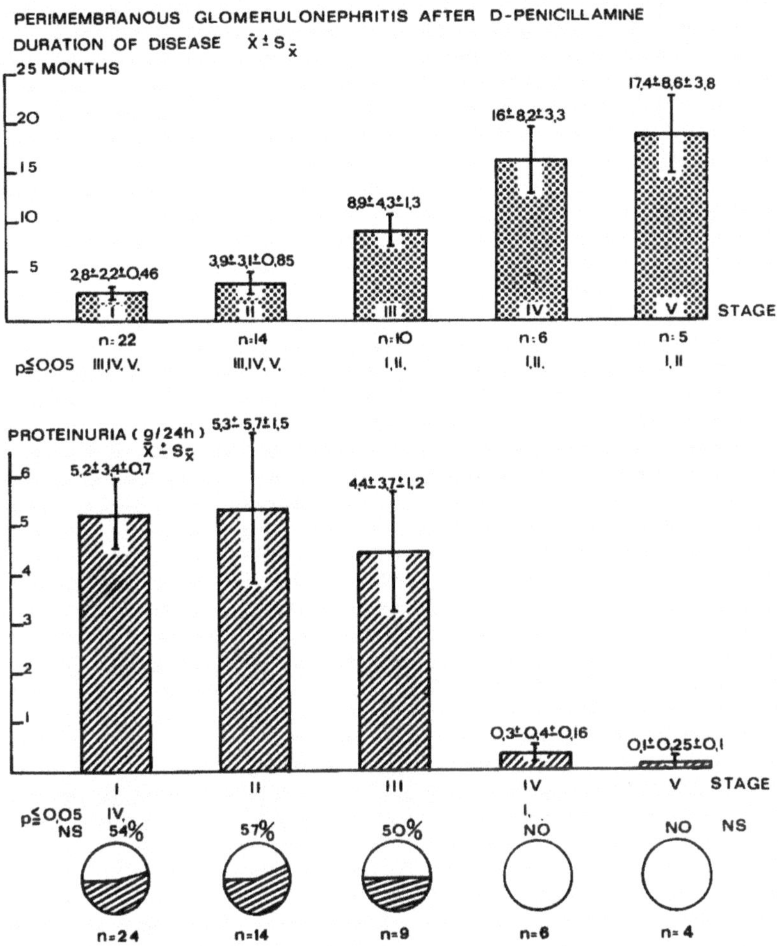

Fig. 3. Penicillamine-associated perimembranous glomerulonephritis. Relationships between duration of the disease, severity of proteinuria, frequency of nephrotic syndrome and the stages I–V, in 60 biopsies of 51 patients (*Gärtner,* Habilitation Thesis, 1977)

f) Course of the Disease and Prognosis

Despite the fact that *Falck* et al. (1979) reported the death of two patients, presenting in one case, renal complications in the form of perimembranous glomerulonephritis with renal vasculitis and, in the other, a MPI, following penicillamine therapy, the prognosis for penicillamine-induced perimembranous glomerulonephritis is nevertheless generally quite favourable. In fact in over 60% of our cases withdrawal of the penicillamine therapy resulted in a disappearance of the proteinuria in the course of the following year. Our morphological observation of the disease process in serial renal biopsies also permits us to state that the prognosis for penicillamine-induced perimembranous glomerulonephritis is much more favourable than that of idiopathic perimembranous glomerulonephritis (*Hallauer* et al. 1974; *Lüttgen* et al. 1975; *Gärtner*, Habilitation Thesis, 1977; *Neild* et al. 1979). Thus in 9 out of 10 of our cases with serial renal biopsies there was an improvement after a period of one year not only in clinical symptoms but also in the morphological changes of the basement membrane; that is, a repair process had occurred.

g) Pathogenesis

Other authors (*Bachmann* et al. 1975; *Dixon* et al. 1975; *Hamilton* 1975) have reported that both the frequency and the severity of the proteinuria were dependent upon the dosage and duration of penicillamine therapy, which they claimed to indicate a toxic effect of penicillamine. However, results from our group do not confirm these findings or conclusions. Thus one group of our patients developed, following a short period of administration of penicillamine at low dosage, a severe proteinuria or nephrotic syndrome. Our results seem to be comparable with those of *Sternlieb* (1966) and *Bacon* et al. (1976). Additionally *Zimmermann* and *Friedrich* (1977) also failed to demonstrate any toxic effects of D-penicillamine when administered in therapeutically effective doses.

Just as aminonucleoside nephrosis may be regarded as a model for drug-induced nephropathy in animals, so penicillamine nephropathy may be similarly looked upon as a correlate of this disease in humans.

In conclusion it seems highly probable that the pathogenetic basis of penicillamine nephropathy lies with an immunological mechanism involving the development of an immune-complex glomerulonephritis of the chronic serum sickness type. However, the nature of the deposited antigen present in penicillamine-induced perimembranous glomerulonephritis has not been established. Since penicillamine has a low molecular weight it can perhaps only function as a hapten. Indeed it is plausible that penicillamine or one of its breakdown products (e.g., penicilloic acid, penicilloyl aldehyde) binds to an autologous protein, thus forming the full antigen. Since a number of our patients, like those of *Helmke* et al. (1975), developed antinuclear factors (that is; antibodies to denatured DNA) during penicillamine therapy, with some individuals even developing the clinical symptoms of SLE, one cannot exclude the possibility that penicillamine elicits the production of autoantigens.

Taken together the following findings argue in favour of immune complex formation being the pathogenetic mechanism of penicillamine nephropathy:

1) The results of animal experiments (*Seelig* et al. 1977), which reveal that following penicillamine administration one can observe an immune-complex glomerulonephritis with the granular deposition of IgG and C_3 along the glomerular basement membrane and in the mesangium. In these experiments the intensity of the immunohistologically identifiable deposits, which is correlated with the quantitiy of immune complexes, was dependent upon the dosage of penicillamine administered. Upon withdrawal of the penicillamine both the clinical symptoms and the immunofluorescent deposits disappeared.
2) The constant and characteristic immunohistological pattern of an immune-complex glomerulonephritis of the perimembranous glomerulonephritis type with the cor-

roborating electron-microscopic picture. A nephrotoxic pathomechanism, as for instance in aminonucleoside nephrosis, does not lead to these morphological changes.

3) The temporal relationship between penicillamine therapy and the appearance of renal symptoms, which contra-indicates a mere coincidental occurrence of perimembranous glomerulonephritis.
4) The lack of a correlation between duration of therapy and dosage of penicillamine administered, on the one hand, and either the severity of the proteinuria or morphological changes at the time of biopsy on the other.
5) The reversibility of both the clinical and the morphological findings upon withdrawal of penicillamine, which also points to a limited amount of antigen.
6) The demonstration of circulating antibodies against penicillamine or its metabolites (penicilloic acid or penicilloyl aldehyde); the positive reaction to penicillamine-polylysine in the intracutaneous test as well as the demonstration of D-penicillamine antibodies in positive ring tests (*Amos* 1968; *Lüttgen* et al. 1975).

2. Glomerular Lesions Associated with Gold Preparations

a) Introduction

Used for many years in the treatment of RA (rheumatoid arthritis), a therapy with gold preparations in the form of organic salts of gold (aurothiopolypeptide = Auro-Detoxin, aurothioglucose = Auriothan, sodium aurothiomalate = Tauredon) can be associated clinically with the appearance of renal symptoms, in addition to other side-effects, which include alterations of the skin and the development of thrombocytopenia.

b) Frequency of Renal Side-Effects

The frequency of appearance of renal symptoms in the form of proteinuria following the administration of gold salts has been variously reported (*Hartfall* et al. 1937: 1–3%; or *Meyboom* 1975: 12.5%).

c) Clinical Findings

As reported by other authors (*Lee* et al. 1965; *Silverberg* et al. 1970; *Katz* and *Little* 1973; *Törnroth* and *Skrifvars* 1974; *Watanabe* et al. 1976) 30 of our biopsied cases had developed proteinuria during a period of chrysotherapy, which manifested itself as a nephrotic syndrome in over one third of these cases (*Gärtner*, Habilitation Thesis, 1977). In general the character of the disease at the time of biopsy resembled that of a penicillamine-induced nephropathy.

d) Morphological Findings

In all of the cases examined we could clearly identify morphological changes typical of perimembranous glomerulonephritis, corresponding to the reports of other investigators (*Lee* et al. 1965; *Silverberg* et al. 1970; *Strunk* and *Ziff* 1970; *Katz* and *Little* 1973; *Törnroth* and *Skrifvars* 1974; *Watanabe* et al. 1976). As in penicillamine nephropathy, but in contrast to idiopathic PGN, small and often segmentally deposited immune deposits were evident. However, the basement membrane transformation processes were identical with those of idiopathic PGN (*Silverberg* et al. 1970; *Katz* and *Little* 1973; *Törnroth* and *Skrifvars* 1974). A differential diagnostic demarcation of gold-induced PGN is possible by the detection of gold granules. In this context we are in agreement with other authors in having been able electronmicroscopically to detect lysosomal gold granules in the tubular epithelial cells (*Silverberg* et al. 1970; *Katz* and *Little* 1973; *Watanabe* et al. 1976) as well as occasionally in the glomerular epithelial cells (*Strunk* and *Ziff* 1970; *Vaamonde* and *Hunt* 1970; *Watanabe* et al. 1976) and in mesangial cells (*Silverberg* et al. 1970; *Strunk* and *Ziff* 1970; *Katz* and *Little* 1973) (Fig. 4). However, neither we nor other authors (*Silverberg* and *Ziff* 1970) have been able to detect gold particles in the subepithelial or intramembranous deposits using either the electron microscope or X-ray microanalysis (*Watanabe* et al. 1976).

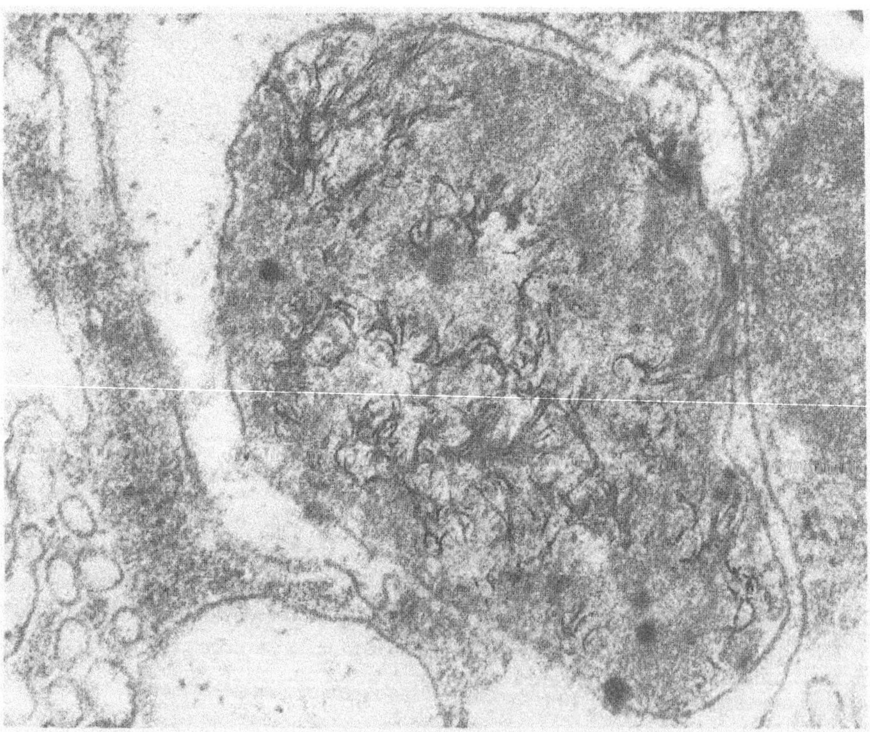

Fig. 4. Perimembranous glomerulonephritis following gold therapy: Electron micrograph demonstrating the presence of gold particles in lysosomes of the proximal tubular epithelium. X 625 000

e) Clinical and Morphological Correlations

As also reported by *Törnroth* and *Skrifvars* (1974) our results indicate that there is no influence of either the total gold dosage administered or the duration of gold therapy upon either the severity of the morphological renal changes or the degree of proteinuria at the time of biopsy. These results, which argue against a nephrotoxic action of gold salts, confirm the report of *Silverberg* et al. (1970), in as much as these authors could show no correlation between the severity of the renal symptoms and either the amount of gold administered or the blood and urine gold levels. In contrast we have previously established (*Gärtner*, Habilitation Thesis, 1977) that a correlation does exist between the duration of the disease and the degree of the basement membrane transformation, as it does in both penicillamine-associated and idiopathic PGN. Moreover, the duration of the disease in the individual stages is comparable to that of penicillamine-associated PGN, i.e. markedly shorter than for idiopathic PGN.

f) Course and Prognosis of the Disease

In addition to our results (*Gärtner*, Habilitation Thesis, 1977) those of other authors (*Lee* et al. 1965; *Silverberg* et al. 1970; *Strunk* and *Ziff* 1970; *Vaamonde* and *Hunt* 1970; *Katz* and *Little* 1973; *Törnroth* and *Skrifvars* 1974) indicate that both the clinical and morphological alterations may be reversed upon withdrawal of the therapy.

g) Pathogenesis

Several lines of evidence argue against a coincidental appearance of a PGN during gold therapy. Thus there is the close temporal relationship between the initiation of the therapy and the appearance of renal symptoms as well as the fact that both the clinical and morphological changes are reversible upon withdrawal of the drug. However, perhaps the strongest evidence is the induction of PGN by gold salts in animals (*Nagi* et al. 1971). Whilst the pathogenesis of gold-induced PGN is still largely unclear, the morphological picture of an immune-complex nephritis and the lack of any influence of both the duration of therapy and the gold dosage upon the severity of the morphological and clinical pictures suggest an immunological pathomechanism. In addition there is the serological demonstration of various antibodies and antigen-antibody systems in one patient with a gold nephropathy (*Palosuo* et al. 1976), which also supports the foregoing contention. One obvious explanation of this condition, which has not to date been verified, is that gold behaves as a hapten and generates the production of antibodies; there thus being the deposition of gold protein-antibody complexes in the glomerular subepithelium. An alternative hypothesis also involves an immunological pathomechanism where there is the development of an autologous immune-complex nephritis of the Heymann nephritis type. In this instance it is postulated that gold, in the form of its soluble salt, has a direct toxic effect upon tubular structures (mitochondria), which in turn leads to the production of autoantigens. Subsequently there would be immune complex formation with the resulting production of a PGN. Again, several pieces of evidence support such a hypothetical pathomechanism, namely: the destructive effect of gold upon mitochondria (*Struve* and *Galle* 1970), the persistent demonstration of gold particles in the tubulo-epithelium (*Yarom* et al. 1975; *Viol* et al. 1977), and the observation of tubular necrosis following the administration of high doses of gold (*Derot* et al. 1954; *Nagi* et al. 1971).

3. Glomerular Lesions Produced by Mercury (Mercury Nephropathy)

a) Introduction

Mercury compounds, like other heavy metals (gold), have been used as therapeutic agents, most notably in mercury diuretics and mercury-containing ointments. Like gold preparations, mercury-containing medications are known to produce side-effects, the most noticeable being renal damage, alterations of the skin and damage to the bone marrow (*Derow* and *Wolff* 1947; *Zollinger* 1955; *Becker* et al. 1962; *Mandema* et al. 1963; *Cameron* and *Trounce* 1965; *Silverberg* et al. 1967). Particularly during the last few years reports have been accumulating concerning the appearance of a nephrotic syndrome in young female Africans following the use of a mercury-containing bleaching cream (*Barr* et al. 1972; *Kibukamusoke* et al. 1974).

b) Frequency of Renal Side-Effects

The incidence of a nephrotic syndrome has been assessed at 4% (*Kanzantzis* et al. 1962) and proteinuria has been reported to occur in 16% of the cases (*Young* 1960).

c) Clinical Findings

Our estimation of the clinical picture of mercury nephropathy is in agreement with that of other authors (*Becker* et al. 1962; *Barr* et al. 1972; *Kibukamusoke* et al. 1974) in that the condition is characterised by a severe proteinuria or nephrotic syndrome.

d) Morphological Findings

In the two cases which we have examined the morphological changes were generally consistent with a PGN, with the basement membrane alterations being particularly pronounced and indistinguishable from those of idiopathic PGN. Furthermore, both the morphological and clinical course of mercury-associated nephropathy are more unfavourable when compared with either gold- or penicillamine-associated PGN. Thus, in addition to the basement membrane changes one patient had also developed interstitial nephritis with tubular necrosis, degenerative tubular alterations with tubular atrophy, and interstitial fibrosis with infiltration of mononuclear cells. It was these alterations which had led to the raised serum creatinine value and the increasing

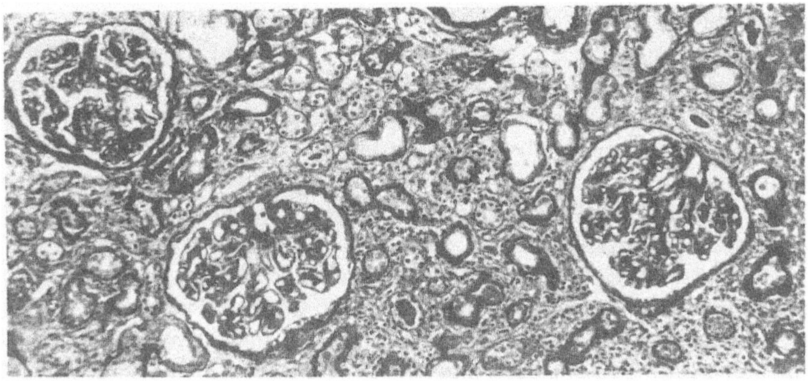

Fig. 5. Mercury-associated perimembranous glomerulonephritis showing an interstitial fibrosis and interstitial infiltration as well as tubular atrophy and degenerative tubular changes. PAS reaction X 144

renal insufficiency in this patient (Fig. 5). These changes in the interstitium, which are apparent in mercury nephropathy but which are absent in both penicillamine and gold nephropathies, are possibly the expression of a different pathomechanism.

e) Pathogenesis

On the basis of animal experiments some authors earlier thought that the renal symptoms produced by mercury compounds were attributable to a direct nephrotoxic effect of the heavy metal upon the tubuli (*Zollinger* 1955; *Gritzka* and *Trump* 1968). However, it is now realised that mercury compounds may produce renal damage via various mechanisms. Thus, besides the direct toxic effect of high doses of mercury compounds upon the tubuli, lower doses over longer periods produce glomerular changes for which an immune pathomechanism seems to be responsible. This immune pathomechanism may be triggered in various ways: *Bariéty* et al. (1971) reported the production of a mercury-induced immune-complex glomerulonephritis of a PGN type in Wistar rats, whilst *Sapin* et al. (1977) found an anti-basement-membrane glomerulonephritis with a linear fluorescence pattern in another strain of rat. Moreover, *Roman-Franco* et al. (1978) observed glomerular changes, where, in addition to antiglomerular basement membrane antibodies with a linear fluorescence, there were also deposits of immune complexes in the glomeruli with a granular fluorescence pattern. These findings appear to be the consequence of a glomerulopathy which proceeds in two phases. The first phase seem to be an anti-basement-membrane glomerulonephritis, whilst in the second phase there is the superimposition of an immune-complex glomerulonephritis. A likely candidate for the antigen in the second phase seems to be altered subendothelial elements of the glomerular basement membrane (*Hinglais* et al. 1979). Finally, following the administration of mercury to animals *Weening* et al. (1978) succeeded in demonstrating the presence of antinuclear antibodies which had subsequently formed immune complexes, these complexes having become deposited along the glomerular basement membrane and in the mesangium. Which of these immune mechanisms of mercury-induced nephropathy elucidated in animal systems is responsible for mercury nephropathy in man is uncertain at the present. However, it is certain that all of the mercury-induced glomerular lesions known in man may be viewed as immune-complex glomerulonephritis, although it remains an open question as to how the mercury contributes to the generation of the antigen. Two possible mechanisms may be proposed: the first is that mercury acts directly as a hapten, and the second is that the heavy metal elicits indirectly an immune mechanism. In the second mechanism it might be suggested that mercury causes the release of tubular autoantigens via toxic tubular damage. These autoantigens subsequently lead to a PGN of the Heymann nephritis type with a concomitant deposition of immune complexes in the interstitium producing an additional autologous interstitial immune-complex nephritis (*Andres* and *McCluskey* 1975). These proposals are supported, above all, both by our observation of interstitial inflammation processes [as remarked upon earlier by *Freeman* et al. (1962)] and our demonstration of electron-dense deposits within the interstitium, as well as the unfavourable clinical course of the disease, a fact which has also been reported by *Morel-Maroger* and *Verroust* (1975).

4. Glomerular Lesions Associated with Trimethadione (Tridione) and Distraneurine Therapy

a) Clinical Findings

Administration of trimethadione both in humans, as a therapy for petit-mal epilepsy in children, and in rats (*Heymann* et al. 1960) may lead to the appearance of a nephrotic syndrome, as noted by many authors (*Barnett* et al. 1948; *Nabarro* and *Rosenheim* 1952; *Haugen* 1957; *Bar-Khayim* et al. 1973). Our investigations also reveal the appearance of a nephrotic syndrome in one patient who had been treated for one month with trimethadione for petit-mal epilepsy.

b) Morphological Findings

Light and electron microscopical as well as immunohistological results reveal the morphological picture of renal changes characteristic of a perimembranous glomerulonephritis, as has also been noted by other investigators (*Rosenblum* et al. 1959; *Bar-Khayim* et al. 1973).

Possibly the morphological changes reported by *Bergstrand* et al. (1962), who noted in addition to a minimal focal cell proliferation an irregular thickening of the glomerular capillary wall, might also represent a PGN.

c) Pathogenesis

On the basis of the morphological findings one might postulate that the pathomechanism of trimethadione-induced renal damage lies with an immune process. Perhaps this drug acting as a hapten could cause the development of a self-limiting (since the amount of antigen available is defined) immune-complex glomerulonephritis of the serum sickness type. In favour of this notion is the observation made both in this group and elsewhere that following cessation of therapy there ensues a favourable course of the disease (*Nabarro* and *Rosenheim* 1952; *Haugen* 1957; *Hooft* et al. 1962; *Bar-Khayim* et al. 1973).

The pathogenetic mechanisms which lead to the development of a PGN in cases of distraneurine addiction are unclear, although they may also involve hapten effects.

5. Glomerular Lesions Associated with Captopril

a) Introduction

Captopril (Lopirin), through its ability to inhibit converting enzyme, is employed as an effective antihypertensive drug in modern medicine. However, in addition to its antihypertensive properties, captopril has a number of side-effects which include skin rashes, fever and loss of taste. During 1979 this list of side-effects was further extended to include renal symptoms following observations made on two patients receiving captopril therapy (*Prins* et al. 1979; *Hoorntje* et al. 1979).

b) Clinical and Morphological Findings

Both cases exhibited an acute nephrotic syndrome which appeared to be the consequence of morphological glomerular changes characteristic of an early stage of PGN, since it was possible to demonstrate subepithelial electron-dense deposits and a segmental, granular immunofluorescence pattern along the glomerular basement membrane. Besides IgG deposits one could also recognise deposits of IgA, IgM and C_3. In one of these cases it was reported that the clinical symptoms disappeared following the cessation of captopril therapy.

c) Pathogenesis

On the basis of the foregoing findings we feel that a causal relationship between the administration of captopril and the appearance of an immune-complex glomerulonephritis has been established. Since captopril is a peptide it is possible that it may act directly as an antigen rather than as a hapten.

6. Glomerular Lesions Produced by Sulphadiazine-Silver Therapy

Finally one might consider the case report of *Owens* et al. (1974) where it was observed that a patient who had been treated with sulphadiazine-silver therapy for severe burns had developed a nephrotic syndrome with the morphological correlate of an immune-complex GN. However, whether this immune-complex glomerulonephritis was the result of the basic disease (burns antigens) or rather a product of the sulphadiazine-silver therapy remains unaswered.

7. Glomerular Lesions Associated with Drug-Induced Systemic Lupus Erythematosus (SLE) with Secondary Renal Involvement

a) Introduction

Shortly following the first description of the erythematosus cell phenomenon by *Hargraves* (1969) came the report of an appearance of SLE in association with drug therapy. In this latter context, SLE may be induced by the most various range of therapeutic agents, which may have quite different structures and effects as well as totally different patterns of metabolic degradation. The following groups of drugs are known to be able to trigger SLE:

I. *Antiarrhythmics*
   1. Procainamide
   2. Practolol

II. *Antibiotics*
   1. Sulphonamides
   2. Penicillin
   3. Tetracycline
   4. Streptomycin
   5. Para-aminosalicylic acid
   6. Griseofulvin
   7. Isoniozid

III. *Anticonvulsives*
   1. Hydantoin derivatives: trimethadione, diphenylhydantoin, mephenytoin, phenytoin, trioxidone
   2. Succinamide: ethosuximide
   3. Barbiturates: primidione
   4. Others: carpamazepin, pheneturide

IV. *Antihypertensives*
   1. Guanoxan
   2. Hydralazine
   3. Methyl-DOPA
   4. Reserpine

V. *Thyrostatics*
   1. Methylthiouracil
   2. Propylthiouracil

VI. *Miscellaneous*
   1. Chlorpromazine
   2. D-penicillamine
   3. Methylsergit
   4. Contraceptives
   5. Phenylbutazone

Whilst the appearance of antinuclear factors (ANF or ANA) is observed in almost all patients receiving the above-mentioned drugs [procainamide: *Henningsen* et al. (1975): 83%; *Lee* and *Chase* (1975): 50–74%, isoniazid: *Lee* and *Chase* (1975): 25%] the manifestation of clinical symptoms of SLE is more rare [procainamide: *Harpey* (1974): 12–25%; *Henningsen* et al. (1975): 29%; *Bernstein* (1979): 10–30%; hydralazine: *Lee* and *Chase* (1975): 2–21%]. In fact in the instance of patients who developed antinuclear antibodies during the course of methyl-DOPA therapy no clinical symptoms of SLE were apparent. All the above-named drugs frequently elicit the production of antinuclear antibodies, although the specificity of these antibodies may vary:

1. Procainamide (Blomgren et al. 1972): Antibodies are directed against denatured DNA (singel-stranded DNA), nucleohistone, the cell membrane of erythrocytes and IgG, whilst anti-procainamide antibodies are only rarely found.

2. Hydralazine (Lee and Chase 1975): Antibodies against deoxyribonucleoprotein, native DNA [identified by *Hahn* et al. (1972) as being present in all patients treated with hydralazine] and hydralazine itself.

3. Isoniazid (Lee and Chase 1975): Antibodies directed against soluble nucleoprotein (antibodies to nucleoprotein and whole nucleus).

4. Hydantoin (Lee and Chase 1975): Antibody to soluble nucleoprotein.

The clinical criteria for the diagnosis of drug-induced SLE are the same as those for the diagnosis of idiopathic SLE. Thus, for a drug to be considered as being the cause of SLE the following points must be fulfilled (*Lee* and *Chase* 1975):

1) Prior to the administration of the drug these must be no symptoms of SLE.
2) The therapeutic agent must be administered over a definite period of time (approximately 3 weeks to 2 years).
3) Following the withdrawal of the drug therapy there should be an improvement in the clinical situation within days, whilst the serological findings could persist for months or years.
4) Renewed administration of the drug should lead immediately, that is within hours or days, to a reappearance of clinical symptoms.

The frequency of appearance of a SLE syndrome following drug administration is dependent upon the type of therapeutic agent given. Likewise the type of clinical symptoms manifested and the severity of the clinical picture of the disease are also drug-type-dependent.

Therefore, a particular drug may elicit either the full picture of SLE or merely an oligo- or monosymptomatic form of the disease. The most frequent incidences of drug-induced SLE syndrome are noted during procainamide (4–9%) and hydralazine (2–21%) therapy (*Blomgren* et al. 1972). Moreover, the manifestation of the disease is independent of both the dose of the drug given and the duration of therapy. In general, however, from the total population of patients receiving hydralazine, procainamide, practolol or D-penicillamine, one percent will develop the clinical manifestations of an SLE syndrome (*Lee* and *Chase* 1975). The clinical picture of drug-induced SLE exhibits certain marked differences to that of idiopathic SLE: thus for instance a procainamide-induced SLE syndrome is less severely pronounced, less feverish, and shows less frequent skin and renal symptoms, although there is a more frequent pleuropulmonary involvement (*Blomgren* et al. 1972; *Lee* and *Chase* 1975). However, the greatest difference lies in the frequency of renal manifestations, which in the case of idiopathic SLE has been estimated at between 70 and 80% (*Muehrcke* et al. 1957; *Rothfield* et al. 1963; *Pollak* et al. 1964; *Zweimann* et al. 1968), whereas the incidence of renal involvement in cases of drug-induced SLE is much lower. *Blomgren* and co-workers (1972) have explained these differences by the fact that in drug-induced SLE there is only rarely a production of anti-native-DNA antibodies; the native DNA being supposed to represent the relevant nephritogenic antigen since in idiopathic SLE anti-native-DNA antibodies represent the predominant component of glomerular immune complexes (*Koffler* et al. 1971). A similar interpretation has been put forward by *Henningsen* et al. (1975), who could demonstrate that in general the ANF found in idiopathic SLE reacted exclusively with native DNA and were, moreover, complement-binding.

Hitherto the preponderance of individual reports concerning the appearance of renal symptoms with a drug-induced SLE syndrome have referred to the following drugs:

1) Hydralazine: *White* (1966); *Alarcón-Segovia* et al. (1967)
2) Anticonvulsives (Tridione, Maliasin, Zentropil, Neo-Citrollamin) (*Jacobs* 1963; *Thönes* et al. 1972)
3) Thyreostatics (propylthiouracil): *Amrhein* et al. (1970)
4) Penicillamine: *Elsas* et al. (1971); *Brass* et al. (1976).
5) Procainamide: *Castleman* and *McNeely* (1968); *Rutherford* (1968); *Günther* et al. (1969), *Whittingham* and *McKay* (1970); *Whitle* and *Ainsworth* (1976); *Zech* et al. (1979).

b) Clinical Findings

The clinical symptoms associated with drug-induced SLE with renal involvement are identical with those associated with idiopathic SLE, and are characterised by a severe proteinuria mostly in the form of a nephrotic syndrome.

c) Morphological Findings

The morphological glomerular changes occurring in drug-induced SLE correspond to those seen in idiopathic SLE, that is, glomerulonephritis of the immune-complex type. Thus *Thönes* et al. (1972) have reported two cases of a drug-induced SLE with renal manifestations. One of these patients presented the typical picture of a perimembranous glomerulonephritis, whilst the other revealed a mesangio-proliferative glomerulonephritis with focal/segmental accentuation. These morphological findings are identical to those seen in idiopathic SLE, this being particularly noticeable in the second case, with signs of activity in the form of a focal/segmental accentuation being present (*Pollak* et al. 1964) and with the simultaneous appearance of deposits on diverse glomerular structures, e.g. in subepithelial, subendothelial and intramembranous positions, as well as within the mesangium. The presence of an immune-complex glomerulonephritis has been verified both by immunohistological and electron microscopical findings.

There exist further reports of an immune-complex glomerulonephritis being associated with a procainamide induced SLE syndrome. In one instance the immune-complex glomerulonephritis took the form of a PGN (*Castleman* and *McNeely* 1968; *Günther* et al. 1969; *Whittingham* and *McKay* 1970), whereas other authors reported changes representing a mesangio-proliferative glomerulonephritis with focal/segmental accentuation and with the concomitant deposition of immune complexes in both the mesangium and subendothelium (*Whittle* and *Ainsworth* 1976; *Zech* et al. 1979).

Moreover, *Zech* et al. (1979) further described the presence of interstitial changes with a pronounced lymphoplasma-cell infiltration, typical of idiopathic SLE. *Brass* et al. (1976) have also indicated similar morphological changes in their patients suffering from a D-penicillamine glomerulopathy. In all cases these changes have been described as constituting a mesangioproliferative glomerulonephritis with irregular thickening of the walls of the glomerular capillary loops and with a marked mononuclear-cell infiltration of the interstitium. Consideration of the light microscopical and immunofluorescence findings, as well as the fact that antinuclear factors were detected in practically all these patients, leads to the conclusion that one is dealing here with the renal manifestations of a penicillamine-induced SLE syndrome.

We were also able to detect amongst our patients with a D-penicillamine-associated PGN some who exhibited the clinical symptoms of SLE syndrome and who were positive for antinuclear antibodies. Following withdrawal of D-penicillamine both the clinical and the serological findings progressively disappeared.

d) Pathogenesis

The pathogenesis of both drug-induced SLE and its associated immune-complex glomerulonephritis is uncertain although a number of possibilities have been proposed. In addition to genetic factors such as a sex-dependent predisposition to the disease (*Siegel* et al. 1967) and the increased tendency for the condition to appear within one family, there is the suggestion that procainamide and hydralazine may form complexes with DNA. It is this drug-DNA complex which then acts as a full antigen and induces antibody synthesis, the antibody being capable of cross-reacting with native DNA. Furthermore, it is assumed that cross-reactivity will also occur with analogous antigenic structures of procainamide and DNA. Moreover, procainamide, like many drugs, may bind to cell membrane structures and thus lead to the formation of the corresponding autoantibodies (*Bluestein* et al. 1979). The antigenic efficiency of these drugs is probably enhanced by a defective metabolic degradation, which is seen as a genetically determined slow rate of acetylation (*Perry* et al. 1970; *Woosley* et al. 1978).

However, the critical role in the immune-complex pathogenesis of drug-induced SLE syndrome seems to be played by the complexing of the drug with catabolically released DNA (*Grabar* 1974), the drug-DNA complex provoking antibody formation (*Alarcón-Segovia* et al. 1969).

It is a characteristic of both idiopathic and drug-induced SLE that one finds various types of antigens present which result in the formation of both qualitatively and quantitatively different immune complexes. This accounts for the fact that in drug-induced SLE there may also appear various types of immune-complex glomerulonephritis. It explains in addition why in individual cases there are diverse sites of immune-complex deposition within the glomeruli and why immune complexes are frequently observed in the interstitium.

8. Glomerular Lesions Produced by Heroin (Diacetylmorphine)

a) Introduction

Although the addictive drug heroin cannot be classified as a therapeutic agent, in view of its current social significance the opportunity will be taken here to discuss the known glomerular changes associated with heroin addiction.

b) Frequency of Renal Side-Effects

Friedman et al. (1974) have estimated that 1% of drug addicts develop a nephropathy.

c) Clinical Findings

The clinical manifestations are in most cases a severe proteinuria or nephrotic syndrome, with haematuria only being rarely observed.

d) Morphological Findings

Although basically all forms of a glomerulonephritis have been observed in instances of drug addiction, a significant incidence of glomerular changes, consistent with those of a focal sclerosing glomerulonephritis have been reported (*Rao* et al. 1974; *Eknoyan* et al. 1975; *Grishman* et al. 1976; *Churg* and *Grishman* 1978). In addition to focal sclerosis one also observes a proliferation of epithelial cells, the latter also showing evidence of severe degenerative changes; they may also become partially detached from the glomerular basement membrane with the resulting cleft becoming filled with fibrillar basement-membrane-like material (*Grishman* et al. 1976). It is possible that the findings of *Kilcoyne* et al. (1972), which were described as a focal membrano-proliferative glomerulonephritis, might represent similar changes to those cited above. This seems more certain since the immunofluorescence results obtained by *Kilcoyne* et al. (1972), of an irregular deposition of IgM and C_3 in the glomeruli, are identical to those reported by *Salomon* et al. (1972) and *Friedman* et al. (1974).

Grishmann et al. (1976) take the view that the imposing renal changes observed in drug addicts, which are often evident as a focal sclerosing glomerulonephritis, represent a particular phase of a single disease process. This process may manifest itself in its least severe form as a minimal proliferating intercapillary glomerulonephritis, whilst its other extreme is a focal-global sclerosing glomerulonephritis.

e) Pathogenesis

The pathogenesis of these glomerular changes has still to be clearly established. However, the fact that the morphological picture bears a remarkable resemblance to that of experimental aminonucleoside nephrosis has lead *Grishmann* et al. (1976) to suppose a toxic drug action. Further evidence contra-indicates an immunological pathomechanism since glomerular changes characteristic of a PGN, which is a typical example of an immune-complex glomerulonephritis, have not generally been observed. In fact, not a single drug addict was to be identified amongst 160 patients presenting PGN (*Ehrenreich* et al. 1975). Other evidence, however, is rather unsupportive of a nephrotoxic mechanism since administration of morphine sulphate to animals did not induce any glomerular changes (*Marchand* et al. 1963). Other reports might lead us to suppose an immune pathomechanism for heroin-induced glomerular damage. Thus it is known that 25–75% of heroin addicts develop elevated IgM titres which are independent of the solvent employed (*Ryan* et al. 1972; *Cushman* 1974), whereas addicts who inhale the drug through the nose show normal IgM levels. In addition it has been observed that when heroin was substituted by methadone the IgM levels returned to normal values. However, whether these results permit one to invoke an immunological pathomechanism for heroin-associated glomerular lesions seems to us highly questionable.

If one accepts these latter contentions as being indicative of an immune pathomechanism, one could suggest that the glomerular changes might be interpreted as representing an immune-complex glomerulonephritis, whereby in addition to heroin itself other antigens such as bacteria, virus and non-specific factors (solvent/carrier) play a vital role. That heroin could function as a hapten is supported by the evidence that morphine can form complexes with 7 S-gamma globulin (*Ryan* et al. 1972).

9. Glomerular Lesions Associated with the Inhalation of Volatile Hydrocarbons

a) Introduction

Finally one may point to a disease form which is elicited not by a pharmaceutical preparation in the true sense of the word, but rather by chemical compounds to which many humans, and especially those in particular professions, are exposed in our present western environment. One is referring here to volatile hydrocarbons, which may lead, under certain conditions to the induction of a clinical picture consistent with a Goodpasture syndrome. *Beirne* and *Brennan* (1972) on investigation of 8 cases of Goodpasture syndrome could identify 6 of these as having had prior contact with hydrocarbon-containing solvents. The results of *Zimmermann* et al. (1975) which have been supported by the work of *Lagrue* (1976) and *Ravnskov* et al. (1979) also point to the fact that all patients exhibiting a glomerulonephritis have had a significantly higher exposure to hydrocarbons than have control groups of patients. *Klavis* and *Drommer*

(1970) were able to induce a Goodpasture-like syndrome in rats following petrol intoxication, although no immunohistological examination was performed during this study.

b) Clinical Findings

Goodpasture syndrome typically begins with a cough, shortness of breath and haemoptysis, and can proceed to pulmonary bleeding, with the simultanous appearance of severe renal symptoms in the form of a haematuria, proteinuria, oliguria and a rapidly developing renal insufficiency. The disease picture generally proceeds within weeks or months to death due to uraemia or pulmonary bleeding. Serologically one may identify circulating antiglomerular basement membrane antibodies.

c) Morphological Findings

The morphological findings in the kidney are generally those of a rapidly progressive glomerulonephritis, that is, a glomerulonephritis which proceeds with 80–100% crescent formation, whereby the necrotic regions and crescents may have different ages. Immunohistological examination reveals a brilliant linear fluorescence of the glomerular basement membrane with IgG deposits. C_3 deposits, however, are not observed in all cases, but when present they are frequently arrayed in a discontinuous pattern.

d) Pathogenesis

The pathogenetic principle lying at the source of a Goodpasture syndrome is probably an autoimmune mechanism, there being primary damage to the alveolar basement membrane of the lung by the inhalation of volatile hydrocarbons. The altered basement membrane then acts as an autoantigen, inducing autoantibody production, with these autoantibodies being able to cross-react with the glomerular basement membrane. In a more recent study involving 4 patients with a PGN (*Ehrenreich* et al. 1977), an autoimmune mechanism was proposed which is perhaps dependent upon damage to the tubular epithelium by volatile hydrocarbons with the subsequent release of endogenous tubular antigens.

10. Indirect Effects Via Electrolyte and Water Imbalance: Glomerular Changes Associated with Laxative and Diuretic Abuse

The glomerular changes apparent following laxative or diuretic abuse are characterised by a shrinkage of the capillaries of the glomerular convoluted loops, with a concomitant increase of the mesangial matrix caused by a hyalinisation or sclerosis of the mesangium. Furthermore, one may observe focal hyalinisation and less commonly the encroachment of the proximal tubular epithelium onto the parietal layer of the Bowman's capsule.

Thus it is that the glomerular changes appearing as a result of the misuse of laxatives or diuretics do not present lesions in the normal sense of the word. Rather one is observing an adaptive process which is the consequence of the chronic water and electrolyte deficiency, and which is mainly focussed upon the tubuli. This process will be discussed in more detail in relationship to hypokalaemic nephropathy in the section B of part II chapter 5.

Conclusions

For a successful drug therapy a knowledge of the side-effects of the drug is an absolute prerequisite. Of greatest importance in instances of drug-induced damage is which essential organs are affected. The kidneys represent one such instance and because of their involvement in both the elimination and secretion processes their morphological structures are particularly predisposed to drug-induced damage. Above all, therefore, one must reckon with the appearance of glomerular lesions in addition to tubulo-interstitial damage as a consequence of the filtration process and the fact that the kidney has a relatively large endothelial surface.

From the point of view of pathogenic mechanisms, one can consider both a toxic and an immunological process as being responsible for the triggering of the glomerular lesions. The clinical symptoms are independent of the pathogenic mechanism and are in general characterised by proteinuria or a nephrotic syndrome.

Glomerular lesions which are provoked by toxic damage, as is for instance the case in aminonucleoside nephrosis in animal experiments, are generally unknown in humans, since the required dose to produce toxic damage in animal experiments is far in excess of that required for a therapeutic effect in human medicine.

In contrast, immunological pathomechanisms are of the greatest importance because of the predilection of glomerular structures to immunological reactions. Thus, in favour of an immunological pathomechanism one might cite the lightmicroscopical, immunohistological and electronmicroscopical findings which reveal in the majority of cases an immune-complex glomerulonephritis, whereas the appearance of an anti-basement-membrane glomerulonephritis is only seldom observed. In addition the appearance of the morphological changes following a latent period, the lack of dependence between both the clinical and the morphological changes and the dose of the drug administered and the duration of therapy, and the general reversibility of the changes following the cessation of the therapy, also favour an immune pathomechanism.

Most frequently the drugs under investigation trigger an immune reaction in the glomeruli which is a type III hypersensitivity reaction. This process reveals itself as an immune-complex glomerulonephritis of the PGN type, as is especially evident in penicillamine and gold therapy.

It is possible to propose two mechanisms which might be responsible for the generation of this immune-complex glomerulonephritis of the PGN type. The first is deposition of circulating immune complexes, the second is in situ immune complex formation. Thus the drug may either act as a hapten or it may induce an autoimmune mechanism.

Infrequently an instance of drug-dependent glomerular damage is produced by an autoimmune mechanism, analogous to a type II hypersensitivity reaction, which leads to an anti-basement-membrane glomerulonephritis.

The prognosis for the majority of these glomerular lesions, which are induced by diverse drugs, is favourable upon cessation of the therapy. This is because the quantity of antigen is limited and as a consequence the degree of immune reaction is also restricted, there thus being a reversibility of the clinical and morphological findings.

References

Abraham EP, Chain E, Baker W, Robinson R (1943) Penicillamine: A characteristic degradation product of penicillin. Nature (London) 151: 107

Alarcon-Segovia D, Wakim KG, Worthington JW et al (1967) Clinical and experimental studies on the hydralazine syndrome and its relationship to systemic lupus erythematosus. Medicine 46: 1–33

Alarcon-Segovia D (1969) Drug induced lupus syndromes. Mayo Clin Proc 44: 664–681

Amos H (1968) Detection of antibodies in penicillamine sensitivity. Postgrad med J Suppl II/14: 27–28

Amrhein JA, Kenny FM, Ross D (1970) Granulocytopenia, lupus-like syndrome and other complications of propylthiouracil therapy. J Pediatr 76: 54–63

Andres GA, McCluskey RT (1975) Tubular and interstitial renal disease due to immunologic mechanisms. Kidney int 7: 271–289

Bachmann F, Frind W, Genth E, Hartl PW (1975) Nebenwirkungen unter D-Penicillamintherapie. Untersuchung iher Abhängigkeit von Tagesdosis, Gesamtdosis und Therapiedauer. Aus: Jüngste Fortschritte mit D-Penicillamin. G Braun, Karlsruhe, pp 187–188

Bacon PA, Tribe CR, Mackenzie JC, Verrier-Jones J, Cumming RH, Amer B (1976) Penicillamine nephropathy in rheumatoid arthritis. Quart J Med 180: 661–684

Bariety J, Druet Ph, Laliberte F, Sapin C (1971) Glomerulonephritis with γ- and β1C-globulin deposits induced in rats by mercuric cloride. Amer J Pathol 65: 293–302

Bar-Khayim Y, Teplitz C, Garella S, Chazan JA (1973) Trimethadione (Tridione)-induced nephrotic syndrome. Amer J Med 54: 272–279

Barnett HL, Simons DJ, Wells RE jr (1948) Nephrotic syndrome occurring during Tridione therapy. Amer J Med 4: 760–764

Barr RD, Rees PH, Cordy PE, Kungu A, Woodger BA, Cameron HM (1972) Nephrotic syndrome in adult Africans in Nairobi. Brit Med J 2: 131–134

Batsford SR, Rohrbach R, Riede UN, Sandritter W, Kluthe R (1976) Effects of D-penicillamine administration to rats, induction of renal changes: preliminary communication. Clin Nephrol 6: 394–397

Becker CG, Becker EL, Maher JF, Schreiner GE (1962) Nephrotic syndrome after contact with mercury. Arch Intern Med 110: 178–186

Beirne GJ, Brennan JT (1972) Glomerulonephritis associated with hydrocarbons. Arch Environ Health 25: 365–369

Bergstrand A, Bergstrand CG, Engstrom N, Herrlin KM (1962) Renal histology during treatment with oxazolidine-diones (trimethadione, ethadione, and paramethadione). Pediatrics 30: 601

Bernstein RE (1979) Procainamide, acetylprocainamide and drug induced lupus erythematosus. Lancet II: 1076

Blomgren StE, Condemi JJ, Vaughan JH (1972) Procainamide-induced lupus erythematosus. Am J Med 52: 338–348

Bluestein HG, Zvaifler NJ, Weisman MH, Shapiro RF (1979) Lymphocyte alteration by procainamide: Relation to drug-induced lupus erythematosus syndrome. Lancet II: 816–819

Borowsky BA, Kessner DM, Hartroft WS, Recant L, Koch MB (1961) Aminonucleoside-induced chronic glomerulonephritis in rats. J Lab Clin Med 57: 512–521

Brass H, Genth E, Hartl PW, Bauerdick H, Buss H, Lapp H, Heintz R (1976) Die D-Pencillamin-Glomerulopathie. Med Welt 27: 2151–2153

Cameron JS, Trounce JR (1965) Membranous glomerulonephritis and the nephrotic syndrome appearing during mersalyl therapy. Gyn Hosp Rep 114: 101–107

Castleman B, McNeely BU (1968) Case reports of the Massachusetts General Hospital. N Engl J Med 278: 1167–1173

Caulfield JP, Farquhar MG (1978) Loss of anionic sites from the glomerular basement membrane in aminonucleoside nephrosis. Lab Invest 39: 505–512

Caulfield JP, Reid JJ, Farquhar MG (1976) Alterations of the glomerular epithelium in acute aminonucleoside nephrosis. Lab Invest 34: 43–59

Churg J, Grishman E (1978) Heroin nephropathy. Proceedings Vth international congress of nephrology, June 18–23, Montreal. Karger, Basel, p 57–59

Cushman P (1974) Hyperimmunoglobulinemia in heroin addition. Some epidemiologic observations, including some possible effects of route of administration and multiple drug abuse. Amer J Epidem 99: 218–224

Day AT, Goldring JR (1974) Hazards of penicillamine therapy in the treatment of rheumatoid arthritis. Postgrad Med J Suppl 2: 71–73

Derot M, Kahn A, Mazalten A, Peyrafolrt J (1954) Nephrite anurique aigue mortelle apres traitement aurique, chrysocyanose associee (fatal anuric nephritis with associated chrysocyanosis following gold therapy). Bull Soc Med Hop Paris 70: 234–239

Derow HA, Wolff L (1947) Oral administration of mercupurin tablets in ambulatory patients with chronic congestive heart failure. Amer J Med 3: 693–703

Di Marco A (1967) Daunomycin and related antibiotics. In: Gottlieb D, Schaw PD (eds) Antibiotics mechanism of action. Springer, Berlin Heidelberg New York

Dische FE, Swinson DR, Hamilton EBD, Parsons V (1976) Immunopathology of penicillamine induced glomerular disease. J Rheumatol 3/2: 145–155

Dixon FJ, Feldman JD, Vazquez JJ (1961) Experimental glomerulonephritis. The pathogenesis of a laboratory model resembling the spectrum of human glomerulonephritis. J exp Med 113: 899–920

Dixon AStJ, Davies J, Dormandy TL, Hamilton EBD, Holt PJL, Mason RM, Thompson M, Weber JCP, Zutshi DW (1975) Synthetic D(-) penicillamine in rheumatoid arthritis. Ann rheum Dis 34: 416–421

Edgington ThS, Glassock RJ, Dixon FJ (1968) Autologous immune complex nephritis induced with renal tubular antigen. J exp Med 127: 555–571

Ehrenreich T, Porush JG, Churg J, Glabman S, Goldstein MH, Grishdan E, Yunis SL (1975) Membranous nephropathy: classification, natural history, pathology and treatment. VIth international congress of nephrology, Florence, June 8–12

Ehrenreich T, Yunis StL, Churg J (1977) Membranous nephropathy following exposure to volatile hydrocarbons. Environmental Research 14: 35–45

Eknoyan G, Györkey F, Dichoso C, Györkey Ph (1975) Nephropathy in patients with drug addiction. Virch Arch A Path Anat and Histol 365: 1–13

Elsas LJ, Hayslett JP, Spargo BH, Durant JL, Rosenberg LE (1971) Wilson's disease with reversible renal tubular dysfunction. Ann Int Med 75: 427–433

Empire Rheumatism Council (1960) Gold therapy in rheumatoid arthritis: Report of a multicentre controlled trial. Ann Rheum Dis 19: 95–119

Falck HM, Törnroth T, Kock B, Wegelins O (1979) Fatal renal vasculitis and minimal change glomerulonephritis complicating treatment with penicillamine. Acta Med Scand 205: 133–138

Farquhar MG, Palade GE (1961) Glomerular permeability: II. Ferritin transfer across the glomerular capillary wall in nephrotic rats. J Exp Med 114: 699–715

Ferris ThF, Morgan WS, Levitin H (1961) Nephrotic syndrome caused by probenecid. New Engl J Med 265: 381–383

Freeman RB, Maher JF, Schreiner GE, Mostofi FK (1962) Renal tubular necrosis due to nephrotoxicity of organic mercurial diuretics. Ann intern Med 57: 34–43

Frenk S, Antonowicz I, Craig JM, Metcoff J (1955) Experimental nephrotic syndrome induced in rats by aminonucleoside. Renal lesions and body electrolyte composition. Proc Soc Exp Biol Med 89: 424–427

Friedman EA, Sreepada Rao TK, Nicastri AD (1974) Heroin-associated nephropathy. Nephron 13: 421–426

Gärtner H-V (1977) Die perimembranöse Glomerulonephritis – Prototyp einer Immunkomplexnephritis – Eine klinisch-morphologische Studie. Habilitationsschrift, Tübingen

Gärtner HV, Neild GH, Bohle A, Hallauer W, Hoppe-Seyler G, Lüttgen FM, Schollmeyer P (1975) Perimembranöse Glomerulonephritis nach Penicillamintherapie. Klin Wschr 53: 835–837

Gerhartz H (1967) Chemotherapie der akuten Leukämien. Dtsch med Wochenschr 92: 2371–2375

Germuth FG jr, Rodriguez E (1973) In: Immunopathology of the renal glomerulus: Immune complex deposit and antibasement membrane disease. Little, Brown and Company, Boston

Gibson T, Burry HC, Ogg C (1976) Goodpasture syndrome and D-penicillamine. Ann Int Med 84: 100

Glassock RJ, Edgington ThS, Watson JI, Dixon FJ (1968) Autologous immune complex nephritis induced with renal tubular antigen. II. The pathogenetic mechanism. J exp Med 127: 573–587

Grabar P (1974) "Self" and "not-self" in immunology. Lancet I: 1320–1322

Grishman E, Churg J, Porush JC (1976) Glomerular morphology in nephrotic heroin addicts. Lab Invest 35: 415–424

Gritzka TL, Trump BF (1968) Renal tubular lesions caused by mercuric cloride. Electron microscopic observations: degeneration of the pars recta. Amer J Pathol 52: 1225–1277

Gros H, Zwirner K (1975) Klinische Untersuchungen mit D-Penicillamin bei der Behandlung von Leberkrankheiten. Aus: Jüngste Forstschritte mit D-Penicillamin. G Braun, Karlsruhe, pp 109–111

Günther R, Asamer H, Dittrich P (1969) Das reversible Procainamid-induzierte Lupuserythematodes-Syndrom. Dtsch Med Wochenschr 94: 2338–2342

Hahn BH, Sharp GC, Irvin WS, Kanton OS, Gardner CA, Bagby KM, Perry HM, Osterland CK (1972) Immune response to hydralazine and nuclear antigens in hydralazine-induced lupus erythematosus. Ann Intern Med 76: 365–374

Hallauer W, Gärtner HV, Kronenberg KH, Manz G (1974) Immunkomplexnephritis mit nephrotischem Syndrom unter Therapie mit D-Penicillamin. Schweiz Med Wschr 104: 434–438

Hamilton EBD (1975) Klinische Untersuchung von Penicillamin in zwei Dosierungen bei der rheumatoiden Arthritis. Aus: Jüngste Fortschritte mit D-Penicillamin. G Braun, Karlsruhe, pp 59–62

Hargraves MM (1969) Discovery of the LE cell and its morphology. Mayo Clin Proc 44: 579–599

Harkin JC, Recant L (1960) Pathogenesis of experimental nephrosis. Electron microscopic observations. Amer J Path 36: 303–314

Harpey JP (1974) Lupus-like syndromes induced by drugs. Ann Allergy 33: 256–261

Hartfall StJ, Garland HG, Goldie W (1937) Gold treatment of arthritis. Lancet II: 838–842

Haugen HN (1957) Tridione nephropathy. Acta Med Scand CLIX: 375–380

Helmke K, Velcovsky HG, Federlin K (1975) Klinische und prognostische Bedeutung antinukleärer Faktoren bei einer D-Penicillamin-Therapie. Dtsch Med Wochenschr 100: 2198–2203

Henningsen B, Maintz J, Basedow M, Harders H (1973) Nephrotisches Syndrom durch Penicillamin. Dtsch Med Wochenschr 98: 1768–1772
Henningsen NCh, Cederberg Å, Hanson A, Johansson BW (1975) Effects of long-term treatment with procainamide. Acta med scand 198: 475–482
Hertz Ph, Yager H, Richardson JA (1972) Probenecid-induced nephrotic syndrome. Arch Path 94: 241–243
Heyman W, Hackel DB, Harwood S, Wilson SGF, Hunter JLP (1959) Production of nephrotic syndrome in rats by Freund's adjuvants and rat kidney suspensions. Proc Soc exp Biol (NY) 100: 660–664
Heyman W, Hackel DB, Hunter JLP (1960) Trimethadione (Tridione) nephrosis in rats. Pediatrics 25: 112–118
Hinglais N, Druet Ph, Grossetete J, Sapin C, Bariety J (1979) Ultrastructural study of nephritis induced in Brown Norway rats by mercuric chloride. Lab Invest 41: 150–159
Hooft C, van Acker K, Deneve V (1962) Clinical and histological course of the nephrotic syndrome during trimethadione (Neoabsentol-) therapy. Helv Paediat Acta 4/5: 329–340
Hoorntje StJ, Weening JJ, Kallenberg CGM, Prins EJL, Donker AJM (1979) Serum-sickness-like syndrome with membranous glomerulopathy in patient on captopril. Lancet II: 1297
Huskisson EC (1975) Ein Vergleich zwischen Gold und Penicillamin bei der rheumatoiden Arthritis. Aus: Jüngste Fortschritte mit D-Penicillamin. G Braun, Karlsruhe, pp 67–77
Jacobs JC (1963) Systemic lupus erythematosus in childhood. Pediatrics 32: 257–264
Jaffe IA, Treser G, Suzuki Y, Ehrenreich Th (1968) Nephropathy induced by D-penicillamine. Ann intern Med 69: 549–556
Jaffe IA (1974) The treatment of rheumatoid arthritis with D-penicillamine. Symposium Berlin, 1973. In: Ott VR, Schmidt KL (eds) Der Rheumatismus, Bd 42. Dietrich Steinkopff, Darmstadt, pp 84–94
Kallenbach H, Schattenfroh C (1961) Endoxan-Nebenwirkungen bei Langzeitbehandlung, zugleich ein tierexperimenteller Beitrag zur Theorie der sog. seriösen Entzündung der Leber. Langenbecks Arch Klin Chir 296: 517–527
Katz A, Little AH (1973) Gold nephropathy. An immunopathologic study. Arch Pathol 96: 133–136
Kazantzis G, Schiller KFR, Asscher AW, Drew RG (1962) Albuminuria and the nephrotic syndrome following exposure to mercury and its compounds. Quart J Med 31: 403–418
Kibukamusoke JW, Davies DR, Hutt MSR (1974) Membranous nephropathy due to skin-lightening cream. Brit Med J 2: 646–647
Kilcoyne MM, Daly JJ, Gocke DJ, Thomson GE, Meltzer JI, Hsu KC, Tannenbaum M (1972) Nephrotic syndrome in heroin addicts. Lancet I: 17–20
Klavis G, Drommer W (1970) Goodpasture-Syndrom und Benzineinwirkung. Arch Toxikol 26: 40–55
Koffler D, Agnello V, Thoburn R, Kunkel HG (1971) Systemic lupus erythematosus: Prototype of immune complex nephritis in man. J Exp Med 134: 169–179
Kortge P, Palme G, Merker HJ (1961) Licht- und elektronenmikroskopische Untersuchungen am Glomerulum bei der Aminonucleosidnephrose der Ratte. Z Ges Exp Med 135: 167–182
Kreiter H, Begemann H, Rastetter J (1968) Erfahrungen mit Daunomycin und Cytosin-Arabinosid bei der Behandlung akuter myeloischer Leukämien. Med Klinik 63: 2058–2066
Kronenberg KH, Schöll A, Schmülling RM, Gärtner HV (1972) Glomeruläre Frühveränderungen bei der Daunomycin-Nephrose. Verh Dtsch Ges Path 56: 602–606
Lachmann PJ (1968) Nephrotic syndrome from penicillamine. Postgraduate med J Suppl II/14: 23–27

Lagrue G (1976) Hydrocarbon exposure and chronic glomerulonephritis. Lancet I: 1191

Lannigan R, Kark R, Pollack VE (1962) The effect of a single intravenous injection of aminonucleoside of puromycin on the rat kidney: A light- and electron-microscope study. J Pathol Bacteriol 83: 357–362

Lee RE, Vernier RL, Ulstrom RA (1961) The nephrotic syndrome as a complication of perchlorate treatment of thyrotoxicosis. New Engl J Med 264: 1221–1226

Lee JC, Dushkin M, Eyring EJ, Engleman EP, Hopper J jr (1965) Renal lesions associated with gold therapy. Light and electron microscopic studies. Arth and Rheumat 8: 1–13

Lee StL, Chase PH (1975) Drug-induced systemic lupus erythematosus: A critical review. Seminars in Arthritis and Rheumatism 5: 83–103

Lerner R, Dixon FJ (1966) Transfer of ovine experimental allergic glomerulonephritis (EAG) with serum. J Exp Med 124: 431–442

Lopes VM (1967) Cyclophosphamide nephrotoxicity in man. Lancet I: 1060

Lüttgen FM, Gärtner HV, Lindenmaier K, Babucke G, Kluthe R (1975) Glomerulonephritis nach D-Penicillamintherapie. Nieren- u. Hochdruckkrankh 2: 56–60

Mandema E, Arends A, van Zeijst J, Vermeer G, van der Hem GK, van der Slikke LB (1963) Mercury and the kidney. Lancet I, 8: 1266

Marchand G, Cantin M, Cote M (1963) Evidence for the nephrotoxicity of morphine sulphate in rats. Canad J Physiol Pharmacol 47: 649–655

Metcoff J, Kaiser E, Spargo B (1963) Correlation of ultrastructure and enzyme activities in kidneys of rats with aminonucleoside nephrosis. Proc 2nd Intern Congr Nephrol. Karger, Basel, pp 511–513

Meyboom RHB (1975) In: Dukes MNG (ed) Meyler's side effects of drugs, vol VIII. Excerpta Medica, Amsterdam, p 505

Michael AF, Blau E, Vernier RL (1970) Glomerular polyanion: alteration in aminonucleoside nephrosis. Lab Invest 23: 649–657

Morel-Maroger LJ, Verroust PJ (1975) Clinicopathological correlations in glomerular diseases. Rec Adv in Renal Disease 1: 48–89

Muehrcke RC, Kark RM, Pirani CL, Pollak VE (1957) Lupus nephritis: A clinical and pathologic study based on renal biopsies. Medicine 36: 1–145

Multicentre Trial Group (1973) Controlled trial of D (-)penicillamine in severe rheumatoid arthritis. Lancet I: 275–280

Nabarro JDN, Rosenheim ML (1952) Nephrotic syndrome complicating tridione (troxidone) therapy. Lancet I: 1091

Nagi AH, Alexander F, Barabas AZ (1971) Gold nephropathy in rats – light and electron microscopic studies. Exp and Molecul Pathol 15: 354–362

Neild GH, Gärtner HV, Bohle A (1979) Penicillamine induced membranous glomerulonephritis. Scand J Rheumatology, Suppl 28: 79–90

Nussenzveig I, Villela de Faria C, Lopes de Faria C, Barros Magaldi J (1963) Aminonucleoside induced nephrotic syndrome in human beings: Report of five cases. Proc 2nd Intern Congr Nephrol. Karger, Basel, pp 506–510

Obrecht P, Merker H, Hennekeuser HH, Meuret G, Westerhausen M, Simon A (1970) Klinisch-pharmakologische, cytochemische und feulgen-photometrische Untersuchungen bei unreifzelligen Erwachsenenleukosen unter kombinierter Chemotherapie mit Vincristin, Daunomycin und Prednison. Klin Wochenschr 48: 1281–1291

Okuda R, Kaplan MH, Cuppage FE, Heymann W (1965) Deposition of autologous gamma globulin in kidneys of rats with nephrotic renal disease of various etiologies. J Lab Clin Med 66: 204–215

Owens ChJ, Yarbrough DR, Brackett NC (1974) Nephrotic syndrome following topically applied sulfadiazine silver therapy. Arch Int Med 134: 332–335

Palosuo T, Provost TT, Milgrom F (1976) Gold nephropathy: serologic data suggesting an immune complex disease. Clin exp Immunol 25: 311–318

Perry HM, Tan EM, Carmody S, Sakamoto A (1970) Relationship of acetyl transferase activity to antinuclear antibodies and toxic symptoms in hypertensive patients treated with hydralazine. J Lab Clin Med 76: 114–125

Pollak VE, Pirani CL, Schwartz FD (1964) The natural history of the renal manifestations of systemic lupus erythematosus. J Lab and Clin Med 63: 537–550

Prins EJL, Hoorntje StJ, Weening JJ, Donker ABJM (1979) Nephrotic syndrome in patient on captopril. Lancet II: 306–307

Rao TKS, Nicastri AD, Friedman EA (1974) Natural history of heroin-associated nephropathy. New Engl J Med 290: 19–23

Ravnskov U, Forsberg B, Skerfving St (1979) Glomerulonephritis and exposure to organic solvents. Acta Med Scand 205: 575–579

Roman-Franco AA, Turiello M, Albini B, Ossi E, Milgrom F, Andres GA (1978) Anti-basement membrane antibodies and antigen-antibody complexes in rabbits injected with mercuric chloride. Clin Imm Immunpathol 9: 464–481

Rosenblum J, Sonnenschein H, Minsky AA (1959) Trimethadione (Tridione) nephrosis. AMAJ Dis Child 97: 42–47

Rothfield NF, McCluskey RT, Baldwin DS (1963) Renal disease in systemic lupus erythematosus. New Engl J Med 269: 537–544

Rutherford BD (1968) Procainamide-induced systemic lupus erythematosus. NZ Med J 68: 235–240

Ryan JJ, Parker CW, Williams RC (1972) γ-Globulin binding of morphine in heroin addicts. J Lab Clin Med 80: 155–164

Ryan GB, Karnovsky MJ (1975) An ultrastructural study of the mechanism of proteinuria in aminonucleoside nephrosis. Kid Int 8: 219–232

Salomon MI, Pui Poon T, Goldblatt M, Tchertkoff V (1972) Renal lesions in heroin addicts – a study based on kidney biopsies. Nephron 9: 356–363

Salant DJ, Belok St, Stilmant MM, Darby Ch, Couser WG (1979) Determinants of glomerular localization of subepithelial immune deposits. Lab Invest 41: 89–99

Sapin C, Druet E, Druet P (1977) Induction of anti-glomerular basement membrane antibodies in the Brown-Norway rat by mercuric chloride. Clin Exp Immunol 28: 173–179

Schnall Ch, Wiener JS (1958) Nephrosis occurring during tolbutamide administration. JAMA 167: 214–215

Schöll A, Hiller GW, Gärtner HV, Fischbach H (1974) Fokale Glomerulumläsionen im Spätstadium der Aminonucleosidnephrose (ANN) bei Ratten. Verh Dtsch Ges Path 58: 483

Seelig HP, Seelig R, Fischer A, Maurer R, Safer A, Schnitzlein W (1977) Immunkomplex-Glomerulonephritis nach peroraler Penicillamin-Applikation bei Ratten. Res exp Med 170: 35–55

Shimizu F (1970) Histopathologic and immunological studies on chronic renal lesions in rats induced by aminonucleoside of puromycin. Japan J Exp Med 40: 227–242

Siegel M, Lee SL, Peress NS (1967) The epidemiology of drug induced systemic lupus erythematosus. Arthritis Rheum 10: 407–415

Silverberg DS, McCall JT, Hunt JC (1967) Nephrotic syndrome with use of ammoniated mercury. Arch intern Med 120: 581–586

Silverberg DS, Kidd EG, Shnitka TK, Ulan RA (1970) Gold nephropathy. A clinical and pathological study. Arth Rheumat 13: 812–825

Steblay RW (1962) Glomerulonephritis induced in sheep by injections of heterologous glomerular basement membrane and Freund's complete adjuvant. J Exp Med 116: 253–272

Sternberg SS (1970) Cross-striated fibrils and other ultrastructural alterations in glomeruli of rats with daunomycin nephrosis. Lab Invest 23: 39–51

Sternlieb J (1966) Penicillamine and the nephrotic syndrome. JAMA 198: 1311–1312

Sternlieb J, Scheinberg JH (1964) Penicillamine therapy for hepatolenticular degeneration. JAMA 189: 748–754

Sternlieb J, Bennett B, Scheinberg JH (1975) D-Penicillamine induced Goodpasture's syndrome in Wilson's disease. Ann intern Med 82: 673–676

Strunk StW, Ziff M (1970) Ultrastructural studies of the passage of gold thiomalate across the renal glomerular capillary wall. Arth Rheumat 13: 39–52

Struve J, Galle P (1970) Role of mitochondria in the handling of gold by the kidney: A study by electron microscopy and electron probe microanalysis. J Cell Biol 44: 667–676

Tessmann D, Schill H, Voss J, Hamann H, Engelmann C (1972) Nierenveränderungen nach Behandlung mit Zytostatika (Trenimon, Cyclophosphamid, Imuran). Zbl allg Path 115: 522–531

Thoenes W, Thoenes G, Ansorge R (1972) Drogen-induzierte Lupus-Nephritis. Lichtelektronen- und immunfluoreszenzmikroskopische Untersuchungen. Verh Dtsch Ges Pathol 56: 346–352

Törnroth T, Skrifvars B (1974) Gold nephropathy prototype of membranous glomerulonephritis. Amer J Pathol 75: 573–590

Treser G, Sagel I, Lange K (1964) Specificity of immunofluorescence in experimental and human renal diseases. Proc Soc Exp Biol Med 117: 842–844

Tribe CR, Bacon PA, Mackenzie JC (1975) Eine vorläufige Mitteilung über die Nierenschädigung durch D-Penicillamin-Toxizität. Aus: Jüngste Fortschritte mit D-Penicillamin. G Braun, Karlsruhe, pp 147–150

Vaamonde CA, Hunt FR (1970) The nephrotic syndrome as a complication of gold therapy. Arth Rheumat 13: 826–834

Van Damme BJC, Fleuren GJ, Bakker WW, Vernier RL, Hoedemauer PhJ (1978) Experimental glomerulonephritis in the rat induced by antibodies directed against tubular antigens. V. Fixed glomerular antigens in the pathogenesis of heterologous immune complex glomerulonephritis. Lab Invest 38: 502–510

Vernier RC, Papermaster BW, Good RA (1959) Aminonucleoside nephrosis. I. Electron microscopic study of the renal lesion in rats. J Exp Med 109: 115–126

Viol GW, Minielly JA, Bistricki Th (1977) Gold nephropathy. Tissue analysis by X-ray fluorescent spectroscopy. Arch Pathol Lab Med 101: 635–640

Walshe JM (1956) Wilson's disease. New oral therapy. Lancet I: 25–26

Watanabe I, Whittier FC, Moore J, Cuppage FE (1976) Gold nephropathy. Ultrastructural, fluorescence, and microanalytic studies of two patients. Arch Pathol Lab Med 100: 632–635

Weening JJ, Fleuren GJ, Hoedemaeker PhJ (1978) Demonstration of antinuclear antibodies in mercuric chloride-induced glomerulopathy in the rat. Lab Invest 39: 405–411

Wehner H (1975) Nierenveränderungen bei Behandlung mit Azathioprin. Res exp Med 166: 265–273

White AB (1966) Hydralazine (Apresoline) lupus with total renal failure. J Am Geriatr Soc 14: 361–365

Whittingham S, Mackay IR (1970) Systemic lupus erythematosus induced by procaine amide. Inst Ann Med 4: 358–361

Whittle ThS, Ainsworth StK (1976) Procainamide-induced systemic lupus erythematosus. Arch Pathol Lab Med 100: 469–474

Wilson SGF, Hackel DB, Horwood S, Nash G, Heymann W (1958) Aminonucleoside nephrosis in rats. Pediatrics 21: 963–973

Woosley RL, Drayer DE, Reidenberg MM, Nies AS, Carr K, Oates JA (1978) Effect of acetylator phenotype on the rate at which procainamide induces antinuclear antibodies and the lupus syndrome. N Engl J Med 298: 1157–1159

Yarom R, Stein H, Peters PD, Slavin Sh, Hall ThA (1975) Nephrotoxic effect of parenteral and intraarticular gold. Arch Pathol 99: 36–43

Young E (1960) Ammoniated mercury poisoning. Brit J Derm 72: 449–455

Zech P, Colon S, Labeeuw M, Bernheim J, Blanc-Brunat N (1979) Nephrotic syndrome in procainamide induced lupus nephritis. Clin Nephrol 11: 218–221

Zimmerman StW, Groehler K, Beirne GJ (1975) Hydrocarbon exposure and chronic glomerulonephritis. Lancet II: 199–201

Zimmermann F, Friedrich L (1977) Pharmakologie, Toxikologie und Pharmakokinetik des D-Penicillamines. In: Kreysel HW (ed) D-Penicillamin. Schattauer, Stuttgart, pp 25–46

Zollinger HU (1955) Autoptische und experimentelle Untersuchungen über Lipoidnephrose, hervorgerufen durch chron. Quecksilbervergiftung. Schweiz Z Pathol Bakt 18: 155–169

Zweiman B, Kornblum J, Cornog J, Hildreth EA (1968) The prognosis of lupus nephritis. Ann Int Med 69: 441–462

Drug-Associated Nephropathy

Part II: Tubulo-Interstitial Lesions

A: Acute Interstitial Nephritis, Nephrotoxic Lesions, Analgesic Nephropathy

H. G. LABERKE

I. Introduction 184
II. Acute Lesions of Predominantly (Immuno)Allergic Etiology 184
1. Introduction 184
2. Drugs 185
a) Antibiotics and Other Chemotherapeutic Agents 185
b) Antituberculous Agents 185
c) Diuretics 185
d) Other Drugs 186
3. Acute Interstitial Nephritis 186
a) Definition 186
b) Incidence 186
c) Morphology 187
α) Macroscopic Findings 187
β) Light and Electron Microscopic Findings 187
γ) Fluorescence Microscopic Findings 189
δ) Rare Forms of AIN 190
d) Clinical Aspects 190
III. Acute Lesions Due Predominantly to Nephrotoxic Effects 191
1. Introduction 191
2. Incidence 191
3. Drugs, Morphology, and Clinical Symptoms 192
a) Antibiotics 192
b) Antifungal Agents 193
c) Antituberculous Agents 194
d) Analgesics 194
4. Clinical Aspects 194
IV. Acute Lesions Due to Nephrotoxic and/or (Immuno)Allergic Effects 194
1. Introduction 194
2. Drugs, Morphology, Clinical Symptoms 194
a) Antibiotics 194
b) Antituberculous Agents 195
c) Analgesics 195
3. Clinical Aspects 195
V. Primarily Chronic Tubulo-interstitial Lesions – Analgesic Nephropathy . . . 196
1. Introduction 196
2. Definitions 196
3. Historical Survey 196
4. Analgesic Nephropathy in Different Countries 197
5. Incidence (Clinical Observation, Biopsy, Autopsy) 197
6. Age and Sex 197
7. Morphology 198

a) Macroscopic Findings 198
b) Light and Electron Microscopic Findings 198
c) Fluorescence Microscopic Findings 201
8. Clinical Aspects 201
9. Differential Diagnosis 202
10. Etiology and Pathogenesis 203
11. Primarily Chronic Interstitial Nephritis Not Induced by Analgesic Agents 205
VI. Concluding Remarks 205
References 205

I. Introduction

The diagnostic assumption of drug-induced renal damage presupposes a causal and/or temporal relationship between the ingestion of a particular drug or drugs and the appearance of the symptoms. Demonstration of a causal relationship is often complicated by the ingestion of several potentially nephrotoxic drugs (*McMenamin* et al. 1976).

The diagnosis and etiology, to a large extent, are confirmed when re-exposure to the drug produces similar symptoms and histologic pictures. Confirmation of this sort is rare since re-exposure is avoided if possible.

Data on the incidence of such renal damage depend primarily on the type of cases examined. Clinical data which are not confirmed by biopsy are often unreliable. Many cases are undoubtedly undetected or incorrectly diagnosed. Because of the negative selection and the impossibility of obtaining an exact drug history in retrospect, autopsy material is not a useful indicator of the incidence.

Since the kidneys receive 25% of the cardiac output, they are almost predisposed to drug damage due to the high drug concentration in the tubules after glomerular filtration (*Appel* and *Neu* 1977). Damage is either primarily acute or primarily chronic. A distinction is made below between nephrotoxic and (immuno)allergic damage in the case of primarily acute lesions. A clear distinction between the two pathologic mechanisms is often impossible (cf. text IV, p. 194).

Primarily chronic damage is discussed in the context of analgesic nephropathy. Chronic ingestion of many drugs, the effects of which have not been clinically or experimentally confirmed in relation to renal damage, may possibly also lead to the development of chronic renal insufficiency. Such renal insufficiency may also appear secondarily when acute drug-induced renal damage is undetected and therefore cannot be established later in the drug history or when the damage is so severe that complete restoration of renal function is impossible.

II. Acute Lesions of Predominantly (Immuno)Allergic Etiology

1. Introduction

Many drugs, independent of the dose and hence unforeseeably, lead to renal disease of varying degrees of severity. Although the histologic picture is similar, the symptoms often differ considerably. These symptoms of acute interstitial nephritis (AIN) are being recognized more and more as an entity and therefore are defined as a syndrome.

2. Drugs

Cases of AIN following ingestion of the following pharmacological preparations have been described in the literature:

a) Antibiotics and Other Chemotherapeutic Agents

Penicillins: *Schrier* et al. 1966; *Baldwin* et al. 1968; *Gilbert* et al. 1970; *Colvin* et al. 1974; *Orchard* and *Rooker* 1974; *Milman* 1978; *Richet* and *Mayaud* 1978; *Laberke* and *Bohle* 1980a.

Methicillin: *Schrier* et al. 1966; *Baldwin* et al. 1968; *Simenhoff* et al. 1968; *Gilbert* et al. 1970; *Border* et al. 1974; *Sanjad* et al. 1974; *Woodroffe* et al. 1974b; *Chesney* and *Chesney* 1976; *Olsen* and *Asklund* 1976; *Galpin* et al. 1978; *Richet* and *Mayaud* 1978.

Ampicillin: *Méry* 1970; *Tannenberg* et al. 1971; *Maxwell* et al. 1974; *Ruley* and *Lisi* 1974, *Woodroffe* et al. 1975; *Milman* 1978; *Laberke* and *Bohle* 1980a.

Oxacillin: *Burton* et al. 1974a, *Appel* and *Neu* 1977.

Nafcillin: *Parry* et al. 1973.

Cephalosporins: *Silverblatt* et al. 1973; *Burton* et al. 1974b; *Heptinstall* 1974; *Pasternak* and *Stephens* 1975; *Drago* et al. 1976; *Milman* 1978.

Gentamicin: *Schultze* et al. 1971; *Schrier* 1979; *Laberke* and *Bohle* 1980a.

Kanamycin: *Schreiner* and *Maher* 1965; *Hollenberg* et al. 1970.

Colistin: *Fillastre* et al. 1970; *Appel* and *Neu* 1977; *Richet* and *Mayaud* 1978.

Polymyxin B: *Beirne* et al. 1967; *Appel* and *Neu* 1977.

Chloramphenicol: *Laberke* and *Bohle* 1980a.

Glafenin: *Duplay* et al. 1974, *Mirouze* et al. 1974; *Andrieu* et al. 1976; *Richet* and *Mayaud* 1978.

Carbenicillin. *Appel* and *Neu* 1977; *Appel* et al. 1978.

Sulfonamides: *French* 1946; *Robson* et al. 1970; *Appel* and *Neu* 1977.

b) Antituberculous Agents

Rifampin: *Poole* et al. 1971; *Ramgopal* et al. 1973; *Bundschu* et al. 1974; *Bolt* 1975; *Gabow* et al. 1976; *Appel* and *Neu* 1977; *Kleinknecht* and *Adhémar* 1977; *Rossi* and *Montagna* 1978.

c) Diuretics

Furosemide: *Lyons* et al. 1973; *Fialk* et al. 1974; *Fuller* et al. 1976.

Thiazides: *Lyons* et al. 1973.

Chlorthalidone: *Peskoe* et al. 1978.

d) Other Drugs

Phenylbutazone: *Scheitlin* and *Jeanneret* 1957; *Streicher* 1964; *Kuhlmann* et al. 1978; *Richet* and *Mayaud* 1978.

Phenindione. *Baker* and *Williams* 1963; *Galea* et al. 1963; *Hollman* and *Wong* 1964; *Heptinstall* 1974; *McMenamin* et al. 1976; *Richet* and *Mayaud* 1978.

Allopurinol: *Jarzobski* et al. 1970; *Mills* 1971; *Gelbart* et al. 1977.

Diphenylhydantoin: *Heptinstall* 1976.

Azathioprine: *Sloth* and *Thomson* 1971.

Antipyrine: *Ortuno* and *Botella* 1973.

Phenobarbital: *Faarup* and *Christensen* 1974.

Carbimazol: *Baldamus* 1978.

3. Acute Interstitial Nephritis

a) Definition

AIN is a disease characterized by lesions localized in the region of the renal interstitium and the tubules. The clinical symptoms and findings are fever, acute renal insufficiency accompanied by nausea and vomiting, microscopic hematuria, and sometimes exanthema and blood eosinophilia. The term "acute interstitial nephritis" is based on the fact that the onset of the disease is acute and the initial course often severe (*Heptinstall* 1974). According to the conventional definition, however, the histologic picture (interstitial infiltration of lymphocytes and plasma cells) is identical to that of chronic inflammation. In the pre-antibiotic era, *Councilman* (1898) was the first to describe AIN in association with scarlet fever and diphtheria exclusively as a parainfectious disease. Determination of the exact etiology of the scarlet fever-associated nephritis still observed today (*Laberke* and *Bohle* 1980a) is complicated by drug therapy. At present, however, the etiology of most cases of AIN can be clarified on the basis of the patient's drug history.

Since AIN is defined strictly as nonpurulent inflammation or immunologic reaction, cases with sepsis cannot be included in the concept of this disease (*Baldamus* 1978; *Laberke* and *Bohle* 1980a). Based on our findings, we define the AIN syndrome as renal insufficiency with inflammatory symptoms, i.e., fever, accelerated blood sedimentation rate, nausea and vomiting, microscopic hematuria, exanthema, and blood eosinophilia.

b) Incidence

Given the world-wide use of the drugs listed in II_2, the frequency of AIN is quite low (*Simenhoff* et al. 1968; *Brass* et al. 1974; *Wilkinson* and *Boyd* 1978). It can be assumed that a certain number of cases are not detected (*Heptinstall* 1976; *Edel* 1978) since, on the one hand, AIN is often not diagnosed and/or not known in the clinical setting and, on the other, the diagnosis is often not confirmed by kidney biopsy. AIN was demonstrated in 1.3‰ of the cases in our kidney biopsy material. A considerably higher incidence of AIN has been reported by other authors who however also included cases with primary acute renal failure of longer duration (e.g., due to shock) with scattered lymphocytic interstitial infiltrates in their definition of AIN (*Zollinger* and *Mihatsch* 1978, 1979). In our opinion, neither the clinical course nor the laboratory findings justify including these cases in the concept of AIN.

c) Morphology

α) Macroscopic Findings

Corresponding to the radiologic findings of enlarged kidneys, usually with acute renal failure, post mortem examination shows large, pale or reddened, soft kidneys with smooth, shining surfaces. The cut surfaces exhibit diffuse, fine, grayish-red patches on the parenchyma of the renal cortex resulting partly from the hyperemic capillaries and partly from the interstitial infiltrates.

β) Light and Electron Microscopic Findings

The *interstitium* of the renal cortex varies in volume due to edema and inflammatory infiltrate made up predominantly of lymphocytes and plasma cells (*Baldwin* et al. 1968; *Ruley* and *Lisi* 1974; *Heptinstall* 1976). On the basis of the 30 cases we examined histologically (*Laberke* and *Bohle* 1980a), we established that the course of AIN is more severe and the prognosis poorer with diffuse round cell infiltration (Fig. 1) than with not completely diffuse, patchy infiltration (Fig. 2). Only 25% of the cases showed an accumulation of eosinophilic granulocytes in the infiltrate. It may well be that these cells, suggesting an allergic reaction, were not observable in kidney biopsy material obtained several weeks after the onset of the disease. Neutrophilic granulocytes have been described in the renal interstitium in some cases of methicillin- and phenindione-induced AIN (*Heptinstall* 1974). In a few instances, we observed up to 6% neutrophilic granulocytes following ingestion of tetracyclines, penicillins, and ampicillin. Whether the presence of these cells represents a primarily inflammatory infiltrate or is a sign of a localized resorptive process related to a type of destruction not readily ascertainable with light microscopy is still an open question.

Tubular lesions, demonstrable with light microscopy, were not important histologic alterations in our biopsy material. Signs of the degeneration of tubular epithelial cells, such as flattening, swelling, and occasionally also exfoliation of individual epithelial cells, were observed. Slight tubular damage (*Meadows* 1978), tubular lesions of various degrees of severity (*Baldwin* et al. 1968; *Ruley* and *Lisi* 1974; *Heptinstall* 1976), and extremely severe damage (*Beirne* et al. 1967; *Mayaud* et al. 1975; *Olsen* and *Asklund* 1976) have been described in the literature. Necrosis of the tubular epithelium and ruptures of the tubular basement membrane following sulfonamide therapy (*Robson* et al. 1970) are more likely the expression of nephrotoxic damage. The etiologic agent for the severe tubular destruction associated with methicillin-induced AIN (*Mayaud* et al. 1975) has not been definitely clarified. Since bacteremia has repeatedly been diagnosed in these cases, the damage may well be identical to focal destructive interstitial nephritis due to bacterial infection.

The *glomeruli* while predominantly unaltered, showed a low-grade proliferation of mesangial cells in 25% of our cases. This finding has also been described by other authors (*Woodroffe* et al. 1974b).

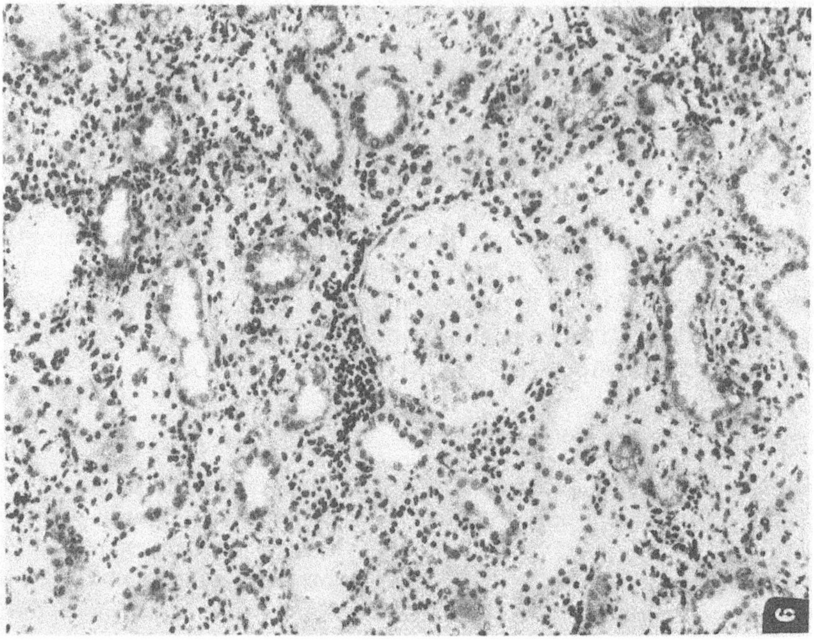

Fig. 1.Acute diffuse interstitial nephritis. Edematously widened interstitium with infiltrates of lymphocytes and plasma cells, preserved tubules, and unaltered glomeruli. (Semi-thin section, Giemsa, X 200)

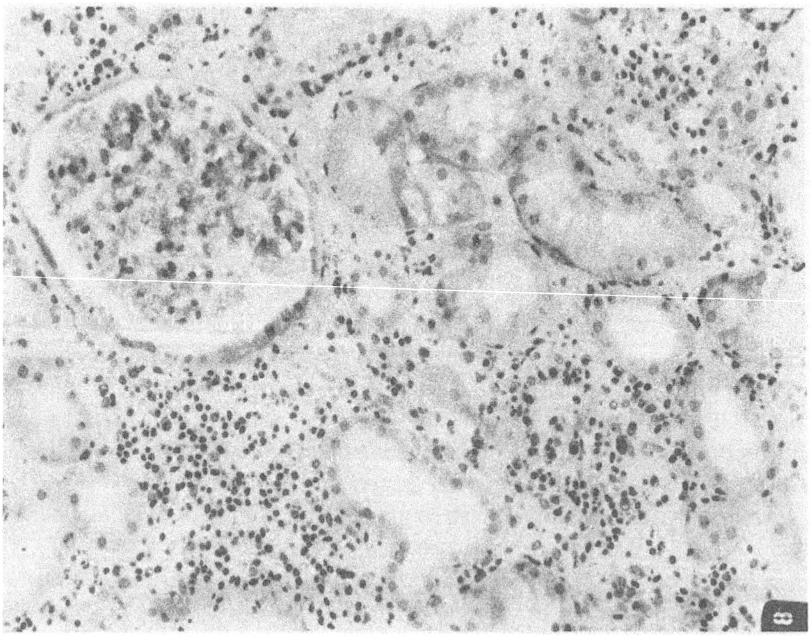

Fig. 2. Acute not completely diffuse interstitial nephritis. Edematously widened interstitium with patchy infiltrates of lymphocytes and plasma cells, preserved tubules, and unaltered glomeruli. (Semi-thin section, Giemsa, X 200)

As a rule, important pathologic alterations are not found in the *renal vessels*. Allergic vasculitides, which some authors have discussed as an independent syndrome (*Méry* and *Fillastre* 1978), usually develop in the context of AIN, following ingestion of various drugs, i.e., Beromycin (*Schrier* et al. 1966; *Laberke* and *Bohle* 1980a), allopurinol (*Jarzobski* et al. 1970), sulfonamides (*French* 1946), and thazides (*Kjellbo* et al. 1965).

γ) Fluorescence Microscopic Findings

Immunohistologic findings were available for some of our patients. The picture of antitubular basement membrane nephritis could be established in two cases. The prognosis for this rare form of AIN is unfavorable.

Unless immunologic processes are actually absent, the inability to demonstrate these processes (*Woodroffe* et al. 1975; *Olsen* and *Asklund* 1976; *Ditlove* 1977; *Galpin* et al. 1978; *Milman* 1978; *Richet* and *Mayaud* 1978) may be due to the fact that they are detected only in biopsy material obtained during the early phase of the disease. The discovery of serum antibodies (IgG, IgM) directed against the benzylpenicilloyl antigen was a great step forward in the pathogenetic clarification (*Baldwin* et al. 1968; *Border* et al. 1974; *Lehman* et al. 1975) of methicillin-induced AIN, which characteristically appears several days after institution of methicillin therapy (*Méry* and *Fillastre* 1978). IgG and dimethoxyphenyl-penicilloyl hapten were demonstrable particularly along the tubular basement membrane (TBM), but also along the glomerular basement membrane (*Baldwin* et al. 1968). *Colvin* and co-workers (1974) found IgG in the renal interstitium as well as granular deposits of C3 along the tubules in cases of penicillin-induced AIN. They interpreted this finding as a cell-mediated immune response. Other authors who detected IgG and C3 after administration of methicillin only along the TBM (*Border* et al. 1974) considered the most probable explanation to be a humoral mechanism (*Steblay* and *Rudofsky* 1973; *Andreas* and *McCluskey* 1975). Other observations indicate that AIN can be triggered by anti-TBM antibodies (*Klassen* et al. 1972; *Andres* et al. 1978; *Ooi* et al. 1978), a finding corroborated by experimental studies with animals (*Lehman* et al. 1974; *Andres* and *McCluskey* 1975; *Klassen* et al. 1977).

Similarly, high concentrations of IgE in the serum (*Ooi* et al. 1974; *Bustamente* and *Laso* 1978; *Milman* 1978) as well as in interstitial plasma cells (*Faarup* and *Christensen* 1974) tend to speak for an (immuno)allergic process. The observation that the histologic picture of AIN closely resembles that of transplant rejection also indicates that (immuno)allergic processes are probably the most frequent pathologic mechanisms (*Nieth* 1968; *Chazan* et al. 1972; *Brass* et al. 1974; *Graber* et al. 1978; *Wilkinson* and *Boyd* 1978; *Zollinger* and *Mihatsch* 1979), particularly because the immunofluorescence microscopic findings are also similar in both cases (*Andres* and *McCluskey* 1975).

Rifampin can lead to renal damage both toxically and through (immuno)allergic processes. The etiology can be clarified by demonstrating specific antibodies against rifampin. Unfortunately, it is seldom possible to demonstrate these antibodies successfully (*Kleinknecht* et al. 1972; *Rampogal* et al. 1973). Intermittent rifampin therapy apparently encourages the development of these processes (*Rampogal* et al. 1973; *Bundschu* et al. 1974).

δ) Rare Forms of AIN

Granuloma-like inflammatory alterations (*Olsen* and *Asklund* 1976; *Wilkinson* and *Boyd* 1978) and the appearance of giant cells (*Wauters* 1977) have been observed on rare occasions. These histologic findings as well as the rare presence of uveitis (*Dobrin* et al. 1975) are important only for the differential diagnosis.

Cases of AIN have been described in association with hepatitis and exfoliative dermatitis (*McMenamin* et al. 1976). The etiology could not be clarified in every case; the acute event appears to have occurred in some cases following administration of phenindione. Cases of AIN in association with exfoliative dermatitis were also reported following allopurinol therapy (*Mills* 1971).

d) Clinical Aspects

The most important clinical symptoms are nausea and vomiting as well as fever and microscopic hematuria. If acute renal failure is present, as is usually the case, the nausea and vomiting are due to increasing retention values. Gross hematuria has also been observed with methicillin-induced AIN (*Méry* and *Fillastre* 1978). The patient often complains of spontaneous flank pain and sensitivity in the regions of both kidneys on percussion. The evaluations of glucosuria and proteinuria vary in the literature (*Beirne* et al. 1967; *Gabow* et al. 1976; *Baldamus* 1978; *Laberke* and *Bohle* 1980a). The deposition of antigen-antibody complexes in the tubular system may well contribute to glucosuria (*Andres* and *McCluskey* 1975).

Temporary anemia is a frequently reported finding in conjunction with AIN; erythrocytes are probably injured by the drug itself or circulating antigens and antibodies. Blood eosinophilia and transient generalized exanthema, both of which suggest an allergic event, are often considered typical symptoms of AIN. When these symptoms are absent, establishment of the diagnosis may be impossible (*Chazan* et al. 1972; *Laberke* and *Bohle* 1980b). The diagnosis is also difficult to establish if the patient is not febrile (*Burton* et al. 1974a; *Orchard* and *Rooker* 1974; *Laberke* and *Bohle* 1980a). The picture of AIN does not include hypertension.

A uniform description of the AIN syndrome is not presented in the literature because the symptoms tend to vary considerably (*Maxwell* et al. 1974; *Ruley* and *Lisi* 1974, *Chesney* and *Chesney* 1976; *Heptinstall* 1976). This variability may well be due primarily to individual differences in the cases examined.

Clinical resolution of AIN occurs in the majority of cases within a few weeks or, in rare cases, months, particularly after institution of steroid therapy (*Simenhoff* et al. 1968, *Gilbert* et al. 1970; *Chazan* et al. 1972; *McMenamin* et al. 1976; *Galpin* et al. 1978; *Milman* 1978; *Wilkinson* and *Boyd* 1978; *Laberke* 1980b).

Studies of larger groups of patients basically tend to indicate a favorable prognosis for AIN (*Baldwin* et al. 1968; *Ruley* and *Lisi* 1974; *Sanjad* et al. 1974; *Simenhoff* et al. 1974, *Olsen* and *Asklund* 1976; *Ditlove* et al. 1977; *Wilkinson* and *Boyd* 1978; *Laberke* and *Bohle* 1980a). Some authors however evaluate the prognosis for AIN more cautiously (*Brass* et al. 1974; *Heptinstall* 1976; *Baldamus* 1978; *Richet* and *Mayaud* 1978). Transitional forms leading to chronic renal insufficiency were observed

(*Mills* 1971; *Woodroffe* et al. 1974b; *McMenamin* et al. 1976; *Laberke* and *Bohle* 1980a). The prognosis for phenindione-induced AIN, sometimes in association with the nephrotic syndrome (*Hollman* and *Wong* 1964), is particularly poor (*Hollman* and *Wong* 1964; *Smith* 1965). A few deaths have been reported (*Galea* et al. 1963; *Baldwin* et al. 1968). We established that the prognosis for AIN is poor when acute renal failure persists for a relatively long period of time. In general, the prognosis for diffuse interstitial inflammation is poorer than that for patchy infiltration.

Establishment of the differential diagnosis (*Laberke* and *Bohle* 1980b) leads to the institution of certain therapeutic measures of particular importance in children when a differentiation must be made between AIN and acute glomerulonephritis (*Haddow* and *Robotham* 1978).

The possibility of mononucleosis (*Woodroffe* et al. 1974a), leptospirosis (*Zollinger* et al. 1971; *Ooi* et al. 1972), or brucellosis (*Dunea* et al. 1969) should be considered in the presence of a histologic picture characteristic for AIN and of the corresponding clinical symptoms. Clarification of the etiologic agents however is becoming more and more difficult in light of the wide variety of therapeutic measures currently available.

III. Acute Lesions Due Predominantly to Nephrotoxic Effects

1. Introduction

While experience has shown that patients with drug-related AIN are often being treated for minor diseases, patients receiving drugs with a potentially nephrotoxic effect are often seriously ill. This explains, at least in part, the presence of toxic renal damage and the less favorable course in cases associated with a severe primary disease. A drug dose lower than that necessary to produce a nephrotoxic effect in a healthy individual is often sufficient to cause renal damage if the dynamics of the renal blood flow are altered, the electrolyte metabolism is disturbed, or dehydration is present. If the patient is already in critical condition, the nephrotoxic side effects could contribute to a considerable worsening of the disease (*Appel* and *Neu* 1977). Furthermore, the symptomatic therapy necessary for such complications represents an additional strain on an already severely ill patient.

Drug-induced damage for the preparations mentioned below is localized in the tubular system and the interstitium.

2. Incidence

Reliable statistics are almost impossible to obtain. Nephrotoxic symptoms have been observed in 2% to 10% of all patients receiving gentamicin (*Hewitt* 1974); 1% to 2% of all deaths occurring in patients receiving tobramycin were attributed to nephrotoxic damage (*Neu* 1976).

The decrease in nephrotoxic complications is due to the development of broad-spectrum antibiotics and increased knowledge of the potential nephrotoxic effect of these drugs.

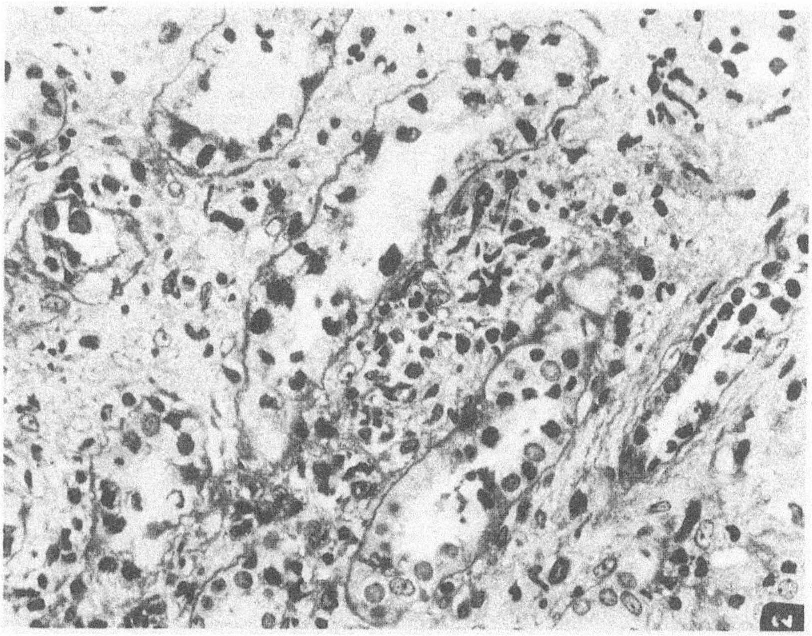

Fig. 3. Degenerative alterations in tubular epithelium with nuclear hyperchromatism and pyknosis as well as vacuolization of cytoplasm following gentamicin ingestion. (Semi-thin section, Giemsa, X 400)

3. Drugs, Morphology, and Clinical Symptoms

a) Antibiotics

Gentamicin can produce acute necrosis in the proximal convoluted tubule (*Kleinknecht* et al. 1973) (Fig. 3). An overdose results in either an oliguric or an anuric condition (*Plager* 1976) or acute nonoliguric renal failure (*Kahn* and *Stein* 1972). Gentamicin is such a valuable antibiotic for severe infections that the relatively low nephrotoxicity must be tolerated (*Méry* and *Fillastre* 1978).

Combined administration of gentamicin and cephalothin enhances the nephrotoxic effect of the drugs, particularly in the presence of a severe primary disease (e.g., hypovolemia, cardiovascular disease). The pathogenesis however has not yet been fully clarified (*Kleinknecht* et al. 1973; *Plager* 1976).

The nephrotoxic effects of and the histologic findings for *tobramycin* and *kanamycin* are similar to those for gentamicin; both apparently bind to the renal parenchyma (*Appel* and *Neu* 1977). Higher concentrations of kanamycin lead to tubular necrosis, the clinical symptoms of which are proteinuria, hematuria, cylindruria, and rising retention values. The maximum concentration capacity is sharply reduced (*Finegold* 1966; *Kreis* 1966). Cases with severe acute renal failure were described by *Hollenberg* and co-workers (1970), who interpreted this finding as the result of an unclarified, local, intrarenal, vasomotor mechanism.

A higher nephrotoxicity for *neomycin* (*Falco* et al. 1969) has been demonstrated, particularly in animal studies (*Einspruch* and *Gónzalez* 1960); apparently the accumulation risk is higher because most of the neomycin is excreted via the kidneys (*Kunin* et al. 1960). The histologic findings and clinical symptoms correspond to those described for kanamycin (*Powell* and *Hooker* 1956).

Streptomycin is reputed to have the lowest nephrotoxicity of the above-mentioned antibiotics (*Méry* and *Fillastre* 1978). Although there is a strong tendency for accumulation (*Appel* and *Neu* 1977), nephrotoxic effects appear only with high drug concentrations.

The incidence of renal complications following administration of *cephalosporins* has been extremely low in the last few years (*Carling* et al. 1975). Reported complications were acute tubular necrosis with an oliguric or anuric course, microscopic hematuria, and pyuria. The development of interstitial edema and mononuclear infiltration in response to overdosage (*Kleinknecht* et al. 1973) as well as unaltered glomeruli and vessels illustrate the similarity of the histologic picture to that of AIN (*Heptinstall* 1979).

The nephrotoxicity of *cephalothin* depends on the current status of renal function, i.e., impaired renal function enhances the nephrotoxic effect (*Pickering* et al. 1970). Some authors however reject the possibility of a nephrotoxic effect and the accumulation risk of cephalothin (*Méry* and *Fillastre* 1978).

An accumulation risk has been established for the *tetracyclines* (*Keenan* et al. 1973). Out-dated tetracycline and/or chemical changes due to long-term storage can damage the proximal tubules in particular. Cases of reversible Fanconi's syndrome have been described (*Gross* 1963). We found histologic alterations in a similar case which were almost identical with the picture of AIN.

Colistin and *polymyxin B* lead to necrosis of the proximal (*Appel* and *Neu* 1977) and also the distal convoluted tubule (*Fillastre* et al. 1970), particularly with pre-existing renal lesions. The clinical findings are proteinuria, cylindruria, and rising retention values (*Price* and *Graham* 1970). Acute renal failure seldom develops after colistin therapy (*Hollenberg* et al. 1970).

The nephrotoxicity of *sulfonamides* is primarily of historical interest. Earlier, microscopic hematuria and gross hematuria, renal colic due to obstructing sulfonamide crystals in the lower urinary tract, as well as oliguric, anuric or even uremic courses were observed (*Dowling* and *Lepper* 1943). The main nephrotoxic effects seen currently are degenerative tubular alterations and interstitial leukocytic infiltrates (*Schreiner* and *Maher* 1965), whereby the infiltrate cells can be interpreted as an expression of a resorptive inflammatory process.

Some French authors (*Duplay* et al. 1974; *Mirouze* et al. 1974) reported that higher doses of *glafenin* (glyceryl-amino-phenquine) can trigger acute renal failure.

b) Antifungal Agents

The nephrotoxic effect of *amphotericin B* is dose dependent; individual differences in tolerance levels have been reported (*Miller* and *Bates* 1969). Histologic alterations, such as necrosis and signs of degeneration in the epithelium of both convoluted tubules, are rare (*Iovine* et al. 1963; *Butler* et al. 1964). Nephrocalcinosis was observed in the tubuli and the interstitium (*Butler* et al. 1964). Thickening of the TBM has been reported (*Reynolds* et al. 1963).

c) Antituberculous Agents

p-Aminosalicylic acid (PAS) rarely causes acute tubular necrosis with acute renal failure (*Pasternack* et al. 1970). Allergic mechanisms may possibly play a role here.

d) Analgesics

Similar alterations have also been observed following high doses of *phenacetin* (p-acetophenetidine) (*Pasternack* et al. 1970). In light of the current understanding of the etiopathogenesis of acute renal failure, it is highly unlikely that the development of acute renal failure can be attributed solely to concomitant hemolysis as *MacGibbon* and coworkers (1960) suggested.

4. Clinical Aspects

Overdosage or drug accumulation must be avoided or treated symptomatically. The prognosis is favorable if renal damage is diagnosed early. A reduction in the nephrotoxic side effects may well be achieved by combining drugs to influence the synergistic effect and, at the same time, to reduce the possible side effects.

IV. Acute Lesions Due to Nephrotoxic and/or (Immuno)Allergic Effects

1. Introduction

A clear-cut differentiation between the two pathologic mechanisms is often impossible in the case of the drugs mentioned below. Given similar histologic findings, the clinical symptoms and their interpretation are often determinative. Dose-dependent damage tends to speak more for nephrotoxic side effects; dose-independent damage, the symptoms of which sometimes first appear days later, for an allergic mechanism.

2. Drugs, Morphology, Clinical Symptoms

a) Antibiotics

Some authors (*Méry* and *Fillastre* 1978) categorically reject the possibility of nephrotoxic side effects for the *penicillins,* while other authors (*Appel* and *Neu* 1977) have clearly demonstrated them. An analysis of cases interpreted as penicillin nephrotoxicity (*Kovnat* et al. 1973) and an evaluation of the described angiitis and glomerulonephritic alterations (*Spring* 1951; *Peters* et al. 1960; *Schrier* et al. 1966) revealed findings indicative of AIN. The same is also true for courses with acute renal failure after one round of penicillin (*Carré* and *Squire* 1956; *Zilberg* 1958); a complete drug history that would exclude the possibility of an allergic process is not always possible with these universally administered drugs. Moreover, a nephrotoxic etiology is questionable, because usually neither a clear-cut overdosage nor pre-existing renal damage was present.

Questionable for the same reasons is the possible nephrotoxic effect of an eventual overdosage of *methicillin* (*Chesney* and *Chesney* 1976).

Both pathologic mechanisms may well be active in the case of *polymyxin B*. Histologic alterations characteristic for AIN and blood eosinophilia were present as well as severe tubular damage, which could be interpreted as the result of nephrotoxicity (*Beirne* et al. 1967). The possibility of an additional toxic component therefore cannot be excluded even for typical cases of AIN with acute renal failure (*Brass* et al. 1974).

b) Antituberculous Agents

Nephrotoxic damage associated with *rifampin* therapy has been reported (*Poole* et al. 1971; *Bundschu* et al. 1974) in cases with an eventual high dosage and no demonstrable antibodies. Cases of AIN attributed to antigen-antibody reactions have been provoked by intermittent rifampin therapy (*Kleinknecht* et al. 1972; *Decroix* et al. 1973). Regardless of the clinical importance of this intermittent therapy, it is not a recommendable therapeutic measure because of the risk of sensitization.

c) Analgesics

Although the incidence is low, nephrotoxic properties due to direct intervention in the metabolism of the tubular cells (*Senft* 1959), influence on the tubular enzymes (*Hörlin* et al. 1955), and disturbance of the tubular transport mechanism (*Yü* 1958) have been reported with *phenylbutazone*. The incidence of allergic reactions however is higher (*Scheitlin* and *Jeanneret* 1957; *Richardson* and *Alderfer* 1963; *Streicher* 1964; *Fillastre* et al. 1969; *Kuhlmann* et al. 1978; *Richet* and *Mayaud* 1978).

3. Clinical Aspects

The discussion of the clinical aspects in II_4 also applies for those cases in which the nephrotoxic and (immuno)allergic mechanisms overlap.

V. Primarily Chronic Tubulo-interstitial Lesions – Analgesic Nephropathy

1. Introduction

The most extensively studied form of primarily chronic tubulo-interstitial lesions is analgesic nephropathy (AN). AN, because of its high incidence, is also of considerable importance. In 1978, approximately 300 million DM were spent for nonprescription analgesics in the Federal Republic of Germany. At the beginning of 1979, 83 preparations containing between 100 and 350 mg of phenacetin were available on the German drug market (*Baust* 1979).

2. Definitions

Analgesic nephropathy is defined as chronic renal disease due to analgesic abuse. The clinical symptoms are anemia, increasing signs of renal insufficiency, hematuria, leukocyturia, hypertension, and colic during the excretion of papillary fragments. The premature aging of the patient is impressive (*Gault* et al. 1968; *Nanra* 1976a). Morphologic alterations in the advanced stage include aseptic papillary necrosis, diffuse interstitial fibrosis, and tubular atrophy of the overlying cortical tissue (*Burry* 1967; *Nanra* 1976b; *Kincaid-Smith* and *Nanra* 1978).

Some authors define analgesic abuse as the ingestion of 0.3 to 1.5 g of phenacetin daily, over a period of one or more years (*Schweingruber* 1955; *Bengtsson* and *Hood* 1965; *Gloor* 1965a). Other authors base their definition on the total analgesic intake, i.e., 2 kg phenacetin/acetaminophen (paracetamol)/acetylsalicylic acid (*Nanra* 1976a) or 2 kg acetylsalicylic acid (*Burry* and *Hopkins* 1977). Some definitions also include a decrease in the creatinine clearance as well as clinical and radiologic findings (*Cove-Smith* and *Knapp* 1973).

3. Historical Survey

At the end of the 1960s, *Kincaid-Smith* (comp. *Dawborn* et al. 1966), in particular, suggested the term "analgesic nephropathy." This term seems appropriate since the exact analgesic and/or respective metabolite inflicting the most damage is still disputed.

Terms such as "Saridon nephritis" (*Zollinger* 1955), expressing the causal relationship between Saridon and nephritis (*Spühler* and *Zollinger* 1953), and "phenacetin kidney" (*Moeschlin* 1957) are basically only of historical interest. Pyelonephritis, in the narrow sense of the word, was identified as a secondary phenomenon and differentiated from chronic sclerosing interstitial nephritis resulting from analgesic abuse (*Kincaid-Smith* 1967).

Murry and *Goldberg* (1978) felt that the term "analgesic abuse" was far too judgmental and therefore suggested "analgesic-associated nephropathy."

4. Analgesic Nephropathy in Different Countries

After AN was first observed by *Spühler* and *Zollinger* (1953) in Switzerland, more and more countries began to recognize its importance. Assuming that the patient records and data are comparable, AN appears to have less significance in the Federal Republic of Germany, the United States, Canada, and Great Britain than in Switzerland and Australia. The causal relationship between analgesic abuse and nephropathy seems to be particularly clear in those countries where a marked decrease in the number of AN-related deaths was observed a few years after phenacetin was eliminated from mixed preparations (Denmark: *Kjaerulff* and *Harvald* 1968; Sweden: *Nordenfelt* 1973).

5. Incidence (Clinical Observation, Biopsy, Autopsy)

Since analgesic abuse is often discovered for the first time after the patient has developed chronic renal insufficiency and since many cases go undetected because the patients tend to deny analgesic abuse or a drug history is unavailable, exact statistics on analgesic abuse cannot be obtained. Moreover, the source of the statistics (clinical observation, biopsy, or post mortem examination) must be taken into consideration.

The incidence of AN is expected to peak in the next few years. The number of AN patients therefore will drop sharply within the next 10 to 20 years when the pharmacologic composition of analgesics is changed and as many analgesic abusers as possible are informed of possible side effects and when it has been established that phenacetin and its metabolites constitute the most important contributory factor for renal damage, a fact currently disputed.

The number of analgesic abusers in the Federal Republic of Germany is estimated at between 2.1% and 10% of all patients with kidney disease (*Bock* 1974). In Australia, 11% to 15% of the general population apparently take various amounts of analgesics daily (*Healy* 1975). Analgesic abuse is considered to be a contributing factor for 10% to 20% of all cases of renal insufficiency and renal failure in long-term dialysis patients and prospective recipients of kidney transplants (*Sheil* et al. 1969; *Kingsley* et al. 1972; *Lawrence* et al. 1973; *Kramer* 1975; *Cove-Smith* and *Knapp* 1978; *Kincaid-Smith* 1979).

The incidence of analgesic abuse in our biopsy material was 0.5%, a figure which corresponds with statistics reported for Great Britain [Switzerland, 1.3%; Denmark, 2.5%; Australia, 20% (*Kincaid-Smith* 1979)].

6. Age and Sex

The average age of the AN patients in our biopsy material ranged between 45 and 55, thus agreeing with the observation that AN occurs most frequently in middle-aged individuals (*Gloor* 1962; *Prescott* 1966a; *Nitzsche* and *Bock* 1970; *Dubach* 1971; *Gault* et al. 1971; *Höffler* et al. 1973; *Gsell* 1974). Signs of AN however have also been reported in the 20- to 30-year-old age group (*Hensler* 1957; *Scheidegger* 1958; *Gsell* 1974; *Ringoir* 1974).

Reports that the incidence of AN is higher in men than in women are rare, e.g., men working with heavy metals in Sweden (*Nordenfelt* and *Ringertz* 1961; *Grimlund* 1963) and a study by *Gault* and co-workers (1971) in which the predominance of men cannot be similarly interpreted. The reported incidence is usually considerably higher in women: 3:1 (*Hensler* 1957; *Koutsaimanis* and *de Wardener* 1970; *Nitzsche* and *Bock* 1970; *Kingsley* et al. 1972; *Haschek* and *Schmidt* 1975) or 4:1 (*Höffler* et al. 1973; *Adams* and *Murray* 1975; *Wagoner* 1976; *Cove-Smith* and *Knapp* 1978; *Kincaid-Smith* 1979). Reports of ratios as low as 2:1 (*Haas* 1956; *Larsen* and *Moeller* 1958; *Lee* et al. 1974; *Bock* and *Nitzsche* 1976; *Laberke* 1980a) or as high as 5:1 (*Lornoy* et al. 1971; *Murray* and *Goldberg* 1975; *Nanra* 1976a) are less frequent.

7. Morphology

a) Macroscopic Findings

Macroscopic findings at the time of autopsy are generally identical to those for the advanced stage of AN; both kidneys are small. Depressed areas of scar tissue representing cortical atrophy overlying the papillae alternate with compensatory hypertrophic areas in the region of the renal columns of Bertin. The cortical parenchyma is narrowed on the cut surface. When papillary necrosis is present, brownish-black papillae and/or papillary defects and sometimes calcification as well as cystic cavities are impressive (*Spühler* and *Zollinger* 1953; *Scheidegger* 1958; *Nanra* 1976b; *Kincaid-Smith* and *Nanra* 1978).

b) Light and Electron Microscopic Findings

The important histologic alterations associated with AN are found in the vessels, tubules, and interstitium. These alterations are discussed below chronologically.

In the early stage of AN, proliferative connective tissue and increased quantities of mast cells appear on the *vessels* of the outer medullary zone (*Gloor* 1961). The capillary basement membrane is uniformly thickened (*Burry* 1978; *Gloor* 1978). Electron microscopic examination of the basement membrane shows a lamellar structure. Necrotic endothelial cells appear somewhat later (*Gloor* 1978). The process then continues until the capillaries of the inner medullary zone are, for the most part, no longer discernible; the vessels of the outer medullary zone are surrounded by collagen.

Since hypertension generally accompanies AN, typical hypertensive alterations are later demonstrable in the cortical vessels (*Uehlinger* 1971; *Lee* et al. 1974).

The impressive thickening of the capillaries near the urothelium (microangiopathy and/or capillary sclerosis) found in 80% of the cases of AN is thought to be pathognomonic (*Gloor* 1978; *Mihatsch* et al. 1978). The papillae and mucosa of the urinary tract have a brown pigmentation due to the deposition of a lipofuscin-like substance. The pigment is also found in the tubular epithelium of the outer medullary zone (*Gloor* 1978). When the cortex shows no pathologic alterations, this finding (Fig. 4) could indicate the presence of early AN. In addition to the kidneys, brown pigmentation has

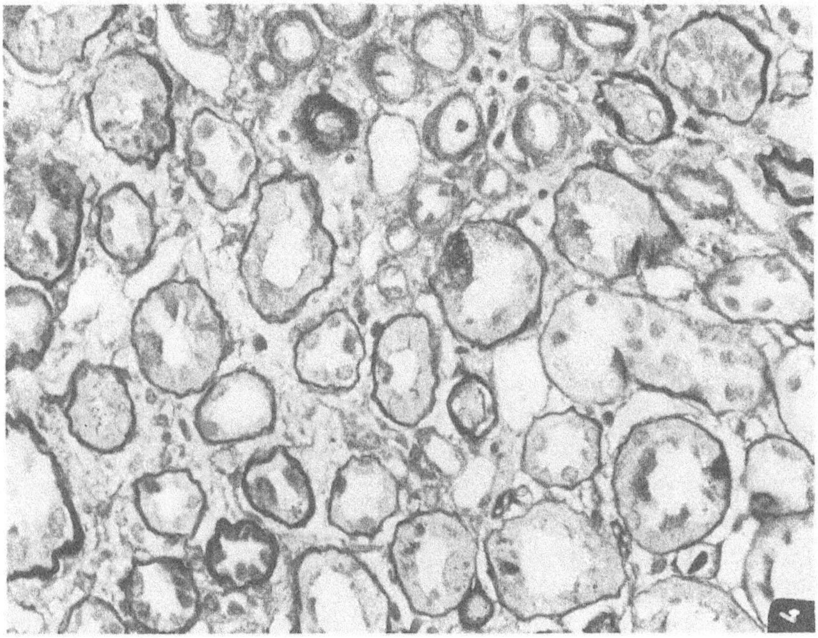

Fig. 4. Early stage of analgesic nephropathy. Lipofuscin-like granules in tubular epithelium of medullary collecting ducts with thickening of vasa recta basement membranes and slight thickening of tubular basement membranes. (Paraffin section, PAS, X 400)

also been reported in the brain, heart, cartilage, and skin (*Gloor* 1965a; *Munck* et al. 1970; *Bianchi* et al. 1972; *Lee* et al. 1974).

Electron microscopic examination in the early stages of AN shows pathologic alterations in the region of the *tubules,* i.e., epithelial cell degeneration and thickened TBM in the medulla and the pyramids (*Gault* and *Muehrcke* 1973). In the more advanced form, the renal medulla shows tubular cell damage and dilation of the tubules in addition to an increasingly thickened TBM. At this point, alterations identical to medullary alterations in the early stage of AN can be observed in the renal cortex. In the advanced stage of AN, there is high-grade atrophy of the tubules and interstitial fibrosis (Fig. 5) overlying the necrotic papillae. In the case of complete papillary necrosis, fissures sometimes develop at the border between intact and necrotic tissue due to cystic dilation of the tubules in the outer medullary zone (*Gloor* 1978).

In the early phase of the disease, circumscribed, usually cell-deficient, fibrosis is found in the *interstitium* of the renal medulla and the papillae (*Gloor* 1974).

The tubules are thought to be compressed by the interstitial fibrosis, thereby resulting in functional impairment (*Uehlinger* 1972). The picture of secondary cortical atrophy overlying the necrotic papillae has occasionally been compared to alterations associated with hydronephrosis (*Sanerkin* 1966; *Kincaid-Smith* 1967; *Burry* 1970).

Bacterial urinary tract infections were observed in the early stages of AN in 10% of all analgesic abuse cases where renal function was not yet detectably impaired

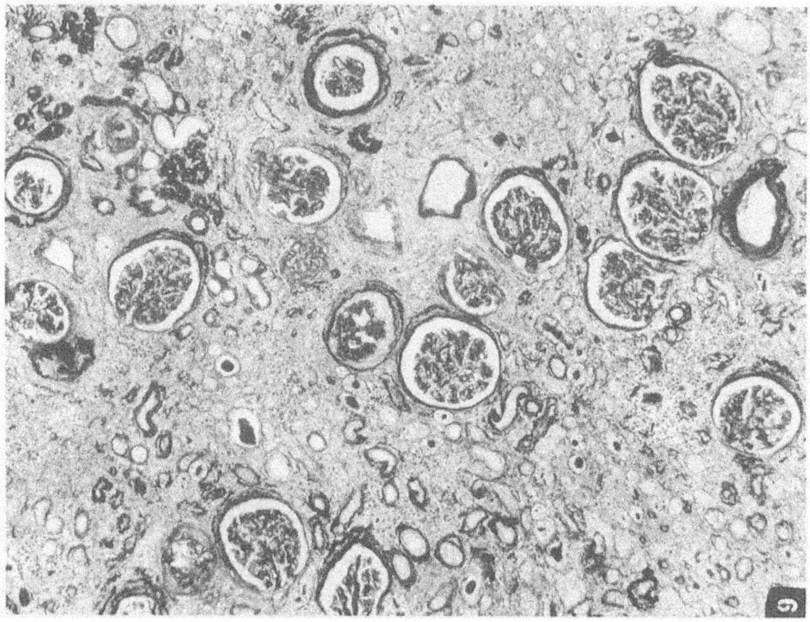

Fig. 5. Late stage of analgesic nephropathy. Diffuse interstitial fibrosis and advanced tubular atrophy with fibrotically thickened Bowman's capsule and essentially preserved glomeruli which lie close together as a result of cortical atrophy. (Paraffin section, PAS, X 80)

(*Gsell* et al. 1968). We however were unable to confirm this observation in our case material; instead, we found a history of urinary tract infection appearing for the first time in the advanced stages of AN. Here the chronic fibrosing character was masked by circumscribed destruction.

The typical grave alterations of the *papillae,* which are nonpathognomonic, are described separately. In general, the alterations are primarily sterile papillary necroses which may provoke inflammatory complications. Papillary necrosis frequently appears in association with AN (*Spühler* and *Zollinger* 1953; *Lindvall* 1960; *Gloor* 1961; *Nordenfelt* and *Ringertz* 1961; *Prescott* 1966a; *Nitzsche* and *Bock* 1970; *Gault* et al. 1971; *Wilson* 1972; *Lee* et al. 1974). Some authors however reported a lower incidence of papillary necrosis, i.e., 25% to 40% of the cases (*Fellner* and *Tuttle* 1969; *Murray* and *Goldberg* 1975, 1978). Differences in the groups of patients studied were apparently responsible for these variations. Papillary necroses were found in 1.7% of all post mortem examinations in Switzerland (*Gloor* 1965a). The reported values for Australia range between 3.7% and 20% (*Jacobs* and *Morris* 1962; *Burry* et al. 1966; *Nanra* et al. 1970; *Arnold* et al. 1973/74; *Nanra* 1976a).

While important alterations are usually not observed in the *glomeruli,* pronounced fibrosis of Bowman's capsule is typical for the more advanced stages of AN (*Gloor* 1961; *Lee* et al. 1974). The glomeruli are surrounded by fibrous tissue and hyalinized in the advanced stage (*Uehlinger* 1971). The natural aging process of the kidney therefore could also be responsible for the isolated hyalinized glomeruli found in elderly AN patients (*Gault* et al. 1971).

c) Fluorescence Microscopic Findings

No positive findings have been obtained with fluorescence microscopy (*Gault* et al. 1971; *Gault* and *Muehrcke* 1973). This absence of positive findings therefore may possibly explain the stabilization or improvement in renal function, even in moderately severe cases, following withdrawal of analgesic intake.

8. Clinical Aspects

The most common reason given for analgesic abuse is headache (*Sarre* and *Rogal* 1964; *Fellner* and *Tuttle* 1969; *Nitzsche* and *Bock* 1970; *Kingsley* et al. 1972; *Lee* et al. 1974; *Haschek* et al. 1975; *Murray* and *Goldberg* 1975). Additional reasons reported were other types of pain, depression and the stimulant effect of some analgesics. Already in 1953, *Spühler* and *Zollinger* established that there are no early symptoms of AN; the disorder therefore is often diagnosed for the first time in the advanced stages of renal insufficiency. The many different symptoms of AN can be divided into renal and extrarenal symptoms (*Gsell* 1974).

Renal symptoms include early reduction in renal concentration capacity (*Gault* et al. 1971; *Cove-Smith* and *Knapp* 1973; *Kramer* 1975) and sodium and potassium depletion, as well as a rise in serum creatinine concentration due to increasing interstitial fibrosis in the advanced stages of AN.

Microscopic and gross hematuria (*Kincaid-Smith* 1979), possibly due to papillary necrosis, nephrolithiasis, hypertensive glomerular damage, and carcinoma of the lower urinary tract are frequent findings. One diagnostically important finding is nonbacterial leukocyturia (i.e., sterile pyuria) (*Pearson* 1967; *Linton* 1972; *Gsell* 1974; *Murray* and *Goldberg* 1978).

Urinary tract infections were reported in 15% to 65% of the cases (*Gault* et al. 1968; *Nitzsche* and *Bock* 1970; *Gloor* 1974; *Haschek* et al. 1975; *Murray* and *Goldberg* 1975; *Kincaid-Smith* 1979). The incidence of such infections increases in direct proportion to the duration and severity of AN. The primary disease is often first diagnosed when urinary tract infection appears (*Gsell* 1974).

Renal hypertension is present in 30% to 60% of all advanced cases of AN (*Fellner* and *Tuttle* 1969; *Kingsley* et al. 1972; *Wilson* 1972; *Bock* 1974; *Murray* and *Goldberg* 1975, 1978).

In regard to the extrarenal symptoms, a medical history of headache, which may not always be the reason for, but rather a sequela of analgesic abuse, is found in 80% to 85% of all cases (*Fellner* and *Tuttle* 1969; *Murray* and *Goldberg* 1975). Pronounced macrocytic non-iron-deficiency anemia may already be observed in the early stages. Clinical examination often shows gray cyanosis due to anemia; sulfahemoglobin, methemoglobin, and inactive hemoglobin are demonstrable (*Schaub* et al. 1953). Toxic components and acidosis, a frequent finding, have been discussed as possible causal factors (*Nissen* and *Friis* 1962; *Uhl* and *Hunstein* 1973); erythropoietin deficiency also plays an additional role in the stage of contracted kidney. Bleeding gastric ulcers developing after salicylate therapy can lead to anemia (*Dawborn* et al. 1966; *Kincaid-Smith* and *Nanra* 1978). Statistics for anemia presented in the literature vary considerably: 25% (*Cove-Smith* and *Knapp* 1978) and 60% to 80% (*Fellner* and *Tuttle* 1969; *Haschek* et al. 1973; *Murray* and *Goldberg* 1975).

Gastrointestinal disorders, such as peptic ulcers, were reported, particularly after salicylate therapy (*Dawborn* et al. 1966; *Murray* and *Goldberg* 1975, 1978; *Nanra* et al. 1978).

Brown pigmentation of the skin is due to deposition of lipofuscin-like pigments (*Berneis* and *Studer* 1969); a similar deposition of pigment in the epithelial cells of the liver (*Gloor* 1965a) is not diagnostically significant. The brown coloration of the urine is attributed to phenacetin metabolites (*Prescott* and *Brown* 1970).

Abnormal emotional behavior has been observed in many individuals with high analgesic intake. It is often difficult to determine whether abnormal behavioral patterns led to analgesic abuse or whether pain and subsequent analgesic abuse precipitated the abnormal behavior. The patients are described as irritable and bad tempered (*Schweingruber* 1955), depressive and anxious (*Kingsley* et al. 1972), as well as emotionally unstable and inflexible.

The diagnostic criteria are derived essentially from the above-mentioned symptoms. A detailed medical and drug history must be taken prior to examination of the patient (*Nanra* 1976a). The correct diagnosis can be made on the basis of the medical and the drug histories, demonstration of phenacetin metabolites in the urine, and radiologic visualization of papillary necrosis. A biopsy is usually necessary when clinical clarification of renal insufficiency is unsuccessful or the severity of renal damage must be established.

Carcinoma of the urothelium is one late complication of AN, developing in approximately 10% of the cases (*Bock* 1973; *Johansson* et al. 1974; *Gloor* 1978). The incidence of carcinoma of the urothelium in individuals with AN is nine times higher than in individuals who do not take analgesics on a regular basis (*Taylor* 1972). Studies of AN patients have shown this causal relationship (*Angervall* 1969; *Bengtsson* et al. 1968, 1975; *Anseline* and *Howarth* 1977).

The prognosis for AN depends on when the diagnosis is established. The condition can stabilize and sometimes even improve if serum creatinine values have not exceeded 2.5 to 3.0 mg% (*Grimlund* 1963; *Nordenfelt* 1972; *Laberke* 1980a).

9. Differential Diagnosis

If papillary necrosis is demonstrated, the possibility of diabetes mellitus, obstructions of the urinary tract, and sickle cell anemia must be excluded in the clinical examination (*Hare* and *Poynter* 1974). A biopsy is necessary when the clinical findings are inconclusive. Since enlarged kidneys with impaired function are found in the acute stage of papillary necrosis, the possibility of acute glomerulonephritis, acute interstitial nephritis, renal vein thrombosis, and infiltrative processes (i.e., plasmacytoma, amyloidosis, leukemia, lymphoma) must be excluded.

Necrotic papillae with cystic structures and irregular defects are also present with renal tuberculosis; pyelogenous cysts, medullary sponge kidney, and absent papillae, with chronic pyelonephritis (particularly chronic juvenile pyelonephritis) and hydronephrosis.

Small kidneys with preserved papillae may be normal (physiologic variation in size) or a sign of bilateral renal artery stenosis, particularly when the patient is hypertensive.

One third of all cases of AN are initially diagnosed as chronic pyelonephritis; the correct diagnosis of another third is established for the first time at the post mortem examination (*Cove-Smith* and *Knapp* 1978). In 1975, *Kramer* noted that the depressed areas on the surface of the AN kidney correspond to the region of the papillae in the state after papillary necrosis; the raised areas, to the calyceal region. With pyelonephritis, the alterations are reversed.

10. Etiology and Pathogenesis

Cortical alterations were originally thought to be the primary lesions; medullary and papillary alterations, the secondary phenomenon (*Spühler* and *Zollinger* 1953; *Thölen* et al. 1956). Damage to the tubular system and the cortical vessels was thought to be due to the toxic effects (*Thölen* et al. 1956; *Gloor* 1978). Cortical alterations were interpreted for the first time in 1965 as the result of medullary and papillary alterations (*Kincaid-Smith* 1965). This opinion was repeatedly substantiated (*Abrahams* et al. 1967; *Burry* 1967; *Clausen* and *Jensen* 1968; *Calder* 1972; *Gloor* 1974; *Wagoner* 1976). Confirmation was also possible with electron microscopic studies (*Gault* et al. 1971) carried out in the earliest phase of AN after a minimum total consumption of 2 kg phenacetin and/or acetylsalicylic acid. Currently, tubular obstruction in the necrotic medulla is thought to be responsible for cortical damage (*Kincaid-Smith* and *Nanra* 1978).

The discussion of whether the renal lesions are produced by phenacetin (*Jacobs* and *Morris* 1962; *Burry* et al. 1966; *Nordenfelt* 1972; *Raaflaub* and *Dubach* 1972; *Gloor* 1978) or its metabolites, e.g., acetophenetidine and acetaminophen (*Raaflaub* and *Dubach* 1972), still continues. Even acetylsalicylic acid (*Nanra* 1976b; *Kincaid-Smith* and *Nanra* 1978) and caffeine (*Boyd* 1959; *Boyd* et al. 1965; *Prescott* 1966b), which is often included in mixed preparations, are assumed to be important etiologic agents. Recently, more significance has been attributed to the toxic effect of acetylsalicylic acid (*Nanra* et al. 1978). Since most drugs consumed are mixed preparations, the question of whether phenacetin or its metabolites are responsible for the renal lesions has not been definitively answered by studies in man or with animals (*Cove-Smith* and *Knapp* 1978; *Murray* and *Goldberg* 1978).

Mixed preparations are even more important when it is assumed that the synergistic effect of phenacetin enhances the toxicity of acetylsalicylic acid (*Nanra* 1976b).

The toxic effect of analgesic agents and their metabolites is intensified by dehydration (*Kincaid-Smith* 1967). Toxicity, anoxia, secretion inhibition, hypocirculation, obstruction of the vasa recta, reduced urine production, competitive inhibitory mechanisms, and decreased prostaglandin synthesis have been discussed as possible pathologic mechanisms (*Heidland* et al. 1967; *Kincaid-Smith* 1967; *Nanra* et al. 1973; *Kincaid-Smith* and *Nanra* 1978; *Dubach* 1979). It is still unclear however how the details of the toxic mechanism are to be understood (*Dubach* 1979). Papillary necrosis has also been reported following therapy with pure aspirin preparations, an observation which complicates the overall evaluation (*Harvald* and *Clausen* 1960; *Prescott* 1966a, 1969; *Murray* et al. 1971; *Duggan* 1974; *Nanra* 1975; *Nanra* et al. 1978).

There are indications that different degrees of "receptivity" for AN may be attributed to individual differences in phenacetin metabolism (*Gsell* 1974).

Immunologic reactions have usually not been demonstrable (*Gault* et al. 1971). Since sensitization processes triggered by phenacetin have been observed (*Rügger* et al. 1973), the possibility of an immunologic process cannot be excluded.

A consideration of the enzyme system of the proximal convoluted tubule and the fact that enzyme activity in the cells of the renal medulla is extremely low suggests that the primary damage is inflicted in the proximal convoluted tubule (*Mitchell* et al. 1977; *Dubach* 1979). The metabolites however are increasingly concentrated toward the medulla and therefore could lead to a toxic effect there. It is possible that, because of reduced blood supply and anaerobic metabolism, the renal medulla reacts more sensitively to noxae than does the renal cortex. Whether primary damage occurs in the vessels (*Nanra* and *Kincaid-Smith* 1972) or in the loops of *Henle* (*Burry* 1968; *Prescott* 1970) is just as disputed as the suggestion that primary damage occurs in the vessels, loops of *Henle*, and the interstitial ground substance (*Gloor* 1965b, 1974).

A genetic factor for AN has been discussed since certain relationships were established between the HL-A antigen and the familial occurrence of AN (*MacDonald* 1976). One possible explanation for the familial occurrence of AN (*Murray* and *Goldberg* 1975) may be that headaches and other conditions leading to analgesic abuse tend to occur more frequently in some families.

Animal studies have not contributed a great deal of information on the pathogenesis of AN. Some animal species appear to be unsuitable as models for AN because of their different metabolic processes (*Murray* and *Goldberg* 1978) and anatomic relationships in the region of the renal papillae (*Shelley* 1978). Since the relative short duration of animal experiments is compensated by high analgesic dosage, the conclusions that can be drawn from the studies are limited (*Studer* 1965; *Shelley* 1978). Mixed analgesic preparations produced papillary necrosis more effectively in animal experiments than did individual drugs (*Molland* 1978). AN could not be induced in rabbits by the administration of analgesic agents alone, but rather developed only after a secondary *E. coli* infection (*Miescher* et al. 1958). Subsequent experiments however indicated that the interstitial infiltrate was not essentially more pronounced in the infected animals (*Miescher* and *Studer* 1961). Phenacetin did not lead to alterations characteristic for AN (*Studer* 1965); comparable lesions sometimes developed after administration of either phenacetin or aspirin (*Clausen* 1965). *Molland* (1978) established that the nephrotoxicity of aspirin is higher than that of phenacetin. The amount of phenacetin consumed by rats did not correlate with the severity of the renal damage (*Saker* and *Kincaid-Smith* 1969).

Regardless of the importance attributed to these animal experiments, they still generally confirm a causal relationship between analgesic intake and renal damage.

11. Primarily Chronic Interstitial Nephritis Not Induced by Analgesic Agents

Bock and co-workers (1973) reported that *antiasthma preparations containing phenacetin* produce clinical and histological pictures identical to AN. Since only two of the 13 antiasthma preparations containing phenacetin listed in Bock's study are currently available in the Federal Republic of Germany, these drugs are not longer significant.

According to *Hestbech* and co-workers (1977), *lithium preparations*, often perscribed for psychiatric disorders, may well be more important now. The cases observed by *Hestbech* were clinical examples of acute intoxication; examination of kidney biopsy material however unexpectedly showed interstitial fibrosis and tubular atrophy, both suggesting chronic processes.

VI. Concluding Remarks

The allergotoxic effects of drugs are often responsible for acute and chronic tubulo-interstitial renal damage. An exact drug history therefore is mandatory. A kidney biopsy may be necessary for etiologic clarification. The histologic alterations, while predominantly nonpathognomonic, are still so typical that a correct diagnosis can be established on the basis of the presence of these alterations together with the clinical data. The prognosis is generally good if use of the drug or drugs is discontinued.

References

Abrahams C, Levin NW, Gecelter L, Rubenstein AH (1967) The diagnosis of analgesic nephropathy by renal biopsy. Med Proc 13: 501–506

Adams FG, Murray RM (1975) The radiological diagnosis of analgesic nephropathy. Clin Radiol 26: 417–427

Andres GA, McCluskey RT (1975) Tubular and interstitial renal disease due to immunologic mechanisms. Kidney Internat 7: 271–289

Andres GA, Brentjens J, Kohli R, Anthone R, Anthone S, Baliah T, Montes M, Mookerjee BK, Prezyna A, Sepulveda M, Venuto R, Elwood C (1978) Histology of human tubulo-interstitial nephritis associated with antibodies to renal basement membranes. Kidney Internat 13: 480–491

Andrieu J, Audebrand C, Chassaigne M, Renier E (1976) Anémie hémolytique et insuffisance rénale imputables à la glafénine. Nouv Presse Med 5: 2394–2395

Angervall L, Bengtsson U, Zetterlund CG, Zsigmond M (1969) Renal pelvic carcinoma in a Swedish district with abuse of a phenacetin-containing drug. Br J Urol 41: 401–405

Anseline P, Howarth VS (1977) A case of transitional cell carcinoma of the renal pelvis, clear cell renal carcinoma, and analgesic nephropathy. Aust NZ J Surg 47: 521–523

Appel GB, Neu HC (1977) Nephrotoxicity of antimicrobial agents. N Engl J Med 296: 663–670, 722–728, 784–787

Appel GB, Woda BA, Neu HC, Parry MF, Silva F, Pirani CL (1978) Acute interstitial nephritis associated with carbenicillin therapy. Arch Intern Med 138: 1265–1267

Arnold L, Collins G, Starmer GA (1973–74) Renal papillary necrosis: the incidence at autopsy in a hospital population in Sidney. Bull Postgrad Comm Med Univ Syd 29: 228–235

Baker SB, Williams RT (1963) Acute interstitial nephritis due to drug sensitivity. Br Med J 1: 1655–1658

Baldamus CA (1978) Akute interstitielle Nephritis. Der Deutsche Arzt 23: 47–56

Baldwin DS, Levine BB, McCluskey RT, Gallo GR (1968) Renal failure and interstitial nephritis due to penicillin and methicillin. N Engl J Med 279: 1245–1252

Baust W (1979) Der vasomotorische Kopfschmerz. Med Welt 30: 761–765

Beirne GJ, Hansing CE, Octaviano GN, Burns RO (1967) Acute renal failure caused by hypersensitivity to polymyxin B sulfate. JAMA 202: 156–158

Bengtsson U, Hood B (1965) Abuse of phenacetin-containing analgesics and renal damage. In: Kass EH (ed) Progress in pyelonephritis. Davis & Co, Philadelphia, pp 297–306

Bengtsson U, Angervall L, Ekman H, Lehmann L (1968) Transitional cell tumors of the renal pelvis in analgesic abusers. Scand J Urol Nephrol 2: 145–150

Bengtsson U, Angervall L, Johansson S, Wahlgvist L (1975) Phenacetin abuse and renal pelvic carcinoma. Int J Clin Pharmacol Biopharm 12: 290–294

Berneis K, Studer A (1969) Ablagerung farbiger Lipide in der Haut als Folge von Phenacetinabusus. Virchows Arch Abt B Zellpath 2: 311–317

Bianchi L, Berneis K, Studer A (1972) Brown discoloration of cartilage in phenacetin abuse. Virchows Arch Abt B Zellpath 10: 339–343

Bock KD (1973) Analgetika-Abusus und maligne Nierenbeckentumoren. In: Haschek H (ed) Internationales Symposium über Probleme des Phenacetin-Abusus. Egermann, Wien, pp 227–233

Bock KD (1974) Häufigkeit und klinische Wertigkeit der arzneimittelbedingten chronischen interstitiellen Nephritis. In: Kluthe R, Oechslen D (eds) Aktuelle Diagnostik von Nierenerkrankungen. 6. Freiburger Tagung über Nephrologie 1974. Thieme, Stuttgart, pp 30–37

Bock KD, Nitzsche T (1976) Laxantienabusus, Plasma-Kalium und chronische interstitielle Nephritis durch Phenacetin-Abusus. Klin Wochenschr 54: 239–241

Bock KD, Nitzsche T, Messer B (1973) Chronische interstitielle Nephritis bei langjährigem Gebrauch phenacetinhaltiger Asthmapulver. Dtsch Med Wochenschr 98: 2234

Bolt HM (1975) Nebenwirkungen von Rifampicin und ihre biochemischen Grundlagen. Dtsch Med Wochenschr 100: 63–65

Border WA, Lehman DH, Egan JD, Sass HJ, Glode JE, Wilson CB (1974) Antitubular basement-membrane antibodies in methicillin-associated interstitial nephritis. N Engl J Med 291: 381–384

Boyd EM (1959) The acute oral toxicity of caffeine. Toxic Appl Pharmacol 1: 250–257

Boyd EM, Dolman M, Knight LM, Sheppard EP (1965) The chronic oral toxicity of caffeine. Canad J Physiol Pharmacol 43: 995–1007

Brass H, Lapp H, Heintz R (1974) Akute interstitielle Nephritis – Mögliche Ursache eines akuten Nierenversagens. Dtsch Med Wochenschr 99: 2335–2340

Bundschu HD, Menz HP, Hayduk K, Schomerus H, Bohle A (1974) Schwere (allergische?) interstitielle Nephritis durch Tuberkulostatica. Verh Dtsch Ges Inn Med 80: 1564–1567

Burry AF (1967) The evolution of analgesic nephropathy. Nephron 5: 185–201

Burry AF (1970) The pathology and pathogenesis of renal papillary necrosis. In: Kincaid-Smith P, Fairley KF (eds) Renal infection and renal scarring. Mercedes Publ Services, Melbourne, pp 335–346

Burry AF (1978) Pathology of analgesic abuse: Australian experience. Kidney Internat 13: 34–40

Burry AF, Hopkins J (1977) Phenacetin and analgesic nephropathy. Med J Aust 1: 879–882

Burry AF, de Jersey P, Weedon D (1966) Phenacetin and renal papillary necrosis: results of a prospective autopsy investigation. Med J Aust 53: 873–879

Burton JR, Lichtenstein NS, Colvin RB, Hyslop NE jr (1974a) Acute interstitial nephritis from oxacillin. Johns Hopkins Med J 134: 58–61

Burton JR, Lichtenstein NS, Colvin RB, Hyslop NE jr (1974b) Acute renal failure during cephalothin therapy. JAMA 229: 679–682

Bustamente J, Laso J (1978) Nefritis intersticial aguda e IgE. Rev Clin Esp 150: 215–216

Butler WT, Bennett JE, Alling DW, Wertlake PT, Utz JP, Hill GJ (1964) Nephrotoxicity of amphotericin B: early and late effects in 81 patients. Ann Intern Med 61: 175–187

Calder IC, Funder CC, Green CR, Ham KN, Tange JD (1972) Nephrotoxic lesions from 5-aminosalicylic acid. Br Med J 1: 152–154

Carling PC, Idelson BA, Casano AA, Alexander EA, McCabe WR (1975) Nephrotoxicity associated with cephalothin administration. Arch Intern Med 135: 797–801

Carré IJ, Squire JR (1956) Anuria ascribed to acute tubular necrosis in infancy and early childhood. Arch Dis Child 31: 512–522

Chazan JA, Garella S, Esparza A (1972) Acute interstitial nephritis. A distinct clinicopathological entity? Nephron 9: 10–26

Chesney RW, Chesney PJ (1976) Methicillin-associated nephritis: clinical rarity or common entity? A review. Clin Pediatr 15: 1013–1017

Clausen E (1965) Histologic changes in the kidneys caused by phenacetin and acetylsalicylic acid, animal experiments. In: Kass EH (ed) Progress in pyelonephritis. Davis & Co, Philadelphia, pp 332–336

Clausen E, Jensen K (1968) Renal biopsies from patients with a high analgesic intake. Histological and bacteriological study. Acta Path Microbiol Scand 72: 219–232

Colvin RB, Burton JR, Hyslop NE jr, Spitz L, Lichtenstein NS (1974) Penicillin-associated interstitial nephritis (letter). Ann Intern Med 81: 404–405

Councilman WT (1898) Acute interstitial nephritis. J Exp Med 3: 393–420

Cove-Smith JR, Knapp MS (1973) Sodium handling in analgesic nephropathy. Lancet II: 70–72

Cove-Smith JR, Knapp MS (1978) Analgesic nephropathy: An important cause of chronic renal failure. Quart J Med New Series XLVII, 185: 49–69

Dawborn JK, Fairley KF, Kincaid-Smith P, King WE (1966) The association of peptic ulceration, chronic renal disease and analgesic abuse. Quart J Med 35: 69–83

Decroix G, Pujet JC, Homberg JC, Feldman A, Kleinknecht D (1973) Insuffisance rénale aiguë due à la rifampicine. Nouv Presse Méd 2: 2093–2095

Ditlove J, Weidmann P, Bernstein M, Massry SG (1977) Methicillin nephritis. Medicine 56: 483–491

Dobrin RS, Vernier RL, Fish AJ (1975) Acute eosinophilic interstitial nephritis and renal failure with bone marrow-lymph node granulomas and anterior uveitis. A new syndrome. Am J Med 59: 325–333

Dowling HF, Lepper MH (1943) Toxic reactions following therapy with sulfapyridine, sulfathiazole and sulfadiazine. JAMA 121: 1190–1194

Drago JR, Rohner TJ jr, Sanford EJ, Engle J, Schoolwerth A (1976) Acute interstitial nephritis. J Urol 115: 105–107

Dubach UC (1971) Urorenale Erkrankungen bei regelmäßiger Einnahme phenacetinhaltiger Analgetica. Dtsch Med Wochenschr 96: 303–305

Dubach UC (1979) Analgesic nephropathy. Contr Nephrol 16. Karger, Basel, pp 65–69

Duggan JM (1974) The analgesic syndrome. Aust NZ J Med 4: 365–372

Dunea G, Kark RM, Lannigan R, d'Alessio D, Muehrcke RC (1969) Brucella nephritis. Ann Intern Med 70: 783–790

Duplay H, Mattei M, Barillon D, Bauza R, Gaillot M, Kermarec J, Duplay MH (1974) Néphritis tubulo-interstitielle aiguë par intoxication à la glafénine. Thérapie 29: 593–597

Edel HH (1978) Interstitielle Nephropathien. Münch Med Wochenschr 120: 1405–1406

Einspruch BC, Gonzalez VV (1960) Clinical and experimental nephropathy resulting from use of neomycin sulfate. JAMA 173: 809–811

Faarup P, Christensen E (1974) IgE-containing plasma cells in acute tubulo-interstitial nephropathy. Lancet II: 718

Falco FG, Smith HM, Arcieri GM (1969) Nephrotoxicity of the aminoglycosides and gentamicin. J Infect Dis 119: 406–409

Fellner S, Tuttle E (1969) The clinical syndrome of analgesic abuse. Arch Intern Med 124: 379–382

Fialk MA, Romankiewicz J, Perrone F, Sherman RL (1974) Allergic interstitial nephritis with diuretics (letter). Ann Intern Med 81: 403–404

Fillastre JP, Morel-Maroger L, Mignon F, Méry JP (1969) Les néphropathies aiguës médicamenteuses. In: Actualités néphrologiques de l'hôpital Necker 1 vol. Flammarion, Paris, p 155

Fillastre JP, Rapin M, Lissac J, Leroux-Robert C, Klein M, Le Gall JR (1970) Insuffisances rénales aiguës survenant au cours des traitements par le méthine sulfonate de colistine. Ann Med Interne (Paris) 121: 817–826

Finegold SM (1966) Toxicity of kanamycin in adults. Ann NY Acad Sci 132: 942–956

French AJ (1946) Hypersensitivity in pathogenesis of histopathologic changes associated with sulfonamide chemotherapy. Am J Path 22: 679–701

Fuller TJ, Barcenas CG, White MG (1976) Diuretic-induced interstitial nephritis. Occurrence in a patient with membranous glomerulonephritis. JAMA 235: 1998–1999

Gabow PA, Lacher JW, Neff TA (1976) Tubulo-interstitial and glomerular nephritis associated with rifampin. Report of a case. JAMA 235: 2517–2518

Galea EG, Young LN, Bell JR (1963) Fatal nephropathy due to phenindione sensitivity. Lancet I: 920–922

Galpin JE, Shinaberger JH, Stanley TM, Blumenkrantz MJ, Bayer AS, Friedman GS, Montgomerie JZ, Guze LB, Coburn JW, Glassock RJ (1978) Acute interstitial nephritis due to methicillin. Am J Med 65: 756–765

Gault MH, Muehrcke RC (1973) Some clinical-pathological correlations in patients with analgesic nephropathy. In: Haschek H (ed) Internationales Symposium über Probleme des Phenacetin-Abusus. Egermann, Wien, pp 11–23

Gault MH, Blennerhassett J, Muehrcke RC (1971) Analgesic nephropathy. A clinicopathologic study using electron microscopy. Am J Med 51: 740–756

Gault MH, Rudwal TC, Engles WD, Dossetor JB (1968) Syndrome associated with the abuse of analgesics. Ann Intern Med 68: 906–925

Gelbart DR, Weinstein AB, Fajardo LF (1977) Allopurinol-induced interstitial nephritis. Ann Intern Med 86: 196–198

Gilbert DN, Gourley R, d'Agostino A, Goodnight SH jr, Worthen H (1970) Interstitial nephritis due to methicillin, penicillin and ampicillin. Ann Allergy 28: 378–385

Gloor F (1961) Die doppelseitige chronische nicht obstruktive interstitielle Nephritis. Ergebn Allg Path Path Anat 41: 63–207

Gloor F (1962) Phenacetinabusus und Nierenschädigung. Schweiz Med Wochenschr 92: 61–67

Gloor F (1965a) Some morphologic features of chronic interstitial nephritis in patients with analgesic abuse. In: Kass EH (ed) Progress in pyelonephritis. Davis & Co, Philadelphia, pp 287–296

Gloor F (1965b) Die doppelseitigen chronischen nicht obstruktiven interstitiellen Nephritiden. Verh Dtsch Ges Path 49: 92–106

Gloor F (1974) Unsere heutigen Vorstellungen über die Morphologie und Pathogenese der Analgetika-Nephropathie. Schweiz Med Wochenschr 104: 785–791
Gloor F (1978) Changing concepts in pathogenesis and morphology of analgesic nephropathy as seen in Europe. Kidney Internat 13: 27–33
Graber ML, Cogan MG, Connor DG (1978) Idiopathic acute interstitial nephritis. West J Med 129: 72–76
Grimlund K (1963) Phenacetin and renal damage at a Swedish factory. Acta Med Scand 174, Suppl 405: 3–26
Gross JM (1963) Fanconi-syndrome (adult type) developing secondary to the ingestion of outdated tetracycline. Ann Intern Med 58: 523–528
Gsell O (1974) Nephropathie durch Analgetica. Papillennekrosen und chronische interstitielle Nephritis durch Mißbrauch phenacetinhaltiger Analgetica. Ergeb Inn Med Kinderheilkd 35: 67–175
Gsell O, Dubach UC, Raillard-Peucker U (1968) Phenacetin abuse and renal disease. Ger Med Mon 13: 257–263
Haas HG (1956) Schmerzmittelmißbrauch. Schweiz Med Wochenschr 86: 401–407
Haddow JE, Robotham JL (1978) Acute interstitial nephritis in children – a process produced by streptococcal infection and by chemotherapeutic agents. A review. J Maine Med Assoc 69: 1–6
Hare WSC, Poynter JD (1974) The radiology of renal papillary necrosis as seen in analgesic nephropathy. Clin Radiol 25: 423–443
Harvald B, Clausen E (1960) Nephrotoxicity of acetylsalicylic acid. Lancet II: 767–768
Haschek H, Schmidt W (1975) Nierenschäden durch Phenacetinabusus. Med Klin 70: 313–321
Haschek H, Porpaczy P, Schmidt W (1973) Medizinische, sozialpolitische und ökonomische Aspekte des Phenacetinmißbrauchs in Österreich. In: Haschek H (ed) Internationales Symposium über Probleme des Phenacetin-Abusus. Egermann, Wien, pp 305–310
Haschek H, Porpaczy P, Schmidt W (1975) Chronischer Kopfschmerz und Phenacetin-Abusus. Münch Med Wochenschr 117: 1959–1960
Healy P (1975) Use of psychotropic drugs in Australia. Mental Health and Drug Education Programme 14: 8
Heidland A, Klütsch K, Spall M, Frohwein H (1967) Klinisch-experimentelle Untersuchungen zur Phenacetinniere. Verh Dtsch Ges Inn Med 73: 1012–1017
Hensler L (1957) Die chronische interstitielle Nephritis. Dtsch Med Wochenschr 82: 202–207
Heptinstall RH (1974) Interstitial nephritis. In: Pathology of the kidney 2nd ed. Little, Brown & Co, Boston, pp 821–836
Heptinstall RH (1976) Interstitial nephritis. A brief review. Am J Pathol 83: 214–236
Heptinstall RH (1979) Lecture in Tübingen 29.1.1979
Hestbech J, Hansen HE, Amdisen A, Olsen S (1977) Chronic renal lesions following long-term treatment with lithium. Kidney Internat 12: 205–213
Hewitt WL (1974) Gentamicin: toxicity in perspective. Postgrad Med J 50, Suppl 7: 55–59
Höffler D, Bittner B, Fiegel P, Köhler H (1973) Phenacetinniere. Dtsch Med Wochenschr 98: 2012–2016
Hörlin W. Linke A, Messmer E (1955) Über die Beeinflussung der Diurese durch Pyramidon, Butazolidin, Irgapyrin. Dtsch Arch Klin Med 201: 690–701
Hollenberg NK, Adams DF, Oken DE (1970) Acute renal failure due to nephrotoxins. N Engl J Med 282: 1329–1334
Hollman A, Wong HO (1964) Phenindione sensitivity. Br Med J 2: 730–732
Iovine G, Berman LB, Halikis DN, Mowrey FH, Chappelle EH, Gierson HW (1963) Nephrotoxicity of amphotericin B: a clinical-pathologic study. Arch Intern Med 112: 853–862

Jacobs LA, Morris JG (1962) Renal papillary necrosis and the abuse of phenacetin. Med J Aust 2: 531–538

Jarzobski J, Ferry J, Wombolt D, Fitch DM, Egan JD (1970) Vasculitis with allopurinol therapy. Am Heart J 79: 116–121

Johansson S, Angervall L, Bengtsson U, Wahlgvist L (1974) Uroepithelial tumors of the renal pelvis associated with the abuse of phenacetin-containing analgesics. Cancer 33: 743–753

Kahn T, Stein RM (1972) Gentamicin and renal failure. Lancet I: 498

Keenan TD, Blacklock H, Little PJ, Bailey RR (1973) Aggravation of renal functional impairment by tetracycline. NZ Med J 78: 164–166

Kincaid-Smith P (1965) In: Kass EH (ed) Progress in pyelonephritis. Davis & Co, Philadelphia, pp 360–361

Kincaid-Smith P (1967) Pathogenesis of the renal lesion associated with the abuse of analgesics. Lancet I: 859–862

Kincaid-Smith P (1979) Analgesic nephropathy in Australia. Contr Nephrol 16. Karger, Basel, pp 57–64

Kincaid-Smith P, Nanra RS (1978) Renal medullary necrosis. In: Hamburger J, Crosnier J, Grünfeld JP (eds) Nephrology. Flammarion Médecine-Sciences Paris, New York London Sidney Toronto, pp 583–594

Kingsley DPE, Goldberg B, Abrahams C, Meyers AJ, Furman KI, Cohen I (1972) Analgesic nephropathy. Br Med J 4: 656–659

Kjaerulff J, Harvald B (1968) Incidensen af papillitis necroticans. Nord Med 80: 1588–1594

Kjellbo H, Stakeberg H, Mellgren J (1965) Possibly thiazide-induced renal necrotising vasculitis. Lancet I: 1034–1035

Klassen J, Milgrom FM, McCluskey RT (1977) Studies of the antigens involved in an immunologic renal tubular lesion in rabbits. Am J Pathol 88: 135–144

Klassen J, Andres GA, Brennan JC, McCluskey RT (1972) An immunologic renal tubular lesion in man. Clin Immunol Immunopath 1: 69–83

Kleinknecht D, Adhémar JP (1977) Les insuffisances rénales aiguës dues à la rifampicine. Méd Mal Infect 7: 117–121

Kleinknecht D, Homberg JC, Decroix G (1972) Acute renal failure after rifampicin. Lancet I: 1238–1239

Kleinknecht D, Ganeval D, Droz D (1973) Acute renal failure after high doses of gentamicin and cephalothin. Lancet I: 1129

Koutsaimanis KG, de Wardener HE (1970) Phenacetin nephropathy, with particular reference to the effect of surgery. Br Med J 4: 131–134

Kovnat P, Labovitz E, Levison S (1973) Antibiotics and the kidney. Med Clin North Am 57: 1045–1063

Kramer P (1975) Analgetikanephropathie. Med Klin 70: 889–895

Kreis B (1966) Kanamycin toxicity in adults. Ann NY Acad Sci 132: 957–967

Kuhlmann U, Fontana A, Briner J, Steinmann U, Siegenthaler W (1978) Akute interstitielle Nephritis mit oligurischem Nierenversagen nach Phenylbutazon-Medikation. Schweiz Med Wochenschr 108: 494–499

Kunin CM, Chalmers TC, Leevy CM, Sebastyen SC, Lieber CS, Finland M (1960) Absorption of orally administered neomycin and kanamycin: with special reference to patients with severe hepatic and renal disease. N Engl J Med 262: 380–385

Laberke HG (1980a) Bedeutung von bakteriellen Harnwegsinfektionen für den Verlauf der Analgetika-Nephropathie. In preparation

Laberke HG (1980b) Acute interstitial nephritis and its treatment. In preparation

Laberke HG, Bohle A (1980a) Acute interstitial nephritis: Correlations between clinical and morphological findings. Clin Nephrol, in press

Laberke HG, Bohle A (1980b) Die akute interstitielle Nephritis: Diagnose und Differentialdiagnose. In preparation

Larsen K, Moeller CE (1958) Nyrelidelse forarsaget af phenacetinmisbrug. Ugeskr Laeg 120: 114–124

Lawrence JR, Disney APS, Clarkson AR (1973) The incidence, cost and some clinical features of analgesic nephropathy in Australia. In: Haschek H (ed) Internationales Symposium über Probleme des Phenacetin-Abusus. Egermann, Wien, pp 311–315

Lee HA, Davidson AR, Burston J (1974) Analgesic nephropathy in Wessex: a clinicopathological survey. Clin Nephrol 2: 197–207

Lehman DH, Wilson CB, Dixon FJ (1974) Interstitial nephritis in rats immunized with heterologous tubular basement membrane. Kidney Internat 5: 187–195

Lehman DH, Wilson CB, Dixon FJ (1975) Extraglomerular immunglobulin deposits in human nephritis. Am J Med 58: 765–786

Lindvall N (1960) Renal papillary necrosis. A roentgenographic study of 155 cases. Acta Radiol (suppl) 192: 1–153

Linton AL (1972) Renal disease due to analgesics. I. Recognition of the problem of analgesic nephropathy. Can Med Assoc J 107: 749–751

Lornoy W, Ringoir S, Lameire N, DeBroe M (1971) Chronische interstitielle Nefritis door Misbruik van Fenacetin-houdende Analgetica. T Geneesk 8: 339–353

Lyons H, Pinn VW, Cortell S, Cohen JJ, Harrington JT (1973) Allergic interstitial nephritis causing reversible renal failure in four patients with idiopathic nephrotic syndrome. N Engl J Med 288: 124–128

MacDonald IM, Dumble LJ, Kincaid-Smith P (1976) HLA-A3, vesico-ureteric reflux and analgesic abuse. First international symposium on HLA and disease. Paris, p 255

MacGibbon BH, Loughridge LW, Hourihune DOB (1960) Auto-immune haemolytic anemia with acute renal failure due to phenacetin and p-aminosalicylic acid. Lancet I: 7–10

Maxwell D, Szwed JJ, Wahle W, Kleit SA (1974) Ampicillin nephropathy. JAMA 230: 586–587

Mayaud C, Kanfer A, Kourilsky O, Sraer JD (1975) Interstitial nephritis after methicillin (letter). N Engl J Med 292: 1132–1133

McMenamin RA, Davies LM, Craswell PW (1976) Drug induced interstitial nephritis, hepatitis and exfoliative dermatitis. Aust NZ J Med 6: 583–587

Meadows R (1978) The interstitial tissues. In: Renal histopathology. A light-, electron- and immunfluorescent microscopic study of renal disease. University Press, Oxford, pp 225–243

Méry JP (1970) Les néphropathies interstitielles aiguës provoquées par les pénicillines. Ann Med Interne (Paris) 121: 811–816

Méry JP, Fillastre JP (1978) The kidney and drugs. In: Hamburger J, Crosnier J, Grünfeld JP (eds) Nephrology. Flammarion Médecine-Sciences Paris, New York London Sydney Toronto, pp 1169–1187

Miescher P, Studer A (1961) Weitere tierexperimentelle Untersuchungen zur Frage der Pathogenese der interstitiellen Nephritis. Schweiz Med Wochenschr 91: 939–943

Miescher P, Schnyder U, Krech U (1958) Zur Pathogenese der interstitiellen Nephritis bei Abusus phenacetinhaltiger Mittel. Schweiz Med Wochenschr 88: 432–437

Mihatsch MJ, Torhorst J, Amsler B, Zollinger HU (1978) Capillarosclerosis of the lower urinary tract in analgesic (phenacetin) abuse. An electron-microscopic study. Virchows Arch Abt A Path Anat 381: 41–47

Miller RP, Bates JH (1969) Amphotericin B toxicity: a follow-up of 53 patients. Ann Intern Med 71: 1089–1095

Mills RM (1971) Severe hypersensitivity reactions associated with allopurinol. JAMA 216: 799–802

Milman N (1978) Acute interstitial nephritis during treatment with penicillin and cephalothin. Acta Med Scand 203: 227–230

Mirouze J, Barjon P, Mion C, Fourcade J, Monnier L, Marty L (1974) Insuffisance rénale aiguë consécutive à l'absorption de glafénine. Thérapie 29: 587–592

Mitchell JR, McMurtry RJ, Stratham CN, Nelson SD (1977) Molecular basis for several drug-induced nephropathies. Am J Med 62: 518–526

Moeschlin S (1957) Phenacetinsucht und -schäden; Innenkörperanämien und interstitielle Nephritis. Schweiz Med Wochenschr 87: 123–128
Molland EA (1978) Experimental renal papillary necrosis. Kidney Internat 13: 5–14
Munck A, Lindlar F, Masshoff W (1970) Die Pigmentierung der Nierenpapillen und der ableitenden Harnwege bei der chronischen sklerosierenden interstitiellen Nephritis ("Phenacetinniere"). Virchows Arch Abt A Path Anat 349: 323–331
Murray TG, Goldberg M (1975) Chronic interstitial nephritis: etiologic factors. Ann Intern Med 82: 453–459
Murray TG, Goldberg M (1978) Analgesic-associated nephropathy in the USA: epidemiologic, clinical and pathogenetic features. Kidney Internat 13: 64–71
Murray RM, Lawson DH, Linton LH (1971) Analgesic nephropathy: clinical syndrome and prognosis. Br Med J 1: 479–482
Nanra RS (1975) Renal papillary necrosis in rheumatoid arthritis. Med J Aust 1: 194–197
Nanra RS (1976a) Analgesic nephropathy. Med J Aust 1: 745–748
Nanra RS (1976b) Pathology, aetiology and pathogenesis of analgesic nephropathy. Aust NZ J Med 6, Suppl 1: 33–37
Nanra RS, Kincaid-Smith P (1972) Chronic effect of analgesics on the kidney. Prog Biochem Pharmacol 7: 285–323
Nanra RS, Chirawong P, Kincaid-Smith P (1973) Medullary ischaemia in experimental analgesic nephropathy: The pathogenesis of renal papillary necrosis. Aust NZ J Med 3: 580–586
Nanra RS, Stuart-Taylor J, de Leon AH, White KH (1978) Analgesic nephropathy: Etiology, clinical syndrome, and clinicopathologic correlations in Australia. Kidney Internat 13: 79–92
Nanra RS, Hicks JD, McNamara JH, Lie JT, Leslie DW, Jackson BJ, Kincaid-Smith P (1970) Seasonal variation in the postmortem incidence of renal papillary necrosis. Med J Aust 1: 293–296
Neu HC (1976) Tobramycin: an overview. J Infect Dis 134, Suppl: 3–19
Nieth H (1968) Akute interstitielle Nephritis. In: Handbuch der Inneren Medizin, vol VIII/2, 5th edition. Springer, Berlin Heidelberg New York, pp 668–679
Nissen NI, Friis I (1962) Further study of the mechanism of reduction of erythrocyte survival time in phenacetin habitus and its relation to phenacetin kidney disorders. Acta Med Scand 171: 125–134
Nitzsche T, Bock KD (1970) Verlaufsbeobachtung bei Kranken mit Nephropathie nach Analgeticaabusus. Dtsch Med Wochenschr 95: 927–934
Nordenfelt O (1972) Deaths from renal failure in abusers of phenacetin-containing drugs. Acta Med Scand 191: 11–16
Nordenfelt O (1973) Mortalität an Niereninsuffizienz nach Beendigung des Phenacetinabusus. In: Haschek H (ed) Internationales Symposium über Probleme des Phenacetin-Abusus. Egermann, Wien, pp 149–156
Nordenfelt O, Ringertz N (1961) Phenacetin takers dead with renal failure. 27 men and 3 women. Acta Med Scand 170: 385–402
Olsen S, Asklund M (1976) Interstitial nephritis with acute renal failure following cardiac surgery and treatment with methicillin. Acta Med Scand 199: 305–310
Ooi BS, Chen BTM, Tan KK, Khoo OT (1972) Human renal leptospirosis. Am J Trop Med Hyg 21: 336–341
Ooi BS, Pesce AJ, First MR, Pollak VE, Bernstein IL, Jao W (1974) IgE levels in interstitial nephritis. Lancet I: 1254–1256
Ooi BS, Ooi YM, Mohini R, Pollak VE (1978) Humoral mechanisms in drug-induced acute interstitial nephritis. Clin Immunol Immunopathol 10: 330–334
Orchard RT, Rooker G (1974) Penicillin-hypersensitivity nephritis (letter). Lancet I: 689
Ortuno J, Botella J (1973) Recurrent acute renal failure induced by phenazone hypersensitivity. Lancet II: 1473–1476

Parry MF, Ball WD, Conte JE jr, Cohen SN (1973) Nafcillin nephritis. JAMA 225: 178–180

Pasternack A, Tallquist C, Kuhlback B (1970) Occurrence of interstitial nephritis in acute renal failure. Acta Med Scand 187: 27–31

Pasternak DR, Stephens BG (1975) Reversible nephrotoxicity associated with cephalothin therapy. Arch Intern Med 135: 599–602

Pearson HH (1967) Residual renal defects in non-fatal phenacetin nephritis. Med J Aust 2: 308–313

Peskoe ST, McMillan JH, Lorch A, Sussman H, Ozawa T (1978) Reversible acute renal failure associated with chlorthalidone therapy: possible drug-induced interstitial nephritis. J Med Assoc Ga 67: 17–18

Peters GA, Moskowitz RW, Prickman LE, Carryer HM (1960) Fatal necrotizing angiitis associated with hypersensitivity to penicillin O and iodides: report of a case. J Allergy 31: 455–467

Pickering MJ, Spooner GR, Quesada A (1970) Declining renal function associated with administration of cephalothin. Southern Med J 63: 426–428

Plager JE (1976) Association of renal injury with combined cephalothin-gentamicin therapy among patients severely ill with malignant disease. Cancer 37: 1937–1943

Poole G, Stradling P, Worlledge S (1971) Potentially serious side effects of high dose twice weekly rifampicin. Br Med J 3: 343–347

Powell LW jr, Hooker JW (1956) Neomycin nephropathy. JAMA 160: 557–560

Prescott LF (1966a) Analgesic abuse and renal disease in North-Eastern Scotland. Lancet II: 1143–1145

Prescott LF (1966b) The nephrotoxicity of analgesics. J Pharm Pharmacol 18: 331–353

Prescott LF (1969) Renal papillary necrosis and aspirin. Scot Med J 14: 82–85

Prescott LF (1970) The absorption, metabolism, excretion and CNS effects of phenacetin. In: Kincaid-Smith P, Fairley KF (eds) Renal infection and renal scarring. Mercedes Publ Services, Melbourne, pp 359–384

Prescott LF, Brown SS (1970) Brown urine: A clue to phenacetin intoxication. Lancet II: 1253

Price DJE, Graham DI (1970) Effects of large doses of colistin sulphomethate sodium on renal function. Br Med J 4: 525–527

Raaflaub J, Dubach UC (1972) Zur Frage der Pathogenese der chronisch-interstitiellen Nephritis nach protrahiertem Schmerzmittelabusus. Klin Wochenschr 50: 489–497

Rampogal V, Leonard C, Bhathena D (1973) Acute renal failure associated with rifampicin. Lancet I: 1195–1196

Reynolds ES, Tomkiewicz ZN, Dammin GJ (1963) The renal lesion related to amphotericin B treatment for coccidioidomycosis. Med Clin North Am 47: 1149–1154

Richardson JH, Alderfer HH (1963) Acute renal failure caused by phenylbutazone. N Engl J Med 268: 809–811

Richet G, Mayaud C (1978) The course of acute renal failure in pyelonephritis and other types of interstitial nephritis. Nephron 22: 124–127

Ringoir S (1974) Aspects cliniques, épidémiologiques et expérimentaux de la néphropathie chronique avec abus d'analgésiques. Thérapie 29: 507–546

Robson M, Levi J, Dolberg L, Rosenfeld JB (1970) Acute tubulo-interstitial nephritis following sulfadiazine therapy. Isr J Med Sci 6: 561–566

Rossi E, Montagna G (1978) Insufficienza renale acuta da Rifampicina. Minerva Medica 69: 3319–3322

Rügger R, Spengler H, de Weck AL, Dubach UC (1973) Immunologische Aspekte der Sensibilisierung auf Phenacetin. Dtsch Med Wochenschr 98: 762–769

Ruley EJ, Lisi LM (1974) Interstitial nephritis and renal failure due to ampicillin. J Pediatr 84: 878–882

Saker BM, Kincaid-Smith P (1969) Papillary necrosis in experimental analgesic nephropathy. Br Med J 1: 161–162

Sanerkin NG (1966) Chronic phenacetin nephropathy. (With particular reference to the relationship between renal papillary necrosis and "chronic interstitial nephritis"). Br J Urol 38: 361–370

Sanjad SA, Haddad GG, Nassar VH (1974) Nephropathy, an underestimated complication of methicillin therapy. J Pediatr 84: 873–877

Sarre H, Rogal U (1964) Nierenerkrankung bei Phenacetinabusus. Dtsch Med Wochenschr 89: 2269–2274

Schaub F, Bühlmann A, Maier C (1953) Blutschäden nach chronischem Phenacetinabusus. Helvet Med Acta 20: 428–432

Scheidegger S (1958) Pathologisch-anatomischer Beitrag zur Frage der chronischen interstitiellen Nephritis im Anschluß an Abusus von phenacetinhaltigen Analgetica. Bull Schweiz Akad Med Wiss 14: 139–153

Scheitlin W, Jeanneret P (1957) Über akute Nierenschädigungen unter Phenylbutazontherapie. Schweiz Med Wochenschr 87: 881–885

Schreiner GE, Maher JF (1965) Toxic nephropathy. Am J Med 38: 409–449

Schrier RW (1979) Acute renal failure. Kidney Internat 15: 205–216

Schrier RW, Bulger RJ, van Arsdel PP jr (1966) Nephropathy associated with penicillin and homologues. Ann Intern Med 64: 116–127

Schultze RG, Winters RE, Kauffman H (1971) Possible nephrotoxicity of gentamicin. J Infect Dis 124: 145–147

Schweingruber P (1955) Probleme der chronischen Vergiftung mit kombinierten Phenacetinpräparaten. Schweiz Med Wochenschr 85: 1162–1166

Senft G (1959) Die Wirkung von Pyrazolon-Derivaten auf den Elektrolyt- und Wasserhaushalt. Naunyn-Schmiedeberg's Arch Exp Path Pharmak 236: 179–182

Sheil AGR, Johnson JR, Storey BG, Charlesworth JA, Sharp A, Sands JR, Stewart JH, May J, Rogers JH, Wright R, Johnston JM, Loewenthal J (1969) Community treatment of end-stage renal failure by dialysis and renal transplantation from cadaver donors. Lancet II: 917–920

Shelley JH (1978) Pharmacological mechanisms of analgesic nephropathy. Kidney Internat 13: 15–26

Silverblatt F, Harrison WO, Turck M (1973) Nephrotoxicity of cephalosporin antibiotics in experimental animals. J Infect Dis 128, Suppl: 367–372

Simenhoff ML, Guild WR, Dammin GJ (1968) Acute diffuse interstitial nephritis. Review of the literature and case report. Am J Med 44: 618–625

Sloth K, Thomsen AC (1971) Acute renal insufficiency during treatment with azathioprine. Acta Med Scand 189: 145–148

Smith K (1965) Acute renal failure in phenindione sensitivity. Br Med J 2: 24–26

Spring M (1951) Purpura and nephritis after administration of procaine penicillin. JAMA 147. 1139–1141

Spühler O, Zollinger HU (1953) Die chronisch-interstitielle Nephritis. Z Klin Med 151: 1–50

Steblay RW, Rudofsky U (1973) Transfer of experimental autoimmune renal cortical tubular and interstitial disease in guinea pigs by serum. Science 180: 966–968

Streicher E (1964) Akutes Nierenversagen nach therapeutischer Anwendung von Phenylbutazon. Dtsch Med Wochenschr 89: 429–436

Studer A (1965) Attempts to induce renal lesions in the experimental animal by analgesics. In: Kass EH (ed) Progress in pyelonephritis. Davis & Co, Philadelphia, pp 307–311

Tannenberg AM, Wicher KJ, Rose NR (1971) Ampicillin nephropathy. JAMA 218: 449

Taylor JS (1972) Carcinoma of the urinary tract and analgesic abuse. Med J Aust 1: 407–409

Thölen H, Voegtli J, Renschler H, Schaeffer A (1956) Ein Beitrag zur Genese der interstitiellen Nephritis. Schweiz Med Wochenschr 86: 946–949, 978–981

Uehlinger E (1971) Das Wesen der chronischen Nierenkrankheit in der Sicht des Morphologen. Bibl Tuberc (Basel) 27: 97–108

Uhl N, Hunstein W (1973) Veränderungen von Blutbildung und Blutbild bei chronischem Phenacetin-Abusus mit Niereninsuffizienz. In: Haschek H (ed) Internationales Symposium über Probleme des Phenacetin-Abusus. Egermann, Wien, pp 209–213

Wagoner RD (1976) Analgesic nephropathy – a continuing problem. Postgrad Med 60: 50–53

Wauters JP (1977) Néphropathie à la phénacétine. Rev Med Suisse Romande 97: 589–593

Wilkinson DG, Boyd DH (1978) Recovery from acute interstitial nephritis. Br Med J 1: 827–828

Wilson DR (1972) Analgesic nephropathy. Can Med Assoc J 107: 715–716

Woodroffe AJ, Row PG, Meadows R, Lawrence JR (1974a) Nephritis in infectious mononucleosis. Quart J Med 43: 451–460

Woodroffe AJ, Thomson NM, Meadows R, Lawrence JR (1974b) Nephropathy associated with methicillin administration. Aust NZ J Med 4: 256–261

Woodroffe AJ, Weldon M, Meadows R, Lawrence JR (1975) Acute interstitial nephritis following ampicillin hypersensitivity. Med J Aust 1: 65–68

Yü TF, Burns JJ, Paton BC, Gutman AB, Brodie BB (1958) Phenylbutazone metabolites: antirheumatic, sodium-retaining and uricosuric effects in man. J Pharmakol Exp Ther 123: 63–69

Zilberg B (1958) Anuria following penicillin administration. S Afr Med J 32: 350–352

Zollinger HU (1955) Chronische interstitielle Nephritis bei Abusus von phenacetinhaltigen Analgetika. Schweiz Med Wochenschr 85: 746

Zollinger HU, Mihatsch MJ (1978) Inflammatory interstitial renal lesions. In: Renal pathology in biopsy. Springer, Berlin Heidelberg New York, pp 407–411

Zollinger HU, Mihatsch MJ (1979) Morphology of acute interstitial nephropathies. Contr Nephrol 16. Karger, Basel, pp 118–125

Zollinger HU, Colombi A, Schiltknecht J (1971) New clinical and ultrastructural aspects in leptospirosis icterohaemorrhagica (Weil's disease): a clinical, light and electron microscopic study. Virchows Arch Abt A Path Anat 354: 336–348

Drug-Associated Nephropathy

Part II: Tubulo-Interstitial Lesions

B: Hypokalemic Alterations

TH. RIEMENSCHNEIDER

I. Introduction 217
II. Drugs 218
1. Substances and Pharmacodynamics 218
2. Causes of Cathartic and Diuretic Drug Abuse 220
III. Renal Morphology 221
1. Tubules 221
a) Vacuolar Alterations 221
b) Degenerative Alterations 222
2. Interstitial Tissue 223
a) Connective Tissue 223
b) Cellular Infiltration 223
3. Juxtaglomerular Apparatus 225
4. Medulla 226
a) Multivesicular Bodies 226
b) Interstitial Cells 227
c) Collecting Ducts 228
5. Glomeruli 228
a) Mesangium 228
b) Glomerular Size 229
c) Other Glomerular Alterations 229
6. Vessels 230
IV. Renal Function 230
1. Urinary Concentration 230
2. Acid Excretion 231
3. Renal Sodium Handling 232
4. Renal Potassium Handling 232
5. Glomerular Filtration Rate 233
V. Conclusions 233
References 235

I. Introduction

In 1956, *Conn* and *Johnson* defined hypokalemic nephropathy as a new entity characterized clinically by potassium depletion and morphologically by vacuolar degeneration of the renal tubules.

The following different pathogenetic factors for hypokalemic nephropathy, which are attributed to a variety of diseases, are:

- Reduced potassium intake, e.g., associated with anorexia nervosa;
- Increased renal loss of potassium, e.g., occurring through the use of diuretics, with ureterosigmoidostomies, with Bartter's, Conn's, Liddle's or Fanconi's syndrome;
- Increased gastrointestinal loss of potassium, e.g., occurring through the use of laxatives and with chronic vomiting of various etiologies.

Based on the data presented in the literature and our observations of 80 cases, the chronic use of cathartic and diuretic drugs is the most common cause of clinically and morphologically confirmed hypokalemia. Hypokalemic nephropathy is usually a drug-associated nephropathy.

Some morphologic alterations related to hypokalemia were first described by *Perkins* and co-workers (1950) as a vacuolization of the proximal and distal renal tubules; *Relman* and *Schwartz* (1956) reported a comparable morphologic picture as the consequence of laxative drug abuse. Nevertheless *Muehrcke* and *McMillan* (1963) seldom demonstrated vacuoles but did frequently observe focal interstitial fibrosis with pyelonephritic infiltrates. Afterwards *Cremer* and *Blümcke* (1977) reported a variety of tubular, interstitial, vascular, and glomerular alterations caused by cathartic and diuretic drugs.

Because of the contradictory data reported by different authors and the relatively low number of cases, it has not yet been possible to make definitive statements about the diagnostic and prognostic relevance of these morphologic findings.

Changes in renal function associated with drug-induced hypokalemic nephropathy were described more uniformly in many individual publications; few comprehensive descriptions however are available (*Relman* and *Schwartz* 1958; *Wolff* et al. 1968; *Bock* et al. 1978).

A survey of the literature and our own experience yielded characteristic morphologic and functional renal parameters for cathartic and diuretic drug abuse, thus providing an example of nontoxic and nonallergic "drug-associated tubulo-interstitial nephropathy."

II. Drugs

1. Substances and Pharmacodynamics

Of all drugs interfering with water, sodium and potassium metabolism, only cathartic and diuretic drugs, when taken over long periods of time, produce an impressive nephropathy (*Hollander* 1963).

Penicillins in doses of 100,000,000 units (*Brunner* and *Frick* 1968), high doses of carbenicillin (*Hoffbrand* and *Stewart* 1970; *Klastersky* et al. 1973), and combinations of antibiotics (*Tattersall* et al. 1972) lead to pronounced potassium depletion, but no definite morphologic alterations have been observed. Carbenoxolone therapy leads to hypokalemia with hypernatremia (*Edmonds* 1977; *Hurley* 1977); renal damage however could not be detected in renal biopsy material. The duration and the extent of the electrolyte shift in these most short and medically supervised therapies is not sufficient to damage the renal parenchyma.

Marked potassium depletion can also occur in the context of tubular necrosis and Fanconi's syndrome following ingestion of amphotericin B (*Butler* et al. 1964; *McCurdy* et al. 1968) and out-dated tetracyclines (*Frimpter* et al. 1973; *Gross* 1963). Franconi's syndrome and tubular necrosis however are due to direct toxic pathologic mechanisms (see Part II A).

The following contact cathartics are the most commonly used:

1. Anthraquinone derivatives characterized as natural vegetable laxatives, such as cascara, senna, and aloe;
2. Diphenylmethane derivatives, primarily phenolphthalein and bisacodyl.

The most frequently reported abuse of cathartic drugs involved preparations containing phenolphthalein (*Schwartz* and *Relman* 1953; *French* et al. 1956; *Relman* and *Schwartz* 1956; *Coghill* and *McAllen* 1959; *Kramer* and *Pope* 1964; *Fleischer* et al. 1969; *LaRusso* and *Gill* 1975); recently the abuse of bisacodyl was also described (*Gossain* and *Werk* 1972).

Chronic ingestion of cascara was reported by *Schwartz* and *Relman* (1953), *Relman* and *Schwartz* (1956), *Aitchinson* (1958), *Houghton* and *Pears* (1958), and *LaRusso* and *Gill* (1975); the use of aloe in some patients, by *Schwartz* and *Relman* (1953) as well as *Relman* and *Schwartz* (1956).

Coghill and *McAllen* (1959) as well as *Truninger* and *Spühler* (1960) reported the abuse of unnamed anthraquinone derivatives.

The pharmacodynamics of contact cathartics, which act exclusively on the large intestine, has not been fully explained. The mode of action for diphenylmethane derivatives appears to be direct by inhibiting water and electrolyte reabsorption from the lumen; so-called emodin must first be split by bacteria from anthraquinone before it can be effective by a comparable mechanism; additionally the motility of the colon seems to be augmented (*Fingl* 1975).

When taken in high doses, these cathartics frequently lead to diarrhea (*French* et al. 1956; *Relman* and *Schwartz* 1956; *Aitchinson* 1958; *Houghton* and *Pears* 1958; *Coghill* and *McAllen* 1959; *DeGraeff* and *Schuurs* 1960) and therefore to high sodium losses, depending on the amount of feces (*Fordtran* and *Dietschy* 1966; *Kunau* and *Stein* 1979). Compared with total body potassium, potassium and bicarbonate losses in the feces are relatively low (*Fordtran* and *Dietschy* 1966).

The diuretics producing nephropathy when taken over long periods of time usually belong to one of the following two groups:

1. Thiazide derivatives, such as hydrochlorothiazide and cyclopenthiazide, and thiazide analogues, such as chlorthalidone;
2. High ceiling diuretic agents, such as furosemide and ethacrynic acid.

Both groups are potent, widely used, and enterally effective saluretic agents.

Thiazides may inhibit active sodium chloride transport in the proximal tubule (*Mudge* 1975). Moreover, high ceiling diuretic agents appear to inhibit sodium chloride reabsorption in the ascending limb of the loop of Henle (*Mudge* 1975).

The consequence is the primary loss of sodium and body water through the kidney (*Venning* et al. 1962). In the distal tubule, secondary potassium depletion is induced in the exchange for sodium ions by increased flow, higher sodium supply, as well as increased electronegativity in the lumen, and later by hyperaldosteronism (*Kunau* and *Stein* 1979).

The severity of the renal damage apparently depends on the duration of the cathartic and diuretic drug intake (*Bock* et al. 1978) and/or the size of the dose (*Hollander* and *Blythe* 1971).

The interval between the beginning of cathartic and/or diuretic drug abuse and corfirmation of the diagnosis is usually difficult to determine for two reasons: the patients often do not admit the true extent of their abuse (see II 2) and the transition from the occasional use of low doses of cathartics and/or diuretics to the regular ingestion of high doses of these drugs cannot be easily defined. *Cremer* and *Bock* (1977) reported the mean interval of hypokalemia for their 14 patients with confirmed cathartic and diuretic drug abuse to be 8.8 years; *Bock* and co-workers (1978), 6.5 years. An average of 9.9 years (1–35 years) elapsed between the beginning of regular drug intake and the time of the kidney biopsy in our cases (*Riemenschneider* and *Bohle* 1980). The quantity of drugs ingested varied considerably from patient to patient and for each individual patient over a period of several years (e.g., *DeGraeff* and *Schuurs* 1960). The effectiveness of the laxative also varied from patient to patient (*Fingl* 1975). *Relman* and *Schwartz* (1956) reported ingestion of cathartic drugs more than 20 times that of the normal dose: *Katz* and co-workers (1972) mentioned the ingestion of 20 furosemide tablets of 40 mg each per day.

Drug-induced deficits in sodium, body water, and potassium are often masked by additional electrolyte losses due to psychogenic vomoting or reduced electrolyte intake in association with anorexia nervosa.

2. Causes of Cathartic and Diuretic Drug Abuse

High doses of cathartic and diuretic drugs are rarely taken over long periods of time simply as a matter of habit (*Houghton* and *Pears* 1958) or for primarily somatic disorders, such as chronic constipation (*Coghill* and *McAllen* 1959) and pronounced premenstrual edema (*Love* et al. 1971; *Katz* et al. 1972).

Excessive amounts of laxatives and diuretics are usually taken by individuals with personality disorders or neurotic tendencies, i.e., depressive (*Kramer* and *Pope* 1964; *Wolff* et al. 1968; *Katz* et al. 1972), hysteric (*Wolff* et al. 1968), hypochondriacal (*Kramer* and *Pope* 1964), or paranoid (*Kramer* and *Pope* 1964) personalities.

Triggering conflict situations may be the loss of a member of the immediate family (*Fuchs* et al. 1977), marital problems (*French* et al. 1956), aversion to obesity of the mother (*Truninger* and *Spühler* 1960; *Kramer* and *Pope* 1964), and the idea of inner purification (*Aitchinson* 1958; *Muller* et al. 1963).

The most common psychosomatic disorder in this context is anorexia nervosa. It was observed in 8 of our 34 patients with cathartic and/or diuretic drug abuse (*Riemenschneider* and *Bohle* 1980) and in 25 of 95 patients reported in the literature. Masochistic and self-destructive tendencies are relatively common. A few patients even submitted to a diagnostic laparotomy (*Katz* et al. 1972; *LaRusso* and *Gill* 1975) or "therapeutic" adrenalectomy (*Muller* et al. 1963) without revealing their excessive use of cathartic or diuretic drugs.

Since patients often conceal their abuse of cathartic and/or diuretic drugs, the correct diagnosis can sometimes be established only be questioning the individual intensively or via spectrophotometric (*French* et al. 1956; *Kramer* and *Pope* 1964; *Fleischer* et al. 1969), gas chromatographic, and mass photometric (*Fuchs* et al. 1977) methods.

It is interesting to note that many of the female patients taking diuretics are engaged in pharmacology- or medicine-related occupations, e.g., medical secretaries (*Kramer* and *Pope* 1964) physician's assistants (*Gossain* and *Werk* 1972), secretaries in phamaceutical sales organizations (*Katz* et al. 1972), and nurses (*Wolff* et al. 1968; *Katz* et al. 1972). This group of individuals has relatively easy access to most prescription diuretics.

III. Renal Morphology

The structural alterations in the kidney due to chronic depletion of sodium, potassium, and body water resulting from excessive cathartic and/or diuretic drug intake present a multifaceted morphologic picture. Lesions in the tubules as well as the cortical and medullary interstitium are of primary functional and prognostic significance. Only adaptive alterations are found in the glomeruli; true lesions are absent. The vascular alterations described are probably not related to the drug abuse.

1. Tubules

a) Vacuolar Alterations

In 1919, *Jaffé* and *Sternberg* first described vacuolar degeneration of the renal tubules as a consequence of Sonne dysentery. *Perkins* and co-workers (1950) first reported the relationship between tubular vacuoles and chronic potassium depletion; *Relman* and *Schwartz* (1956) described similar tubular alterations in connection with the excessive use of laxatives.

Conn and *Johnson* 1956) considered tubular vacuolization in connection with long-standing potassium depletion of various etiologies to be a new entity which they referred to as "kaliopenic nephropathy."

Light microcopic examination of the tubules showed large, empty vacuoles that did not stain for fat or glycogen. Approximately two thirds of the alterations were found in the proximal tubules; one third, in the distal tubules (*Conn* and *Johnson* 1956; *Schwartz* and *Relman* 1967).

Electron microscopic examination showed extracellular vacuoles in the basal compartment of the tubules (*Biava* et al. 1963) and variously sized vesicles in the intracellular space surrounded by a basement membrane (*Muehrcke* and *Rosen* 1964; *Cremer* and *Blümcke* 1977).

A survey of the literature on 34 hypokalemic nephropathies (*Hollander* 1963) showed that tubular vacuoles were present in over 60% of the biopsy specimens. It is interesting however to note that only three cases of cathartic drug abuse (*Relman* and *Schwartz* 1956; *DeGraeff* and *Schuurs* 1960), one case of anorexia nervosa (*Wigley* 1960), one case of ureterosigmoidostomy (*Stamey* 1956), two cases of chronic diarrhea (*Keye* 1952; *Relman* and *Schwartz* 1956), and two cases of unclarified potassium depletion (*France* 1962) were reported. Conn's syndrome was the only cause of hypokalemia in the remaining 25 studies.

Tubular vacuoles have seldom been observed in association with excessive use of laxatives or diuretics: two biopsy specimens (*Relman* and *Schwartz* 1956), one of five patients (*Muehrcke* and *McMillan* 1963), four cases (*Cremer* and *Blümcke* 1977), one case (*Wagner* et al. 1971).

Characteristic vacuoles were found only four times in our 34 biopsy cylinders fixed in 4% buffered formalin, i.e., 17.8% of the biopsy material (*Riemenschneider* and *Bohle* 1980). No vacuoles were described in the cortical tubules for any of the cases reported in another survey of 18 hypokalemic nephropathies of various etiologies (*Muehrcke* 1960).

Tubular vacuoles often appear as artifacts in biopsy specimens fixed with aldehyde of different osmolarities (*Maunsbach* 1966). Similar vacuoles were also observed in connection with mild ethylene glycol or EDTA intoxication (*Hollander* and *Blythe* 1971) and in animal experiments following administration of potassium cyanide (*Langer* and *Thoenes* 1969). These vacuoles were interpreted as a manifestation of an energetic insufficiency of the cells (*Langer* and *Thoenes* 1969).

Because of their rare and inconsistent occurrence, these tubular vacuoles are probably not pathognomonic morphologic lesions caused by excessive cathartic and diuretic drug intake.

b) Degenerative Alterations

More important for the diagnosis and prognosis of cathartic and diuretic nephropathies than the occasional tubular vacuoles appears to be the frequent occurrence of irreversible tubular damage.

Relman and *Schwartz* (1956) reported focal or diffuse tubular atrophy associated with pyelonephritic scars in two patients with excessive laxative intake.

Muehrcke (1963) and *Muehrcke* and *Rosen* (1964), on the basis of a review of the literature and an evaluation of 18 (15) biopsy specimens, demonstrated the high incidence of destructive interstitial nephritides in hypokalemic kidneys.

DeGraeff and *Schuurs* (1960), *Schürholz* and co-workers (1969), *Cremer* and *Blümcke* (1977), and *Wagner* and co-workers (1979) reported in connection with chronic laxative and diuretic intake a dilatation and atrophy of the tubules, flattened tubular epithelium, and thickening of the tubular basement membrane.

Using morphometric methods, we found a significant reduction in the total mean surface of the tubule (27.6%) and the epithelial surface (12.1%) over against normal renal tissue (Figs. 2 and 3). A clear correlation could be established between the degree of tubular atrophy and the relative interstitial volume. *Muehrcke* (1963), using semi-quantitative methods, also described this relationship.

The electron microscopic alterations include focal or diffuse thickening of the tubular basement membrane (*Biava* et al. 1963; *Muehrcke* and *Rosen* 1964; *Cremer* and *Blümcke* 1977); degenerative lesions in the tubular cytoplasm, such as hydropic swelling of the mitochondria and rarefaction of other organelles, were often observed (*Muehrcke* and *Rosen* 1964; *Cremer* and *Blümcke* 1977).

2. Interstitial Tissue

a) Connective Tissue

An increase in interstitial volume due to the increase in collagen fibers was observed in different glomerular, vascular, and interstitial renal diseases (*Bohle* et al. 1977a, b, c; *Grund* et al. 1978; *Mackensen* et al. 1979).

Chronic pyelonephritic alterations with focal interstitial fibrosis were reported by *Relman* and *Schwartz* (1956) in two patients with chronic laxative intake and by *Muehrcke* and *McMillan* (1963) in several cases. Recent bioptic studies have also confirmed the frequency of variously pronounced interstitial fibroses following chronic use of cathartic and diuretic drugs (*Cremer* and *Blümcke* 1977; see also *Schürholz* et al. 1969; *Wagner* et al. 1979). *Mackensen* and co-workers (1979) measured the increased interstitial volume in seven patients with drug-induced electrolyte losses.

Quantitative evaluations showed an increase in interstitial volume in 25 of 33 patients, the mean relative interstitial volume being 17%; normal values are approximately 8.6%.

Electron microscopic examinations confirmed the increase of collagen fibers in the cortical and also the medullary interstitium (*Muehrcke* and *Rosen* 1964).

Investigations carried out by *Bohle* and co-workers (1977a, b, c, 1979; see also IV 5) demonstrated the significance of interstitial fibrosis for an irreversible reduction in the glomerular filtration rate.

b) Cellular Infiltration

Cellular infiltration of renal interstitial tissue is, for the most part, lymphocytic and, to a lesser extent, granulocytic (*Muehrcke* and *McMillan* 1963; *Cremer* and *Blümcke* 1977). The degree of infiltration varies considerably for different biopsy specimens from patients with chronic laxative and diuretic drug abuse.

No inflammatory cells whatsoever were mentioned in the well-documented cases reported by *Relman* and *Schwartz* (1956) or in the short morphologic descriptions presented by *Wolff* and co-workers (1968), *Fleischer* and co-workers (1969), and *Trübestein* and co-workers (1972). In their review of potassium depletion nephropathies of various etiologies, *Kulka* and co-workers (1950) as well as *Jensen* and co-workers (1950) found interstitial infiltrates in only 4 of 50 patients.

By comparison, *Muehrcke* (1960) and *Muehrcke* and *McMillan* (1963) in their investigations of the coincidence of chronic pyelonephritides and potassium deficit in

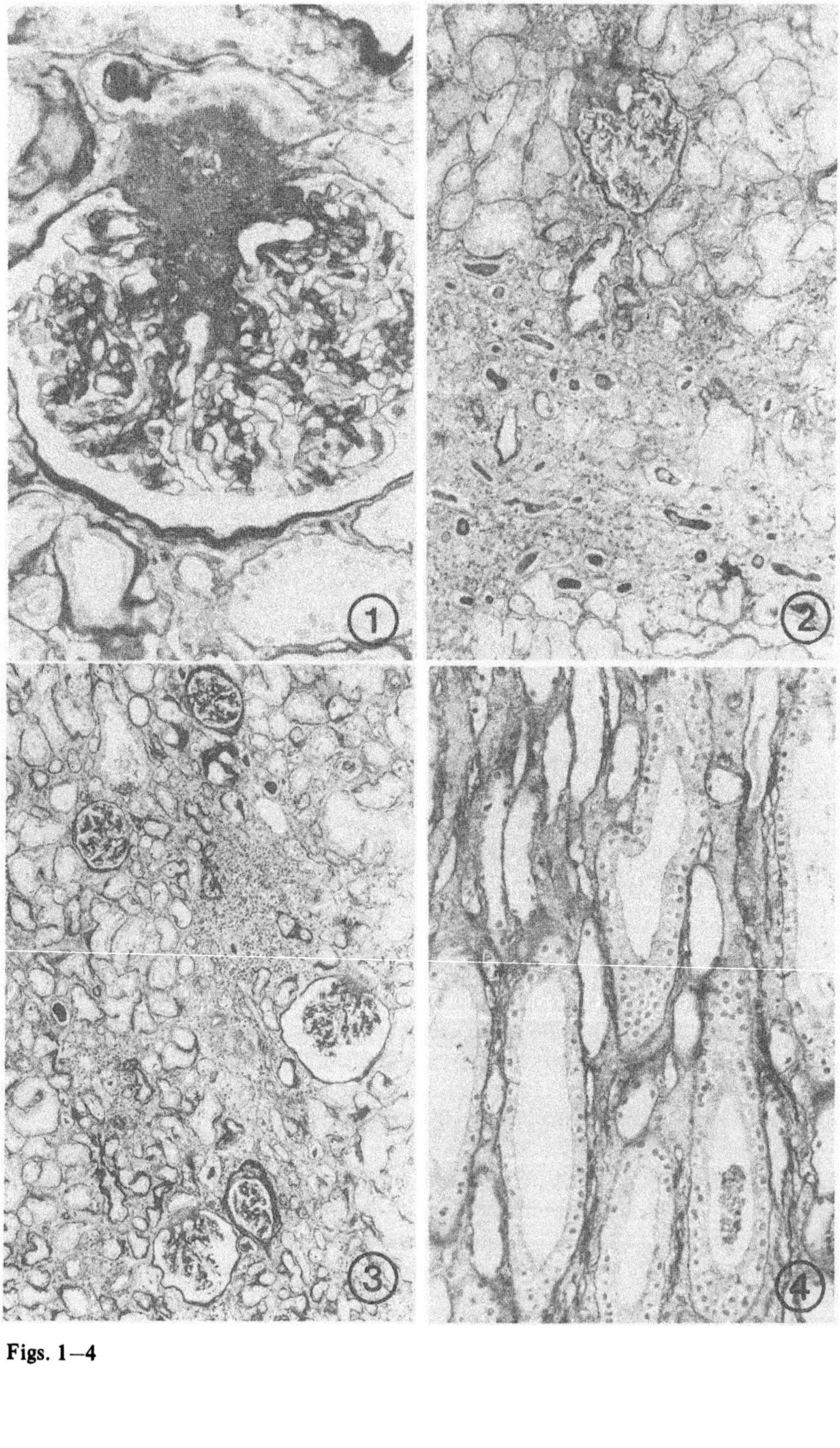

Figs. 1–4

human and animal biopsy material very often found round cell infiltrates. They observed chronic interstitial infiltration in 12 of 18 patients with hypokalemia and in all five of their patients with excessive cathartic and diuretic drug intake, always in connection with interstitial fibrosis.

In other publications on drug-related potassium and sodium depletion, all biopsy specimens showed focal histiocytic infiltrates in the interstitium (*Pollack* et al. 1957; *DeGraeff* and *Schuurs* 1960; *Cremer* and *Blümcke* 1977; *Wagner* et al. 1979).

Lymphocytes were observed in the interstitial tissue in 21 of our 34 biopsy specimens: 16 times in connection with patchy destruction and five times in a more diffuse manner. The infiltrate was always accompanied by marked interstitial fibrosis and often by tubular atrophy (Figs. 2 and 3).

The pathogenesis of the infiltrate is certainly not uniform. Possible causal factors are pyelonephritic episodes as a result of increased susceptibility to infection on the part of the hypokalemic parenchyma (*Muehrcke* and *McMillan* 1963), sclerosing infiltrate as a result of persisting renal failure (*Bohle* et al. 1979), and possibly also interstitial inflammation in reaction to tubular epithelium damage inflicted by hypokalemia.

3. Juxtaglomerular Apparatus

Hypertrophy and hyperplasia of the juxtaglomerular apparatus (JGA) are the characteristic morphologic alterations resulting from a reduction in intravascular pressure and/or volume or from a reduction in the sodium concentration at the macula densa (*Meyer* 1972).

An increase in the size or number of JGA cells therefore is commonly observed with sodium-potassium nephropathy. *Fleischer* and co-workers (1969) and *Cremer* and

←

Fig. 1. Tumorlike hyperplastic juxtaglomerular cell complex consisting of small Goormaghtigh cells, abundant basement-membranelike material, and considerably enlarged macula densa; 44-year-old woman with a 28-year history of excessive cathartic and diuretic drug intake, secondary renal potassium loss for 5 years, and a serum potassium concentration of 2.2 mg/100 ml. (Paraffin section, PAS, × 250)

Fig. 2. Glomerulus with hyperplastic juxtaglomerular apparatus and focal, scantily infiltrated interstitial fibrosis and tubular atrophy; 46-year-old woman with a 20-year history of excessive laxative intake and a serum potassium concentration of 1.9 mg/100 ml. (Paraffin section, PAS, × 100)

Fig. 3. Extensive interstitial fibrosis, focal lymphocytic infiltrate, and predominantly small glomeruli with markedly increased mesangial matrix; 37-year-old woman with a 20-year history of excessive laxative intake, periodic vomiting, and recurrent urinary tract infections. (Paraffin section, PAS, × 80)

Fig. 4. Epithelial cells from the collecting ducts, filled at the apical poles with numberous fine PAS-positive granules, and scattered granules in the loop of Henle and the capillary epithelium; 30-year-old woman with chronic cathartic drug abuse for many years and serum potassium concentration of 2.6 mg/100 ml. (Paraffin section, PAS, × 160)

Blümcke (1977) described hyperplasia and hypertrophy of myoepithelioid cells in six patients with excessive laxative intake. No enlargement of the JGA however was observed in the scant biopsy material available from two patients with pseudo-Bartter's syndrome (*Meurer* et al. 1968; *Trübestein* et al. 1972).

Schürholz and co-workers (1969) and *Helber* and co-workers (1970) each counted the increased number of IGA cells in a biopsy specimen from one patient with excessive laxative intake; *Meyer* (1972), using morphometric methods, found enlarged JGAs in a biopsy specimen from a patient with pseudo-Bartter's syndrome. *Wagner* and co-workers (1979) described the JGA from a patient with diuretic drug abuse as being hypercellular and enlarged.

The epithelial cells of the macula densa as well as the epithelioid and Goormaghtigh cells appear to be increased in number and volume (*Helber* et al. 1970; *Meyer* 1972).

Using morphometric methods, an enormous increase (317%) was determined in the juxtaglomerular cell complexes of biopsy material from 34 of our patients with chronic use of cathartics and diuretics (*Riemenschneider* and *Bohle* 1980) (Figs. 1–3). The enlargement of the section area and therefore of the total JGA volume in pseudo-Bartter's syndrome (*Schürholz* et al. 1969; *Cremer* and *Blümcke* 1977) and true Bartter's syndrome (*Brackett* et al. 1968; *Schmitt* et al. 1973) is the result of a considerable increase in the surrounding basement-membrane-like material, and not just of an increase in the number of cells (see Fig. 1). The true volume of each individual cell seems to be reduced compared with normal renal tissue or renal tissue from patients with Addison's disease (*Christensen* et al. 1976).

The detailed architectonic relationships of the JGA with sodium and potassium depletion have only been studied in serial sections from one patient with Bartter's syndrome (*Christensen* et al. 1976). The Goormaghtigh cell area and the macula densa were hyperplastic; in each case, the contact surfaces of the macula densa and/or the afferent arterioles extended only as far as the Goormaghtigh cells; there was no contact between the macula densa and the afferent arterioles. Microscopically, PAS- and silver-positive granules were observed in the epithelioid cells; electron microscopically, nonspecific lipofuscin bodies and specific secretory granules were demonstrated (*Biava* and *West* 1966; *Schürholz* et al. 1969; *Wagner* et al. 1979), whereby a discrepancy often exists between the low number of secretory granules and hypertrophy and/or hyperplasia of the JGA.

4. Medulla

a) Multivesicular Bodies

One characteristic morphologic alteration occurring in experimentally induced hypokalemia in animals is the accumulation of intracytoplasmic granules in the epithelial cells of the collecting ducts (*Oliver* et al. 1957), the interstitial cells, the endothelial cells of the capillaries, and the epithelial cells of the loop of Henle, i.e., all cell elements of the renal medulla (*Spargo* et al. 1960). The density of the granules increased from the outer medullary zone to the tip of the papilla in relation to the osmotic gradient (*Spargo* et al. 1960). Light microscopic examination indicated that these granules are PAS positive, diastasis-resistant, and argyrophilic (*Spargo* et al. 1960; *France* 1962). Electron microscopic examination showed type II granules (*Maunsbach* 1966) surrounded by a membrane to be "multivesicular bodies" (MVB) consisting of vacuoles, variously sized dense droplets, and membranelike layered inclusions (*Spargo* et al. 1960; *Wilson* et al. 1973). In long-standing hypokalemia, these MVB can extensively replace other organelles (*Sarkar* and *Levine* 1979), but they never destroy the cells themselves. Similar granules were observed in all medullary cells of biopsy material taken from patients with potassium-losing nephritis of unknown origin (*France* 1962; *France* et al. 1973, 1978) and with Bartter's syndrome (*France* et al. 1974; *Verberckmoes* et al. 1976).

Typical PAS-positive granules in the apical section of epithelial cells from the collecting ducts and, to a lesser extent, also in the loops of Henle, endothelial cells from the capillaries, and interstitial cells were found twice in our eight biopsy specimens containing medullary tissue from patients with excessive laxative intake (Fig. 4).

These granules are probably lysosomal inclusions, containing at least five typical enzymes (*Morrison* and *Panner* 1964; *Aithal* et al. 1977), which are also capable of endocytosis (*Panner* 1971). The accumulation of MVB is accompanied by increased phospholipid synthesis (*Wilson* et al. 1973; *Toback* et al. 1976). The MVB disintegrate rapidly after potassium repletion (*Wilson* et al. 1973; *Toback* et al. 1976).

b) Interstitial Cells

A diffuse, Type I hyperplasia of the renomedullary interstitial cells was observed in connection with potassium depletion of unknown origin (*France* et al. 1978) and Bar-- Bartter's syndrome (*France* et al. 1974; *Verberckmoes* et al. 1976). *Lerman* and coworkers (1972) reported nodular hyperplasia in the form of "renomedullary interstitial cell tumors," which, however, in a retrospective study, was usually found in connection with chronic hypoxidosis (*George* and *Zimmermann* 1978).

The interstitial cells appear to be primarily responsible for the synthesis of renal prostaglandins (*Limas* et al. 1976). The activity of prostaglandin synthesis is probably directly proportional to the number of fat droplets in these cells (*Limas* et al. 1976); these droplets contain unsaturated fatty acids and triglycerides associated with prostaglandin synthesis (*Comai* et al. 1974). Morphologically, these granules are totally different from the MVB, staining with oil-red-O, toluidine blue, or *p*-phenylenediamine. The granules are limited by a dense outer zone, but not by a basement membrane (*Bohman* and *Jensen* 1976).

A decrease in the number of lipid droplets was observed with high blood pressure and combined sodium and water depletion (*Bohman* and *Jensen* 1976). The hypotension and the lack of sodium and body water resulting from excessive laxative and diuretic drug intake in association with increased prostaglandin synthesis (*Galvez* et al. 1977; *Nivet* et al. 1978; *Radfar* et al. 1978) suggest that the number of lipid granules may also change with excessive intake of laxatives and diuretics.

c) Collecting Ducts

Another characteristic morphologic alteration found in experimentally induced potassium depletion in rats is the swelling of the epithelial cells in the collecting ducts from the inner zone of the outer medulla (*Oliver* et al. 1957; *MacDonald* et al. 1962; *Woernle* 1969). This type of hyperplasia has not been consistently observed in human biopsy material (*Hollander* and *Blythe* 1971) perhaps because the biopsy cylinders rarely contain medullary tissue.

Additionally, a proliferation of the intercalated cells with "crablike" projections into the lumen of the collecting ducts was observed in potassium depletion and metabolic alkalosis (*Oliver* et al. 1957; *MacDonald* et al. 1962). Impressive scanning electron microscopic findings are dense microplicae on the luminal cell membrane (*Hagège* et al. 1974) and abundant rod-shaped intramembranous particles (*Stetson* et al. 1980); transmission electron microscopy shows an increased density of the microvilli, mitochondria, and free ribosomes (*Hagège* et al. 1974; *Stetson* et al. 1980). It is assumed that, in the presence of base excess and/or hypokalemia, the principal cells of the collecting ducts are transformed into intercalated cells (*Richet* et al. 1970), thus representing an activated form responsible for potassium and bicarbonate reabsorption (*Stetson* et al. 1980).

An impressive increase in intercalated cells was observed in one of our patients with a long history of excessive laxative intake.

5. Glomeruli

The glomerular alterations in chronic abuse of laxatives and diuretics are not true lesions, but rather the result of adaptive processes resulting from body water and electrolyte changes; these alterations therefore are dealt with in this context.

a) Mesangium

A microscopically demonstrable increase in PAS-positive material in the mesangium has sometimes been reported in connection with cathartic and diuretic drug abuse: *Cremer* and *Blümcke* (1977) observed primarily focal mesangial sclerosis and hyalinosis; *Schürholz* and co-workers (1969), a slight, homogeneous enlargement of the mesangium.

Hyperchromatic glomerular syncytium (*Bartter* et al. 1962), increased amounts of basement-membrane-like material (*Brackett* et al. 1968), and focal enlargement of the mesangial matrix (*Fujita* et al. 1977) were observed in Bartter's syndrome.

A mean increase in the mesangial matrix of 22.5% compared to the control cases was determined in 34 biopsy specimens; the relative mesangial surface exceeded normal values in 30 of 34 patients (*Riemenschneider* and *Bohle* 1980) (Figs. 1 and 3). Corresponding to the subjective impression, the material density increased more markedly (47.8%) since the capillary tufts were also smaller (see III 5 b).

An increase in the basement-membrane-like material and collaagen fibers in the neighborhood of the mesangial cells was confirmed by a few electron microscopic studies (e.g., *Brackett* et al. 1968; *Cremer* and *Blümcke* 1977).

b) Glomerular Size

Bartter and co-workers (1962) reported atrophy in 40% of all glomeruli in patients with Bartter's syndrome; *Brackett* and co-workers (1968) however described a maximum increase in the glomerular diameter of 250 μ. To the best of our knowledge, no data are available concerning the size of the glomeruli from patients with pseudo-Bartter's syndrome.

The surfaces of the Bowman's capsules and the capillary convolutions therefore were measured in our biopsy material. The section area showed a significant reduction in the size of the glomerular vascular convolution and Bowman's capsule (mean, 17.5%) (see Fig. 3), compared to normal renal tissue. When the number of cells (see III 5 c) remains constant, the smaller convolutions are responsible for a proportional increase in cell density; an absolute increase in the mesangial matrix (see III 5 a) results in an unproportionally high increase in the material density.

If the volume of the basement membrane and glomerular cells remains constant, the capillary lumina narrow due to the decrease in the volume of the vascular convolution. In agreement with these findings, narrow and bloodless capillaries with pronounced mesangial sclerosis were observed in patients with excessive laxative intake (*Cremer* and *Blümcke* 1977).

c) Other Glomerular Alterations

Jensen and co-workers (1950) observed a sharp increase in the number of glomerular cells due to chronic electrolyte loss associated with ulcerative colitis.

A slight (*Brackett* et al. 1968) and a marked (*Cannon* et al. 1968) proliferation of mesangial cells was also reported in connection with Bartter's syndrome. In our patients with diuretic and cathartic drug abuse, however, the number of glomerular cells remained absolutely constant. In agreement with the subjective impression, the cell density increased by 17.5% due to a decrease in the size of the glomeruli.

Focal glomerulosclerosis accompanied predominantly by periglomerular fibrosis and interstitial collagenization was reported in varying frequencies in patients with cathartic and diuretic drug abuse. *Cremer* and *Blümcke* (1977) observed focal hyalinization in 2% to 22.5% of their cases; *Muehrcke* and *McMillan* (1963), in 3 of 15 patients. Between 2.5% and 61.2% of the glomeruli were hyalinized in our 34 biopsy specimens, even in association with interstitial fibrosis (*Riemenschneider* and *Bohle* 1980).

Wagner and co-workers (1979) reported an extension of the proximal tubule cells onto the parietal layer of Bowman's capsule in a patient with excessive diuretic drug intake. This phenomenon was observed in various types of glomerulonephritis in only

1.7% of the glomeruli (*Wagner* et al. 1979). Proximal tubule epithelium was observed at the site of capsular epithelium in 3 of our 34 cases, i.e., 9%.

6. Vessels

Benign nephrosclerosis with hyalinosis of the intima and the media has been described in a number of cases as a result of excessive intake of laxatives and diuretics.

DeGraeff and *Schuurs* (1960) observed one case of extensive arteriolosclerosis together with splitting of the intima and media. *Muehrcke* and *McMillan* (1963) reported slight hyalinosis of the intima in all patients with cathartic and diuretic drug abuse. *Cremer* and *Blümcke* (1977), slight to moderately severe hyalinosis. In our 34 kidney biopsy specimens, however, only one mild and one moderately severe case of benign nephrosclerosis were detected. Moreover, vascular alterations were never described following enteral potassium and sodium depletion of other etiologies (*Jensen* et al. 1950; *Kulka* et al. 1950; *Perkins* et al. 1950).

Brackett and co-workers (1968) reported hyalinosis of the small arterial vessels in a case of true Bartter's syndrome.

A causal relationship between cathartic or diuretic drug abuse and nephrosclerosis with pre-existing hyponatremia, hypovolemia, and low blood pressure (see Part IV) is highly improbable in regard of pathogenesis.

In addition, *Pasternack* (1970) observed a thickening of the media in arterioles of kidneys and muscles in a patient with anorexia nervosa, vomiting, and diarrhea. This medial hypertrophy was interpreted as an adaptive reaction to chronic reninism (*Pasternack* et al. 1967).

IV. Renal Function

Two processes are apparently responsible for functional disturbances of the kidney due to chronic ingestion of laxatives and diuretics; a dynamic, reversible functional impairment dependent on deficits in available sodium, potassium, and body water, and a static, irreversible functional alteration due to pathomorphologic tubulo-interstitial lesions.

1. Urinary Concentration

One early and typical symptom of hypokalamic nephropathy of different etiologies is the impairment of the concentration function, as demonstrated in concentration tests and following administration of ADH (*Hollander* and *Blythe* 1971). The concentration capacity of the kidneys in patients with excessive laxative intake (*Schwartz* and *Relman* 1953; *Relman* and *Schwartz* 1956; *Pollack* et al. 1957; *Aitchinson* 1958; *Truninger* et al. 1960) and diuretic drug abuse (*Katz* et al. 1972; *Fuchs* et al. 1976; *Wagner* et al. 1979) therefore is also markedly impaired, the maximal specific weight usually being below 1015.

The concentrating ability of the kidneys in some patients following chronic use of laxatives is completely restored after the electrolyte metabolism has returned to normal (*Relman* and *Schwartz* 1956; *Hollander* and *Blythe* 1971). The repair phase ranged from a few months to several years (*Hollander* and *Blythe* 1971). Total restoration of the concentration capacity was probably no longer possible with some patients (*Pollack* et al. 1957; *Aitchinson* 1958; *Hollander* and *Blythe* 1971). The extent of the concentration defect depends on the severity and the duration of the potassium deficit (*Hollander* and *Blythe* 1971).

Only a potassium deficit appears capable of causing a reversible reduction in the concentration capacity, as experimentally induced hypokalemia in man has shown (*Rubini* 1966).

Since the experimental findings are different, the pathogenesis of the impairment in concentration capacity can only be hypothesized. Possible causal factors are:

- Reduced solute concentration in the medulla (*Manitus* et al. 1960) due either to reduced sodium transport in the ascending limb of the loopof Henle (*Buckalew* et al. 1967), e.g., due to reduced oxidative metabolism of the tubules, or to increased blood supply to the medulla, e.g., due to increased prostaglandin synthesis (*Nivet* et al. 1978; *Radfar* et al. 1978).
- Reduced TmH_2O resulting from an ADH deficit following chronic hypokalemic stimulation of the neurohypophyseal system (*Kleeman* and *Maxwell* 1959; *Berl* et al. 1977) or from ADH antagonism due to high production of prostaglandins (*Anderson* et al. 1975; *Galvez* et al. 1977).

The cause of the frequently observed, irreversible concentration loss must be sought in the tubulo-interstitial lesions. The damaged tubules with atrophic epithelium and thickened basement membrane do not appear to be capable of reabsorbing adequate amounts of sodium; in addition, osmotic diuresis may also be present due to advanced cathartic and diuretic nephropathy. *Striker* and co-workers (1970) established a significant correlation between interstitial fibrosis or tubular atrophy and concentration defects.

2. Acid Excretion

Various degrees of metabolic alkalosis in plasma have been determined with cathartic and diuretic drug ingestion in association with chronic sodium and potassium deficits; *Cremer* and *Bock* (1977) found a base excess of 4 units; *Bock* and co-workers (1978), 6 units; *Wolff* and co-workers (1968), 9 units. The mean sodium carbonate concentration was 29 mval/l. The cause appears to be the compensatory penetration of H^+ ions into the intracellular space and an increased loss of H^+ ions in the exchange with sodium in the distal tubules (*Kunau* and *Stein* 1979). The excretion of tritratable acid in the urine is usually within the range of normalcy in patients with cathartic and diuretic drug abuse (*Wolff* et al. 1968), but it is still too high in relation to the extracellular excess of alkali (*Schwartz* and *Relman* 1967). Ammonium excretion however also increases sharply in the presence of a marked potassium deficit and inhibited production of aldosterone (*Tannen* et al. 1970). The increase in glutaminase activity in connection with hypokalemia (*Iacobellis* et al. 1955) is one possible causal factor.

The "paradoxical aciduria' then is due to an overly high concentration of hydrogen in the distal tubule, a direct consequence of elevated H^+ ion secretion and an indirect result of increased NH_4^+ ion production.

3. Renal Sodium Handling

The excretion of sodium through the kidneys is a dynamic process dependent on the amount of laxatives and diuretics ingested and the sodium supply. This process can be divided into three phases.

In the initial phase, renal sodium and body water losses following administration of diuretics are high, even though serum and total body concentrations of sodium are still within the range of normalcy (*Jahrmärker* 1960; *Venning* et al. 1962). Renal losses in patients with carthartic drug abuse are low already in the initial phase (*Coghill* and *McAllen* 1959); considerable sodium however is lost through watery diarrhea (*French* et al. 1956; *Aitchinson* 1958; *Houghton* and *Pears* 1958; *DeGraeff* and *Schuurs* 1960; *Fordtran* and *Dietschy* 1966).

In the second phase, the values for total body sodium are lowered, while serum sodium concentration is still normal (*Schwartz* and *Relman* 1953; *Fuchs* et al. 1977) or decreased (*Coghill* and *McAllen* 1959; *Bock* et al. 1978). Sodium excretion is usually far below normal in such cases, i.e., often under 10 mval/l. Sodium conservation due to secondary hyperaldosteronism or a reduced glomerular filtration rate (see IV 5) is intact, providing the tubulo-interstitial lesions are not too far advanced in the sense of a salt-losing kidney.

In the third phase of sodium and potassium repletion through increased iatrogenic supply or following withdrawal of cathartic and diuretic drug intake, sodium excretion often continues to be low (*Coghill* and *McAllen* 1959) because of a delay in the adaptation of the glomerular filtration rate or the aldosterone production. Edema often develops in ankles and eyelids as a result of the temporary excess of sodium and a hypothetical disturbance in permeability due to the potassium deficit (*Schwartz* and *Relman* 1953; *Coghill* and *McAllen* 1959; *DeGraeff* and *Schuurs* 1960; *Love* et al. 1971). This, in turn, stimulates the patient to renewed cathartic and diuretic drug intake (*DeGraeff* and *Schuurs* 1960; *Kramer* and *Pope* 1964) and the physician to order a kidney biopsy to clarify the cause of the edema.

4. Renal Potassium Handling

Potassium losses through the kidney due to chronic cathartic and diuretic drug intake can be extremely elevated in the first phase, depending on the dose (*Coghill* and *McAllen* 1959; *Venning* et al. 1962; *Katz* et al. 1972), in extreme cases, up to one third of the total body potassium (*Schwartz* and *Relman* 1953). Mean values for serum potassium without preceding therapy, were approximately 2.5 mval/l (*Schwartz* and *Relman* 1953; *Aitchinson* 1958; *Houghton* and *Pears* 1958; *Coghill* and *McAllen* 1959;

Litchfield 1959; *DeGraeff* and *Schuurs* 1960; *Wolff* et al. 1968; *Fleischer* et al. 1969; *Love* et al. 1971; *Gossain* and *Werk* 1972; *Katz* et al. 1972; *LaRusso* and *Gill* 1975; *Fuchs* et al. 1977; *Bock* et al. 1978; *Wagner* et al. 1979). Potassium excretion in this phase was usually low (*Wolff* et al. 1968), but dependent on sodium supply and aldosterone concentration. In a few cases, potassium-losing nephritis developed after chronic drug abuse; histologic examination showed pronounced tubulo-interstitial lesions (*DeGraeff* and *Schuurs* 1960).

Potassium as well as sodium excretion increases gradually in the repletion phase (*Coghill* and *McAllen* 1959; *Love* et al. 1971), but hyperkalemia does not develop since the potassium rapidly shifts into the intracellular space.

5. Glomerular Filtration Rate

On the average, the glomerular filtration rate associated with cathartic and diuretic nephropathy was lowered, the mean being 45.7 ml/min (*Cremer* and *Bock* 1977) or 49.4 ml/min (*Bock* et al. 1978), corresponding serum creatinine concentration was 1.53 mg% (*Riemenschneider* and *Bohle* 1980) or 1.58 mg% (*Wolff* et al. 1968). A low glomerular filtration rate was also confirmed in individual publications (*Relman* and *Schwartz* 1956; *Litchfield* 1959; *Trübestein* et al. 1960; *Wagner* et al. 1979). The glomerular filtration rate rose to normal values in a few cases after equalization of the electrolyte deficit (*Relman* and *Schwartz* 1956; *Litchfield* 1959).

Bock and co-workers (1978) reported a correlation between the decrease in the glomerular filtration rate and the persistence of hypokalemia. A highly significant correlation between the glomerular filtration rate and relative interstitial volume was also established in our cases.

There are two possible etiologic factors responsible for the reduction in the glomerular filtration rate. The perfusion of the glomeruli is lowered due to the sodium deficit (see IV 3), reduced blood volume (*Wolff* et al. 1968), usually low blood pressure (*Wolff* et al. 1968; *Cremer* and *Bock* 1977), and compensatory high plasma renin (*Cremer* and *Bock* 1977; *Bock* et al. 1978). This condition is reversible after equalization of the water and electrolyte deficits. The second causal factor for irreversible reduction of the glomerular filtration rate appears to be the frequent occurrence of interstitial fibrosis and tubular atrophy. Correlations between increasing interstitial volume due to sclerosis and decreasing glomerular filtration rate were established for many glomerular (*Bohle* et al. 1977a, b, c), vascular (*Grund* et al. 1978), and interstitial (*Mackensen* et al. 1979) renal diseases. A serie of biopsies from one patient which could demonstrate the development of interstitial fibrosis in the presence of a falling glomerular filtration rate is unfortunately not available.

V. Conclusions

The pathogenetic evolution of cathartic and diuretic nephropathy begins with a chronic disturbance in water and electrolyte metabolism, followed by disturbances in renal function, and, finally, morphologically detectable lesions. Since the morphology and pathogenesis differ essentially from toxic and immunoallergic processes, a special section is devoted to them.

The *diagnosis* of diuretic and cathartic drug abuse can be established by intensive questioning of the patient, but in many cases it can only be made by biochemical demonstation of these drugs in the urine and feces since the patients often stubbornly deny their excessive use of laxatives and diuretics.

The tentative diagnosis is often based on the typical *clinical constellation:* almost 90% of the patients are female with an average age of 35, are often underweight with a progressive transition to anorexia nervosa, and have consistently low serum potassium concentrations, as an expression of a latent sodium deficit. The patients are hypotensive, and the serum and urinary renin concentrations are frequently elevated. Renal function disturbances are reduced maximal concentration ability, overly high excretion of titerable and nontiterable protons in their relation to the metabolic alkalosis, and, frequently, a reduced glomerular filtration rate.

A typical combination of *morphologic findings* related to hypokalemia and hyponatremia can be demonstrated, although no pathgnomonic pattern is present. The most impressive alteration in this regard is the consistent hyperplasia and hypertrophy of the juxtaglomerular apparatus with an increase in the surrounding basement-membrane-like substance and epithelioid transformation of the Goormaghtigh cells. The increase in the mesangial matrix and decrease in the size of the capillary convolution are diagnostically important. The appearance of "multivesicular bodies" in all cell elements of the renal medulla is rare, but characteristic for potassium and sodium-deficit nephropathy. Vacuolar degeneration of the proximal renal tubules occurs relatively seldom and its appearance is nonspecific. As a result, it cannot be considered typical for cathartic and diuretic nephropathy.

The *severity* of the irreversible *renal lesions* developing in the course of cathartic and diuretic drug abuse can be estimated clinically on the basis of the glomerular filtration rate after the electrolyte deficit has equalized and morphologically on the basis of the extent of interstitial fibrosis. Interstitial fibrosis is the most important factor controbuting to the reduction of the glomerular filtration rate, as measurements in regard to this and many other renal disorders have illustrated.

Atrophy of the tubules and thickening of the basement membrane develop parallel to the interstitial sclerosis.

The *prognosis* for cathartic and diuretic nephropathy appears to depend on the dose of the ingested drug, the individual sensitivity, and the duration of the abuse. The glomerular filtration rate certainly decreases and interstitial fibrosis increases in direct proportion to the duration of hypokalemia.

The progression of the nephropathy can be slowed down by withdrawal of the drug intake or, at least, by electrolyte equalization.

References

Aitchinson JD (1958) Hypokalaemia following chronic diarrhoea from overuse of cascara and deficient diet. Lancet II: 75–76

Aithal HN, Toback FG, Dube S, Getz GS, Spargo BH (1977) Formation of renal medullary lysosomes during potassium depletion nephropathy. Lab Invest 36: 107–113

Anderson RJ, Berl T, McDonald KM, Schrier RW (1975) Evidence for an in vivo antagonism between vasopressin and prostaglandin in the mammalian kidney. J Clin Invest 56: 420–426

Bartter FC, Pronove P, Gill JR, MacCardle RC (1962) Hyperplasia of the juxtaglomerular complex with hyperaldosteronism and hypokalemic alkalosis. Amer J Med 33: 811–828

Berl T, Linas SL, Aisenbrey GA, Anderson RJ (1977) On the mechanism of polyuria in potassium depletion. The role of polydipsia. J Clin Invest 60: 620–625

Biava CG, Dyrda I, Genest J, Benscosme SA (1963) Kaliopenic nephropathy. Lab Invest 12: 443–453

Biava CG, West M (1966) Fine stucture of normal human juxtaglomerular cells. II. Specific and nonspecific cytoplasmic granules. Amer J Path 49: 955–979

Bock KD, Cremer W, Werner U (1978) Chronic hypokalemic nephropathy: A clinical study. Klin Wschr. 56 (Suppl I): 91–96

Bohle A, Bader R, Grund KE, Mackensen S, Neunhoeffer J (1977a) Serum creatinine concentration and renal interstitial volume. Analysis of correlations in endocapillary (acute) glomerulonephritis and in moderately severe mesangioproliferative glomerulonephritis. Virchows Arch A Path Anat and Histol 375: 87–96

Bohle A, Christ H, Grund KE, Mackensen S (1979) The role of the interstitium of the renal cortex in renal disease. Contr Nephrol 16: 109–114

Bohle A, Glomb D, Grund KE, Mackensen S (1977b) Correlations between relative interstitial volume of the renal cortex and serum creatinine concentration in minimal changes with nephrotic syndrome and in focal sclerosing glomerulonephritis. Virchows Arch A Path and Histol 376: 221–232

Bohle A, Grund KE, Mackensen S, Tolon M (1977c) Correlations between renal interstitium and level of serum creatinine. Morphometric investigations of biopsies in perimembranous glomerulonephritis. Virchows Arch A Path Anat and Histol 373: 15–22

Bohman SO, Jensen PKA (1976) Morphometric studies on the lipid droplets of the interstitial cells of the renal medulla in different states of diuresis. J Ultrastruc Res 55: 182–192

Brackett NC, Koppel M, Randall RE, Nixon WP (1968) Hyperplasia of the juxtaglomerular complex with secondary aldosteronism without hypertension (Bartter's syndrome). Amer J Med 44: 803–819

Brunner FP, Frick PG (1968) Hypokalaemia, metabolic alkalosis, and hypernatraemia due to massive sodium penicillin therapy. Brit med J 4: 550–552

Buckalew VM, Ramirez MA, Goldberg M (1967) Free water reabsorption during solute diuresis in normal and potassium depleted rats. Amer J Physiol 212: 381–386

Butler WT, Bennett JE, Alling DW, Wertlake PT, Utz JP, Hill GJ (1964) Nephrotoxicity of amphotericin B. Ann Int Med 61: 175–187

Cannon PJ, Leeming JM, Sommers SC, Winters RW, Laragh JH (1968) Juxtaglomerular cell hyperplasia and secondary hyperaldosteronism (Bartter's syndrome): a reevalution of the pathophysiol. Medicine (Balt) 47: 107–131

Christensen JA, Bader H, Bohle A, Meyer DS (1976) The structure of the juxtaglomerular apparatus in Addison's disease, Bartter's syndrome and in Conn's syndrome. Virchows Arch A Path and Histol 370: 103–112

Coghill NF, McAllen PM (1959) Electrolyte losses associated with taking of purges investigated with aid of sodium and potassium radioisotopes. Brit med J 1: 14–19

Comai K, Prose P, Farber SJ, Paulsrud JR (1974) Correlation of renal medullary prostaglandin content and renal interstitial cell lipid droplets. Prostaglandins 6: 375–379

Conn JW, Johnson RD (1956) Kaliopenic nephropathy. Amer J Clin Nutrit 4: 523–528

Cremer W, Blümcke S (1977) Zur Morphologie der kaliopenischen Nephropathie beim Menschen. Nieren u Hochdruckkrankh 2: 71–78

Cremer W, Bock KD (1977) Symptoms and course of chronic hypokalemic nephropathy in man. Clin Nephrol 7: 112–119

DeGraeff J, Schuurs MAM (1960) Severe potassium depletion caused by the abuse of laxatives. Acta med Scand 166: 407–422

Edmonts CJ (1977) Carbonoxolone, diuretic treatment, and body potassium. Brit med J 1: 775

Fleischer N, Brown H, Graham DY, Delena S (1969) Chronic laxative-induced hyperaldosteronism and hypokalemia simulating Bartter's syndrome. Ann Int Med 70: 791–798

Fingl E (1975) Laxatives and cathartics. In: Goodman LS, Gilman A (eds) The pharmacological basis of therapeutics. MacMillan and Co, pp 976–986

Fordtran JS, Dietschy JM (1966) Water and electrolyte movement in the intestine. Gastroenterology 50: 263–285

France R (1962) Intracellular granules of the renal medulla in potassium depletion. Trans Amer Clin Climat Ass 74: 211–230

France R, Gray ME, Stone WJ, Swift LL (1978) Intracellular granules of the renal medulla in a case of potassium depletion due to renal potassium wasting. Amer J Pathol 91: 299–312

France R, Shelley WM, Gray ME (1974) Abnormal intracellular granules of renal papilla in a child with potassium depletion (Bartter's syndrome) and renal tuberous sclerosis. Hopkins med J 135: 274–285

France R, Stone WJ, Michelakis AM, Island DP, Merill JM, Tolleson WJ (1973) Renal potassium wasting of unknown cause in a clinical setting of chronic potassium depletion: Report of a case. South Med J 66: 115–128

French JM, Gaddie R, Smith N (1956) Diarrhoea due to phenolphthalein. Lancet I: 551–553

Frimpter GW, Timpanelli AE, Eisenmenger WJ, Stein HS, Ehrlich LI (1963) Reversible "Franconi syndrome" caused by degraded tetracycline. JAMA 184: 111–113

Fuchs C, Hunnemann DH, Scheler F (1977) Hyperreninismus ohne Aldosteronismus bei Diuretika-Abusus. Deut Med Wschr 37: 1319–1322

Fujita T, Sakaguchi H, Shibagaki M, Fukui T, Nomura M, Sekiguchi S (1977) The pathogenesis of Bartter's syndrome. Functional and histologic studies. Amer J Med 63: 467–474

Galvez O, Bay WH, Roberts BW, Ferris TF (1977) The hemodynamic effects of potassium deficiency in the dog. Circ Res (Suppl I) 40: 11–15

George J, Zimmermann HO (1978) Noduläre Hyperplasie der interstitiellen Zellen des menschlichen Nierenmarkes: Folge chronischer Hypoxydose? Verh dtsch Ges Path 62: 353

Gossain VV, Werk EE (1972) Surreptitious laxation and hypokalemia. Ann Int Med 76: 671

Gross JM (1963) Fanconi syndrome developing secondary to the ingestion of outdated tetracycline. Ann Int Med 58: 523–528

Grund KE, Mackensen S, Grüner J, Neunhoeffer J, Bader H, Bohle A (1978) Renal insufficiency in nephrosclerosis. Correlations between morphological and functional papameters. Klin Wschr 56: 1147–1158

Hagège J, Gabe M, Richet G (1974) Scanning of the apical pole of distal tubular cells under differing acid-base conditions. Kidney Int 5: 137–146

Helber A, Meyer D, Schürholz J, Bohle A (1970) Zur Struktur und Funktion des juxtaglomerulären Apparates. Dtsch med Wschr 45: 2280–2287

Hoffbrand BI, Stewart JDM (1970) Carbenicillin and hypokalemia. Brit med J 4: 746
Hollander W Jr (1963) The nephropathy of potassium depletion. In: Strauss MB, Welt LG (eds) Diseases of the kidney. Little, Brown, Boston
Hollander W, Blythe WB (1971) Nephropathy of potassium depletion. In: Strauss MB, Welt LG (eds) Diseases of the kidney. Sec. edition, vol II. Little, Brown, Boston, pp 933–972
Houghton BJ, Pears MA (1958) Chronic potassium depletion due to purgation with cascara. Brit med J 1: 1328–1330
Hurley B (1977) Acute renal failure associated with carbenoxolone treatment. Brit med J 4: 1442
Iacobellis M, Muntwyler E, Griffin GE (1955) Kidney glutaminase and carbonic anhydrase activity and tissue electrolyte composition in potassium-deficient dogs. Amer J Physiol 183: 395–400
Jaffe RH, Sternberg H (1919) Über die vacuololäre Nierendegeration bei chronischer Ruhr. Virchows Arch path Anat 227: 313–319
Jahrmärker H (1960) Störungen des Wasser- und Elektrolythaushalts bei diuretischer Therapie. Klin Waschr 38: 351–359
Jensen EJ, Baggenstoss AH, Bargen JA (1950) Renal lesions associated with chronic ulcerative colitis. Amer J Med Sci 219: 281–290
Kannegiesser H, Lee JB (1971) Role of outer renal medullary metabolism in the concentrating defect of potassium depletion. Amer J Physiol 220: 1701–1707
Katz FH (1975) Self-administration of diuretics. Ann Int Med 83: 575–576
Katz FH, Eckert RC, Gebott MD (1972) Hypokalemia caused by surreptitious self-administration of diuretics. Ann Int Med 76: 85–90
Keye JD (1952) Death in potassium deficiency. Report of a case including morphologic findings. Circulat 5: 766–770
Klastersky J, Vanderkelen B, Daneau D, Mathieu M (1973) Carbenicillin and hypokalemia. Ann Int Med 78: 774–776
Kleeman CR, Maxwell MH (1959) Contributory role of extra-renal factors in the polyuria of potassium depletion. New Engl J Med 260: 268–271
Kramer P, Pope CE (1964) Factitious diarrhea induced by phenolphthalein. Arch Int Med 114: 634–636
Kulka JP, Pearson CM, Robbins SL (1950) A distinctive vacuolar nephropathy associated with intestinal disease. Amer J Path 26: 349–377
Kunau RT, Stein JH (1979) Disorders of potassium metabolism. In: Earley LE, Gottschalk CW (eds) Strauss and Welt's Diseases of the kidney. 3rd edition, vol II. Little, Brown, Boston, pp 1581–1625
Langer KH, Thoenes W (1969) Zur Genese "optisch leerer Vacuolen" im Epithel des energetisch insuffizienten proximalen Nierentubulus. Verh dtsch Ges Path 53: 394–401
LaRusso NF, Gill DB (1975) Surreptitious laxative ingestion. Mayo Clin Proc 50: 706–708
Lerman RJ, Pitcock JA, Stephenson P, Muirhead EE (1972) Renomedullary interstitial cell tumor (formerly fibroma of renal medulla). Human Path 3: 559–568
Limas C, Limas CJ, Gesell MS (1976) Effects of indomethacin on renomedullary interstitial cells. Lab Invest 34: 522–528
Litchfield JA (1959) Low potassium syndrome resulting from the use of purgative drugs. Gastrenterology 37: 483–488
Love DR, Brown JJ, Fraser R, Lever AF, Robertson JIS, Timbury GC, Thomson S, Tree M (1971) An unusual case of self-induced electrolyte depletion. Gut 12: 284–290
MacDonald MK, Sabour MS, Lambie AT, Robson JS (1962) The nephropathy of experimental potassium deficiency. An electron microscopic study. Quart J Exp Physiol 47: 262–272

Mackensen S, Grund KE, Sindjić M, Bohle A (1979) Influence of the renal cortical interstitium on the serum creatinine concentration and serum creatinine clearance in different chronic sclerosing interstitial nephritides. Nephron 24: 30–34

Manitus A, Levitin H, Beck D, Epstein FH (1960) On the mechanism of impairment of renal concentrating ability in potassium deficiency. J Clin Invest 39: 684–692

Maunsbach AB (1966) The influence of different fixatives and fixation methods on the ultrastructure of rat kidney proximal tubule cell. J Ultrastruc Res 15: 242–282

McCurdy DK, Frederic M, Elinton JR (1968) Renal tubular acidosis due to amphotericin B. New Engl J Med 278: 124–131

Meurer KA, Kaufmann W, Steiner B, Schürholz J, Streicher E (1968) Zur Differentialdiagnose des Bartter-Syndroms. Med Welt 52: 2886–2893

Meyer D (1972) Morphometrische Untersuchungen an juxtaglomerulärem Apparat und Macula densa menschlicher Nieren bei verschiedenen Erkrankungen. In: Veröffentlichungen aus der morphologischen Pathologie. Fischer, pp 1–83

Morrison AB, Panner BJ (1964) Lysosome induction in experimental potassium deficiency. Amer J Path 45: 295–303

Mudge GM (1975) Drugs affecting renal function and electrolyte metabolism. In: Goodman LS, Gilman A (eds) The pharmacological basis of therapeutics. MacMillan and Co, pp 809–847

Muehrcke RC (1960) Prolonged potassium deficiency and chronic pyelonephritis in man and animals. In: Quinn EL, Kass EH (eds) Biology of pyelonephritis. Little, Brown, Boston, pp 581–603

Muehrcke RC, McMillan JC (1963) The relationship of "chronic pyelonephritis" to chronic potassium deficiency. Ann Int Med 59: 427–448

Muehrcke RC, Rosen S (1964) Hypokalemic nephropathy in rat and man. Lab Invest 13: 1359–1373

Muller AF, Manning EL, Holder J (1963) Hypokaliämie, Aldosteronausscheidung und primärer Hyperaldosteronismus. Schweiz med Wschr 36: 1265–1272

Nivet H, Grenier B, Rolland JC, Lebranchu Y, Dray F (1978) Raised urinary prostaglandins in patient without Bartter's syndrome. Lancet I: 333–334

Panner BJ (1971) Ultrastructural and histochemical observations on developing lysosomes in experimental hypokalemia. Lab Invest 25: 53–59

Pasternack A (1970) Anorexia nervosa, secondary aldosteronism and angiopathie. Acta med Scand 187: 139–143

Pasternack A, Perheentupa J, Launiala K, Hallman K (1967) Kidney biopsy findings in familial chloride diarrhoea. Acta Endocrin 55: 1–9

Perkins JG, Petersen AB, Riley JA (1950) Renal and cardiac lesions in potassium deficiency due to chronic diarrhea. Amer J Med 8: 115–123

Pollack VE, Flagg GW, Muehrcke RC, Kark RM (1957) Potassium depletion following self-induced diarrhea and vomiting, treated by prolonged psychotherapy. Clin Res Proc 5: 194–195

Radfar N, Gill JR, Bartter FC, Bravo E, Taylor AA, Bowden RE (1978) Hypokalemia, in Bartter's syndrome and other disorders, produces resistance to vasopressors via prostaglandin overproduction. Proc exp Biol Med 158: 502–507

Relman AS, Schwartz WB (1956) The nephropathy of potassium depletion. A clinical and pathological entity. New Engl J Med 255: 195–203

Relman AS, Schwartz WB (1958) The kidney in potassium depletion. Amer J Med 24: 764–773

Richet G, Hagège J, Gabe M (1970) Correlations entre les transfers de bicarbonate et l la morphologie du segment terminal du nephron chez le rat. Nephron 7: 413–429

Riemenschneider Th, Bohle A (1980) To be published

Rubini ME (1961) Water excretion in potassium-deficient man. J Clin Invest 40: 2215–2224

Sarkar K, Levine DZ (1979) Ultrastructural changes in the renal papillary cells of rats during maintenance and repair of profound potassium depletion. Brit J exp Path 60: 120–129

Schmidt P, Kopsa H, Kronenberg KH, Meyer D, Zazgornik J, Kotzaurek R, Neumann E (1973) Bartter-Syndrom im Erwachsenenalter. Dtsch med Wschr 98: 723–726

Schürholz J, Schmid HJ, Meyer D, Bohle A (1969) Light and electron microscopic investigations of the juxtaglomerular apparatus in a patient with a "pseudo-Bartter"-syndrome. Progr Nephrol 21: 312–321

Schwartz WB, Relman AS (1953) Metabolic and renal studies in chronic potassium depletion resulting from overuse of laxatives. J Clin Invest 32: 258–271

Schwartz WB, Relman (1967) Effects of electrolyte disorders on renal structure and function. New Engl J Med 276: 383–389

Spargo B, Straus F, Fitch F (1960) Zonal renal papillary droplet change with potassium depletion. Arch Pathol 70: 599–631

Stamey TA (1956) The pathogenesis and implications of the electrolyte imbalance in ureterosigmoidostomy. Surg Gynec Obstet 103: 736–758

Stetson DL, Wade JB, Giebisch G (1980) Morphologic alterations in rat medullary collecting duct following potassium depletion. Kidney Int 17: 45–56

Stricker GE, Schainuck LI, Luther RE, Benditt EP (1970) Structural-functional correlations in renal disease. Part I: A method for assaying and clarifying histopathologic changes in renal disease. Human Pathol 1: 615–630

Tannen RL (1970) The effect of uncomplicated potassium depletion on urine acidification. J Clin Invest 49: 813–827

Tattersall MHN, Battersby G, Spiers ASD (1972) Antibiotics and hypokalaemia. Lancet I: 630–631

Toback FG, Ordóñez NG, Bortz SL, Spargo BH (1976) Zonal changes in renal structure and phospholipid metabolism in potassium-deficient rats. Lab Invest 34: 115–124

Trübestein GK, Werning C, Stadelmann O, Kuhlmann U, Stiehl D, Schweikert HU, Siegenthaler W (1972) Bartter- und Pseudo-Bartter-Syndrom. Münch med Wschr. 114: 635–640

Truninger-Rathe I, Spühler O (1960) Sekundärer Hyperaldosteronismus bei zyklischen Ödemen als Folge von chronischem Laxativabusus bei einem Fall von Anorexia mentalis. Schweiz med Wschr 38: 1061–1064

Venning EH, Dyrenfurth I, Dossetor JB, Beck JC (1962) Effect of chlorothiazide upon aldosterone excretion and sodium and potassium balance in essential hypertension. J Lab Clin Med 60: 79–85

Verberckmoes R, van Damme B, Clement J, Amery A, Michielsen P (1976) Bartter's syndrome with hyperplasia of renomedullary cells: Successful treatment with indomethacin. Kidney Int 9: 302–307

Wagner PK, Pippig L, Thoenes W (1979) Zur Histopathologie der Niere beim Pseudobartter-Syndrom durch chronischen Diuretikaabusus. Klin Wschr 57: 135–142

Wigley RD (1960) Potassium deficiency in anorexia nervosa with reference to renal tubular vacuolation. Brit med J 2: 110–113

Wilson H, Spargo B, Getz GS (1973) Changes in kidney medullary phospholipid metabolism in the potassium-deficient rat. Part I. Amer J Path 71: 295–306

Woernle M (1969) Beitrag zur kaliopenischen Nephropathie. Inaugural-Dissertation, Tübingen

Wolff HP, Henne G, Krück F, Roscher S, Vecsei P, Braun JJ, Düsterdieck G, Lever AF, Robertson JIS (1968) Psychosomatische Syndrome mit gastrointestinalem und/oder renalem Kalium- und Natriumverlust, Hyperreninämie und sekundärem Aldosteronismus. Schweiz med Wschr 48: 1883–1892

Drug-Induced Damage to the Embryo or Fetus

(Molecular and Multilateral Approach to Prenatal Toxicology)

D. NEUBERT, H. J. BARRACH and H.-J. MERKER

Introduction 242
I. Definitions 243
II. Special Aspects Discriminating Prenatal Toxicology from Other Toxic Situations 245
1. Mechanisms Responsible for the Triggering of an Abnormal Prenatal Development 245
a) Contribution of Mutagenic and Teratogenic Effects 245
b) Significance of Proliferation and Differentiation Processes 247
2. Special Pharmacokinetic Aspects of Prenatal Toxicology 249
3. Special Contribution of Maternal Factors 251
a) Deprivation of Maternal Components Vital to the Embryo 252
b) Alteration of Nutritional Supply by Drugs 252
c) Alteration of Uterine Blood Flow by Drugs 253
d) Alteration of the Susceptibility of the Conceptus to Drugs Caused by Pathologic Changes Occurring in the Maternal Organism 256
4. Special Outcome of an Embryotoxic Action 257
a) The "Litter" Effect 257
b) Correlation of Teratogenicity and Embryomortality 259
III. Organotropic Effects in Prenatal Toxicology 266
1. Problem of "Phase Specificity" 266
2. Problem of "Drug Specificity" 271
3. Problem of "Dose Specificity" 273
4. Problem of "Species Specificity" 273
IV. Special Problems of Dose-Response Relationships in Embryotoxicity 274
1. Change in the Outcome of an Embryotoxic Effect with Increased Doses 274
2. Selection of Appropriate Parameters for Evaluating a Dose-Response Relationship 275
3. Additional Confounding Factors which may Complicate the Establishment of Dose-Response Curves 278
4. Some Aspects of Teratogenic Effects of Drug Combinations 279
5. Problem of a "No-Effect Level" Existing in Prenatal Toxicology 282
V. Specificity of a "Teratogenic" Effect and Possible Modes of Teratogenic Actions 283
1. Specificity of a "Teratogenic" Effect 284
2. An Attempt to Classify a Teratogenic Action 285
3. Malformation-Like Abnormalities Induced Prior to or After the Classic "Critical Phase" or Organogenesis 287
4. Significance of Cell Necroses for the Induction of Congenital Structural Abnormalities 291
5. Significance of Changes Within the Blastema for the Induction of Abnormalities 299
6. Induction of Structural Anomalies Without Prior Occurrence of Necroses 305

7. Some Biochemical and Pharmacologic Aspects of Teratogenic Actions ... 309
   a) Biochemical Effects of 6-AN in the Embryo ... 309
   b) Effect of Ambient Temperature on the Teratogenic Effect of 6-AN. ... 312
   c) Distribution of Malformations of the Extremities ... 314

VI. Abnormalities Produced in Organ Culture and Applicability of Organ Culture Techniques in Teratology ... 317

VII. Concluding Remarks ... 321

VIII. Glossary on Terms Used in Prenatal Toxicology ... 323

References ... 324

Introduction

The exclusion of possible toxicologic hazards is still encumbered with the evaluation of three problems involving major difficulties: carcinogenicity, "teratogenicity," and mutagenicity. In this paper we will survey some aspects of a modern approach to studying problems of prenatal toxicology, suggesting multilateral ways of handling these problems and, possibly, overcoming the difficulties involved. So far, research in prenatal toxicology has suffered from the inability to incorporate basic pharmacologic and toxicologic, as well as biochemical and altrastructural, aspects. Until recently, routine screening of possible teratogenic effects and "basic research" into abnormal mammalian development were mostly confined to applying simple macroscopic, morphological techniques.

Since the toxicologic situation resulting in a teratogenic effect is particularly complex, our basic knowledge in this field can only be improved if the problem is systematically approached on a large scale and tackled from a variety of different angles.

The following abbreviations are used:

6-AN	= 6-aminonicotinamide	6-ANADP	= 6-aminonicotinamide-analogue of NADP
6-MP	= 6-mercaptopurine		
6-MPr	= 6-mercaptopurine riboside	TCDD	= 2,3,7,8-tetrachlorodibenzo-p-dioxin
6-MeMPr	= 6-methylmercaptopurine riboside	2,4,5 T	= 2,4,5-trichlorophenoxyacetic acid
Triton WR 1339	= polymer of octylphenol-polyethylenglycolether-formaldehyde	G-6-PD	= glucose-6-phosphate dehydrogenase
		6-P-GD	= 6-phosphogluconate dehydrogenase
ara-C	= cytosine arabinoside	GSSG	= oxidized glutathione
BUdr	= 5'-bromodeoxyuridine	NS	= nicotinic acid
		NA	= nicotinamide
Endoxan	= cyclophosphamide	PrPP	= phosphoribosyl pyrophosphate
HU	= hydroxyurea		
NAD	= nicotinamide-adenine dinucleotide	ppp	= pentose phosphate pathway
NADP	= nicotinamide-adenine dinucleotide phosphate	GSSG-Red.	= glutathione reductase

Some of the special aspects of "teratology" have been summarized and discussed before from a different point of view (*Bass* et al. 1977; *Krowke* and *Neubert* 1977; *Neubert* and *Barrach* 1978; *Neubert* et al. 1980; *Barrach* et al. 1980). In this paper we will analyze some of the parameters which, jointly, form the picture of a "teratogenic" action.

I. Definitions

In the field of developmental toxicology – and more specifically in "prenatal toxicology" – the nomenclature used by previous investigators has caused considerable confusion. Although toxicologists would agree that the terms *toxic* and *lethal* are not synonymous, several investigators in teratology have used the term embryo*toxic* to characterize an embryo*lethal* effect, discriminating it against a *teratogenic* effect. Such incorrect nomenclature is misleading because it may imply that a teratogenic effect or a growth retardation is not the result of a toxic effect, thus disregarding the basic principles of pharmacology and toxicology. A *toxic* event interfering with prenatal development can certainly manifest itself in many ways.

In accordance with the terminology used in all other fields of toxicologic research, we have suggested a nomenclature (*Neubert* et al. 1973; *Bass* et al. 1977) to be used in *prenatal toxicology* which equally takes into account the special situation of prenatal development (Fig. 1).

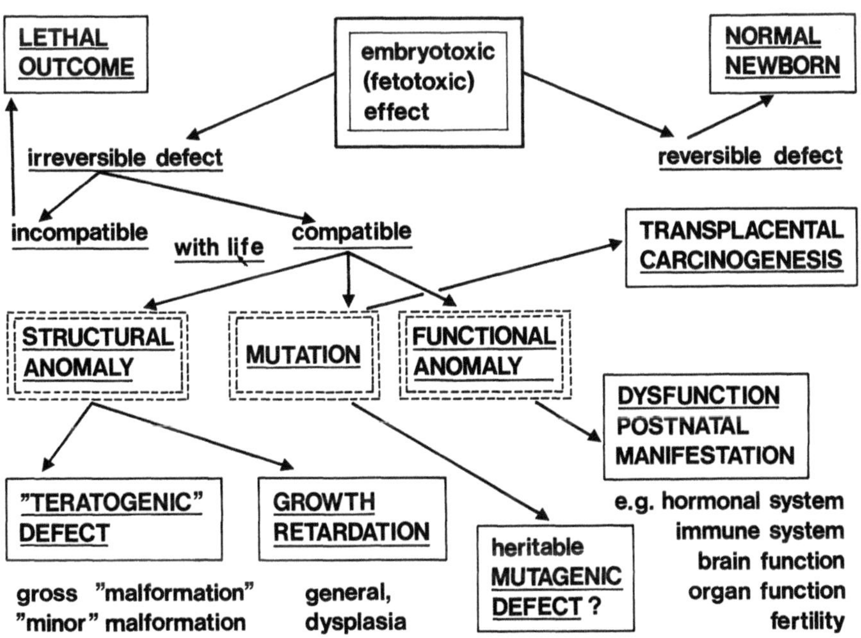

Fig. 1. Variable outcome of an embryotoxic effect in mammals

"Embryotoxic" (fetotoxic) is the most comprehensive term covering every kind of chemical, physical, or biologic interference with prenatal development. Such an embryo- or fetotoxic event may attack the developing organism at any stage from the zygote up to birth.

The embryotoxic lesion can be reversible or irreversible. Due to the high capacity of embryonic tissue to restore a lesion, many defects are apparently "repaired" during the prenatal period, resulting in a completely normal organism (restitution ad integrum).

An irreversible lesion, on the other hand, may be either incompatible or compatible with life. If incompatible with further development, an *embryolethal* (fetolethal) effect ("embryo-" or "fetomortality," resorption, abortion, stillbirth) is the outcome.

Consequences of a lesion compatible with prenatal life may be a structural (morphological) anomaly, a mutation, or a functional anomaly. A *"growth retardation"* may affect the whole organism ("small-for-date-baby" – either mature or immature) or only one or several organ systems (hypoplasia). Such growth retardation frequently is the most evident, and sometimes the only symptom indicating that a toxic effect has occurred.

So far, major attention, rightly or wrongly, in prenatal toxicology has been focused on *teratogenic effects.* They should be understood to be congenital, morphological (structural) abnormalities and are often called "congenital malformations." In addition to the well-known "gross malformations" or major abnormalities, "minor anomalies" – diversely defined by various authors – have recently become of interest. The term "minor anomalies" refers to abnormalities which are close to the physiologic variability, but which may arise more frequently as the result of a drug-induced toxic action (e.g., "neonatal alcohol syndrome," so-called DPH syndrome, etc., cf. Sect. II.4).

More recently, prenatally induced abnormalities which are not obviously associated with clearly visible structural defects have gained considerable interest and attention. These may be called *"congenital functional anomalies"* or prenatally induced dysfunctions, and they manifest themselves – sometimes late – postnatally. The systems which may be affected include brain (dysfunction and learning inabilities), the hormonal or immune systems, other organ systems, sexual function and fertility, and even life expectancy. Such functional defects, when analyzed in detail, may be found to be combined with structural defects on the microscopic level, but they may likewise represent defects on the "molecular level."

Mutations may also be induced during the prenatal period. These may affect the germ cells, but somatic mutations are more likely to occur. The significance of such somatic mutations – chromosomal aberrations or point mutations – for the induction of teratogenic effects is still in question. Somatic mutations may also be considered the initation of *transplacental carcinogenesis.* This has not only clearly been demonstrated in animal experiments but, unfortunately, has also been observed in humans treated in utero with diethylstilbestrol (*Herbst* et al. 1971, 1974, 1975). Transplacental carcinogenesis should be considered a clear-cut example of an embryo- or fetotoxic effect. The association of this type of carcinogenesis with other embryo- or fetotoxic manifestations is still far from being understood.

For convenience, we have supplemented this review with a glossary of the terms frequently used in "teratology" (cf. Sect. VIII).

II. Special Aspects Discriminating Prenatal Toxicology from Other Toxic Situations

A prenatally induced toxic event differs in a number of aspects from a toxic effect acting on an adult organism. Basic parameters ruling embryotoxic actions are of utmost importance when possible hazards for man as well as the cause and mode of action of abnormal prenatal development are being evaluated. Some aspects which deserve attention will now be discussed.

Two basic problems must be scrutinized:

a) the mechanism responsible for the triggering of an abnormal prenatal development;

b) special toxicologic problems involved with drug-induced embryotoxic effects, such as special contribution of maternal factors, pharmacokinetics, and outcome of an embryotoxic event.

Our knowledge of all of these parameters is fragmentary and much more systematic research is needed before we can claim to understand the peculiarities of the mode of action of embryotoxic agents.

1. Mechanisms Responsible for the Triggering of an Abnormal Prenatal Development

Research in prenatal toxicology is complicated by a number of aspects discriminating this type of toxicologic situation from others possibly arising in the adult organism. Two of these aspects are particularly important in this respect: (1) the final outcome, a "malformation," may be produced by two entirely different types of mechanism; and (2) some characteristic peculiarities distinguish embryonic metabolism from that occurring in the majority of tissues of an adult organism.

a) Contribution of Mutagenic and Teratogenic Effects

Principally, two causes can be visualized initiating abnormal embryonic or fetal development (Fig. 2):

The first is an *inheritable gene defect*, which, at a critical stage of development, prevents a certain gene from being properly expressed, thereby upsetting the sequence necessary for normal embryonic development. The event leading to such a defect is a *mutagenic effect.* It either originates in the *parental germ cells* "spontaneously" or is induced by mutagenic chemicals or radiation. Although of supreme interest and significance, especially with regard to a connection existing between mutagenicity and teratogenicity, these mutagenic aspects of toxicology will not be included in this survey as they are not directly relevant to the problem of drug-induced embryotoxic effects.

The second cause is *interference* by chemicals, radiation, or other agents which differentiation processes and cell interactions which, occurring *during prenatal development*, result in an impairment of typical reactions necessary for normal development. The *intrinsic problems of "teratology"* or *prenatal toxicology* are reflected by such a type of interaction.

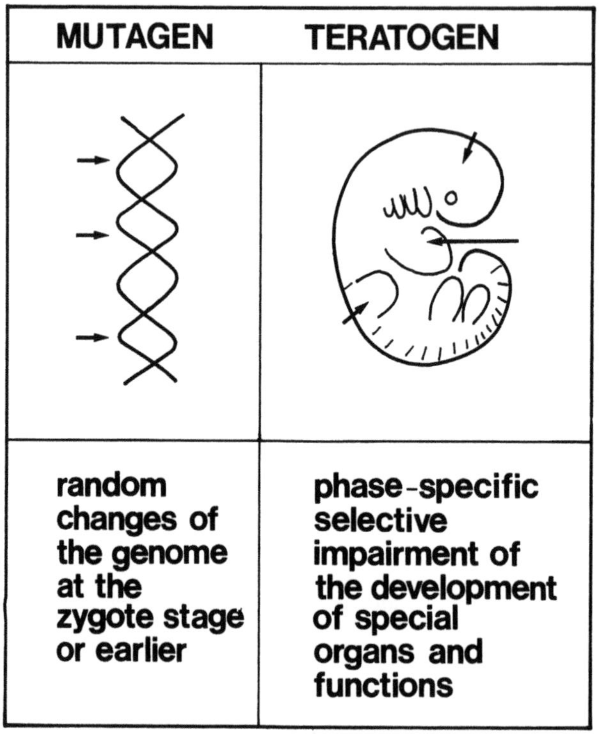

Fig. 2. Differences between "mutagenic" and "teratogenic" effects

The injury may result from a direct impairment with the genome and transcriptional processes or may be caused at a later stage of gene expression, e.g., on the level of translation or during the formation of a component essential in the sequence of developmental events. The anomaly resulting from this drug-induced abnormal development can be manifold. It may be called a *phenocopia* (*Landauer* 1959; *Lenz* 1973) if the defect resembles a malformation syndrome known as an inheritable genetic defect.

For a long time, it was generally believed that malformations were predominantly caused by a gene defect and therefore preponderantly represented typical inheritable diseases. While a certain percentage of congenital abnormalities may actually be attributed to mutations in the parental germ cells, our main concern now has to be directed to drugs and environmental factors causing such effects by interacting with prenatal development – and not via a mutation in the germ cell. *Therefore, teratologic research is much more complex than mutation research because the number of factors that may give rise to abnormal prenatal development is definitely higher than that of agents causing mutations in germ cells.* However, the genetic background and the additional factors affecting the developing embryo continue to be of considerable significance and importance.

For the reasons given, it is necessary to discriminate between a *mutagenic effect* (in this connection preferentially one already present in the zygote) and a *"teratogenic effect"* – or better, embryo- or fetotoxic effect – *which should be defined as a toxic effect occurring at a later developmental stage than the zygote and possibly even later than implantation.*

It should be pointed out that there is a principal difference between the result of a mutagenic effect hitting the germ cells and a teratogenic effect (Fig. 2). A mutagenic effect is a random event rarely resulting in an increased occurrence of a certain type of malformation, but in general raising the "background level" of all possible abnormalities caused by an impairment of diverse parts of the genome. Furthermore, many, if not the majority, of chromosomal aberrations are not compatible with successful embryonic development generating a viable newborn. They result in embryo- or fetomortality. Owing to the special toxicologic circumstances of drug-induced embryotoxic effects, well-defined abnormalities can be produced at a high frequency in experimental animals as well as in man, e.g., as demonstrated with the effects of thalidomide.

The question arises whether a drug-induced teratogenic effect may be expected to be inheritable. This is highly unlikely since a teratogenic event at the embryonic target and a mutagenic event in the embryonic germ cell exactly corresponding to the "phenocopia" produced by the teratogenic agent would have to coincide. To render this at all possible, the "teratogenic agent" likewise would be required to possess mutagenic properties inducing mutations in the germ cells of the developing embryo or fetus. A variety of different gene defects caused by such an action would be expected to occur, giving rise to many different types of abnormalities in the F_2-generation. Little is known from experimental animal studies on the probability of such an event taking place, and no information whatsoever is available with regard to humans.

b) Significance of Proliferation and Differentiation Processes

Mammalian embryonic tissues are distinguished, particularly during the stage of organogenesis, by two special metabolic characteristics: (1) the rate of proliferation is extremely high as compared with other mammalian tissues; and (2) a great variety of differentiation processes take place, both on the cellular and on the morphogenetic (cf. Sect. VIII) level.

During the early stages of organogenesis, the embryo *proliferates* at an extremely rapid rate. Within the first 10–11 days of gestation the DNA content of the mouse or rat embryo is increased approximately one million times (Fig. 3). Since the rate of DNA replication is comparatively low during the preimplantation stages, an increase in DNA content of 1000 times is achieved within 2 or 3 days of the early phase of organogenesis. From day 11 (mouse) or 13 (rat) of gestation on, the rate of DNA increase per 24 h slows down to twofold, or even lower values at later stages. Therefore, it is not surprising that many agents known to interfere with DNA replication have been found to possess a teratogenic potential. But questions still exist as to the mode of the teratogenic action of such compounds, and other points of attack, such as RNA metabolism, often cannot be ruled out completely (cf. *Krowke* and *Neubert* 1977).

However, we favor the assumption that an interference with *differentiation* processes may be a preferred mode of action of agents with a teratogenic potential. We distinguish two different types of differentiation processes:

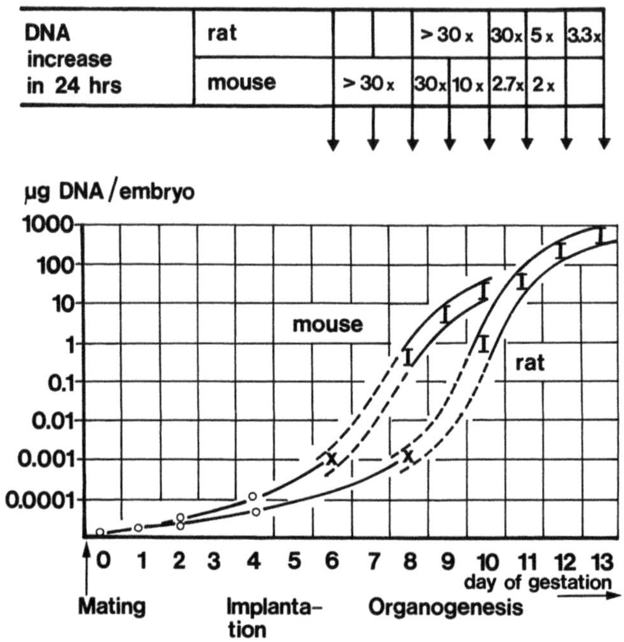

Fig. 3. Increase in DNA content during the early stage of gestation and the organogenesis phase in mice and rats

1. The term *"differentiation at the cellular level"* is used by us for processes leading to new cell capabilities: e.g., the transition from blastema cells to chondroblasts, which can produce extracellular substances typical for cartilage, the "induction" of new or more prominent enzymes within a cell, or the "induction" of a specific change in cell behavior, etc.

2. The term *"differentiation at the morphogenetic level"* is used by us for processes leading to the formation of specific tissue structures or organ anlagen: e.g., the formation of a specific inner or outer "shape" of an organism, or the fact that cartilage is not only formed as such, but in the form of specific cartilaginous bone anlagen.

The biochemical elucidation of the main events involved in differentiations has, so far, only partly been achieved. Differentiations may be expected to be triggered by a change in the gene expression of the cells. These changes can be monitored by the modern methods of molecular biology at the transcriptional and translational levels. But the sequence of the following events which finally give rise to the modification in cell shape or function are largely unknown.

The importance of the induction of cell death as a cause for a structural abnormality will be discussed later (Sect. V.4). Some of the events that may be responsible for the induction of an abnormal prenatal development are compiled in Figs. 4 and 5.

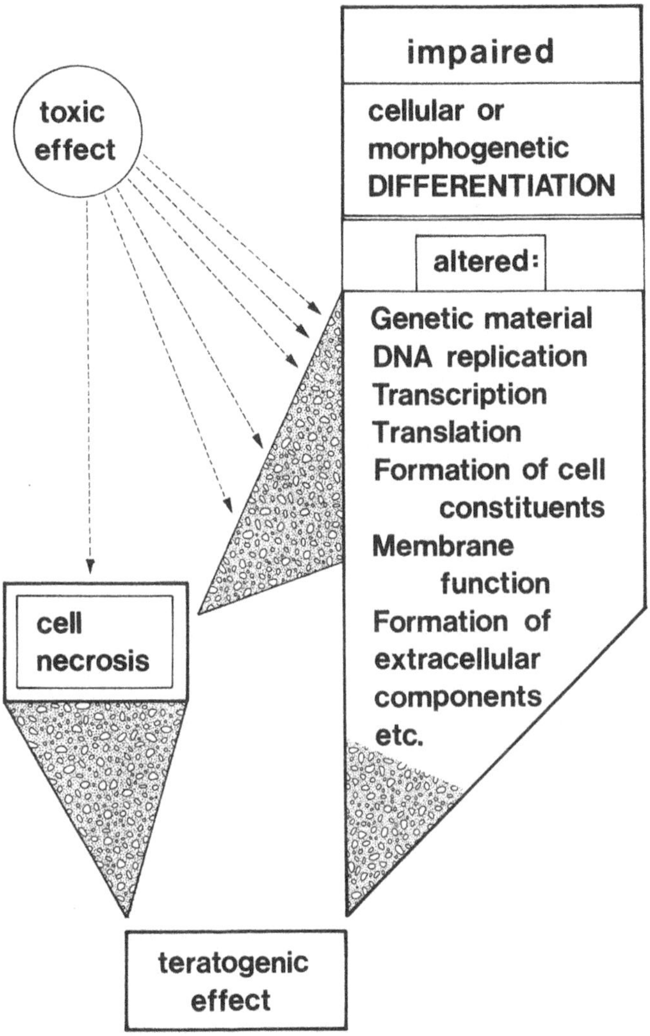

Fig. 4. Hypothetical scheme on the modes of action responsible for the induction of teratogenic effects. A teratogenic effect can apparently be caused by the action of one of two possible mechanisms: via cell death and via mechanisms not resulting in cell necroses. In principle, the effect is triggered by an impairment of cellular or morphogenetic differentiation processes

2. Special Pharmacokinetic Aspects of Prenatal Toxicology

The kinetics of drug absorption and elimination processes of the two-component system mother/embryo are much more complex than those of an adult organism (*Neubert* 1978). For an evaluation, two major difficulties have to be taken into account:

a) The embryonic compartment frequently is not easily accessible to measurements.

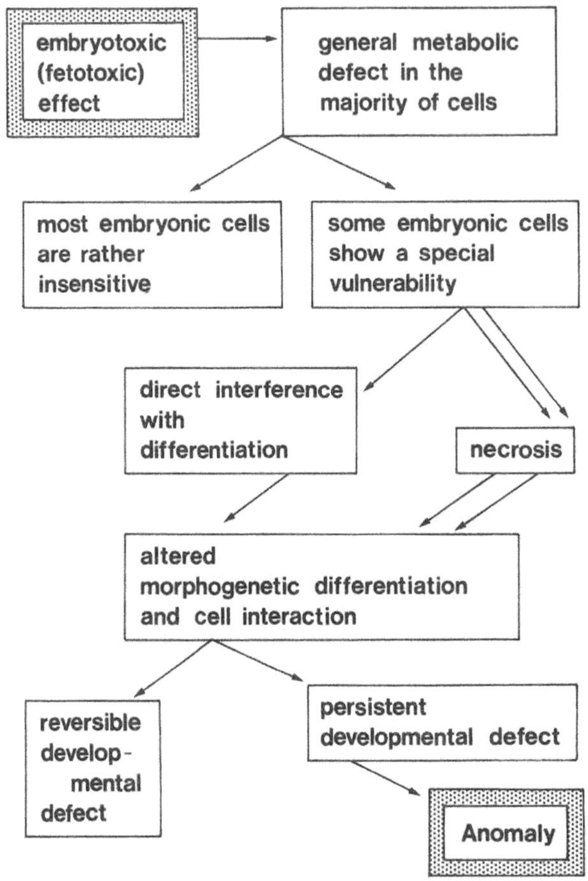

Fig. 5. Schematic presentation of the sequence of events leading to a structural or functional anomaly

b) Considerable variation of the drug concentration reaching the embryo is to be expected depending on the developmental stage under investigation.

The majority of studies performed so far in experimental rodents have been confined to a circumscribed single stage of development, such as preimplantation, implantation, histiotrophic nutrition, function of the yolk sack placenta, and early or late stages of the function of the hemochorial placenta. Information in humans has predominantly been obtained at the end of pregnancy and during delivery, with little information available at the most important stage, that of organogenesis.

The role of pharmacokinetic factors in prenatal toxicology has been discussed in detail at a recent symposium, and a good review of the literature has been published in its proceedings (*Neubert* et al. 1978). For this reason, only a few aspects are mentioned here.

Three different pharmacokinetic situations may arise during a drug-induced, embryotoxic action:

a) The chemical has an embryotoxic potential and reaches the embryo at a concentration sufficient to induce a toxic effect.

b) The chemical has *no* embryotoxic potential, but is converted in the maternal compartment into a stable embryotoxic agent that may penetrate into the embryo or fetus.

c) The chemical has *no* embryotoxic potential and the mother is *not able* to produce the stable toxic metabolite, but can only supply an inactive form of the drug to the embryo. In this case, the conversion of the substance into a short-living embryotoxic metabolite has to be accomplished in the embryo or fetus itself.

Many examples of each of the three situations are known in experimental teratology. Situation (a) apparently applies to chemicals, such as *N*-nitrosourea; cyclophosphamide is a good example for situation (b); and teratogenic effects produced by 6-mercaptopurine and 6-aminonicotinamide positively arise via mechanism (c).

Considerable difficulty may be caused by species differences existing between the predominatly used rodent and lagomorpha experimental animals, on the one hand, and primates on the other hand. While the pharmacologically and toxicologically important cytochrome P_{450}-type drug-metabolizing enzyme system develops its activity in rodents perinatally or even clearly postnatally, this system is already operative in primates during the fetal and even the embryonic periods – in humans as early as in the 6th to 7th week of gestation (cf. *Nau* and *Neubert* 1978).

The cytochrome P_{450}-type system not only "inactivates" toxic chemicals in the mammalian organism, but is likewise able to "activate" or "toxify" a variety of chemicals which otherwise would be harmless for mammals. By these enzymes, a variety of mutagens and carcinogens are "activated" in the adult organism to become toxic metabolites. For this reason, it is possible that primate fetuses or embryos have the capacity to activate certain chemicals to embryotoxic substances which cannot be converted by the rodent fetus due to a deficiency of the enzyme systems needed. *Therefore, a negative result in rodent species does not generally indicate that the chemical is "safe" for primates – including man. This applies not only to the usual embryo- or fetotoxic effects, but also to transplacental carcinogenesis.*

3. Special Contribution of Maternal Factors

In addition to the pharmacokinetic factors mentioned by which the maternal organism may greatly contribute to the outcome of a possible embryotoxic action, other maternal factors may be involved with the triggering of abnormal prenatal development. In principle, three different types of such "indirect" interference with prenatal development can be visualized:

a) an alteration of the maternal food supply to the conceptus due to a deficiency of such components vital to the embryo in the maternal organism;

b) an alteration of the nutritional supply of the mother to the conceptus or an impairment of uterine blood supply induced by drugs;

c) an alteration of the susceptibility of the conceptus to certain drug actions by a concomitantly induced pathologic situation, such as malnutrition in the mother or another pathologic metabolic situation.

a) Deprivation of Maternal Components Vital to the Embryo

Since the development of the embryo or fetus in each gestational stage critically depends on the supply of vital components provided by the maternal organism, interference with the maternal metabolism or nutrient supply may be visualized as "indirectly" interfering with prenatal development. Fortunately, the maternal organism frequently tries to supply the embryonic compartment with the vital components as long as possible, even under conditions of "malnutrition." However, there are ample experimental data that, for example, a vitamin deficiency of the maternal organism can trigger an abnormal prenatal development. Inducing malformations by vitamin deficiency in experimental animals was actually one of the first techniques applied in experimental teratology (e.g., *Warkany* and co-workers 1943, 1948). Another well-known example of a maternal metabolic deficiency causing abnormal embryonic development is a zinc or a magnesium deficiency (*Hurley* and co-workers 1961, 1966, 1970, 1971, 1973, 1977).

b) Alteration of Nutritional Supply by Drugs

It has been known for some time that, at certain stages of prenatal development, drugs may be able to interfere with the transport of nutrients from the mother to the embryo. The teratogenic effect of *trypan blue* is often considered to represent a classic example for this kind of an "embryonic malnutrition." Although the diazo dye has been reported to induce metabolic changes in the maternal organism (*Christie* 1966), such an effect is not made responsible for the teratogenic action. The extensive studies from the laboratories of *Beck* and *Lloyd* suggested that this dye, which is only teratogenic before a chorioallantoic placenta begins functioning, acts in rodents by affecting the extraembryonic (inverted yolk sack) membranes, and thereby the "histiotrophic nutrition," which is the utilization of macromolecules broken down by hydrolytic enzymes for the nutrition of the embryo. Trypan blue is teratogenic at appropriate doses when given on day 8.5 of pregnancy in the rat, but not when given on day 11.5 or later. Earlier studies performed with light microscopic techniques (*Gillman* et al. 1948) or with the radioactively labeled dye (*Wilson* et al. 1963) seemed to indicate that trypan blue does not penetrate into the embryonic tissue. But the results of more recent studies cast doubts on this. Small amounts of trypan blue *do* apparently reach the embryo (*Davis* and *Sauter* 1977; *Dencker* 1977), and electron microscopic investigations (*Schmidt* 1979) also support the theory of a direct action of the dye on embryonic development. Other drugs with high molecular weight (like the non-ionic detergent Triton WR 1339) which also are teratogenic exclusively in early stages of embryonic development (e.g., days 6–7 of pregnancy in the mouse) may act via a similar mechanism by interfering with histiotrophic nutrition (*Schultz* et al. 1966). But *Tuchmann-Duplessis* (1970) has called attention to the fact that Triton WR 1339 in addition induces other metabolic changes within the maternal organism, such as hyperlipemia and hypercholesteremia, which may equally well be connected with the teratogenic and embryolethal potential of this drug. The mechanism of action would, in any case, be indirect.

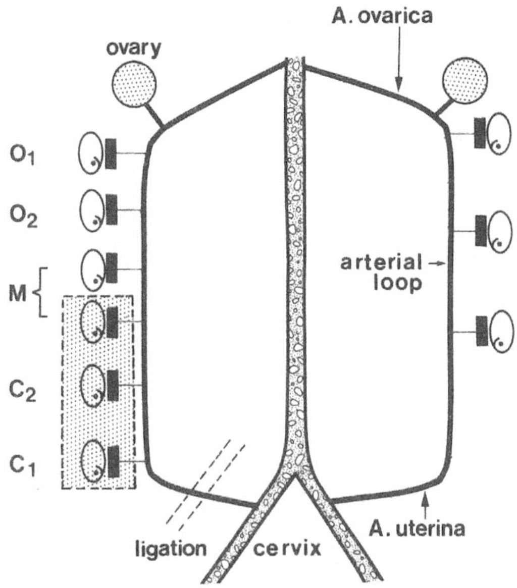

Fig. 6. Scheme of the uterine blood supply in rodents. The scheme gives the nomenclature used for localizing the position of a fetus within the uterine horn. The dotted area indicates the position of the embryos most severely affected by a ligation of the A. uterina (modified from: *Epping* 1972).
(O = close to ovary; C = close to cervix; M = middle position.)
For the data presented in this paper the following nomenclature is used for indicating the implantation site within the uterine horn:
5 fetuses per horn: O_1-O_2-M_1-C_2-C_1
6 fetuses per horn: O_1-O_2-M_2-M_3-C_2-C_1
7 fetuses per horn: O_1-O_2-M_2-M_1-M_3-C_2-C_1
8 fetuses per horn: O_1-O_2-O_3-M_2-M_3-C_3-C_2-C_1
9 fetuses per horn: O_1-O_2-O_3-M_2-M_1-M_3-C_3-C_2-C_1
This nomenclature is based on the assumption of an even distribution of the implantation sites within the uterine horn and allowing one-third of the space available to each of the "ovarial section" (O); the "middle section" (M); and the "cervical section" (C). Only the uterine horns with five or more implantation sites were evaluated in these studies

c) Alteration of Uterine Blood Flow by Drugs

The blood supply along the rodent uterus is guaranteed by a rather complex system (cf. Fig. 6). A cascade of two arteries, A. uterina (or iliolumbar artery) and A. ovarica furnish both horns of the uterus; thus the amount and quality of blood reaching the individual embryo may not be exactly the same. It was, in fact, found (*Barr* and *Brent* 1970; *Epping* 1972) that a ligation of a uterine artery results in anoxia and subsequently in the death of embryos depending on their location in the uterus (close to the ovary or close to the cervix). More detailed data obtained in our laboratory are shown in Table 1. When the A. uterina is ligated on day 11 of pregnancy in the rat, fetomortality cannot be observed before day 13 of gestation and lethality is confined to the

Table 1. Fetomortality in the rat after ligation of the arteria uterina on one site on day 11 of pregnancy

Day of gestation	Fetomortality/ implantation sites Σ [litters]	%	O_1	O_2	O_3	M_2	M_1	M_3	C_3	C_2	C_1	Σ O	Σ M	Σ C
12	5/51 [9]	9.8% Res.	9 (1)	9 (1)		5	5 (1)	5		9 (1)	9 (1)	18 (2) 11%	15 (1) 7%	18 (2) 11%
13	12/51 [8]	23.5% Res.	8 (1)	8	1	7 (1)	3 (2)	7 (1)	1 (1)	8 (2)	8 (4)	17 (1) 6%	17 (4) 24%	17 (7) 41%
14	20/44 [7]	43.5% Res.	7 (1)	7 (1)	2 (1)	4 (1)	4 (1)	4 (3)	2 (2)	7 (5)	7 (5)	16 (3) 19%	12 (5) 42%	16 (12) 75%
20	45/108 [17]	41.7% Res.	17 (4)	17	2	13 (3)	10 (3)	13 (6)	2 (2)	17 (10)	17 (17)	36 (4) 11%	36 (12) 33%	36 (29) 81%
Control 20	3/60 (12)	5.0% Res.										24 (1)	12 (1)	24 (1)

The arteria uterina supplying one of the uterine horns was ligated in pentobarbital anesthesia on day 11 of gestation. The fetuses developing in the other uterine horn served as controls. The animals were killed at the times following ligation as indicated. Only horns with five or more implantation sites were evaluated. For nomenclature of the uterine positions, cf. Fig. 6. The number of dead fetuses is given in parenthesis under the total of implantation sites. (*Epping, J., Neubert, D.*, unpublished data)
(O = close to the ovary; C = close to the cervix; M = middle position).
The χ^2-test gives the following results:
$P > 0.05$: Σ controls → 12-O; Σ-12; 13-O; 14-O; 13-M; 20-O
P 0.01–0.05 : 13-O → 13-C
$P < 0.01$: Σ controls → Σ-13; 13-C; 14-C; 14-M; 20-M; 20-C; Σ-14;
14-C → 14-O; 20-O → 20 C; 20-M → 20-O; 20-O → 20-M

fetuses located at the cervical site of the uterine horn. On day 14 of gestation, dead fetuses are also found at a significantly higher percentage in the middle positions of the uterine horn. No significantly increased number of resorptions could be detected in these studies at the ovarial site of the uterine horns, even on day 20 of pregnancy. Although ligation was performed at a developmental stage susceptible to the induction of "malformations," *no* clear-cut gross structural anomalies could be observed in the surviving fetuses developing in the endangered positions of the uterine horns after ligation (*Epping* 1972). Since the blood supply to the embryo and fetus changes considerably during pregnancy – the supply apparently becoming more critical at later stages of development – the result of an interference with the uterine blood circulation varies depending on the stage of pregnancy (*Franklin* and *Brent* 1964; *Bruce* 1972). The results of these experiments indicate that the importance of a hypoxia or "malnutrition" for the induction of gross, structural abnormalities should not be overemphasized, at least for the developmental stage studied.

In addition to the "clamping" experiments, a possible effect of various vasoactive agents on prenatal development has extensively been studied. Virtually all such agents have been shown to induce embryo- or fetomortality. However, it is still difficult to judge whether teratogenic effects reported in some of these studies can be attributed to an "indirect" action of the agents – generated via an effect on the maternal organism. Ergotamine has been demonstrated to induce embryomortality in mice, rats, and rabbits when applied at doses toxic to the pregnant females (*Grauwiler* and *Schön* 1973). No clear-cut dose-response relation was found to exist. The results were explained by an impairment of blood supply to the uterus and placenta resulting from vasoconstriction, probably caused either by stimulation of α-receptors or by the uterotonic action of the drug. Ergotamine apparently reaches the embryo only at small concentrations. It is of major significance that in these extensive studies *no* increased rate of malformations induced during the organogenesis period could be observed. Only minor anomalies (retarded ossifications, some deformed vertebral arches, and a somewhat increased rate of abnormalities of the ossification of sternebrae) were noticed with the highest doses in mice and rats. No drug-related abnormalities were seen in rabbits. Ergotamine, at a dose of 2.5 mg/kg (i.v.), was found to reduce the transplacental passage of ^{3}H-l-leucine by 87% 3 h after injection. After this treatment embryomortality amounted to 63% (*Leist* and *Grauwiler* 1974).

In various publications the results of experiments with the agents serotonin, angiotensine, bradykinin, and 5-hydroxytryptamine are reported. These studies are attempted to further elucidate the significance of changes in the maternal blood supply for the inductions of embryotoxic effects. All these agents had the common result of increasing the rate of resorptions, but the teratogenic effects caused by these vasoactive agents varied. While angiotensin was not significantly teratogenic in mice (*Thompson* and *Gautier* 1969), clear-cut morphological, gross malformations, such as omphalocele, myelocele, meningocele, and micrognathia, were reported in golden hamsters after treatment with this substance (*Geber* 1969). 5-hydroxytryptamine was also clearly able to induce gross structural abnormalities in the surviving fetuses after injection into pregnant rats (*Reddy* et al. 1963). Under these experimental conditions, the transfer of ^{23}Na into uterine tissues was drastically decreased; a direct effect on the developing fetus, however, could not be completely excluded (*Marley* et al. 1967).

Therefore, it cannot generally be concluded from a drug-induced embryotoxic effect per se that the drug involved *directly* interferes with developmental processes of the embryo. Since the function of the extra-embryonic membranes as well as the type of placentation vary considerably in different mammalian species, extensive variations may be expected in the susceptibility of different species of experimental animals to teratogens affecting the histiotroph (*Beck* 1975).

Summarizing, it may be stated that embryotoxic effects, such as embryolethality or growth retardation, can be induced by vasoactive agents affecting the maternal organism (e.g., the uterine vessels). However, the question as to whether clear-cut gross abnormalities may also be produced "indirectly" by alteration of maternal hemodynamic parameters is still difficult to answer. Discriminating whether a drug reaches embryonic tissues at a well-defined concentration and interferes with typical differentiation processes or whether it acts indirectly by upsetting the maternal metabolism or the nutrition of the embryo or fetus still provides important information if experimental data of one species are extrapolated to another one – including extrapolation to the conditions probably existing in humans.

d) Alteration of the Susceptibility of the Conceptus to Drugs Caused by Pathologic Changes Occurring in the Maternal Organism

While the two types of contribution of maternal factors mentioned so far are rather convincing and have been studied in experiments to some extent, the significance of a third aspect is still rather obscure. This aspect refers to the possible modification (and here, of course, predominantly an amplification) of a drug-induced, teratogenic effect caused by an alteration in the maternal nutritional status or another abnormality in the maternal metabolism including the hormonal status.

Taking into account the difficulties we are faced with when trying to evaluate the effect of a single teratogenic factor in animal models or in man it is obvious why, up to now, an analysis of such rather complex situations has rarely been attempted. But for a satisfactory toxicologic evaluation with relevance to humans it is also essential to know whether an amplification of a teratogenic hazard in a certain population at risk is to be expected. The answer to this question is highly important if a drug which does not induce prenatal toxic effects in a well-nourished population is supposed to trigger embryotoxic effects when applied to undernourished mothers. Since the percentage of people suffering from malnutrition on this planet is very high, it is of considerable importance to find an answer to this question. But much more information is still needed and much more experimental work as well as epidemiological research will have to be performed before we will be able to give a satisfactory answer.

Similarly, diabetes and other metabolic abnormalities are known to generate "risk pregnancies" and could be expected to aggravate the hazard produced by certain drugs given during pregnancy. But again, no risk evaluation is possible for an additional drug consumption in such a group of women with the data – experimental or epidemiological – available.

Fever has also been suspected to represent a risk factor for the embryo or fetus (*Edwards* and *Wanner* 1977). No data are available to answer the question whether fever might potentiate the action of a teratogenic agent present at a subthreshold dose.

4. Special Outcome of an Embryotoxic Action

One of the most intriguing aspects of research in prenatal toxicology is the fact that the outcome of a drug-induced toxic effect is quite variable, even if a genetically homogeneous population of experimental animals is used and a well-defined dose is applied at a defined gestational stage. If, as predominantly done in experimental research, polytocous animals like rodents or lagomorpha are used, the litters, and even the members of the same litter, very often respond in a variety of ways. In principle, the following types of outcomes (frequently within the same litter) can be observed when evaluated shortly before birth (cf. Fig. 1).:

a) an apparently normal development;
b) growth retardation;
c) gross structural abnormalities or malformations;
d) lethality (resorption, abortions, stillbirths).

From a toxicologic point of view these variations may be classified as resulting from two different situations:

1. a variation among different litters (interlitterial), and
2. a variation within the members of the same litter (intralitterial).

The varying response of different individuals to a given pharmacologic or toxic stimulus is a well-known fact in pharmacologic research. Part of this variability is certainly due to a difference in the genetic background and it should be reduced by using experimental animals of an inbred strain. Inbred animals still show a variability in a pharmacologic or toxicologic response, indicating that much of the "biological variation" is caused by individual factors which may even vary within the same individual. For example, circadian fluctuations, including food uptake and hormone production, have been shown to modify the pharmacokinetics of some drugs in adult animals. Similar types of variation are also likely to occur in teratology, as in other fields of pharmacology and toxicology.

a) The "Litter" Effect

A variation in response to a drug also occurs within the members of the same litter. Such an intralitterial variation is the rule rather than the exception in teratological research. Five parameters may be blamed for such a variance in the susceptibility to a certain embryotoxic drug:

a) The embryos are not uniformly exposed to the identical drug concentration.

b) The embryos do not uniformly receive the identical amount of nutritional supply.

c) The embryos, at a given time, are not uniformly at the identical developmental stage.

d) The genetic background of the fetuses may be different, especially if an outbred strain is used.

e) Other "individual" factors contribute to the difference in susceptibility.

Few studies have been performed to clarify the question of whether or not embryos developing in different positions of the uterine horn are likely to receive differ-

Table 2. Uptake of radioactivity from the uterine vessels by rat embryos (day 12 of gestation) at different positions within the uterine horn

Compound injected	Uptake and incorporation of radioactivity (dpm/μg DNA) into rat embryos in the uterine position (M ± S.D.):			
	Σ	$O_1 + O_2$	$M_3 + M_1 + M_2$	$C_1 + C_2$
^{14}C-glucose	490 ± 75 (146)	465 ± 79 (48)	515 ± 84 (50)	489 ± 81 (48)
^{32}P inorganic phosphate	521 ± 51 (146)	505 ± 84 (48)	538 ± 55 (50)	519 ± 52 (48)

t-test gives the following results:

	for ^{14}C:		for ^{32}P:	
M → O		Δ 11% - P < 0.0027 ***		Δ 7% - P < 0.0027 ***
Σ → M		Δ 5% - P = 0.06 *		Δ 3% - P = 0.06 *
Σ → O		Δ 5% - P = 0.06 *		Δ 3% - P = 0.06 *
C → O		Δ 5% - P > 0.1		Δ 3% - p > 0.1
C → M		Δ 5% - P > 0.1		Δ 4% - P > 0.05

*** = highly significant; * = borderline significance

Pregnant Wistar rats received on day 12 of pregnancy intravenously 1 mCi/kg of both ^{14}C-glucose (spec. act.: 200 μCi/μmole) and ^{32}P inorganic phosphate (50 μCi/nmole). Three hours later the total radioactivity of the two radioisotopes was measured in individual embryos (for method cf. *Krowke* et al. 1971). Only uterine horns with five or more embryos were evaluated. For nomenclature of the uterine positions, cf. Fig. 6 (O = close to ovary; C = close to cervix; M = middle position). Positions O_3 and C_3 were not included in the evaluation since the number was too small. The number of embryos evaluated is given in parentheses. DNA was measured with the *Burton* (1965) method. In the case of ^{14}C, 31% was found to be acid soluble, in the case of ^{32}P, 76%. The DNA content of the embryos was 121 ± 15 μg/embryo ent "doses" of a chemical offered via the maternal circulation. Some data obtained in our laboratory which may contribute to answering this question are compiled in Table 2. A mixture of two radioisotopes (^{14}C-glucose and ^{32}P-phosphate) was injected into rats on day 12 of pregnancy. Three hours later the uptake and incorporation of these "physiologic" precursors into fetuses developing in different positions of the uterine horns were studied. The fetuses developing in the middle positions of the uterine horns apparently received an increased average amount of 11% of ^{14}C-glucose and of 7% of ^{32}P-phosphate compared with those located at the ovarial site of the horns, and this difference was statistically highly significant. However, the biologic and toxicologic significance of this finding should not be overestimated since the standard deviations themselves of embryos developing in identical positions of the uterine horn were 10%–17%. We would like to conclude from these data that, with regard to a toxicologic evaluation, embryos developing at different sites of the rat uterus may be considered to receive a random share of components from the maternal circulation and that a difference in "dosing" cannot be the major reason for variations in the response of the different members of a litter to an embryotoxic chemical or agent.

The third of the items mentioned may be of higher significance, especially if random-bred animals are used for teratologic studies. There is no doubt that the gestational stage of the embryos developing within the same uterus of a rodent is not completely "synchronized." When counting the number of somites within one litter at the stage of organogenesis, a variance of ± 1–2 somites was the rule at a 35- to 45-somite stage in random-bred rats or mice, even though the mating period was confined to 1–2 h. Different random-bred rodent mothers may deliver their fetuses during a period of 12 h or even more. The deviation in the number of somites at a given developmental stage may be reduced to some extent by using inbred strains of these rodents which may deliver their fetuses during a period of a few hours. However, an embryotoxic drug still leads to a varying outcome among the embryos or fetuses of a single litter, even if inbred animals are used.

At present, we therefore favor the idea that a variety of other "individual" factors also determine the outcome of a teratogenic effect in a given embryo or fetus – similarly as in a pharmacologic or toxicologic experiment performed in the postnatal period. At the moment, we cannot define the factors which may be responsible for the outcome of an embryotoxic event, an outcome which may vary from a lethal effect to a complete restitution.

b) Correlation of Teratogenicity and Embryomortality

One may attempt to describe dose-response relationships in prenatal toxicology as follows: high doses of an embryotoxic drug may lead to mortality, whereas intermediate doses may result in teratogenic effects and the lowest effective range may cause growth retardation. However, the situation is *not* as simple as that!

There certainly is more than a quantitative difference between teratogenicity and embryolethality. With a given teratogen, it is completely feasible to obtain 100% malformations, such as cleft palates or abnormalities of the extremities, etc., without observing embryo- or fetomortality. Similarly, although malformed offspring often are

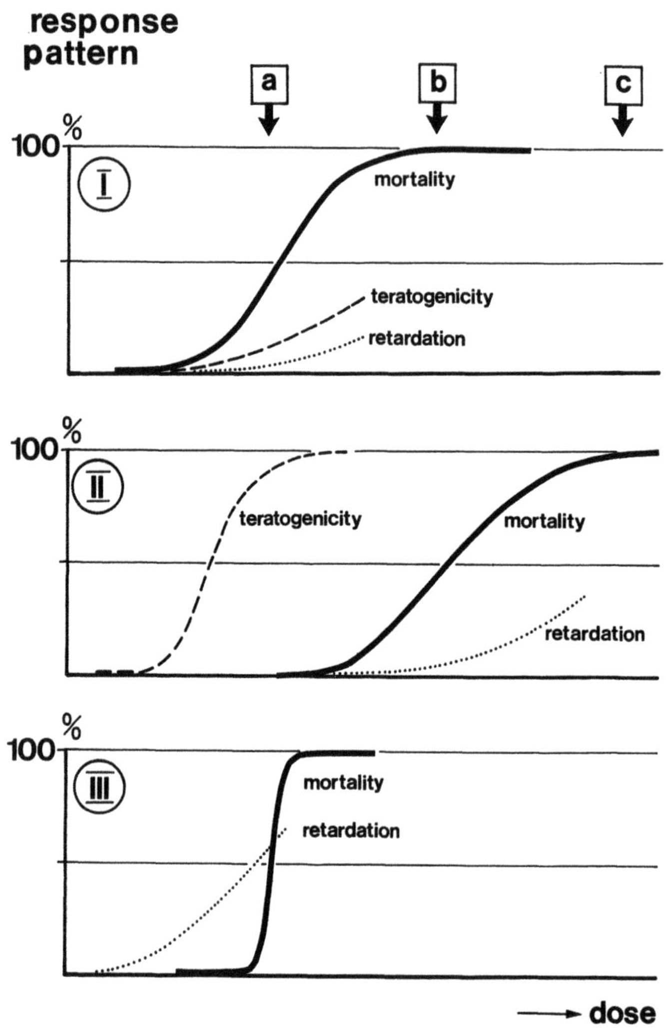

Fig. 7. Hypothetical response pattern of an embryotoxic action. The three different effects: teratogenicity, embryomortality, and retardation, have to be evaluated separately. They may show quite different dose-response relationships. Depending on the response pattern (I, II, or III) and the dose applied (a, b, or c), the outcome of an embryotoxic effect varies considerably

growth-retarded, such a growth retardation is not necessarily linked with a gross malformation; and, conversely, a severe growth retardation may be present without any apparent structural abnormality.

The steepness of the dose-response curves for the three parameters, growth retardation, malformation, and mortality, varies considerably with the embryotoxic drug used, and these three parameters are not necessarily interlinked.

The principle situations governing a given embryotoxic effect are given schematically in Fig. 7:

I. If response pattern I exists (as is frequently the case in experimental "teratology"), a dose-dependent increase of all three parameters mentioned is observed with doses between (a) and (b). The slope of the dose-response curves may, of course, greatly vary with different agents belonging to this class.

II. An agent acting according to pattern II is able to produce structural (and possibly functional) anomalies at a dose range where no embryo- or fetomortality or even growth retardation is observed. An illustration of this type of pattern is the action of glucocorticoids in rodents. The pattern may be modified for some agents in such a way that the dose-response curve for retardation is located more closely to the left of the graph, so that retardation is seen with the higher teratogenic doses, possibly without embryomortality.

III. If the toxic event interferes with prenatal development according to pattern III of Fig. 7, no malformations are induced with any dose; however, growth retardation and embryolethality occur. An example of such a reaction pattern has been reported by *Bass* and *Oerter* (1975, 1977) using chloramphenicol and thiamphenicol in rats. In this example, the dose-response curve for embryomortality is unusually steep. This causes us to ask if teratogenicity may only be expected at an extremely small dose range which, under experimental conditions, may be almost impossible to select. As yet, very extensive studies using this model performed by *Bass* and co-workers have failed to reveal any teratogenicity.

Thorough biochemical investigations by *Bass* and his group have revealed that this type of embryotoxic action is produced by an interference with mitochondriogenesis and a breakdown in energy metabolism (*Bass* 1975).

These results of studies with chloramphenicol and earlier data published by *Tuchmann-Duplessis* (1970) clearly indicate that embryolethality may be caused by a toxic mechanism other than teratogenicity. Therefore, dose-response relationships in prenatal toxicology have to be evaluated separately for the three parameters, growth retardation, teratogenicity and embryo- or fetomortality, if conclusions are to be drawn with regard to mechanisms of action.

Three additional aspects are worth mentioning in this respect:

1. From the points discussed previously it is understandable and often observed in experimental "teratology" that even for a given embryotoxic drug (as depicted in Fig. 7) the type of the abnormality pattern might not be constant under different experimental conditions. By simply varying the scheme of drug application, the frequency of embryomortality may be changed without greatly altering the frequency of malformations (cf. Fig. 8). Similar results can be obtained by giving, in addition to the embryotoxic drug, a treatment which may, for example, antagonize the rate of embryolethality without interfering with the induction of malformations.

The possibility of achieving such results was demonstrated by *Roussell* and *Tuchmann-Duplessis* (1968) and *Tuchmann-Duplessis* (1970), who subjected animals under study for embryotoxic effects of the non-ionic detergent Triton WR 1339 to an additional treatment (cf. Table 3). By simultaneous treatment with Triton WR 1339 and progesterone, the number of resorptions was reduced toward the normal rate; however, the frequency of malformations was apparently increased. Simultaneous treatment with Triton WR 1339 and nicotinic acid, on the other hand, completely reduced the induction of anomalies with much less effect on embryolethality. The results again

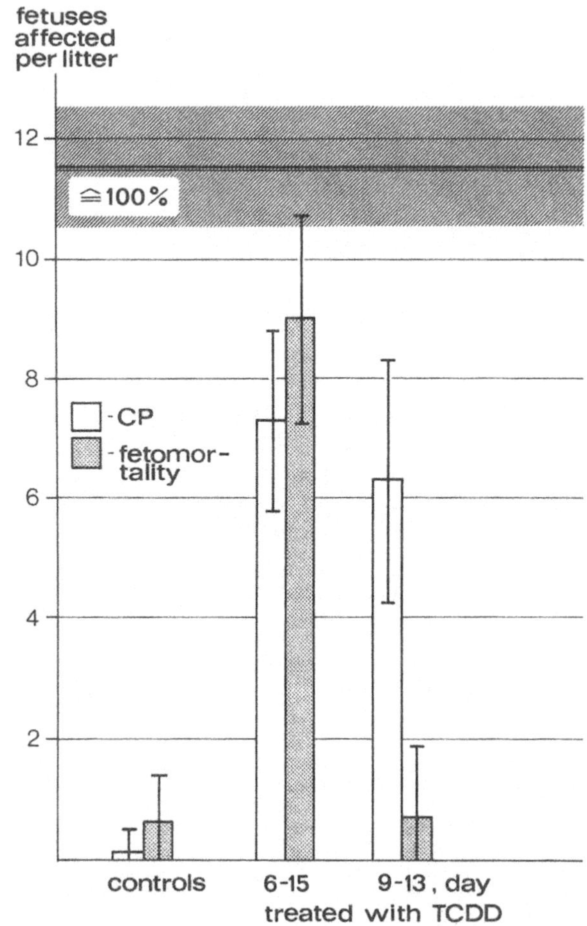

Fig. 8. Comparison of a teratogenic effect (CP = cleft palate) and fetomortality produced by 2,3,7,8-tetrachlorodibenzo-*p*-dioxin (TCDD). Pregnant NMRI mice (10 per group) received TCDD (9 μg/kg daily) orally during the days of pregnancy indicated. Depending on the time of treatment the relationship of teratogenicity and fetomortality can be altered drastically

emphasize the point that dose-response relationships of teratogenicity and embryo- or fetomortality have to be evaluated and considered separately.

2. The variability in the outcome of an embryo- or fetotoxic effect among various litters or within a single litter renders the evaluation and interpretation of experimental data difficult. Often, the data presented in the literature are very poorly documented and it may therefore be hard, and sometimes impossible, to evaluate the results properly and allow a satisfactory risk evaluation. Statistical evaluations of the data are also rendered difficult by the fact that different litters often respond in a variety of ways to an embryotoxic agent.

Extensive discussions have been published on the problem of whether the litter or the pregnant animal or the total of the fetuses in one experimental group should be

Table 3. Evidence for a dissociation of teratogenic and embryolethal effects in mice (Data of *Roussel* and *Tuchmann-Duplessis* 1968; *Tuchmann-Duplessis* 1970)

Treatment	On day of pregnancy	Percentage of Resorptions	Gross abnormalities
Triton WR 1339 400 mg/kg	5– 7	53%	21%
Triton WR 1339 + Novacyl 3 g/kg	5– 7	40%	0
Triton WR 1339 + progesterone 5 mg/day	5– 7 5–16	15%	44%
Control	–	15%	0

Novacyl = *n*-oxy-nicotinic acid
The dose of Triton WR 1339 was identical in all the experimental series

considered as the unit for statistical calculations (*Weil* 1970; *Healy* 1972; *Becker* 1974; *Kalter* 1974; *Staples* and *Haseman* 1974). In our opinion, it is impossible to find a satisfactory solution to these questions, since both types of reference have advantages and disadvantages, under certain conditions. The data given should be as complete as possible to allow a clear-cut evaluation. This means that, for fetomortality as well as for teratogenicity, *both* the data based on the single litter ($\bar{M}$ ± S.D.) *and* the number of total fetuses evaluated should be indicated. An example and a suggestion for such an evaluation is given in Tables 4 and 5.

It can be seen from this fictitious example (which actually represents part of a genuine experimental series performed on a larger scale, but which, for the sake of clarity, is given here in a condensed form – Table 5) that some litters from the treated series contain only normal fetuses and others a varying number of resorptions and abnormal fetuses. A low rate of resorptions and of abnormalities is also found in the control group. This is a usual situation in experimental teratology. It can also be seen from the table that one litter of the treated group consists only of resorptions. This litter should not be included with the others, but should be evaluated separately. An example of a presentation and evaluation of the data shown in the fictitious experiment (Table 5) is given in Table 4. All the information pertinent to the experiment can be taken from this compilation of the data – including the standard deviation of the effects seen in different litters. With these data available every scientist can decide for himself which type of statistical analysis is preferable to him.

We very strongly feel that data which have not been published in this or a similar way should not be considered in a safety evaluation since the conditions of the experiment and of the results are impossible to judge. It should be kept in mind that no regulatory agency would be willing to accept data from industrial laboratories if they are as fragmentarily documented and inaccurately performed as are results given in papers published by some university laboratories.

Table 4. Example of the compilation and evaluation of data from a test for prenatal toxicity (Data were taken from the example given in Table 5)

	Parameter evaluated	Treated			Animals	Control			
a	Pregnant female mice (n)	12				10			
b	Litters with resorptions only (n)	1				0			
c	Total implantation sites (n) (-b)	109	(100)			100	(100)		
d	Total living fetuses (n)	82				96			
e	Total resorbed or dead fetuses (n) (-b)	27	(18)			4			
f	Implantation sites (n)*/litter, with (b) excluded	11.0 ± 1.6				11.1 ± 1.8			
g	Living fetuses (n)*/litter, with (b) excluded	82 ± 2.6				9.6 ± 1.7			
h	Resorptions (n)*/litter, with (b) excluded	1.8 ± 2.2				0.4 ± 0.6			
i	Living fetuses % (per litter)*, with (b) excluded	82 ± 24%				96 ± 8%			
k	Resorptions % (per litter)*, with (b) excluded	18 ± 23%				4 ± 6%			
l	Litters with resorptions/total litters	8/12		=	67%	4/10		=	40%
m	Litters with resorptions *only*/total litters	1/12		=	8%	0/10		=	0
n	Abnormalities**	16				2			
o	(structural variations)	0				0			
p	(retardations)	0				0			
q	(gross abnormalities, malformations)	16				2			
r	Abnormalities/living fetuses (% per litter)*	15 ± 24				2 ± 4			
s	Total abnormalities/total living fetuses	16/82		=	20%	2/96		=	2%
t	Litters with abnormalities/total litters, (b) excl.	4/10		=	40%	1/10		=	10%
u	Fetal weight (living fetuses)*	1.30 ± 0.14				1.25 ± 0.17			

n = number
* ($\bar{M}$ ± S.D.)
** to be specified separately

Table 5. Fictitious example of the outcome of testing for prenatal toxicity

Fetuses	Treated animals A	B	C	D	E	F	Control animals G	H	I	K	L
1	R	A	x	A	R	R	A	R	R	x	x
2	R	A	x	A	R	x	x	x	R	x	x
3	R	R	x	A	R	x	x	x	x	x	x
4	R	R	x	A	R	x	x	x	x	x	x
5	R	R	x	A	R	x	x	x	x	x	x
6	R	x	x	A	x	x	x	x	x	x	x
7	R	x	x	x	x	x	x	x	x	x	x
8	R	x	x	x	x	x	x	x	x	x	x
9	R	x	x	x	x	x	x	x	x	x	x
10		x	x	x		x	x	x	x	x	
11		x	x	x			x	x		x	
12		x	x				x	x			
13			x					x			

(R) resorptions : 9/55 = 16%
(A) abnormalities : 8/55 = 15%
x = normal fetuses

resorptions : 3/55 = 6%
abnormalities: 1/55 = 2%

3. For the evaluation of a possible hazard to man, all kinds of abnormal prenatal development are significant if they occur with a dose well below that toxic to the maternal organism. When a drug is administered at a dose which drastically interferes with the maternal organism, "unspecific" effects can frequently be observed in the embryo or fetus (cf. Sect. V.2). These may consist of an increased incidence of prenatal mortality or of growth retardation. Gross morphological anomalies are rarely seen under such conditions. Nevertheless some borderline abnormalities or structural variations which may also occur in controls may be found, and they are hard to interpret from a toxicologic point of view. This general experience again points to a considerable "specificity" in the triggering of malformations which represents much more than an indication of a general toxic effect on the fetus.

A growth retardation, however, even if it is not accompanied by gross malformations, represents a dangerous effect since it is known that small-for-date newborns experience a higher risk of prenatal mortality and possibly also of an abnormal postnatal development than fully grown and mature babies. The term "apparently normal at birth" used in this connection has to be defined more clearly. This refers to experimental studies as well as to observations made in man. It is a well-known fact that in the human population only about 50% of abnormalities can be discovered at birth. If, in experimental studies or observations in humans, parameters like mental and sexual development, the status of hormonal or immune systems, other functional deviations in special organ systems, or even transplacental carcinogenesis are included, the percentage of anomalies detectable at birth may, under certain conditions, represent only a small fraction. With the usual technique of evaluating fetuses after a cesarian section close to term, members of a litter in which embryotoxic effects occurred should, therefore, only be classified as "apparently normal." The treatment certainly has induced effects in the majority of the embryos or fetuses. Although these embryotoxic effects, as judged by macroscopic criteria, have been largely reversible, it cannot be excluded that functional lesions have occurred. These may manifest themselves postnatally or may lead to an alteration in metabolism or function manifesting itself only by the increased susceptibility of the newborn – or even adult – to toxic lesions, including, possibly, carcinogenesis.

For this reason, more emphasis has to be placed on revealing prenatally induced lesions which manifest themselves only (sometimes late) postnatally. This applies to experimental studies as well as to observations made in children exposed in utero to drugs or other toxic actions. It is fair to stress the point that, in spite of many encouraging results published in this new field of prenatal toxicology, no routine procedures are available today in experimental research which allow screening for such functional anomalies and permit the prediction of possible hazards to humans. We are even further from excluding them.

III. Organotropic Effects in Prenatal Toxicology

Every *pharmacologic* effect originates from the general principle that various cell types or organ functions do not respond uniformly qualitatively and quantitatively to a given drug concentration, but show considerable variation in susceptibility. The same principle holds for *toxicologic* actions of a drug. The preference of a drug action for a certain organ or organ function is called "organotropy" or "organotropic effect." As in carcinogenesis and other areas of toxicology, there also exists a high degree of organotropy in teratology. Some aspects of this selectivity in the teratogenic action of certain drugs will be discussed in the following section.

Because of theoretical as well as practical reasons, we will focus the discussion of organotropic actions in prenatal toxicology on three different aspects of organ specificity, namely:

1. The problem of "phase specificity";
2. The problem of "drug specificity";
3. The problem of "dose specificity."

Together with the additional problem of "species specificity," they represent especially important and unique aspects of prenatal toxicity.

1. Problem of "Phase Specificity"

It is well recognized now that prenatal development consists of a great number of consecutive steps leading to the formation of organ anlagen and finally to differentiated cells and tissues. Therefore, it is not surprising that a toxic effect hitting the developing organism may interfere with quite different induction and differentiation processes depending on the developmental stage at which the interference is operative. It is a well-established observation that the same drug or the same interfering agent (such as

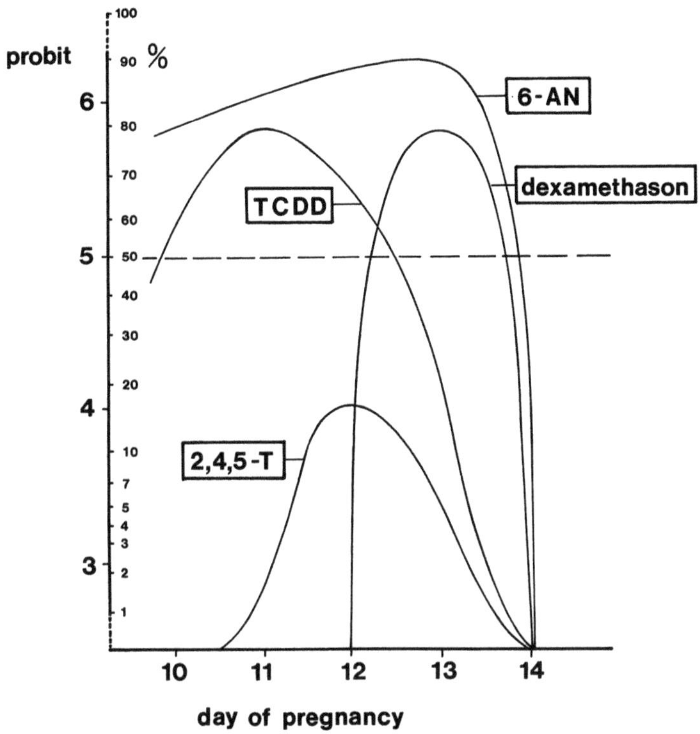

Fig. 9. Time course of the susceptibility of NMRI mice to the induction of cleft palate by different agents. The following doses were given: 6-AN = 12 mg/kg; dexamethasone = 40 mg/kg; tetrachlorodibenzodioxin = 30 μg/kg; 2,4,5-trichlorophenoxyacetic acid = 300 mg/kg. Differences in the period of maximum susceptibility suggest differences in the mode of action of the various compounds in inducing cleft palate

X-rays) can lead to quite different abnormalities if introduced at different stages of gestation.

The term "phase specificity" describes the capacity for, or the possibility of, inducing the occurrence of a certain type of abnormality or a certain malformation syndrome at a given stage of gestation in a given species or strain. Beyond this critical phase, it is not possible to induce the same typical abnormality; however, other abnormalities can still be produced. Thus, a polydactyly does not occur in mouse embryos if a teratogen is given on day 13 of gestation or later, and cleft palate cannot be induced at a gestational stage later than day 14, after the closure of the palatal shelves. The sensitive periods for inducing special types of abnormalities may be as short as 1 day or may extend over many days. Cleft palate in the mouse, for example, can result from a drug treatment administered between days 8 and 13 of gestation, which is about one-third of the total gestational period. Some data on the induction of cleft palate, obtained with the mouse strain NMRI used in our laboratory, are compiled in Fig 9. It can be seen that each compound exhibits a rather characteristic time pattern at which cleft palate can be produced. This finding indicates that apparently quite different mechanisms of action may lead to the same final outcome: the anomaly cleft palate.

The extent of the period of susceptibility to the induction of cleft palate may be explained by compiling the processes participating in the formation of the definite palate. The development begins with the formation of the palatal shelves which need to reach a certain size for a successful closure of the palate. The expansion of the shelves is at first ruled by the activity of proliferation, i.e., the number of cells, but later on also by the amount of produced intercellular substance, i.e., collagens and proteoglycans. The number of factors involved with the ensuing elevation of the shelves is still higher: degree of polymerization and capability of the shelf proteoglycans for water binding; proliferation and formation; behavior of epithelial cells; arrangement and contraction ability of mesenchymal cells; growth and three-dimensional shape of the cranial base; dorsal flexion of the head; movements of lower jaw; growth of mandibula; and alteration of the position of the tongue and activation of tongue mobility. Finally, the contact of the elevated shelves not only has to be accomplished, but also secured. This includes contact of the epithelia by adhesion, development of special cell contacts, loss of epithelium by activation of the lysosomal systems, and, furthermore, the development of a cohesive bond of connective tissue and a bone plate (*Ferguson* 1978; *Larsson* 1962; *Babiarz* et al. 1979; *Greene* and *Kochhar* 1975; *Ross* and *Walker* 1967; *Walker* and *Fraser* 1956; *Ross* and *Walker* 1972).

A closer analysis shows that the formation of an organ anlage or a skeletal system consists of a large number of single steps. Figure 10 illustrates the sequence of events involved with skeletogenesis of the extremities in a simplified form. Each of the steps consists of many single events. The complex structure is rendered evident, for instance, by studying the synthesis, secretion, and extracellular maturation of collagen.

The sequence of events in the development of the extremity, the so-called critical phase (e.g., of the mouse, days 8–12), includes the migration of cells in the limb bud, its proliferation, the formation of the blastema with the corresponding pattern formation, and the differentiation and production of intercellular substance (i.e., the beginning of cartilage formation). It is almost impossible for all these steps to be impaired by *one* teratogenic noxa, or for *all* teratogens to interfere with the same step. However, it seems reasonable to assume that, depending on the mechanism of action of the compound administered, actually only one of the steps is predominantly affected.

These considerations may be confirmed by teratologic investigations. There are, in fact, substances, such as acetazolamide, known to act in the mouse only on day 9, a long time before formation of the blastema (*Holmes* and *Trelstad* 1979). Others, in particular alkylating substances or those interfering with nucleic acid metabolism, are effective only on days 11 or 12 or as late as day 14 (*Brummet* and *Johnson* 1979). Thus, it may be postulated that the so-called classic "critical phase" consists of many single critical phases either forming a sequence or proceeding in an overlapping or synchronous way.

Each of these critical phases can be interfered with only if a teratogenic noxa having the appropriate mechanism of action is present at the relevant developmental stage. Hence, the following rules may be formulated:

1. The classical "critical phase" frequently consists of several, or even many, single critical subphases.

2. The type of malformation is determined by the time of the application of the drug as well as by its mechanism of action.

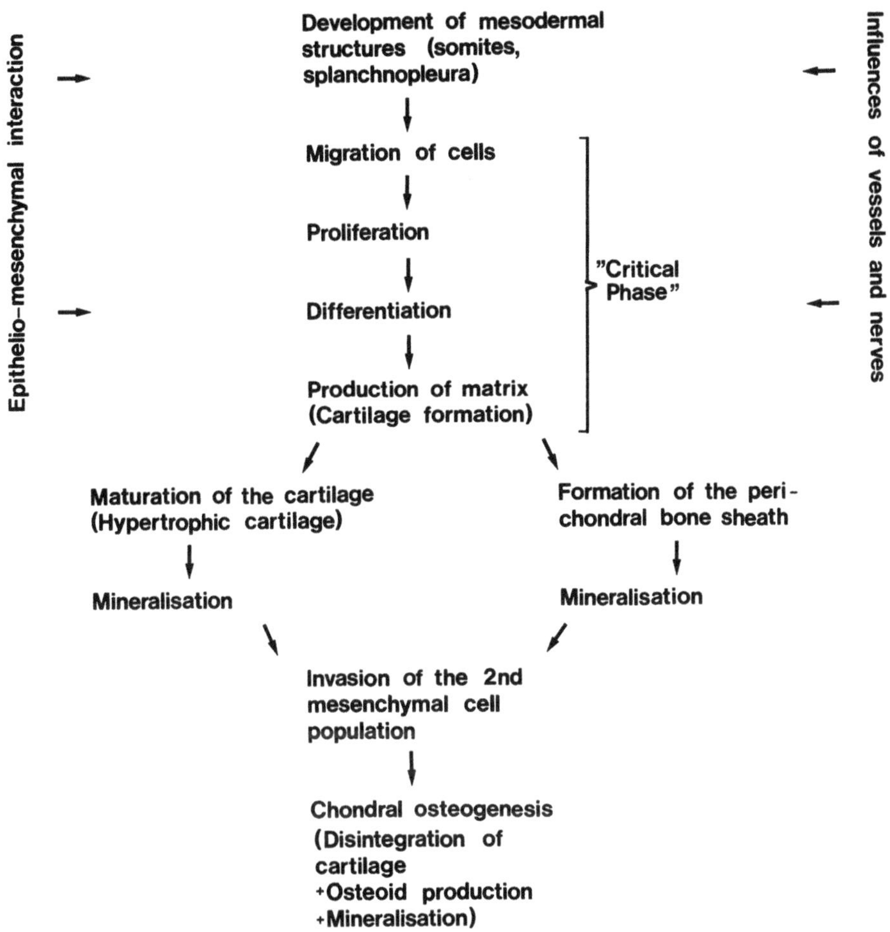

Fig. 10. Scheme of some principle events occurring during differentiation of limb buds in mammals

In teratologic research an example of a malformation that can be triggered over an extended period of gestation, such as the inducibility of cleft palate, is an exception rather than the rule. In general, a typical, well-defined abnormality can be induced only during a far shorter interval.

As an additional example, we would like to present an effect which can be produced only within a few hours of prenatal development. We observed that treatment of mice with the well-known teratogenic agent retinoic acid (which at different stages of prenatal development may cause numerous abnormalities) induces a rupture of the stomach and a "ballooning" of the abdomen (Fig. 11) in newborn mice when given on day 11, at 13.00 hours, of pregnancy. Although the mechanism of this teratogenic action has not yet been completely disclosed, the abnormality and death of the newborn is probably caused by a tracheo-oesophagal fistula, which, when the newborn starts breathing, allows air to be pumped into the stomach via a valve mechanism. When the

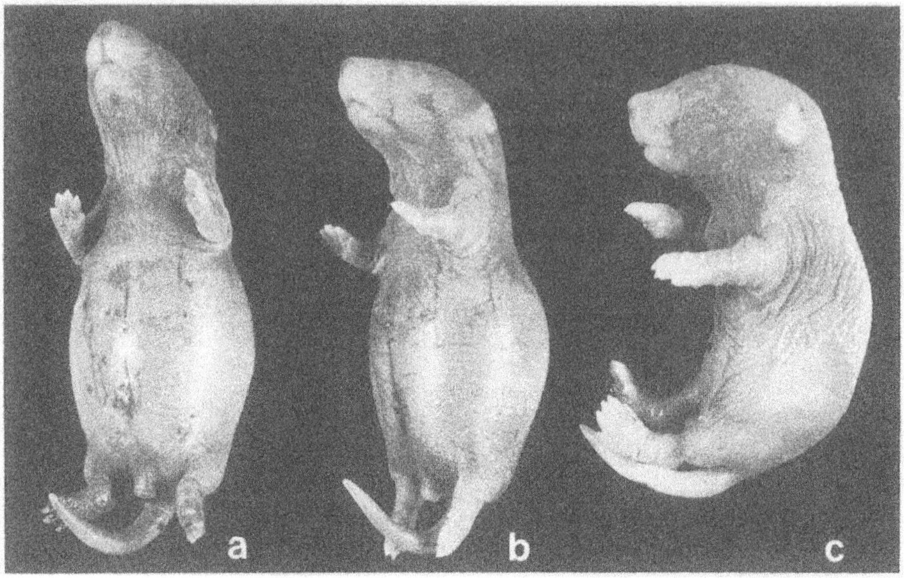

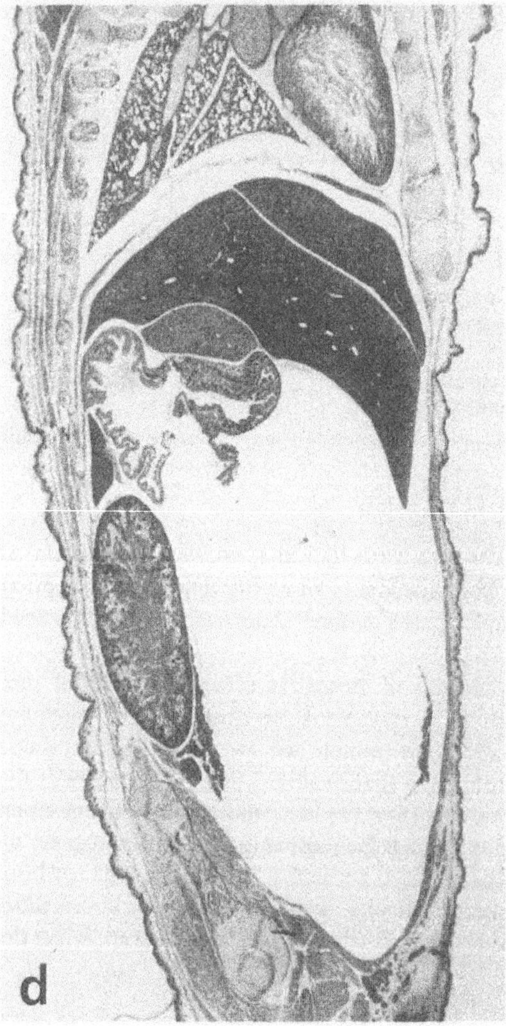

Fig. 11a–d. Newborn mice. Postnatal "ballooning" and subsequent rupture of the stomach and distended, air-filled abdomen. NMRI mice were treated with a single oral dose (100 mg/kg) or retinoic acid (in vegetable oil) at 13.00 hours of day 11 of pregnancy.

a, **b**, and **d** = newborn of treated mothers

c = newborn of controls.

d = histologic section. The ruptured stomach, abdomen filled with air, and displaced organs can be recognized sensitive gestational phase during which the anomaly can be induced is studied, it is found that, with the mouse strain used, this teratogenic effect is not seen if the chemical is administered either at 10.00 h or at 16.00 h of the same day.

These observations are interesting for two reasons: (1) the defect can apparently be induced only during a very short period of gestation – less than 6 h of day 11 of gestation; and (2) a routine evaluation of fetuses obtained by cesarean section on day 18 of gestation is unlikely to disclose the defect since the prenatally induced lesion manifests itself only postnatum.

2. Problem of "Drug Specificity"

The recognition of the phenomenon of "phase specificity" could imply that it is just the developmental stage which determines the outcome of an embryotoxic effect and not the type of chemical or teratogenic agent used. According to our present experience, such a conclusion is only justified when considering a certain group of teratogens which may be called "general" or "universal" teratogenic agents (cf. Sect. V.2). These universal teratogenic agents generally inhibit basic metabolic processes which are of crucial importance to all the different proliferation and differentiation events occurring during embryonic development. The points of attack of such agents may be reactions of nucleic acid metabolism, mitotic events, or important steps of protein synthesis.

Another class of teratogenic agents exists: "specific teratogenic agents" (cf. Sect. V.2), which only exert their toxic effects at a well-defined developmental period and which give rise only to a few types of abnormality, or even a single malformation, or to a typical malformation syndrome. At present, it is difficult to judge whether the "universal" or the "specific" teratogenic actions comprise the majority of teratogenic hazards. In experimental research, the compounds used have often been selected because of their ability to interfere with certain basic parameters of cell metabolism, such as nucleic acid synthesis. Therefore, many results of experimental studies seem to indicate that most teratogenic actions belong to the "universal" class. On the other hand, the suspicion aroused by epidemiologic observations in humans seems to associate well-defined and circumscribed single abnormalities with drug actions.

Very often, an agent may act in an intermediate way, i.e., it acts at several, but not the majority of the stages of embryonic development, thus producing an abnormality pattern fairly specific for the respective compound under defined experimental conditions. It should also be stressed that compounds which would be classified as "universally" acting may not necessarily produce strictly the same abnormality pattern. This becomes evident if a time sequence of the inducibility of abnormalities is studied. Figure 12 gives an example of results obtained in mice with different agents which may all be classified as "universally" acting. The proportion of the fore- and hindlimbs affected by various teratogenic chemicals on days 9–11 of gestation was studied. The results indicate that 6-aminonicotinamide (6-AN) is much more effective in producing abnormalities of the extremities when given on day 9 than it is on day 10 of pregnancy. Cytosine arabinoside (ara-C) behaves quite differently, the effect being much more pronounced if the drug is given on day 10 of pregnancy. The teratogenic

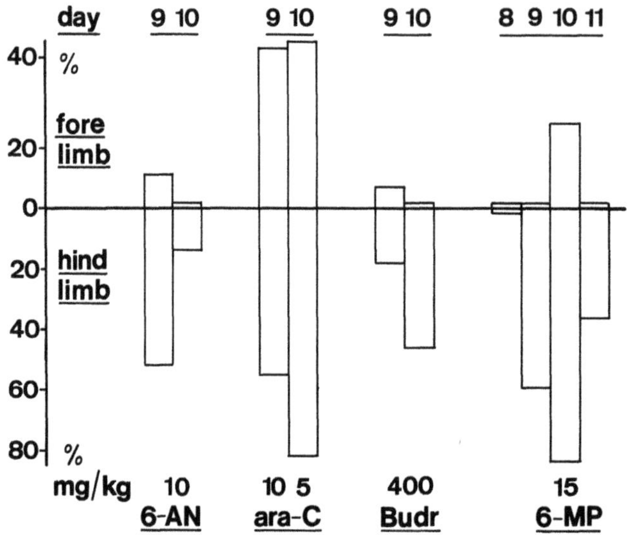

Fig. 12. Frequency of abnormalities of the limbs produced by various agents applied at different stages of pregnancy in NMRI mice. 6-AN = 6-aminonicotinamide; ara-C = cytosine arabinoside; BUdr = 5'-bromodesoxyuridine; 6-MP = 6-mercaptopurine. The frequency of abnormalities induced at the fore- or hindlimbs on day 9 or 10 of pregnancy varies greatly with different chemicals ("drug specificity")

effect of bromo-desoxyuridine (BUdr) and that of 6-mercaptopurine (6-MP) are also more pronounced if the compounds are given to pregnant animals on day 10 rather than on day 9 of pregnancy. Furthermore, 6-AN preferentially affects the hindlimbs (this will be discussed in more detail in Sect. V.7.c). In our mouse strain, ara-C and 6-MP affect both fore- and hindlimbs, but again, the hindlimbs to a greater extent. Since forelimbs develop somewhat earlier than the hindlimbs, all the effects compiled in Fig. 12 can hardly be explained by a phase specificity. The examples shown in Fig. 12 clearly demonstrate the phenomenon which we choose to term drug specificity.

The phenomenon of drug specificity can be illustrated with a variety of additional compounds. It is well-known that in experimental studies with glucocorticoids only cleft palate can be induced in rats and mice and no other types of abnormality are seen in other organ anlagen if these compounds are given to pregnant animals, even at extremely high doses. This class of drugs apparently interferes rather specifically with the closure of the palatal shelves. The basic developmental event interfered with apparently does not play a major role in morphogenetic events occurring at other organ anlagen. It should, therefore, be possible to find additional substances which specifically interfere with another single differentiation process in a given organ anlage and which then would give rise only to a well-defined single abnormality. Screening of a large variety of compounds, as now routinely performed, will definitely provide additional illustrations of this kind in the near future. Compounds of this type may turn out to be valuable tools for the elucidation of certain morphogenetic differentiation processes which are still imperfectly understood today.

3. Problem of "Dose Specificity"

The type of abnormality observed after application of a given chemical depends not only on the gestational stage during which the compound acts and on the specific properties of the chemical, but also on the dose given. It is a well-known fact in pharmacology that low doses of a compound produce only a few pharmacodynamic actions. At higher doses, this specificity of action is generally lost and additional actions appear. The same holds in teratology. At low doses only one type of abnormality may predominate, and when the dose is increased further types of abnormality may occur. It is important to notice that the same also holds true if effects on one single organ anlage are evaluated. With many compounds it can clearly be shown that low doses may exclusively produce polydactyly, for example. Higher doses of the same compound given at the same time of pregnancy may induce reduction abnormalities at the phalanges and the long bones, and amelia may result if the dose is further increased (*Neubert* and *Barrach* 1977). With many teratogenic actions, a typical malformation pattern can only be expected at a certain dose range. If individuals are exposed to different dose regimes, the same compound may induce rather different types of abnormalities. This is also to be expected in the human situation.

The phenomenon of "dose specificity" may sometimes render the evaluation of dose-response relationships difficult. This will be discussed in more detail in Sect. IV.

4. Problem of "Species Specificity"

It is well-documented in teratologic literature that different species may respond to the same teratogenic action in a variety of ways. This is also a well-known fact in other fields of pharmacology and toxicology. Such findings have been used as an argument that teratologic data obtained in animal species cannot be extrapolated to the situation possibly existing in humans. This is a poor argument with respect to teratologic research, as it is – in such a generalized form – for other fields of toxicology and pharmacology. The phenomenon of species specificity, on the other hand, underlines the importance of using more than one species for a risk evaluation with relevance to humans and for establishing and using model systems which mimic a special situation in the human organism as closely as possible. Very often, apparent differences in the susceptibility of different animal species, also possibly man, may be resolved by including pharmacokinetic data in the evaluation and the design of experiments. A risk evaluation of this kind has been attempted by *Bass* (1978) for chloramphenicol and thiamphenicol. It is essential for such an evaluation that pharmacokinetic data as well as information on the mechanism of the toxic action are available.

It is fair to conclude that, at the moment, many of the species differences in teratologic response have not been resolved since the mechanisms of the teratogenic action are still obscure or poorly understood. The best example in this respect is the typical malformation syndrome induced by thalidomide in primates, which can only be unsatisfactorily reproduced in other animal species, e.g., in rodents.

IV. Special Problems of Dose-Response Relationships in Embryotoxicity

Teratogenic actions are dose dependent like all other pharmacologic and toxicologic actions. No exception has been found to the rule – nor can one be expected – that a reduction of the dose of a teratogenic agent will reduce the severity and frequency of the resulting abnormalities. But there are a number of special aspects which have to be considered when attempting to evaluate a dose-response relationship in the field of prenatal toxicology:

1. The outcome of an embryotoxic effect may be variable if the dose is increased.
2. Appropriate parameters have to be selected for establishing a dose-response relationship.
3. Additional confounding factors which may render establishment of dose-response relationships difficult must be considered.

1. Change in the Outcome of an Embryotoxic Effect with Increased Doses

It has already been discussed (cf. Sect. II.4) that an embryotoxic action generally triggers several different kinds of interferences of embryonic development, such as teratogenicity, embryolethality, and growth retardation, which have to be considered and evaluated separately. Since a rather independent dose-response relationship may be expected for each of these events (Fig. 7), these different toxic parameters may interfere with each other when a quantitative evaluation is attempted. For example, if a certain frequency of structural abnormalities is observed at a certain dose, embryomortality also may increase considerably when the dose is increased. This will invariably lead to a situation in which a high percentage of the fetuses do not survive until term, the period at which the outcome of an embryotoxic effect is routinely evaluated. Since, in the majority of the studies, the frequency of malformations is only estimated within the living fetuses and no consideration is given to malformations which occurred in resorbed embryos a teratogenic action can hardly be evaluated. Results from such experiments may give rise to misleading interpretations if quantitative conclusions are drawn or if the outcome of such an experiment is compared with that of other experimental series. In principle, dose-response relationships should not be considered – or should at least be expressed with utmost caution – with respect to teratogenic effects if the embryo- and fetomortality exceeds 50% of the implantation sites. In many publications this principle has not been considered and conclusions have been drawn from the results which are not justified from the experimental data. If it is necessary to establish a dose-response relationship at a dose range where considerable embryo- or fetomortality occurred, the data obtained at the end of pregnancy have to be supplemented with results of studies in which the fetuses or embryos are evaluated at earlier stages of development. These considerations are of special importance if experiments with drug combinations are to be performed.

Besides embryomortality, growth retardation increasing with dose could also render the quantitative interpretation of data difficult. With increasing doses not only may an increased number of abnormalities be expected, but also signs of retarded development may occur at a high frequency. Very often such retardations are hard to distinguish from gross abnormalities, if, for example, bone development is to be

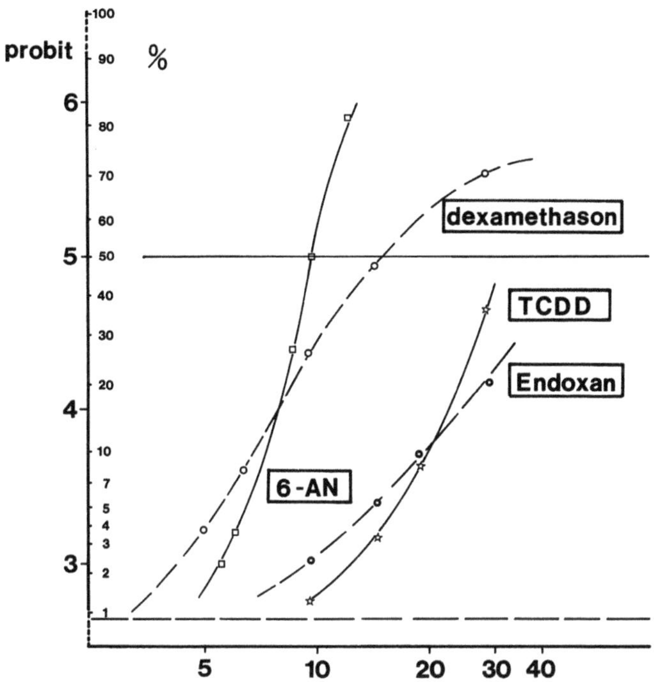

Fig. 13. Dose-response relationship of the induction of cleft palate in NMRI mice by various teratogenic agents given on day 13 of pregnancy. The dose-response curves show a rather different slope. X-axis = μg/kg for TCDD; mg/kg for the other agents

studied. Information on one or even both of the following parameters may clarify the situation: (1) analysis of the developmental stage 1 day prior to the stage normally examined in a given experiment (since growth retardations seldom exceed 1 day); and (2) outcome of an experiment in which pregnancy has been prolonged artificially for 1 or 2 days.

Frequently, dose-response curves in teratology show a steep slope. This may also complicate the evaluation of growth response relationships if only a few doses have been used for the experiment. In Fig. 13, the example given for 6-AN shows that incidence of a teratogenic effect rises from almost 0% of cases to almost 100% when the dose is only doubled. Many other drugs may not show such an extreme dose-response effect. But generally in prenatal toxicology, many doses have to be used if a clear-cut dose-response relationship is to be established and quantitative aspects of a drug action are to be discussed.

2. Selection of Appropriate Parameters for Evaluating a Dose-Response Relationship

From the foregoing it is obvious that not all parameters are equally suited for a quantitative evaluation of dose-response relationships in prenatal toxicology. But it has been

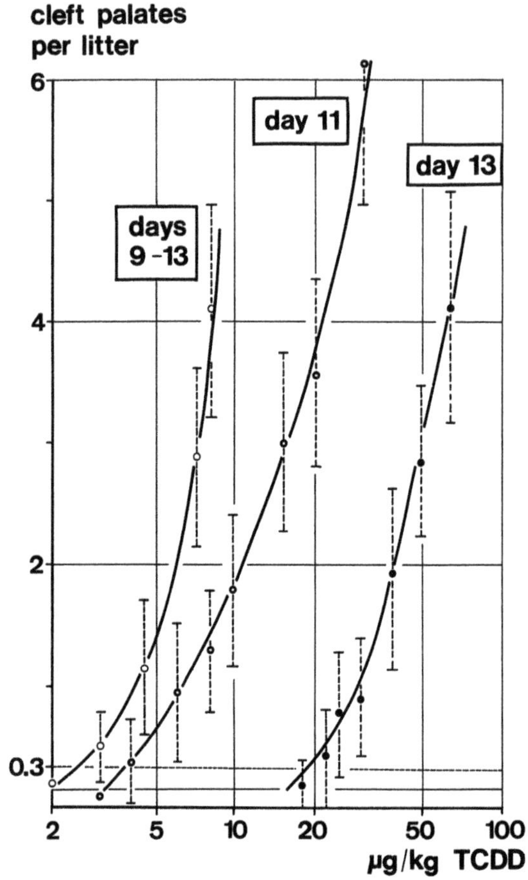

Fig. 14. Cleft palate frequency after application of TCDD to NMRI mice. TCDD was given orally either over 5 days or as a single application. M ± S.D. of 10–20 litters per dose. Values < 0.3 are not significantly different from controls under the experimental conditions used. The dose-response curves are nearly parallel, but a higher susceptibility to lower doses is obvious on day 11 of gestation

well documented that dose-response curves can be obtained for teratologic parameters in a similar way as in other fields of toxicology. In all cases typical, sigmoid-shaped curves have been found, and it is advisable to plot the data on a scale, e.g., probit of the effect versus logarithm of the dose, in order to obtain reasonably linear curves.

Single abnormalities have to be evaluated in a quantitative way. For many reasons it is not very helpful to give data on "total malformation rates." If clear-cut and defined structural abnormalities are selected, such as cleft palate frequency or number of anomalies at the extremities, in many instances useful quantitative information can be obtained. Some examples of such quantitative evaluations are given in Figs. 13, 14, and 15. It may be advisable not only to plot the data for the total number of fetuses examined but also to include an examination of the dose-response relationship of data based on the individual litters (Fig. 14). Often, the dose-response curves for these two

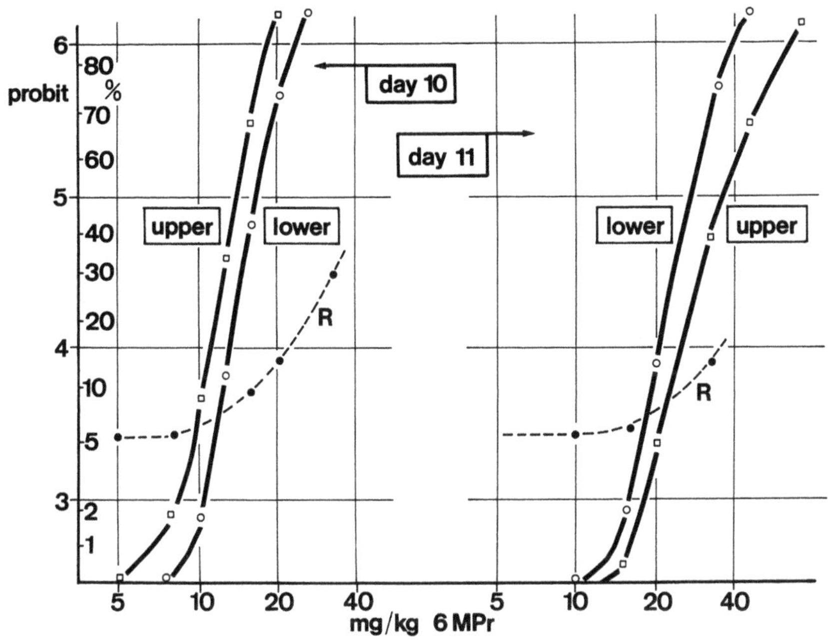

Fig. 15. Dose-response relationship of the induction of limb anomalies by 6-mercaptopurine riboside (6-MPr). 6-MPr was given s.c. to NMRI mice as a single dose either on day 10 or on day 11 of pregnancy. Each point represents the average of 10–20 litters. The defects (aplasia or defect of the long bones and defects of the paw skeleton) were evaluated after cesarean section on day 18 of pregnancy, "clearing" of the fetuses and staining with alizarine red. In this graph the sum of the abnormalities at the extremities (number of affected fetuses) is plotted (probit scale) against the dose (log scale)

methods of evaluation will be fairly parallel, but this might not always be the case and important conclusions may be drawn from such a deviation.

The quantitative evaluation can be used to compare the slopes of dose-response curves obtained with different drugs able to induce the same kind of abnormality (Fig. 13). Such an evaluation is essential if data from experiments with drug combinations (cf. Sect. IV.4) are to be analyzed (*Neubert* et al. 1973; *Neubert* and *Dillmann* 1972). A quantitative analysis of the kind described may also be useful if the time course of teratologic events is to be analyzed in more detail (Figs. 14 and 15). Often, from a quantitative evaluation, additional information can be obtained on the phase specificity of a teratogenic effect. An example of such a change in susceptibility is given in Fig. 15 for the effect of 6-mercaptopurine riboside on limb development. Since the forelimbs develop earlier than the hindlimbs, the upper extremities may be expected to be more susceptible to a teratogenic effect at earlier developmental stages and the lower extremities at later stages. This phenomenon is clearly shown in Fig. 15: both the dose-response curves are shifted toward the higher doses when studying day 11 of gestation instead of day 10 in the mouse. But the effect is much more pronounced for the upper than for the lower extremities. It is important to remember that *not* all teratogenic agents show this change in susceptibility for fore- and hindlimbs. The phenomenon of drug specificity may be more pronounced than that of phase specificity. The effect of 6-AN on limb development, as described in Sect. V.7, is a good example of such a specific action on one limb. But clear-cut dose-effect relationships can be obtained for the effects on limb development of both the agents mentioned (6-MP as well as 6-AN).

Summarizing, it can be stated that if the appropriate parameters are selected a quantitative evaluation of data on embryotoxicity is possible in many instances. Since it may only be possible to establish dose-response curves for teratologic data within a certain dose range (due to confounding factors), it may be necessary to have available data on doses clustered close together.

3. Additional Confounding Factors which may Complicate the Establishment of Dose-response Curves

A quantitative evaluation of data obtained in studies on embryotoxicity is sometimes rendered difficult and may be impossible if important information is lacking. A few examples shall be given here.

a) Establishing a dose-response relationship on teratologic effects might be comparatively easy in a low dose range if the teratogenic effect occurs at doses far below those affecting the maternal organism. The situation may be much less favorable if a "weak" teratogenic effect is to be evaluated at doses which interfere with maternal functions. In such a situation often no clear-cut dose-response relationship can be established and the lack of a dose-response relationship may even provide a clue that "unspecific" teratogenic actions play the predominant role. A drastic interference with maternal metabolic parameters and a resulting inhibition of proliferation processes (growth retardation) may even lead to situations where the teratogenic effect is found to be smaller at higher doses than in a lower dose range.

b) Considerable experience is necessary for evaluating results of teratologic experiments in which a combination of teratogenic agents is used. *No quantitative conclusions should be attempted on the teratogenic effect of drug combinations if no clean and clear-cut dose-response curves for the actions of the single components are provided by the author.* This is the same criterion as would hold in other fields of toxicology. Many confounding factors may contribute to the outcome of a combination experiment, and it is essential that many such additional factors are taken into account for an interpretation of the data. This will include the fact that two agents may influence each other's pharmacokinetics in the maternal compartment. Such an interference may especially be expected at higher doses of one of the drugs and may lead to a nonlinear supply of the components to the embryo. A similar difficulty will arise if a compound at higher doses interferes with the supply of a vital nutritional component supplied from the mother to the fetuses or if it affects the uterine blood supply at higher doses.

The availability of further data – especially on pharmacokinetics – is essential in the course of a quantitative evaluation in order to reach a valid conclusion. Research in prenatal toxicology can no longer be restricted to purely morphological, descriptive studies, but must incorporate the information obtained by various other modern methods: micromorphological, biochemical, analytical, and others.

4. Some Aspects of Teratogenic Effects of Drug Combinations

Consideration should be given to the possibilities of a teratogenic potential being created by a combination of drugs or other teratogenic agents acting simultaneously or in sequence. An analysis of the teratogenic action of more than one agent may give valuable information on two different levels:

1. It could provide data on the toxic potential of drug combinations or combinations of drugs with environmental agents to which humans may be exposed.
2. It could provide additional data on the toxic potential of a substance that may not show up when the agent is tested in isolation, but is amplified when the individual exposed to this agent is exposed to a second agent, possibly at a "subthreshold dose."

Little attention has thus far been given to either of these problems in experimental teratology. The reasons are obvious: few, if any, teratogenic actions have been analyzed completely from the molecular lesion through the impairments of the morphogenetic differentiations involved to the elucidation of all possible outcomes – including those functional abnormalities which manifest themselves late postnatally. Furthermore, in the majority of the routine testing for possible teratogenic hazards, only a few doses are tested and only a limited number of animals are used; this does not allow for a sophisticated evaluation of dose-response relationships. A study of the teratogenic potential of a drug is further complicated by the fact that the different kinds of mechanisms that may lead to a synergistic or antagonistic action have to be analyzed in detail with a variety of methods, including biochemical and pharmacokinetic techniques. This can today successfully be done in only a few laboratories.

In teratology, as in all other fields of toxicology, a combination of agents can produce three different situations with respect to teratogenic effects. The effect caused by one teratogenic agent is:

1. not modified by the second agent;
2. reduced by the second agent (antagonism);
3. exaggerated by the second agent (synergism).

An *antagonistic* effect may be of considerable interest when attempting to reduce a teratogenic potential in humans, and an additional clue may be provided on the possible mode of the teratogenic effect. But the possibility of two agents having a *synergistic* teratogenic action may still be of greater significance for the evaluation of possible risks for humans. It should be realized that, scientifically, a sophisticated analysis of synergistic actions is most difficult to accomplish. This is especially so in teratologic research, since the outcome of an embryotoxic action may be manifold and can be varied by modifying the experimental conditions (cf. Sect. II.4.b).

Two synergistic effects should be differentiated from each other:

1. An additive effect:

in the simplest case, the sum of effects (expressed as percentage effect) is observed if two agents are applied at a given dose.

2. An over-additive effect ("potentiation"):

an effect of more than the sum of the single effects (again expressed as percentage effect) is observed. The simplest case would occur if one of the agents has no measurable effect of its own – since $x + o > x$ always indicates on over-additive effect.

The situation is complex since two different kinds of mechanisms could give rise to an over-additive effect:

Table 6. Dose-response relationship of some teratogenic agents. The frequency of inducing cleft palate in NMRI mice was evaluated; application on day 13 of pregnancy

Teratogen	Slope of dose-response curve tg α	"Just teratogenic dose"** mg/kg	"Just non-teratogenic dose"** mg/kg	ED_{50} (cleft palate) mg/kg
6-AN	7.6	7.5	7.0	10
TCDD	2.3	0.015	0.012	0.04
Endoxan	1.5	15	10	60*
Dexamethasone	1.4	4	2	20
2,4,5-T	0.8	250	150	2000*

* No ED_{50} can be measured owing to maternal toxicity; the figures were extrapolated
** For definition of "just teratogenic" and "just non-teratogenic," see text

a) The second agent could interfere with the metabolism of the first, teratologically active one, thus increasing the effective concentration of the teratogen. This is exclusively a pharmacokinetic effect and the resulting action is the same as that of a higher dose of the active chemical.

b) Both of the agents have a teratogenic potential, probably with a different point of attack. Because of experimental and statistical difficulties, a convincing effect is demonstrated most easily if both agents are given at a dose which does not induce a measurable effect and a clear-cut and significant teratogenic effect arises.

A differentiation of the two possible types of over-additive effects and an analysis of the mode of action is essential in teratologic research, since the significance of the two situations for a risk evaluation in humans may be quite different. Situation (a) may be of much less significance for humans and it has to be shown that an effect similar to that caused by the "teratologically inactive" agent (e.g., an induction of activating enzymes) can also be obtained in humans. Situation (b) may be of considerable importance if the effect is obtained with comparatively small doses of the agents to which humans are likely to be exposed. We must stress the point that, in experimental research on the possible synergistic effect of teratogenic agent, *each type* of abnormality has to be evaluated separately (cf. Sect. IV.2). Only in this manner can valid conclusions be drawn.

In recent years, we have performed combination experiments with agents known to have a potential for inducing cleft palates in rodents (*Neubert* and *Dillmann* 1972; *Neubert* et al. 1973). Dose-response curves were established for all of the agents involved, using at least five doses with a minimum of 15 litters per dose and 30 litters at the doses close to the detectable limit of the effect. A dose is defined by us as having a "non-measurable effect" when there is no significant difference between treated animals (30 litters) and controls (1000 litters). In each case only those agents were included which produced only negligible embryomortality at the doses used for the evaluation. In Table 6 the values obtained in this way are compiled and the slope of the dose-effect curve (tg α) is given. It is obvious that the slope of the dose-response curves is very different for the agents used. All data were obtained on day 13 of pregnancy with

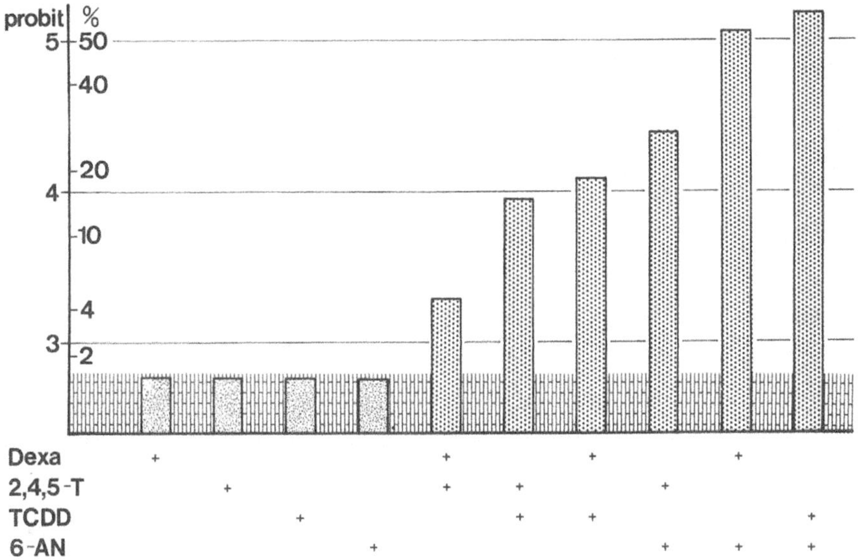

Fig. 16. Teratogenic effect of the combination of two chemicals in mice. Only cleft palate frequency was evaluated in NMRI mice. In each group at least 12 litters were evaluated. All chemicals were administered at 12.00 hours of day 13 of pregnancy at "just non-teratogenic" doses (cf. text for definition and Table 6).
Dexa = dexamethasone; 1 mg/kg s.c.
2,4,5-T = 2,4,5-trichlorophenoxyacetic acid; 75 mg/kg orally
TCDD = 2,3,7,8-tetrachlorodibenzodioxin; 6 μg/kg orally
6-AN = 6-aminonicotinamide; 3.5 mg/kg s.c.
Endoxan = cyclophosphamide; 5 mg/kg s.c.
A clear-cut "over-additive" effect is obvious

NMRI mice since the agents had to be given simultaneously. This period is not the time of highest susceptibility for some of the agents (cf. Fig. 9).

Using this background information, combination experiments were performed, the results of some of which are shown in Fig. 16. The effects observed are over-additive in the majority of the cases tested. This may indicate different points of attack of the agents used in inducing cleft palate.

In further studies combinations of up to five agents have been tested and clear-cut over-additive actions were observed even when using all of the agents at doses considerably lower than those which alone would not produce a detectable effect (Fig. 17).

We have, furthermore, attempted to establish a common principle which may govern the effects studied with our model. When considering the data given in Table 6 and Fig. 13, a correlation appears to exist between the frequency of cleft palate induced by the combination of two chemicals each given at a "just nonteratogenic" dose and the slope of the dose-response curves of the two chemicals involved. A linear relationship is obtained if the frequency of cleft palate induction (probit scale) is plotted against the product of the tg α-values (log scale) of the two chemicals combined (Fig.

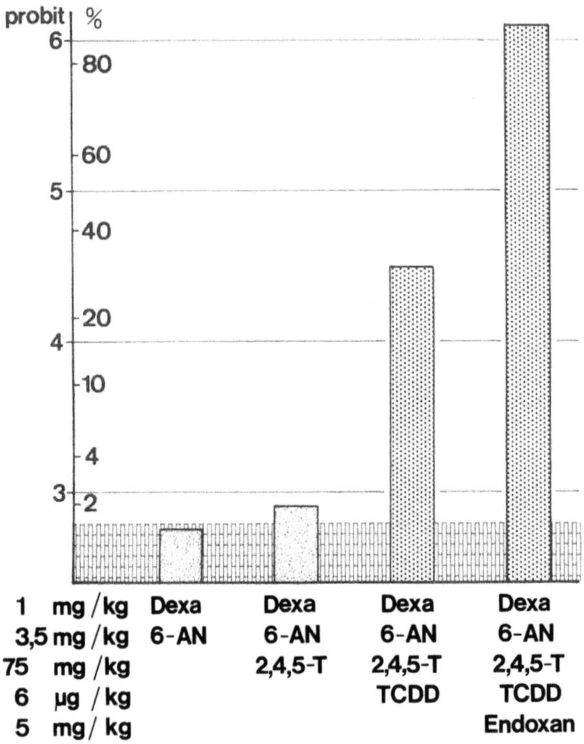

Fig. 17. Teratogenic effect of the combination of up to five chemicals in mice. Only cleft palate frequency was evaluated in NMRI mice. In each group at least 20 litters were evaluated. All chemicals were given at 12.00 hours of day 13 of pregnancy at *one half* of the "just non-teratogenic" dose (cf. text for definition and data compiled in Table 6).
Dexa = dexamethasone; 1 mg/kg s.c.
2,4,5-T = 2,4,5-trichlorophenoxyacetic acid; 75 mg/kg orally
TCDD = 2,3,7,8-tetrachlorodibenzodioxin; 6 µg/kg orally
6-AN = 6-aminonicotinamide; 3.5 mg/kg s.c.
Endoxan = cyclophosphamide; 5 mg/kg s.c.
Although two or three chemicals given at a "subthreshold" dose may not lead to a detectable effect, the addition of a fourth and fifth teratogenic agent induces a greatly enhanced teratogenic effect

18). Although this result at the moment only applies to the model used for our studies, it is interesting that the extent of an over-additive effect can be estimated if the dose-response curves are known for the two components.

5. Problem of a "No-Effect Level" Existing in Prenatal Toxicology

When discussing aspects of dose-response relationships in embryotoxicity, it is of significance to consider the problem of whether or not a "no-effect level" is likely to exist. This question is of importance when a risk evaluation for humans is to be at-

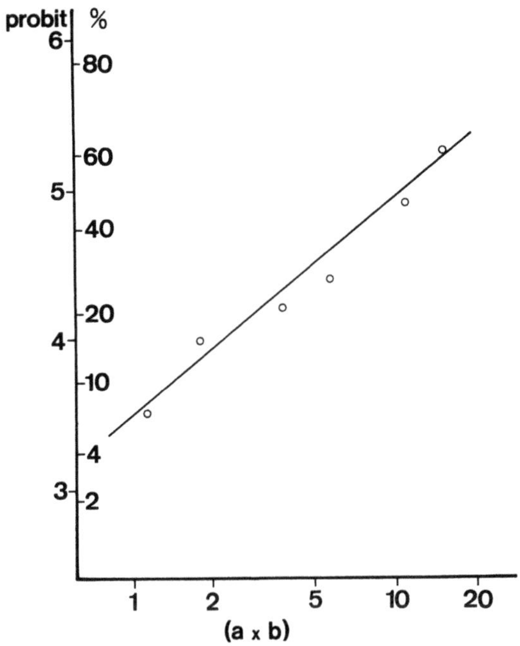

Fig. 18. Attempt to correlate the teratogenic effects obtained with two chemicals administered simultaneously. NMRI mice were treated with a combination of two teratogenic agents on day 13 of pregnancy. Only cleft palate frequency was evaluated. The effect (probit scale) obtained with the combination ("just non-teratogenic doses") of the teratogenic agents (cf. Fig. 16) was plotted against the product of the tg α-values of the dose-response curves (cf. Table 6) of the single agents (log scale). With the model used (cleft palate frequency in mice) the extent of over-additive effects can apparently be estimated from the slope of the dose-response curves

tempted. Since most embryotoxic agents can be expected to affect some enzyme reaction, we favor the assumption that such a "safe level" should exist in teratology. But at such a low dose level it is hard to obtain solid data and even "mego mouse studies" have not been too helpful in this respect. The problem of a "no-effect level" has been discussed by us elsewhere (*Neubert* and *Barrach* 1977), and in the same paper we have given arguments against the suggestion made by *Jusko* (1972) that certain teratogenic actions may not show a lower limit of effectiveness.

V. Specificity of a "Teratogenic" Effect and Possible Modes of Teratogenic Actions

In this chapter, we will discuss some special aspects of prenatal toxicology. Some of these aspects are crucial for a risk evaluation with respect to humans, and to the problem of extrapolating data from experimental findings to the situation possibly existing in man.

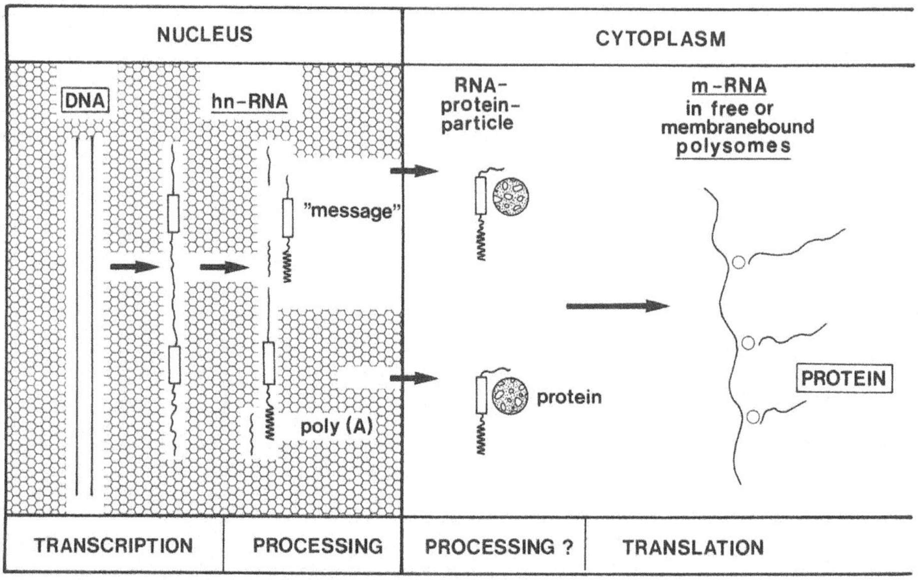

Fig. 19. Scheme of the principle events occurring during transcription and translation. Many of these steps are preferential points of attack for embryotoxic substances

1. Specificity of a "Teratogenic" Effect

It is frequently stated that any given toxic agent, if applied during the prenatal period at a sufficiently high dose, can induce severe structural anomalies. Such statements are even found in respected textbooks on teratology. Although this problem may be the most important one in prenatal toxicology, it is, with the experimental as well as epidemiologic evidence available today, still difficult to solve. We would like to stress the point that not every severe toxic event hitting the maternal organism is generally able to induce malformations. It is well-known to experienced investigators that even doses of a chemical lethal to 50% or more of pregnant animals do not, in the majority of cases, produce malformations in the offspring of the surviving individuals. On the other hand, it is equally well-known that a strong "teratogen" can induce abnormalities in the fetuses at doses far below those toxic to the maternal organism. *Therefore, a teratogenic effect, in the majority of the cases, seems to be a rather specific event produced by an agent able to interfere with prenatal morphogenetic differentiation processes.* Thus, it is not surprising that the majority of the well-known teratogenic agents interfere with processes of replication, transcription, or translation. The point of attack can apparently be any one of the complex steps of transcription or translation (cf. Fig. 19). However, this does not exclude mechanisms of teratogenic action affecting later important stages of the sequence of morphogenetic events. The extent of the impairment achieved greatly depends on the genetic background (Fig. 20).

The specificity of a teratogenic effect seems to be more pronounced than was presumed some years ago. Even with the highly toxic and rather generally acting alkylating agents, a high degree of specificity of the teratogenic effect has recently been es-

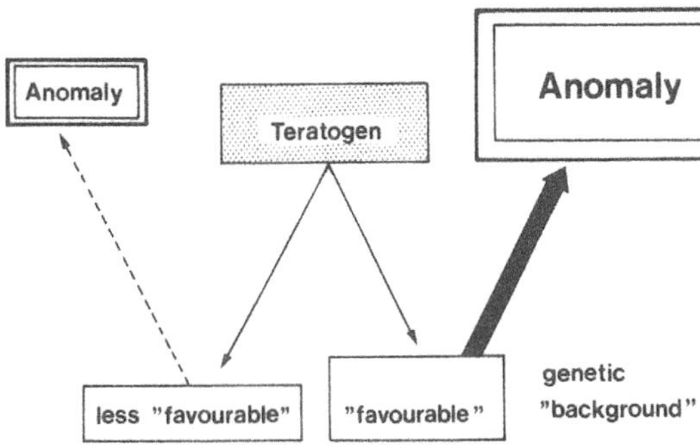

Fig. 20. Importance of the "genetic background" for the susceptibility of an individual to the prenatal induction of anomalies. Genetic background may indicate species differences as well as strain differences in experimental animals or genetic "heterogeneity" in humans

tablished. *Bochert* et al. (1978) demonstrated with a number of different monofunctional alkylating agents that the teratogenic action and alkylation generally do not proceed in a parallel way as established for the alkylation of ^{7}N-guanine. The alkylation of ^{6}O-guanine, on the other hand, is obviously correlated with the teratogenic effect, as has similarly been found for the mutagenic and carcinogenic properties. Additional studies are necessary to reach final solutions to the important problem of the specificity of a teratogenic action and to the question of whether or not it is useful to obtain information on a general teratogenic "potential" of a chemical in a qualitative manner.

2. An Attempt to Classify a Teratogenic Action

With the information available we may attempt to classify a teratogenic action (Tables 7 and 8). We classify a toxic effect capable of inducing a well-defined structural abnormality or a malformation syndrome only at a defined gestational stage as a *"specific" teratogenic action.* In comparison to the maternal toxicity the effect may be characterized as strong or weak (Table 8). An effect produced by an agent capable of inducing numerous and variable effects when applied at different stages of gestation may be classified as a *"universal" teratogenic action.* Again, strong and weak actions of different agents may be discriminated. As mentioned before, an effect caused by a preceding impairment of maternal parameters (cf. Sect. II.3) may be classified as an *"indirect" teratogenic action.* Finally, an effect resulting from an agent highly toxic to the mother may be classified as *"unspecific"*; however, as has already been pointed out (cf. Sect. II.4.b), embryolethal effects or growth retardations may frequently be observed under the latter conditions, gross abnormalities (teratogenic effects) apparently being the exception.

Table 7. Suggestion of a classification of teratogenic actions from a toxicologic point of view

Class	Teratogenic action		*Embryotoxicity* (compared with maternal toxicity)
A	specific	- strong	high
	specific	- weak	low
B	universal	- strong	high
	universal	- weak	low
C	indirect	- strong	high
	indirect	- weak	low
D	unspecific	- weak	low

A = well-defined effect only to be induced at a defined gestational stage
B = agent causing numerous and variable effects depending on the gestational stage of application
C = effect resulting from an impairment within the maternal organism; often an altered supply of nutrients to the embryo
D = effect resulting from a dose of a chemical highly toxic to the mother (gross abnormalities are the exception)

Table 8. Some examples of the classification of teratogenic actions

A Specific	B Universal	C Indirect
Strong	Strong	Strong
Thalidomide (in primates)	*Cyclophosphamide* *X-rays* *6-MPr* *Vit. A*	*Trypan blue?* *Zn deficiency* *Folic acid deficiency*
TCDD ? - →		
Weak	Weak	Weak
Glucocorticoids (in rodents)		*Stress* (mice)
2,4,5-T ? - →		

3. Malformation-Like Abnormalities Induced Prior to or After the Classic "Critical Phase" of Organogenesis

In the discussion of the term "critical" or "sensitive phase," those findings which do not fit into the time scheme hitherto applied must be considered. In this connection, reports by various authors describing the induction of malformations by applying a noxa during the preimplantation stage are of interest, although the reproduction of this effect has not always been successful (*Gottschewski* 1964; *Wilson* 1966; *Spielmann* et al. 1979; *Spielmann* and *Eibs* 1978).

Even a long time after the generally considered critical phase, changes resembling malformations may be produced (Figs. 21 and 22). Our own investigations were successful in obtaining aplasia, drastic shortenings, reductions, and deformations in the vertebral region, the skull, and the skeleton of the extremities of rats by applying substances during the third trimester of pregnancy. Connective tissues and mesenchyma were affected by chemicals, such as lathyrogens like α-aminopropionitrile, or by D-penicillamine or oxytetracycline (*Lix* 1975; *Klingner* 1978; *Merker* 1977; *Merker* et al. 1972, 1975; *Saxen* 1966). Although these are substances having a broad range of action, an explanation of their teratogenic effect essentially has to consider the mesenchymal intercellular substance. This late stage of skeletogenesis is predominantly characterized by the production of osteoid intercellular substances (collagen type I and proteoglycans) as well as mineralization processes. Among others, the lathyrogenic substances influence, by lack of the co-factors Cu and Fe, the activity of proline and lysine hydroxylase and hence the aggregation behavior of collagen (*Levene* et al. 1972; *Nimmi* et al. 1972). It is also possible that, as a secondary effect, the synthesis and secretion of collagen are inhibited (*Lane* et al. 1971).

In order to explain the genesis of such skeletal changes, the methodologic basis of identifying malformations has to be discussed. In teratologic research, malformations of the skeleton are characterized by a complex-type binding of alizarin red to mineralized regions of bone anlagen and a consecutive clearing of the remaining tissues.

A failure to stain does not necessarily signal the absence of the part of the skeleton in question. An impairment of mineralization processes may, in spite of the existence of an osteoid or cartilaginous matrix, be responsible for the failure to stain. We used a double-staining technique where cartilage (alcian blue) as well as bone (alizarine red) are shown. We actually succeeded in demonstrating that, after application of lathyrogenic substances, a cartilaginous pattern may be present although this bone anlage was not detectable in the alizarine red preparation; i.e., an aplasia would have had to be registered (Fig. 23; cf. also Fig. 31). This finding is easily explained by the mechanism of action of lathyrogenic substances. They interfere with the aggregation of collagen and thus the three-dimensional formation of these structures. However, the tertiary and quarternary structures of collagen are a prerequisite for the initiation, localization, and growth of apatite crystals. Oxytetracycline even interferes directly with crystal growth.

Additional mechanisms producing a malformation-like alteration after application of lathyrogenic substances are feasible. The inducing effect of mineralized bone or cartilage matrix should be mentioned here. *Röhnelt* (1975) succeeded in showing that after treatment with diphenylhydantoin the invasions of the second mesenchyma cell

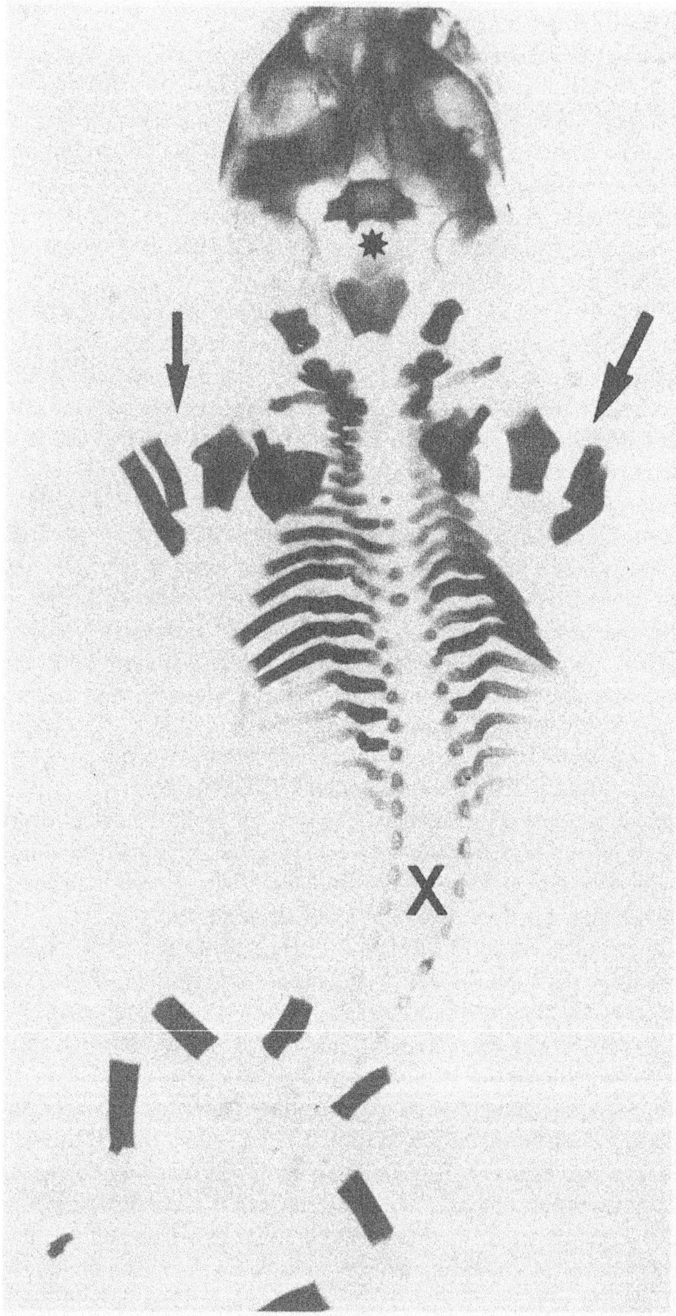

Fig. 21. Rat embryo, day 20 of gestation. Staining with alizarine red. Cleared preparation. 1000 mg/kg D-penicillamine were given daily, i.p., from day 15 to 19 of gestation. Lack of bones in the occipital region (*), striking shortening of humerus, radius, and ulna with deformation (↓), disturbance in the mineralization of the spinal cord anlage (x), deformation of ribs, lack of metatarsalia and metacarpalia

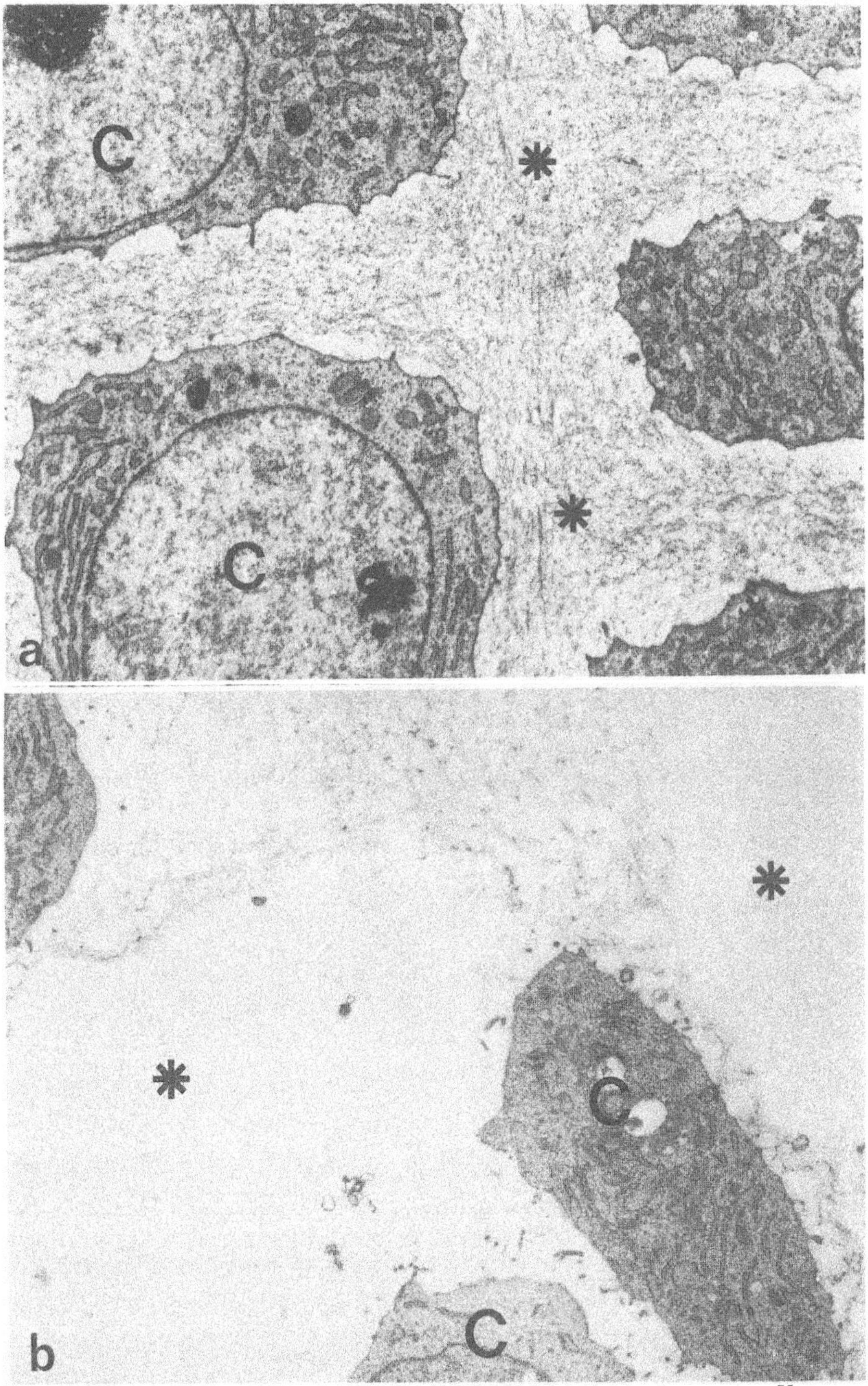

Fig. 22a, b, Rat embryo, day 16 of gestation. Epiphysis from a humerus. **a** Untreated control. Typical cartilage cells (C) with intercellular substance (*). **b** Treated with 1000 mg D-peniciallamine/kg daily, i.p., from day 12 to 15 of gestation. Irregular shape and position of cartilage cells (C). Missing structures of the intercellular space in defined areas (*). × 12,000

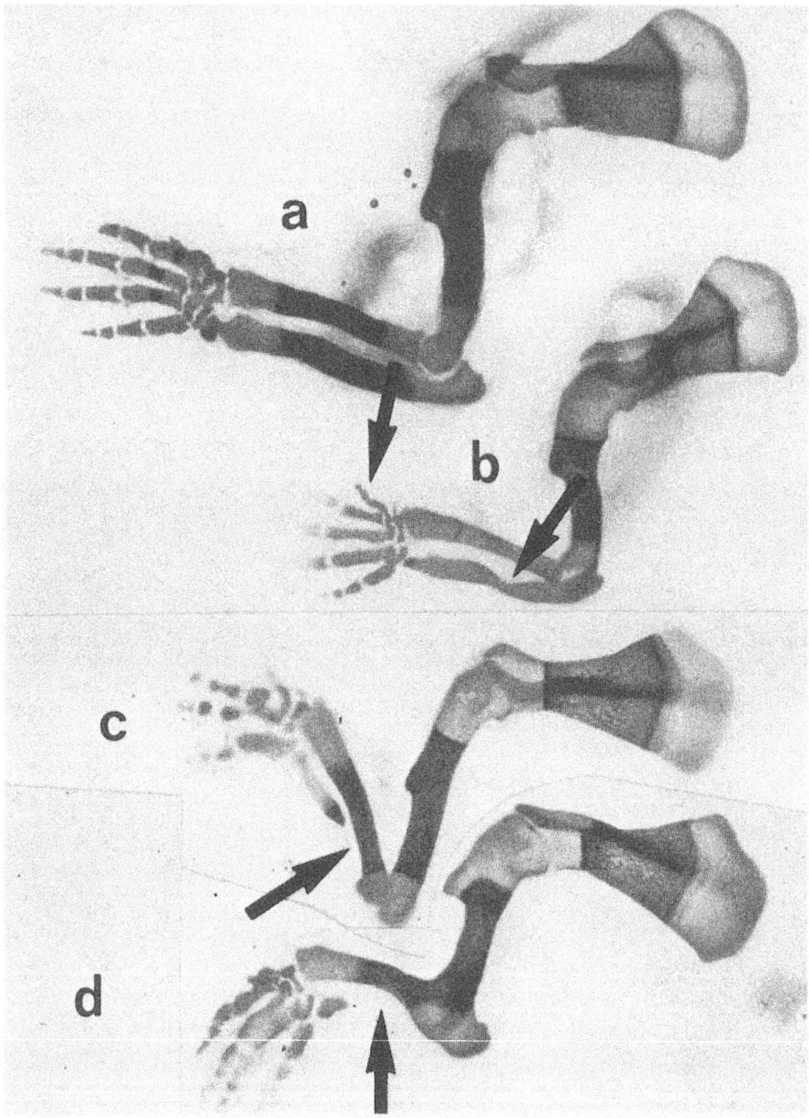

Fig. 23a–d. Rat embryo, day 20 of gestation. Double staining with alizarine red and methylene blue. **a** Control. **b** Treated with 1000 mg D-penicillamine/kg daily, i.p. from day 15 to 19 of pregnancy. Note the shortening of the skeletal anlagen and the lack of a mineralization zone in the ulna (↓) and the distal phalanges (↓). **c** and **d.** Treated with 25 mg/kg 6-MP on day 12 of pregnancy. Pronounced hypoplasia of the ulna (↓)

generation into the cartilaginous bone anlage may be impaired by the altered mineralization in cartilage and in the perichondral bone sheath. Thus, the ensuing chondral osteogenesis is inhibited. Finally, the mechanical significance of the impairment of mineralization may represent an explanation of deformations frequently occurring after treatment with lathyrogenic substances during late pregnancy. When hypertrophic cartilage is formed, mineralized, and finally decomposed in the diaphysis of the cartilage anlagen, this region is not longer capable of resisting mechanical power. Therefore, it must be stabilized by a bone supporter, the perichondral bone sheath. In order to intercept flexure and pressure a systematic incorporation of apatites is necessary. If this process is impaired, as it was in our experiments, drastic deformations may result owing to the onset of load, e.g., early occurrence of muscle contraction.

If mesenchyma-affecting or lathyrogenic substances are applied somewhat earlier, i.e., between the initiation of cartilage formation and of mineralization (days 12–15 in the mouse), malformation-type skeletal changes (hypoplasia, drastic deformations, single aplasia) may likewise be demonstrated. Since the mechanisms discussed (impairment of mineralization and induction) do not exist at this stage or are functionally unimportant, these events must be caused by different factors. In this connection the significance of the cartilaginous matrix for transmitting morphogenetic information should be mentioned. Already, blastemata as well as the evolving cartilaginous anlagen contain information on number, localization, relative size and shape of the resulting bones. Initiated by the process of chondral osteogenesis, the final bone part develops according to the cartilaginous model as the cartilage cells decompose. Owing to this event, the acellular cartilaginous matrix passes on morphogenetic information (*Merker* 1977). Therefore, it is understandable that qualitative and quantitative alterations of the matrix result in smaller and deformed bone parts. The developing bone imitates such shortening or distortion and keeps up this model at least until birth. Rare cases even result in aplasia. Temporary morphological findings seem to indicate that cartilage parts smaller than a certain size decompose or are resorbed later on. The absence of functional load may well be decisive.

When discussing these problems it must be pointed out that there are differences between the classic teratogenic substances, which induce malformations during the so-called critical period, and the lathyrogenic substances discussed above, which are still effective at the end of pregnancy. The usual teratogenic substances are effective at a single dose. They interfere with time-limited, irretrievable developmental steps. The intercellular substance production and the ensuing mineralization, on the other hand, continue after a short-time inhibition. The utmost result is growth inhibition. In order to produce malformation-type effects, the respective substances have to be administered at an adequate dose over a prolonged period of time, at least several days (*Merker* et al. 1975).

4. Significance of Cell Necroses for the Induction of Congenital Structural Abnormalities

The development of a malformation actually needs a mechanism which is more complicated than that involved with the formation of a simple toxic effect. Before a malformation becomes manifest, various prerequisites must have been complied with and attempts of the embryonic organism at recompensation and regeneration must have failed. A scheme of events showing the generation of a developmental abnormality is given in Figs. 4 and 5.

In order to judge and define these problems more accurately, causal genesis of a malformation is discriminated from the formal one. The *causal genesis* corresponds to the so-called primary cause, i.e., the impairment of a specific metabolic step or cellular event by which cell structures and important basic processes are interfered with. The *formal genesis* explains the resulting secondary, tertiary, etc., consequences which finally lead to a significant structurally defective development.

However, a complete clarification of this sequence of teratogenic events has not been accomplished with any substance to date. Although the biomolecular mode of action of a teratogen may be well known, it is still inexplicable why, for example, a cytotoxic teratogen produces necroses only in some cells and at specific locations. Hypotheses must be developed to explain these phenomena: modification of the cell cycle, rate of proliferation, degree of differentiation, blood supply, the existence of gradients, etc. (*Scott* 1978; *Krowke* and *Neubert* 1977; *Neubert* et al. 1971; *Herken* et al. 1978). Our knowledge of the events lying between the molecular lesion (causal genesis) and the finally observed abnormality (impaired morphogenetic differentiation) is even more inferior. Therefore, we may speak of a "black box" which is located between the action of a teratogen and the manifestation of a malformation.

Such a sequence of steps finally leading from the primary cause to the malformation is comparatively well-known with substances having cytotoxic effects. Numerous teratogens act in this way, producing necroses in those parts of the embryo later showing malformations. *Scott* (1978) describes this situation as follows: "The fact that such a wide variety of teratogenic agents produces a cytotoxic response in the embryo has raised the question whether all teratogens act in this manner. Although such a hypothesis is probably not tenable, one is hard pressed to find well-documented cases of teratogenesis without some cytotoxicity." It has frequently been reported that cell necrosis often occurs in the course of a teratogenic event, yet many gaps exist in our understanding of what actually takes place. It is often unknown *why* and *when* a special cell dies. Numerous assumptions have been made concerning the reasons: impaired formation of a vital DNA segment, activation of a latent "code of death," detection of a defective DNA by a controller gene (late replicating DNA), formation of toxic proteins, formation or activation of nucleases, membrane alterations, etc. (*Burki* 1974; *Hassel* and *Pratt* 1977; *Herken* et al. 1978; *Webster* and *Gross* 1970; *Wieland* 1977; *William* et al. 1974; *Scott* 1978). Although all these possibilities present interesting models, they often do not elucidate the actuation itself and the process of the necrosis. The morphology of the necrotic process and the fate of the necroses are much better understood.

The morphological analysis of these cytotoxic effects is complicated by the occurrence of necroses in normal embryonic tissues. This phenomenon is characterized as *physiologic cell death.* Three types of necrosis may be discriminated by electron microscopy (*Schweichel* and *Merker* 1973) in embryonic tissues:

1. Because of its importance, the type of necrosis to be mentioned first is the *shrinkage necrosis* (*Kerr* 1972). It is accompanied by pronounced pyknosis of nuclei, densification of cytoplasm, karyorhexis and, cell fragmentation. Such alterations are predominantly the morphological expression of the physiologic cell death. Shrinkage necroses may, therefore, be found in great number in nonimpaired embryonic tissue.

2. The second type of necrosis, *lysosome-induced necrosis,* is evidently connected with an activation of the lysosomal system. Here, so-called *cytolysosomes* (autophagic vacuoles) are primarily formed, and the cells finally decompose. The assumption is that the damage has been initiated by lysosomal enzymes derived from cytolysomes. Such necroses may be observed in the surface epithelial layers when the palatal shelves are united or the pronephros structures are destroyed.

3. Last is the so-called *swelling* necrosis. It is primarily characterized by a swelling of the membrane-bordered organelles, in particular the mitochondria. Later the entire cell swells, the membranes rupture, and, finally, the nucleus shows signs of pyknosis. This type of necrosis morphologically corresponds to what is termed in pathology "vacuolar degeneration" (*Merker* et al. 1964). However, such altered cells occur only rarely, and always singularly.

Necrosis type 1 is also found with nearly all the cytotoxic teratogens examined to date. Since physiologic cell death predominantly parallels necrosis type 1, the discovery of the inducing factors and process would be of great significance for the understanding of these important events. A promising possibility is the exact morphological analysis of the cytotoxic reaction (*Schweichel* and *Merker* 1973; *Herken* et al. 1978; *Sadler* and *Cardell* 1977). The earliest observable alterations are to be detected via electron microscopy in the nucleus. During the sensitive period, the nuclei contain a homogeneously dispersed karyoplasm with a big and clearly prominent nucleolus. Indistinct densifications of chromatin develop in a limited area at the commencement of the process of necrosis. These heterochromatin plaques become more compact and more clearly distinguishable from the remaining karyoplasm and finally join to build large areas (Figs. 24–27).

Approximately 1 h after the commencement of changes in the nucleus, the first alterations in the cytoplasm are detectable. The cytoplasm becomes electron dense. However, this difference in density is not caused by an incorporation of dense substances but by a concentration of all still unchanged cytoplasmic particles. As densification increases the polysomes disintegrate into single ribosomes. Simultaneously, a star-shaped deformation of the cell occurs, caused by the formation of crude projections and constrictions. Only now do the membrane-bordered organelles, e.g., mitochondria, start swelling. The termination of this necrotic process is the fragmentation of these dense and deformed cells. The nucleus either remains located in a central fragment or also disintegrates. The fragments separately situated in the extracellular space are rapidly phagocytized by intact neighbour cells. Obviously, each embryonic cells is capable during the critical phase of incorporating and intracellularly disintegrating such cell fragments. But they do not alter their morphological behavior in doing so. Neuroepithelial cells, blastema cells, or mesenchyma cells are recognizable as such despite their phagocytic activity. Special phagocytizing cells, characterized by their spherical form, their size, and their number of inclusions, are only found in isolation. The structural transformation of inclusions after phagocytosis indicates lytic activity.

The capability for eliminating cell fragments is so pronounced that, with the usual cytotoxic substances, nearly no extra- or intracellular residues are detectable 48 h after the completion of necroses. There are, however, differences in the time between application of the cytotoxic teratogen and the occurrence of necroses (*Adhami* and *Noack* 1975; *Herken* et al. 1978; *Merker* et al. 1968; *Webster* et al. 1973). Such differences

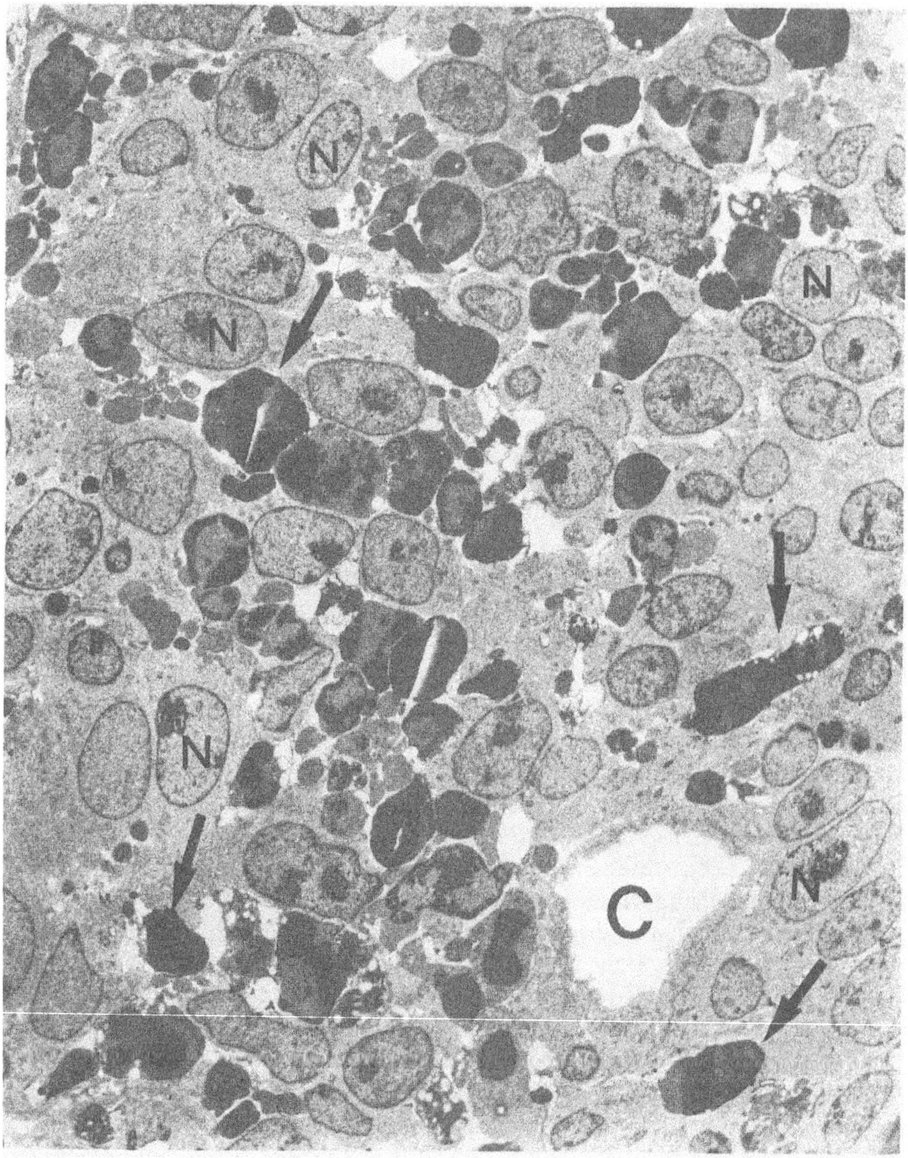

Fig. 24. Rat embryo, day 12 of gestation, 6 h after s.c. application of 25 mg/kg 6-MP. Numerous electron-dense necroses (↓) in the blastema of the humerus analage. Nuclei (N) of undamaged cells with dispersed karyoplasm and prominent nucleolus. C = capillary. X 2,500

Fig. 25a, b. a Rat embryo, day 13 of gestation, 24 h after application of 25 mg/kg 6-MP. Mesenchymal cell from a limb bud with unchanged nucleus (N) and two phagocytotic inclusions (↓). X 10,000. **b** Rat embryo, day 12 of gestation, 6 h after application of 25 mg/kg 6-MP. Mesenchymal cell from a limb bud at the beginning of a shrinkage necrosis with dense karyoplasm (X) and cytoplasm. X 12,000

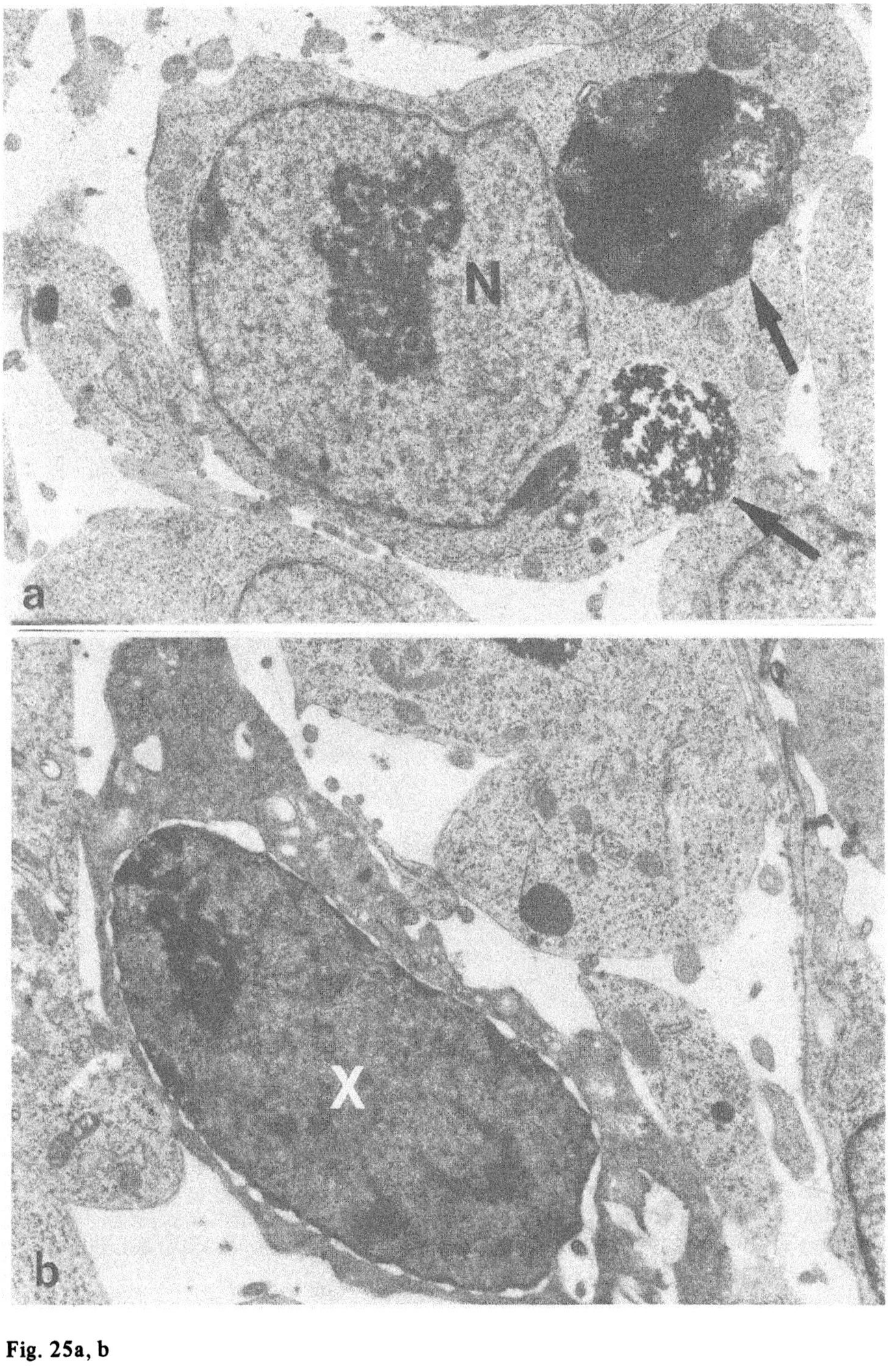

Fig. 25a, b

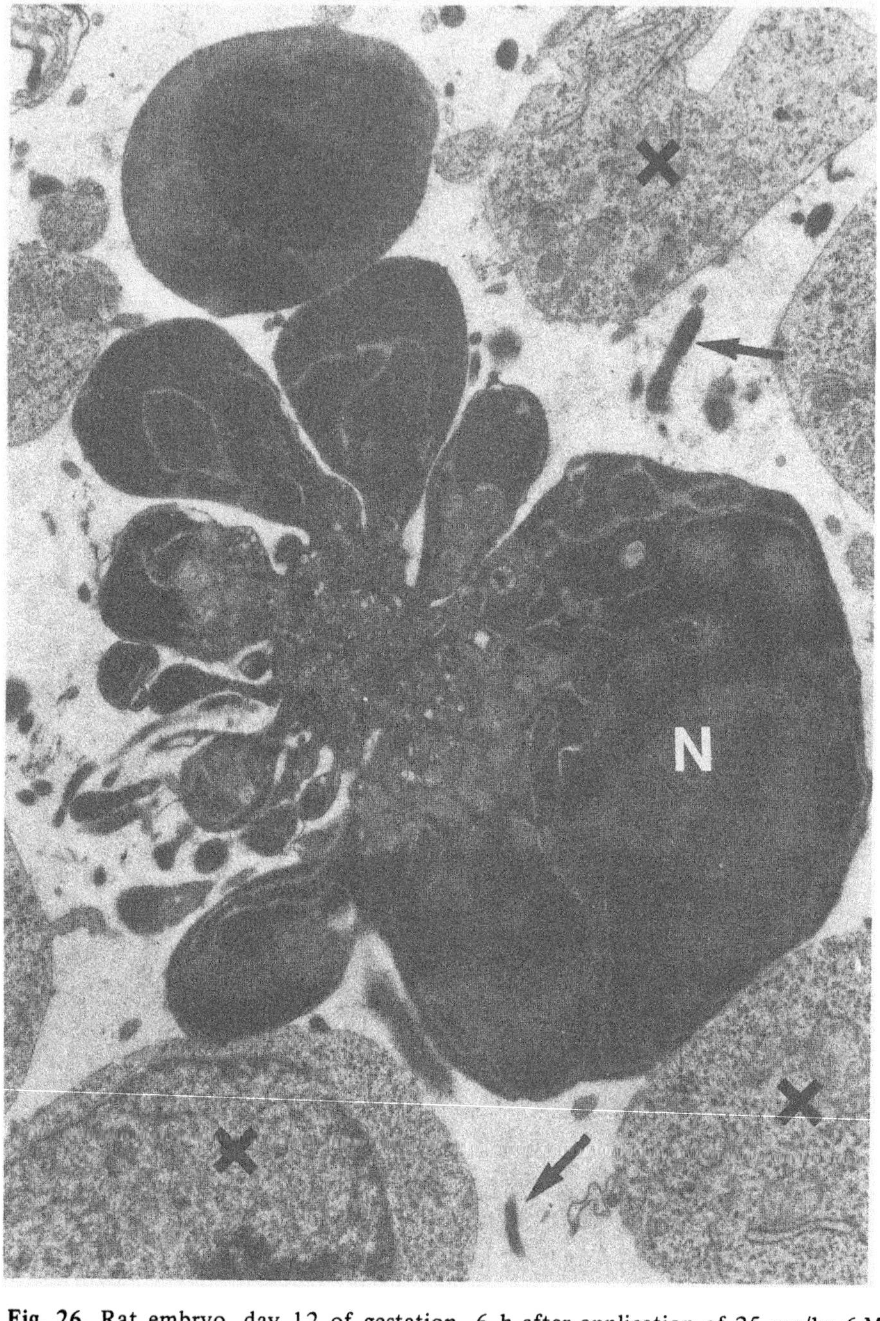

Fig. 26. Rat embryo, day 12 of gestation, 6 h after application of 25 mg/kg 6-MP. Typical shrinkage necrosis of a limb bud blastema cell with dense cyto- and karyoplasm (N) and deformation. In addition, a few free fragments (↓) and undamaged cells (X). × 15,000

Fig. 27a, b. Rat embryo, day 12 of gestation, 12 h after s.c. application of 25 mg/kg 6-MP. **a** Shrinkage necrosis from a limb bud blastema with typical chromatin densifications (X). × 17,500. **b** Fragment of shrinkage necrosis (*) next to an unchanged cell. In the fragment disintegration of polysomes and denser packing of single ribosomes. × 40,000

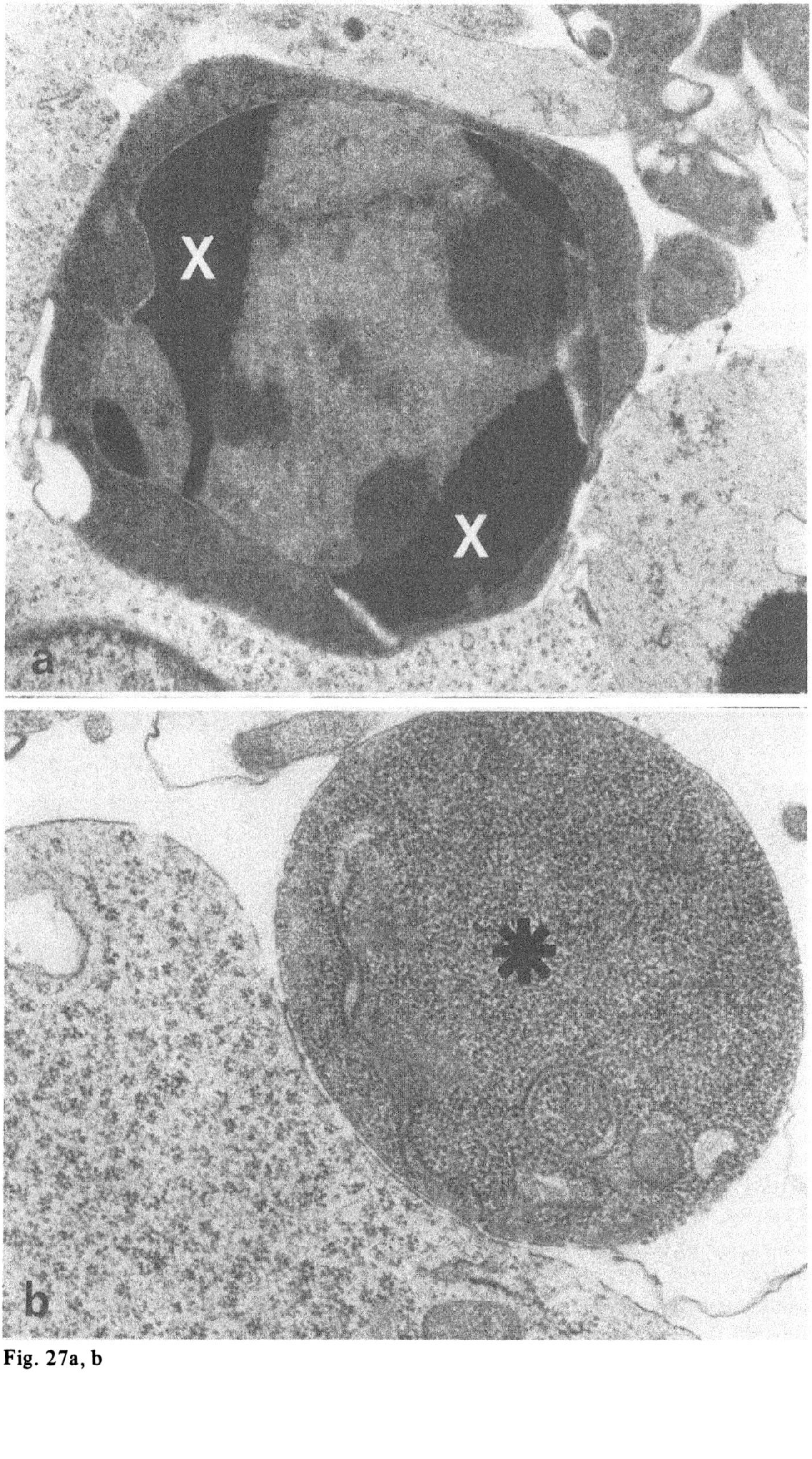

Fig. 27a, b

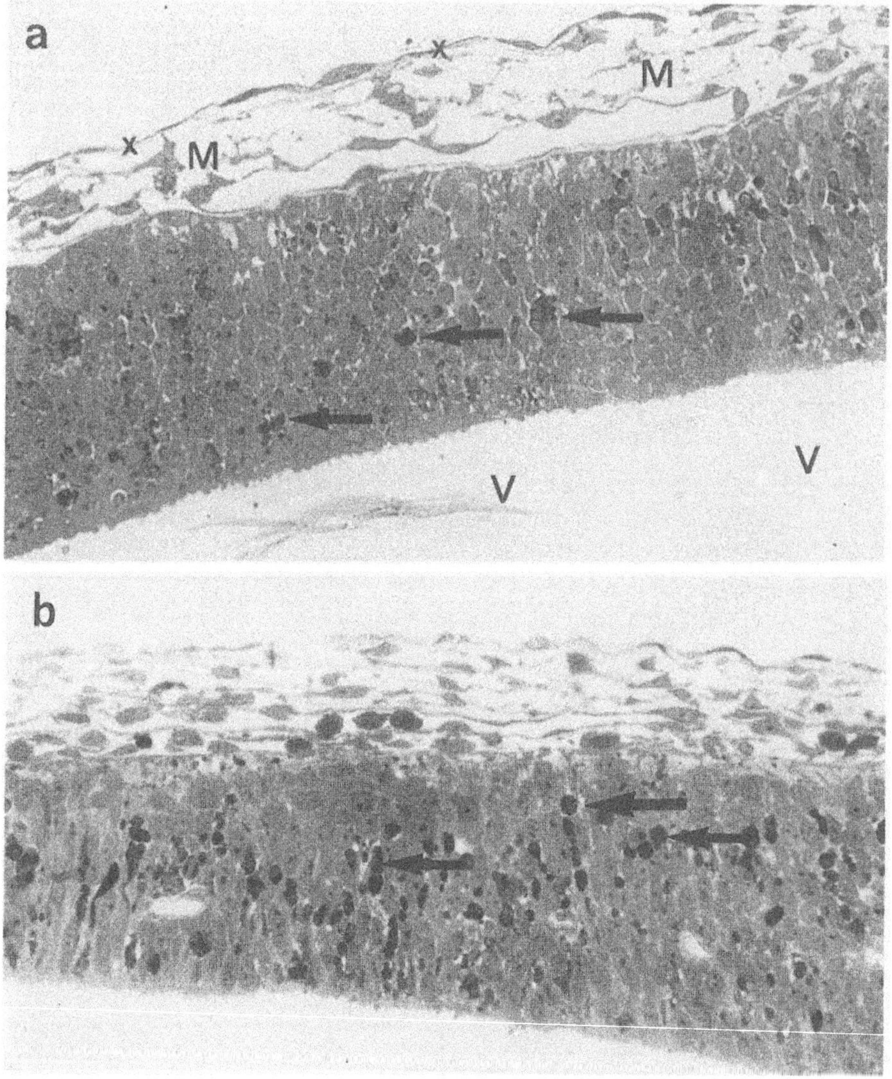

Fig. 28a, b. Mouse embryo, day 11 of gestation. **a** Two hours after i.p. application of 500 mg/kg hydroxyurea. Single necroses (↓) in the neuroepithelium of the telencephalon vesicle. X = ectoderm, M = mesoderm, V = ventricle. **b** Three hours after application of 500 mg/kg hydroxyurea. Numerous necroses (↓) in the neuroepithelium of the telencephalon vesicle

in time are clearly detectable, particularly in the neuroepithelium of the brain anlage. Inhibitors of DNA synthesis, such as hydroxyurea or X-rays, cause a significant increase of necrotic cells as early as 2 h after application (Fig. 28). Alkylating substances, on the other hand, such as cyclophosphamide, show this effect after 5–7 h. Substances such as 6-MP show their cytotoxic effect in the brain only after 20 h. It is assumed that the space of time between the application of a cytotoxic substance and the occurrence of necroses is characterized by the respective mechanism of action.

The phenomenon of differences in time may be explained by the phase specificity of the effect during the cell cycle. Such problems may be tackled by applying autoradiographic techniques. After administration of ^{3}H-thymidine all the cells of the S-phase are labeled. After that, these cells pass the different cyclic phases in the space of time typical for the respective tissue. If the teratogen under investigation is applied simultaneously with, or at different points of time after, the labeling with ^{3}H-thymidine, the cyclic phase at which the substance was effective may be indirectly determined from the proportion of labeled necroses compared with the total number of necroses. Such investigations have been carried out with hydroxyurea (HU) and 6-MP in rats and mice (*Herken* et al. 1978; *Herken* and *Schaefer* 1980). All necroses are labeled after simultaneous application of ^{3}H-thymidine and HU. Consequently, the substance acts during the S-phase, probably via an impairment of DNA synthesis. The rapid occurrence of necroses (as soon as 2 h after injection) suggests that the necrosis itself is induced at the passage from the S- to the G_2-phase or during the G_2-phase. If HU is applied 2–8 h after ^{3}H-thymidine labeling, the proportion of labeled necroses continuously decreases. These findings may be explained by two premises: 1. Labeled cells continuously effuse into the G_2-phase. There no damage occurs. 2. ^{3}H-thymidine is only available for a short space of time. After a given time, these cells are not longer labeled in the S-phase.

Treatment with 6-MP 2–8 h after ^{3}H-thymidine labeling gives quite different results. The proportion of radioactively labeled necroses compared with the total of necroses is, at this stage, uniformly near 90%. If 6-MP acted during the S-phase, the proportion of labeled necroses should decrease; with an action during the G_1-phase, however, it should increase. More suitable would be a short cyclic phase continuously replenished with or passed by labeled cells. If mitosis is excluded (since no biochemically suitable mechanism of action exists), the G_2-phase must be postulated to be the time of effect. According to the calculations by *Herken* and *Schaefer* (1980), nearly 100% of the G_2-cells are labeled 2–8 h after application of ^{3}H-thymidine. With 6-MP, the determination of the phase where the morphologically detectable necrosis proceeds is much more difficult to achieve. Since the cytotoxic reaction manifests itself only after 20 h, a passage of at least one cyclic phase must be assumed to proceed between application of the drug and the formation of necrosis. A further determination by this method is rendered difficult after this lapse of time as it is not to be excluded that the substance itself interferes with the behavior of the cell cycle. Other authors localize the process of necrosis biochemically at the later S- or the G_2-phase (*Horakova* et al. 1974), or morphologically at the G_1-phase (*Adhami* and *Noack* 1975).

5. Significance of Changes Within the Blastema for the Induction of Abnormalities

There is no doubt that our knowledge in the field of the formation of necrosis in embryonic tissues under normal conditions (physiologic cell death) and after application of teratogenic substances is still limited although the cytotoxic reaction is of major consequence for the development of a malformation. According to the findings available at present, this type of impairment of tissue is particularly frequent during the blastema stage (*Scott* 1978). In order to understand the importance of these processes with regard to the formal genesis of many malformations, knowledge of the signifi-

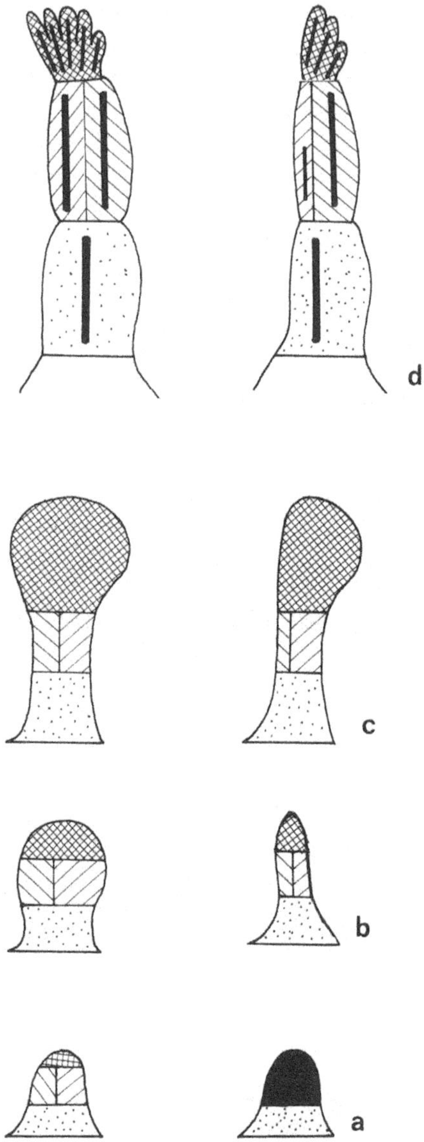

Fig. 29a–d. Spatial relationship between blastemata and skeletal anlage. Schematic representation of normal and disturbed development of limb buds after application of a teratogenic, cytotoxic substance. **a** In the region of necroses (black), **b** less developed blastemata, **c** redistribution of the remaining blastemata, **d** result: normal bone anlagen, hypoplasia and aplasias

cance and fate of the blastema is of great importance. The skeletal blastemata represent densely packed tissue whose cells differentiate to chondroblasts or osteoblasts. With regard to the extremity region, the cartilaginous patterns of the final bones originate from them. As mentioned in the discussion of teratogenic effect of lathyrogenic substances in the critical phase, the blastemata contain all the morphogenetic information on number and localization, as well as relative size and shape of the final bone (*Merker* 1977).

Every interference with this information necessarily changes the respective parameters. According to the information now available the quantitative proportions are of great significance. But this value is clearly influenced by a cytotoxic reaction. The number of blastema cells is decreased in this process. Embryonic attempts at compensation excluded, three possible consequences of the decrease of the number of blastemata are conceivable:

1. The deviation is that small that no morphological effect is detectable.

2. The size of the blastema is clearly reduced, resulting in a diminished cartilage part, a hypoplasia (Fig. 29).

3. The number of blastema cells decreased below a critical value. Cartilage differentiation is discontinued and the respective part of the skeleton is absent (aplasia).

This relationship between size of the blastema and development of the skeleton is, however, modified by two attempts at regeneration and compensation of the embryonic organism:

1. After the termination of the cytotoxic reaction, it is attempted by means of an *increase* in the rate of proliferation to replenish the quantitative loss of blastemata. The increase of labeling and mitotic indices shall be demonstrated with HU taken as an example (Fig. 30). The stimulus of proliferation is induced already with minor impairment of the blastema. This finding may explain the occurrence of *polydactyly* after low doses of cytotoxic teratogens. Obviously, an excessive compensatory attempt results under these conditions. In the region of the hand, the surplus of blastemata is not added to the existing skeletal anlagen. A new ray is formed in accordance with the local morphogenetic conditions.

2. The embryonic organism possesses a second possibility for compensation: redistribution of the blastema. In the extremity segments containing more than one

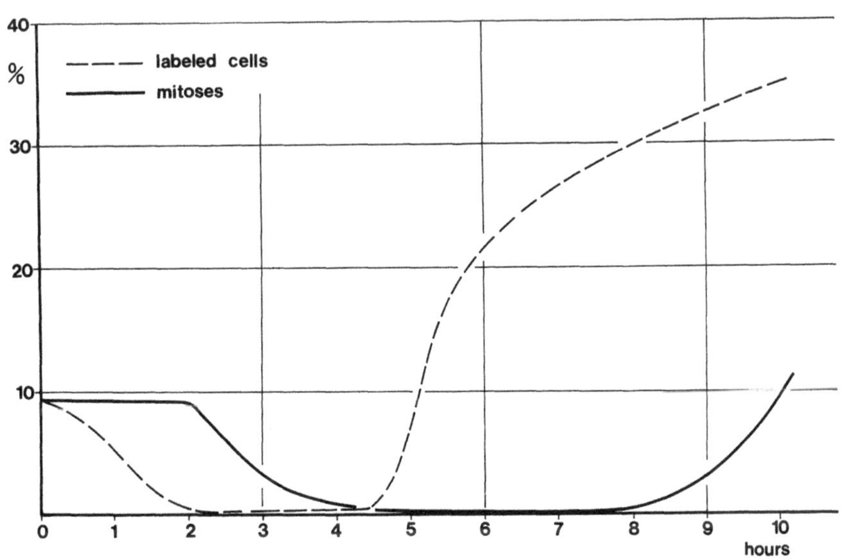

Fig. 30. Percentage of ^{3}H-thymidine-labeled neuroepithelial cells and mitoses after the i.p. injection of 250 mg/kg hydroxyurea to NMRI mice on day 11 of pregnancy. Note the great increase in the labeling index 5 h after the application of the drug (data: courtesy of Dr. *R. Herken*)

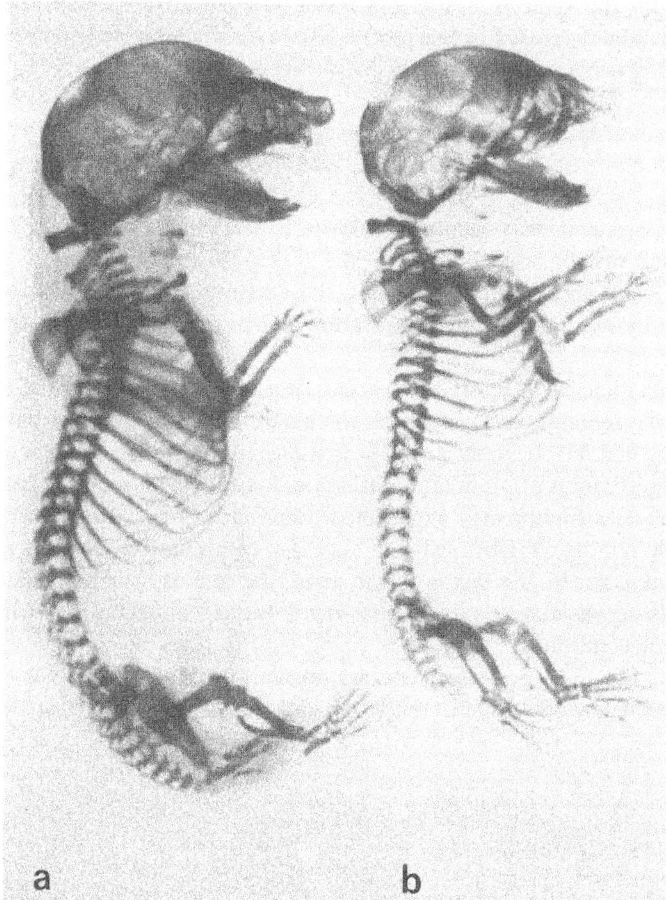

Fig. 31a–d. Rat embryos day 20 of gestation, treated with 20 mg/kg 6-MP on day 12. Double staining with alizarine red and methylene blue. Cleared preparations. **a** and **b** Bone anlagen shorter and thinner. **c** Pronounced disturbance of bone formation, e.g., no mineralization of the fibula (↓). **d** General disturbance of bone formation. Some of the anlagen may be recognized as cartilaginous structures; others are not at all developed

skeletal ray, the decreased amounts of blastema may be distributed to one, or, in the hand region, to less than five rays. The outcome is a *decreased number* of skeletal elements which, nevertheless, have normal size and form. According to the conceptions of classic teratology, the rules applying to this should be characterized by the chromosome-dependent phylogenetic age and behavior (*Grüneberg* 1963). It is known, for example, that the gene-dependent polydactyly predominantly occurs in the radial or preaxial region (*Kocher* 1977).

The frequency of radius aplasias seems to surmount by far that of ulna aplasias. For a long time, ulna aplasias were unknown or rareties worth publishing. But these conceptions were untenable (Fig. 23). By application of 25–50 mg/kg 6-MP on day 12

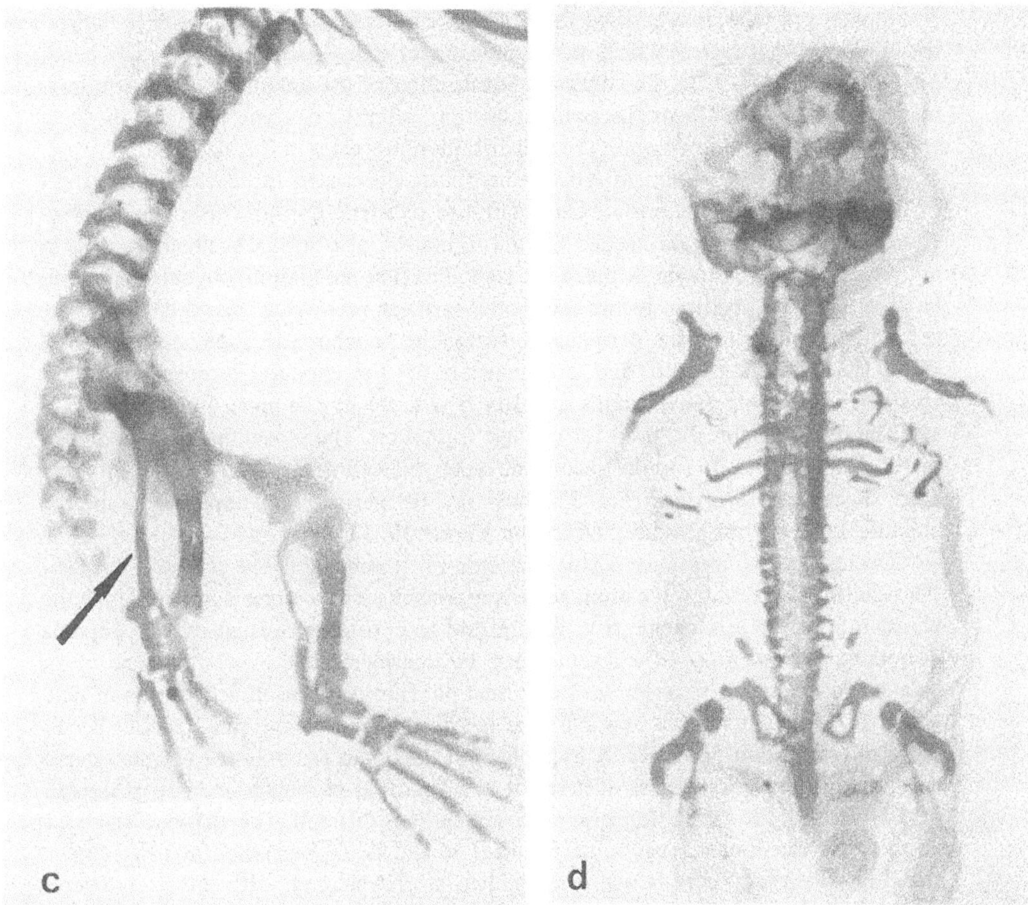

Fig. 31c, d

of pregnancy, a high percentage of ulna aplasias may be induced in the rat (*Merker* et al. 1980). The findings favor a local determination of the blastema distribution and thus the generation of the malformation pattern. These events may easily be explained by conceptions used for the elucidation of the developmental pattern of the extremity skeleton.

As demonstrated in a preceding scheme (Fig. 10), a multitude of single steps have to proceed for the realization of the genetically determined formation of the extremity skeleton. The positional values are considered the inducing factors of pattern formation. The single cell of a limb bud is advised by these values whether it is to continue cell division or whether, and in which direction, it is to differentiate. The positional values may be subjected to direct genetic control. Thus, for example, the number of divisions (mitoses) is supposed to be ruling position. Other authors discuss indirect genetic, i.e., epigenetic, factors. Hence, the formation of the blastema is supposed to be characterized by gradients which depend on, for example, the differing, predominantly peripheral, localization of the vessels in the limb buds.

Similar gradients may also be formed by the production of a substance in the epithelium (epithelial factor) which diffuse into the interior (*Milaire* 1977; *Wolpert* 1969, 1976; *Summerbell* 1973). The changing localization of the aplasias and our own findings with 6-MP rather favor the assumption that, after a cytotoxic reaction, the local epigenetic factors are involved in the redistribution processes in the blastema.

In addition to these quantitative redistribution processes influencing the pattern of the skeleton there obviously exist qualitative redistribution processes. Two mesenchyma cell populations are needed for the formation of a normal skeletal piece. Both are present in the blastema as precursor cells. The first population, obviously accumulated in a central position, forms embryonic cartilage producing type II collagen. The second population – in the periphery – forms the perichondral bone sheath, disintegrates the cartilage anlagen, and is responsible for the chondral osteogenesis. After treatment with 6-MP the blastema quantity is reduced by the great number of necroses. The cells available are used for catilage formation. The remaining quantity of cell material is insufficient for the second mesenchyma cell generation. Hence, a normal piece of cartilage is formed (Fig. 31), however, the perichondral bone sheath and the chondral bone are not produced (*Asisi* and *Merker* 1975).

Owing to the importance of the blastema for number, relative size, and shape of the resulting parts of the skeleton, bone hypoplasias are of certain significance for the elucidation of the teratogenic risk. With regard to cytotoxic substances, a hypoplasia decreasing the quantity of blastema may be considered the elemental stage of an aplasia and, therefore, of a genuine malformation. However, this direct relation of teratogenicity and extent of a hypoplasia is heavily blurred by the simultaneous occurrence of retardation processes. A hypoplasia of the bones can only then be considered an inhibition of skeletogenesis if it is not in proportion to weight and size of the embryo. However, the evaluation of a proportionality is difficult. The length of the bone anlagen is a one-dimensional value, whereas weight is an expression of three-dimensionality. However, there is one bone which, after treatment with some teratogenic substances, shows an ultraproportional growth retardation: the mandibula. Our experiments showed that after application of 16 mg/kg 6-MP, the increase of length of this bone is lower than that of the maxilla. Under the experimental conditions, the reduction of weight gain does not correspond with the foreshortening of the mandibula, even though allowance is made for the three-dimensional basis of this value (*Westermann* 1980).

For the time being these findings can be explained by a localized effect. In fact, 6-MP seems to have a "blastemotrope" effect. In the limb buds, for example, after application of this substance, the necroses are exclusively localized in the region of the blastema (*Merker* et al. 1975). Epithelium, vascular wall cells, and cellular components of the nerves are morphologically not affected. A reduction in weight after application of 6-MP would thus to a large extent be based on a reduction of the blastema or its derivatives.

The more significant growth reduction of the mandibula, as compared to that of the maxilla, still requires further evaluation. Probably the preferential reaction of the mandibula can be explained by its more rapid growth during the sensitive period. Thus the behavior of the mandibula is a model well suited for the registration of blastema damages after application of cytotoxically effective substances. These considerations are an affirmation of many teratologic experiences. Numerous teratogenic or embryotoxic substances are known to have a shortening effect on the lower jaw.

6. Induction of Structural Anomalies Without Prior Occurrence of Necroses

There is no doubt that many teratogenic substances are cytotoxic. Localization and quantity of the resulting necroses make it possible to construct a dose-effect curve and an explanation of the formal genesis of the malformations which occur. There are certainly also substances which have a teratogenic effect, but which *do not* produce any necroses (cf. Figs. 4 and 5).

According to our experience, 6-AN is an example of this group of substances. This example is, furthermore, suitable for demonstrating species differences in teratogenic effect as well as difficulties existing when attempting to elucidate the cause of teratogenic effects on the basis of micromorphological findings. After application of this substance *to rats* on day 12 of pregnancy, dilatations of the perinuclear cistern occur after approximately 24 h (*Merker* et al. 1970; *Merker* and *Novak* 1970; *Neubert* et al. 1971). This ballooning can reach extreme dimensions in the course of which the cytoplasm is pressed together to a narrow border at the periphery (Figs. 32 and 33). The nucleus lies like an island in the developing cavity. It still, however, has contact with the surrounding on one location in the region of nuclear pores, i.e., where the outer nuclear membrane joins the inner one. The number of nuclear pores as well as quantity and size of the cytoplasmic organelles decrease considerably under these conditions, although they do not show any signs of a morphologically detectable damage. Also, with the help of the electron microscope, no damage to cell organelles could be detected. The severe changes disappear slowly, and 5 days after application of 6-AN they can only be detected sporadically. Besides these cytotoxically extraordinary findings, the localization of these changes is striking. The partially extreme ballooning of the perinuclear cisterna is detected in the rat only in cells originating from the ectodermal germ layer: epidermis, CNS, PNS, and also the mesenchyma of the head, originating from the neural crest. Furthermore, a time-dependent process can be observed. On days 10–13 of pregnancy, at a dose of 10 mg/kg, all cells show a more or less pronounced characteristic symptom of an effect of 6-AN. Afterward, the portion of cells with a swelling of the perinuclear cistern decreases continuously. According to the experiments made by us until now, these striking morphological findings can be detected only in the rat.

Opposed to this, the described alterations of the volume of the perinuclear cisterna do *not* develop in the *mouse* after application of 6-AN at the equivalent time.

When examining the teratogenic effect of 6-AN, one finding is particularly striking. In the rat, the animal species with marked microscopic changes, no gross malformations can be detected in the limbs of the Wistar strain used in our studies. However, in mice (NMRI strain used in our studies) which do not show any changes at the cytologic level, severe limb malformations develop. As can be seen from the results of these studies compiled in Fig. 34, a large variety of structural abnormalities is induced by 6-AN.

From these findings two conclusions can be drawn:

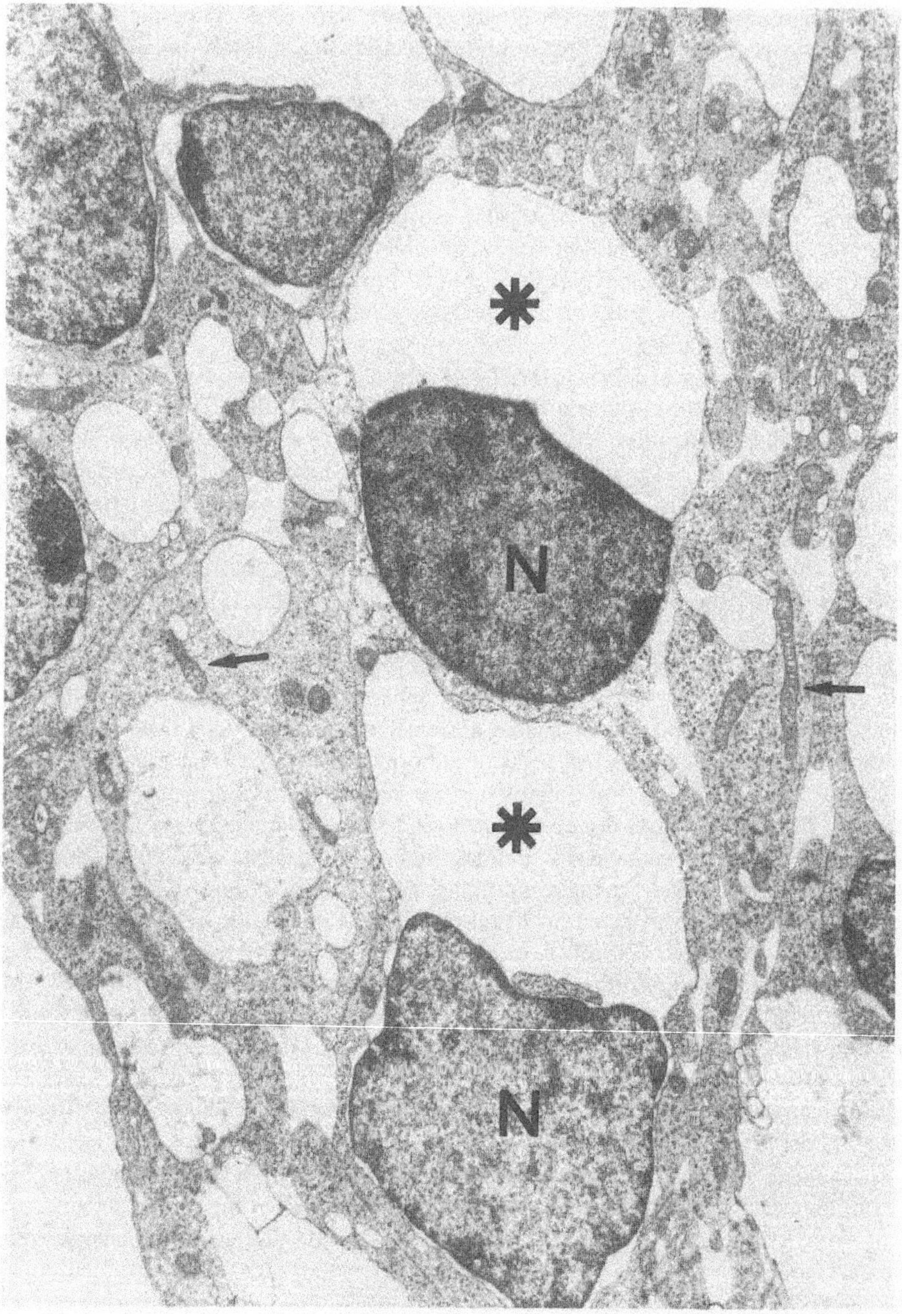

Fig. 32. Rat embryo, day 14 of gestation, 48 h after s.c. application of 10 mg/kg 6-AN. Pronounced dilation of the perinuclear cisterna (*) in neuroepithelial cells of the brain anlage. Other cell organelles, e.g. mitochondria (↓), unchanged. N = nucleus. × 12,500

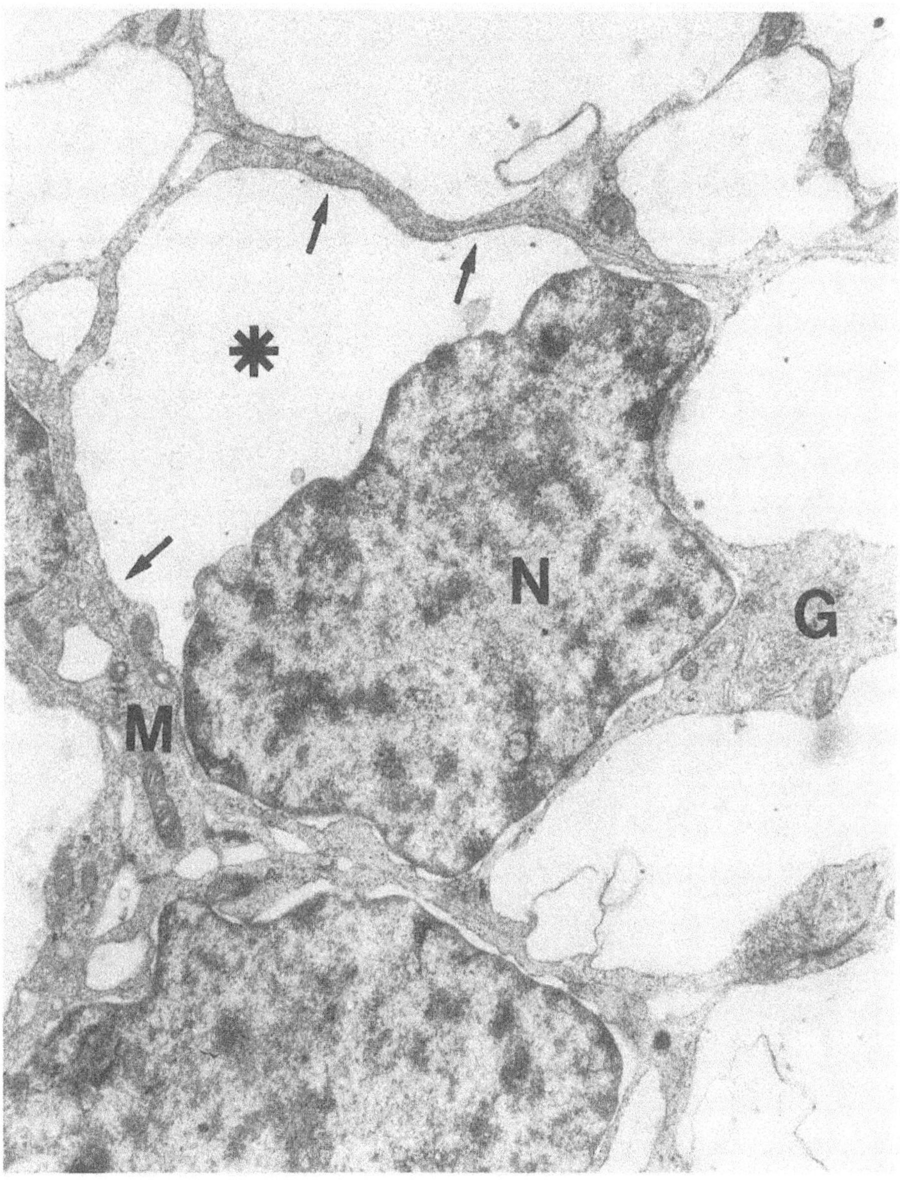

Fig. 33. Rat embryo, day 16 of gestation, 3 days after s.c. application of 10 mg/kg 6-AN. Pronounced dilation of the perinuclear cisterna (*) in epithelial cells of a dental anlage. The cytoplasm in the periphery is condensed to a narrow limbus (↓). Golgi apparatus (G) and mitochondria (M) unchanged. N = nucleus. × 15,000

1. The morphological procedure has not yet developed to a point where each primary cause of malformation can be identified. In the unfavorable cases, such as that just described, only the final steps of the abnormal formal genesis can be detected.

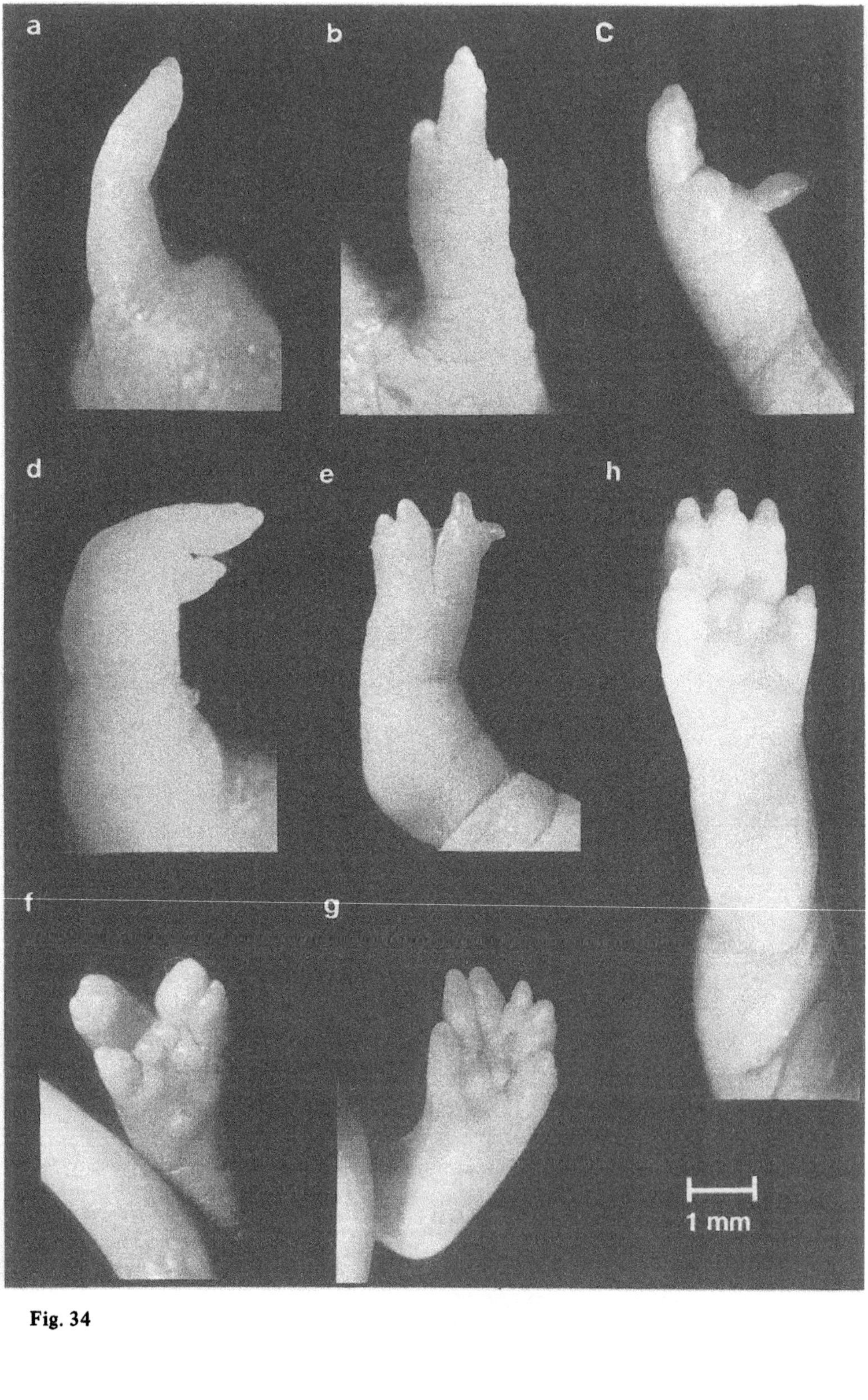

Fig. 34

2. Every morphologically detectable change cannot generally be related causally and linearly to the malformation which occurred. One cause can result in several effects.

7. Some Biochemical and Pharmacologic Aspects of Teratogenic Actions

It has been one of the aims of various groups at our institute working on this problem to correlate biochemical lesions with the resulting teratologic defects. Only a few aspects of this work can be mentioned here. Again, 6-AN is chosen as an example.

a) Biochemical Effects of 6-AN in the Embryo

Extensive studies (*Barrach* 1973) have been performed by our group to define the biochemical lesion in the embryo caused by 6-AN administered during pregnancy. 6-AN is an analogue of nicotinamide. In lieu of the nicotinamide moiety, 6-AN is incorporated into the pyridine nucleotides of the mammalian organism, thus giving rise to NAD^+ or $NADP^+$ derivatives (*Dietrich* et al. 1958). The derivatives 6-ANAD or 6-ANADP are not able to perform hydrogen transport and are capable of inhibiting a number of hydrogenase reactions (*Brunnemann* 1964; *Coper* and *Neubert* 1964). In the adult organism, the incorporation of 6-AN into NAD or NADP molecules normally proceeds via an "exchange reaction" catalyzed by the enzyme NAD-glycohydrolase (E.C. 3.2.2.5) (Fig. 35); however, we have not been able to detect this enzyme in embryonic tissues. Therefore, it is fair to assume that the analogue is formed within the embryonic tissues via the reactions of de novo synthesis of NAD and NADP (Fig. 35).

We have found (*Köhler* et al. 1970; *Barrach* 1973) that the 6-AN analogue of NADP (6-ANADP) strongly inhibits 6-phosphogluconate dehydrogenase (E.C. 1.1.1.44) of embryonic tissues (Table 9) and also, to a much lesser extent, some other NADP-dependent enzymes. The inhibition is strictly competitive (Fig. 36). A similar effect has been found in adult tissues by *Herken* et al. (1974). The pentose-phosphate pathway is completely blocked after this enzyme inhibition, as can be seen from the excessive accumulation of 6-phosphogluconate (Table 10). This effect has again been found in adult tissues (*Herken* et al. 1969).

A calculation of the degree of inhibition of 6-phosphogluconate dehydrogenase, and thereby of the pentose phosphate pathway, depending on the degree of substitution of NADP by 6-ANADP, is given in Fig. 37. Studies on the incorporation of ^{14}C-glucose labeled either in the 1-position or in the 6-position (Fig. 38) have confirmed the assumption that the oxidative part of the pentose-phosphate pathway is complete-

---

Fig. 34. Limb abnormalities produced in NMRI-mice by 6-AN. A single dose of 15 mg/kg 6-AN was given s.c. on day 9 of pregnancy. The fetuses were evaluated on day 18 of gestation. A wide variety of gross anomalies of the limbs is produced by the antimetabolite, from reduction abnormalities of several or some bone anlagen to polydactyly. Often rather bizarre structures result

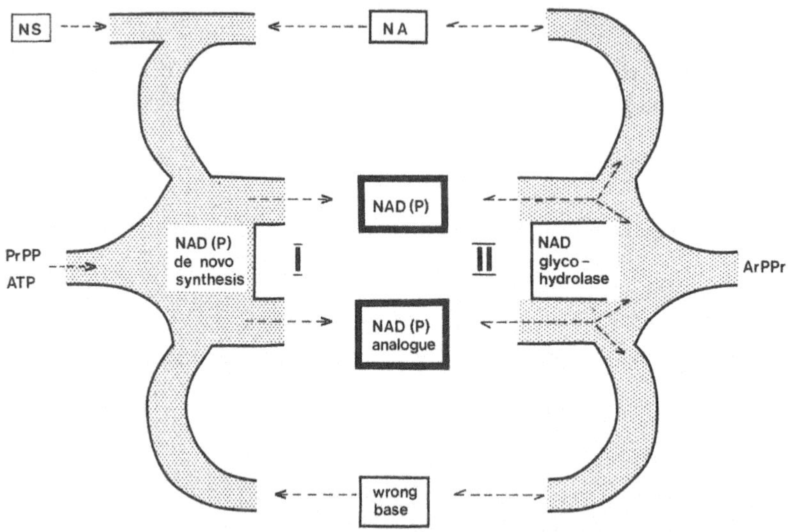

Fig. 35. Two pathways for the formation of pyridine nucleotide analogues in mammalian tissues. While pathway II [using an "exchange reaction": base analogue + NAD(P) = nicotinamide + analogue-AD] predominates in tissues of an adult animal, embryonic tissues are apparently deficient of this pathway and the toxic analogue has to be formed via the steps (reaction I) of the de novo synthesis of NAD(P)

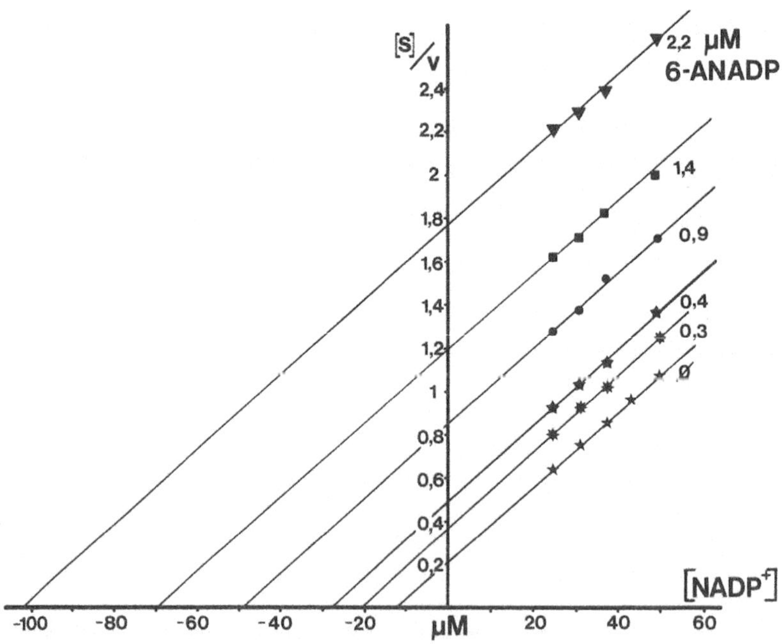

Fig. 36. Competitive inhibition of 6-phosphogluconate dehydrogenase by the 6-AN analogue of NADP (= 6-ANADP). The parallel lines indicate a competitive type of inhibition by 6-ANADP. The points of the intersection with the X-axis indicate the corresponding "K_p"-values (cf. Table 9). v = μmoles NADPH + H^+-formed x mg protein^{-1} x min^{-1} [S] = μM $NADP^+$

Table 9. Comparison of K_m and K_i values for different soluble enzymes from the cytosol of rat embryos on day 13 of gestation

	μM NADP K_m	μM 6-ANADP K_i	
G-6-PD	14.0 ± 1.5	26.4 ± 6.4	n = 11
6-P-GD	11.3 ± 0.5	0.4 ± 0.1	n = 13
GSSG-Red.	5.5 ± 0.1	3.4 ± 0.3	n = 6

The cytosol fraction of an embryo homogenate was passed over a Sephadex G 25 column. Of the three enzymes studied, the 6-P-GD is most sensitive to inhibition by 6-ANADP. Estimation of K_m and K_p according to *Wilkinson* (1961).

K_i values were calculated according to *Dixon* and *Webb* (1958), using the relationship:

$$K_i = \frac{1 \cdot K_m}{K_p - K_m}$$; $K_p \triangleq$ "K_m" (cf. Fig. 28) obtained with one inhibiting 6-ANADP concentration (i).

n = number of sets of experimental data used per inhibiting concentration (at least four values each)

Table 10. 6-P-Gluconate concentration in rat embryos

Control	2 h	3 h	4 h	10 h	14 h	24 h	50 h
0.74 ± 0.19	8 ± 3	50	87 ± 11	260 ± 30	230	120	8 ± 1

5 mg 6-AN/ng was injected i.p. into the female rats on day 13 of pregnancy. After indicated number of hours, the gluconate concentration in the fetuses was measured. Values are expressed in ng 6-P-gluconate/μg DNA

ly blocked while the "lower" part of the cycle is still operative. But, as can also be seen from the data given in Fig. 38, secondary changes occur after a few hours and the metabolic defect is no longer confined to the oxidative part of the pentose-phosphate pathway. Apparently, nearly all nucleic acid synthesis reactions are impaired at this point.

Three aspects are interesting in this respect:

1. 6-AN certainly does not impair metabolic reactions selectively in the embryo. Similar metabolic defects are likewise induced in many adult organs. Thus, the dose necessary to induce a teratogenic action is rather close to the dose toxic to the mother.

2. The metabolic block in the embryo caused by 6-AN is reversible. While proliferation processes are inhibited for nearly 2 days (Fig. 39), growth continues after this period at essentially the normal rate. The growth retardation induced, for example, on day 11 of gestation, is not compensated and is constantly carried on until birth.

3. Although all our data indicate that the biochemical lesion induced by 6-AN is very similar in the rat and the mouse, only mice showed severe teratogenic lesions in our studies.

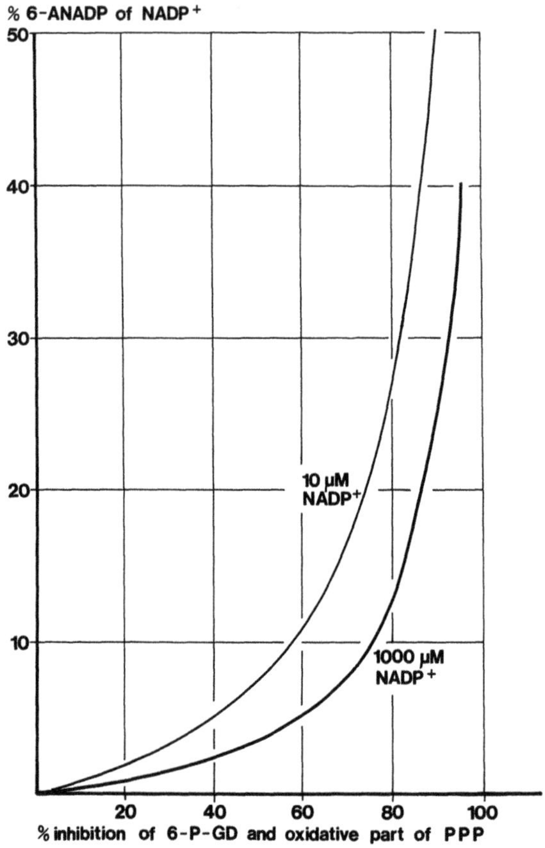

Fig. 37. Calculation of the inhibition of 6-phosphogluconate dehydrogenase by the 6-AN analogue of NADP from kinetic data obtained with fetal rat tissues. The data were obtained by using the relationship:

$$\frac{v_i}{v} = \frac{K_i(K_m + S)}{i \cdot K_m + K_i(K_m + S)}$$ and the K_m- and K_i-values of Table 9

b) Effect of Ambient Temperature on the Teratogenic Effect of 6-AN

6-AN has extensively been used as a model substance in teratologic research, but varying results were obtained in the different laboratories. We would like to mention one aspect where a teratogenic action is altered via a modification of pharmacologic properties inherent to the drug.

It has been found in pharmacologic experiments that many compounds may alter the capacity for temperature regulation. Under the influence of such substances the body temperature drops if the mammalian organism is kept in an environment of low temperature. Actually, this phenomenon, well-known to occur with neuroleptic phenothiazines, has clinically been used for a controlled hypothermia in (neuro-)surgery.

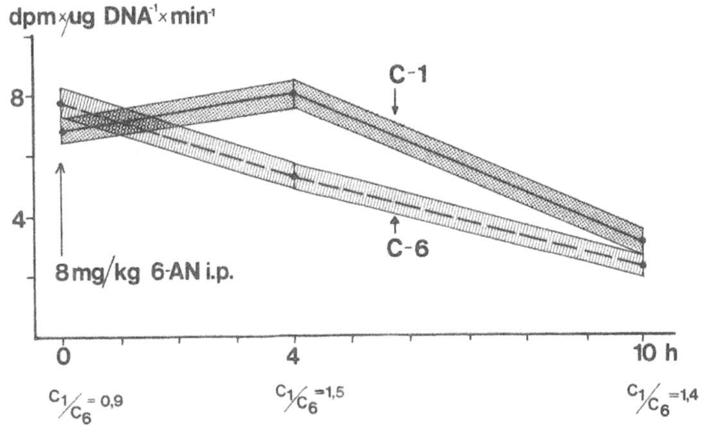

Fig. 38. Incorporation of ^{14}C-glucose into the ribose moiety of RNA. 8 mg/kg 6-AN were given in vivo. ^{14}C-incorporation was measured with intact embryos incubated in vitro. The data indicate the blockade of the oxidative part of the pentose phosphate pathway during the first 4 h following the injection (increase of C_1/C_6). After this period, secondary changes occur and other steps of the glucose metabolism are inhibited as well (from: *Barrach* 1973)

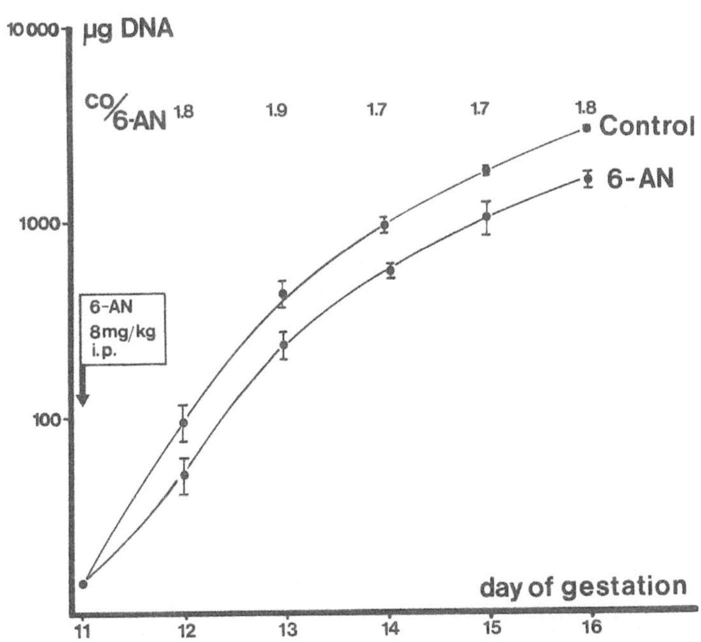

Fig. 39. Growth retardation of rat embryos after application of 6-AN. The proliferation is largely inhibited during the first 24 h; the retardation is not compensated, but is continued at a constant level up to birth (from: *Barrach* 1973)

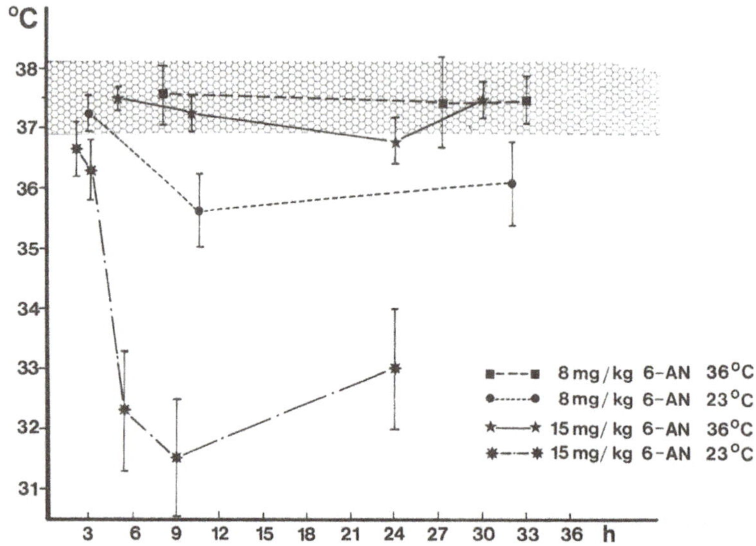

Fig. 40. Body temperature of pregnant mice after treatment with 6-AN. Groups of ten NMRI mice each were treated with 6-AN i.p. and kept at the ambient temperature indicated. 6-AN drastically decreases body temperature if the animals are kept at room temperature or at 23°C

It has been found (*Coper* et al. 1971) that 6-AN is also capable of interfering with temperature regulation in rodents. Under the conditions of a teratologic experiment, the temperature of animals varies with ambient temperature (Fig. 40). If no precautions are taken and the animals are kept at a normal room temperature, the decrease in body temperature will significantly reduce the extent of the teratogenic effect (Table 11). The body temperature can be raised to a normal level by keeping the animals at an increased room temperature (36°C). Under these conditions, the frequency of abnormalities observed is significantly increased – 98% instead of 73%. Moreover, the patterns of abnormality induced at the two different degrees of temperature vary. This is an example showing that, in order to avoid misinterpretations, all pharmacologic parameters must be considered when planning a teratologic experiment.

c) Distribution of Malformations of the Extremities

It is generally assumed that a teratogenic effect hits a pair of organ anlagen in a random way. In many teratologic experiments, the abnormalities actually occur at an approximately equal frequency in the right and left extremities. A teratogenic action favoring one side of the body has rarely been reported. *Tucci* et al. (1978) briefly mentioned the preference for the left hindlimb after treatment with theophylline.

6-AN may again serve as an example for demonstrating such an effect. We treated NMRI mice with varying doses of 6-AN on day 9 or 10 of pregnancy. Surprisingly (Table 12), a clear-cut preference for the position of left hindlimb was noted when

Table 11. Effect of ambient temperature on the teratogenic action of 6-aminonicotinamide (6-AN). 6-AN was given to NMRI mice s.c. on day 9 of pregnancy. The abnormalities were evaluated following a cesarean section on day 18, "clearing" of the fetuses and staining of the skeleton with alizarine red

Abnormalities	Affected/ total number of	10 mg/kg 6-AN 23°C	10 mg/kg 6-AN 36°C	Untreated 23°C	Untreated 36°C
Palate (cleft pal.)	Litters	1/23 = 4%	6/30 = 20%	6/85 = 7%	0/15
	Fetuses	11/209 = 5%	10/226 = 4%	6/901 = 1%	0/118
Forelimb	Litters	1/23 = 4%	13/30 = 43%	0/85	0/15
	Fetuses	1/209 = 1%	28/226 = 12%	0/901	0/118
Hindlimb	Litters	10/23 = 43%	25/30 = 83%	0/85	0/15
	Fetuses	24/209 = 11%	114/226 = 50%	0/901	0/118
Vertebrae	Litters	20/23 = 87%	30/20 = 100%	1/85 = 1%	0/15
	Fetuses	123/209 = 59%	215/226 = 95%	1/901	0/118
Ribs	Litters	3/23 = 13%	9/30 = 30%	2/85 = 2%	0/15
	Fetuses	8/209 = 4%	14/226 = 6%	2/901	0/118
Tail	Litters	11/23 = 49%	10/30 = 33%	13/85 = 15%	0/15
	Fetuses	29/209 = 14%	40/226 = 18%	13/901 = 1%	0/118
Number of:					
Pregnant females		23	32	85	15
Females with living fetuses		23	30	85	15
Females with abnormal fetuses		22	30	20	0
Living fetuses		209	226	901	118
Abnormal fetuses		153 (73%)	221 (98%)	22 (2%)	0

evaluating the effect on limb development. This effect was found to be independent of the time of application of the teratogenic drug and occurred with the two ambient temperatures studied. In the five experimental series given in Table 12, the *left hindlimb* was affected in 88%–100% of the malformed fetuses, singly or in combination; the *left forelimb* in 2%–4% only. At present, we do not have any explanation for this interesting effect. The results of these experiments indicate that the interpretation of findings in teratologic research is sometimes rather difficult. Two aspects may be worth mentioning: (1) The effect can likewise be obtained with a different mouse strain (*C57BL*), but to a lesser degree. (2) Other teratogenic substances have not been found to show such preference for one paw in the same mouse strains.

Table 12. Distribution of malformations at the extremities produced by 6-AN in mice

Day					9		9		9		10		10	
Dose (mg/kg)					15		10		10		10		10	
Temperature					23		23		36		23		36	
	Left hind paw	Right hind paw	Left front paw	Right front paw	n	%	n	%	n	%	n	%	n	%
Only	+				42	61	27	79	77	52	7	78	17	71
Hind paw		+			1	1	0	0	1	1	0	0	0	0
Affected	+	+			7	10	4	12	37	25	2	22	5	21
Only			+		0	0	0	0	1	1	0	0	0	0
Front paw				+	5	7	1	3	4	3	0	0	0	0
Affected			+	+	1	1	0	0	0	0	0	0	0	0
Hind and	+			+	8	12	2	6	8	5	0	0	1	4
Front paws	+		+		0	0	0	0	1	1	0	0	0	0
Affected		+		+	1	1	0	0	1	1	0	0	0	0
– double		+	+		0	0	0	0	0	0	0	0	0	0
– triple	+	+		+	4	6	0	0	14	9	0	0	0	0
	+	+	+		0	0	0	0	0	0	0	0	1	4
	+		+	+	0	0	0	0	1	1	0	0	0	0
		+	+	+	0	0	0	0	1	1	0	0	0	0
– all	+	+	+	+	0	0	0	0	3	2	0	0	0	0
Total no. of fetuses					167	100%	302	100%	277	100%	166	100%	166	100%
No. of fetuses malformed (and % malformed fetuses)					69	41%	34	11%	149	66%	9	5%	24	14%

NMRI mice were treated with a single s.c. dose of 6-AN at the stage of pregnancy indicated. The animals were kept at room temperature (23°C) or at 36°C. Fetuses were evaluated on day 18 of gestation. The distribution of malformations of the extremities is shown. In 90%–100% of the malformed fetuses, the *left hind* paw is affected, either alone or in combination with abnormalities at other limbs; the *left front* paw is affected in 2%–4% of the abnormal fetuses only

VI. Abnormalities Produced in Organ Culture and Applicability of Organ Culture Techniques in Teratology

It has been mentioned several times in this review that the induction of abnormalities in the embryo or fetus represents a rather complex situation since many maternal factors have to be controlled or taken into consideration and since many basic parameters of mammalian prenatal development are still poorly understood. It therefore seems desirable to develop simpler model systems which would allow us to study and to evaluate some of the basic processes of prenatal development and the interference by embryotoxic substances in a more approachable way and in the absence of some of the confounding factors. A model system to be used for this purpose would have to be complex enough to permit the study of typical morphogenetic differentiation processes, and yet simple enough to be used on a large-scale basis and in a very reproducible way. For the reasons mentioned, cell and tissue culture systems are not sophisticated or complex enough for such studies.

Two techniques have been used extensively in teratology in recent years and have given satisfactory results for the study of several problems when applied in a critical way:

1. The use of organ culture techniques for the study of typical prenatal morphogenetic differentiation processes; and
2. The in vivo culture of whole embryos over a certain period of time.

Both of these methods have a number of advantages and disadvantages, and the use of both of these techniques allows the coverage of different stages of prenatal development. In general, the cultivation technique using whole embryos works satisfactorily at comparatively early stages of embryonic development, until early organogenesis. Organ culture techniques can be applied successfully during the developmental period following this early stage and they mostly cover late organogenesis. Since several reviews on this topic have been published by us and by some other investigators (*Barrach* et al. 1975; *Cockroft* 1977; *Kochhar* 1975; *Neubert* and *Barrach* 1977a; *Neubert* et al. 1976; *New* 1973) the applicability of these techniques will only be discussed briefly here.

We have used the technique of organ culturing limb buds (*Neubert* and *Barrach* 1977b) from different mammalian species (*Lessmöllmann* et al. 1975) quite extensively in our laboratory in recent years, culturing about 40,000 limb buds in vitro. We have applied different toxicologic, biochemical, morphological and micromorphological, immunohistologic, and other methods to the study of the development of cartilaginous bone anlagen in these systems and the effect of drugs on these morphogenetic differentiations. A survey of the biochemical results obtained will be given elsewhere (*Barrach* et al. 1980), and the applicability of this technique and of in vitro tests in general is also discussed in detail in another paper (*Neubert* 1980; *Neubert* and *Barrach* 1980; *Barrach* and *Neubert* 1980).

We feel that the in vitro techniques mentioned are extremely valuable for studying the mechanism of teratogenic actions and for obtaining further information on processes of morphogenetic differentiation in mammalian tissue. In our opinion, however, these techniques are less suitable for a "screening" of drugs for a possible teratogenic potential since only a few parameters of prenatal development can be studied. Certain

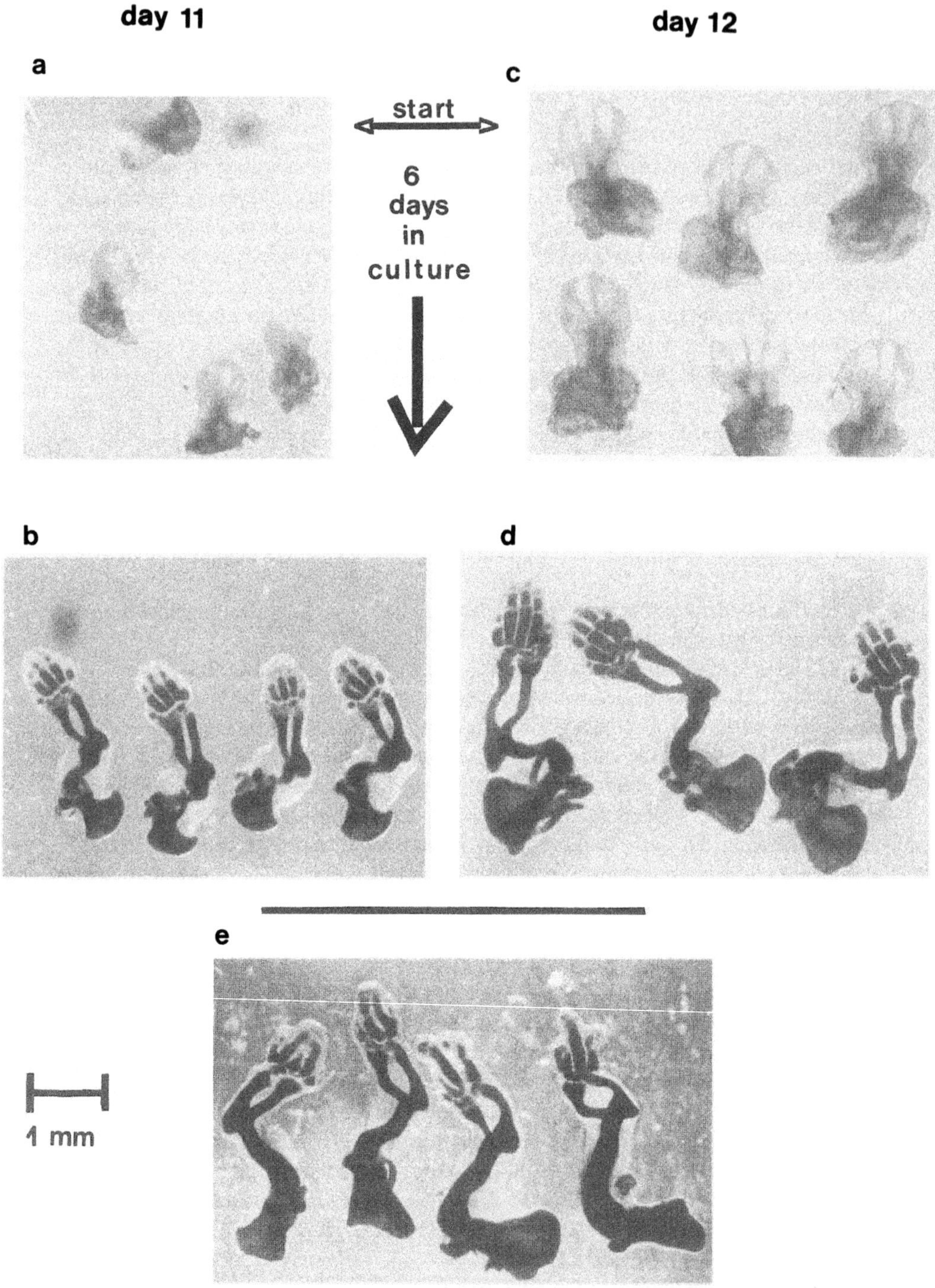

Fig. 41a–e. Organ culture of mouse limb buds. Limb buds from 11-day-old (**a**) or 12-day-old (**c**) mouse embryos were cultured in a chemically defined medium (cf. *Neubert* and *Barrach* 1977; *Barrach* et al. 1978; *Neubert* et al. 1978). Cartilaginous bone anlagen of the extremities can be evaluated after 6 days (**b**) and (**d**) in organ culture. The cartilage is stained with alcian blue. Photograph (**e**) gives an example of an abnormality induced by adding a teratogen to the culture medium

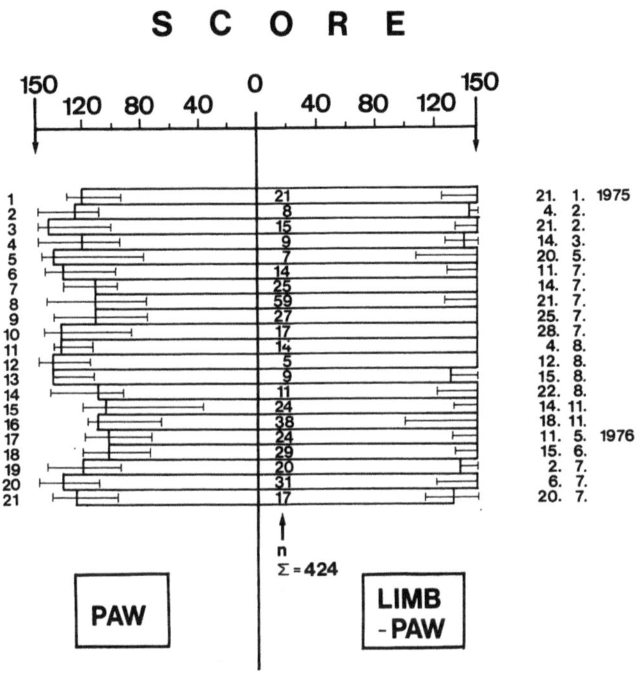

Fig. 42. Variation of the differentiation of limb buds in organ culture. Compilation of a number of control experiments performed over a period of 1 1/2 years with early 11-day-old mouse embryos in a suspension culture. At the stage used in these studies not all of the phalanges developed. A complete paw skeleton is obtained when the culture is started with 12-day-old mouse embryos

effects produced by the "specific" teratogenic agents will only show up in an in vitro system if the right differentiation process is studied.

We have been able to standardize our organ culture system and consider it a routine procedure in our laboratory (*Neubert* et al. 1974a). Starting with limb buds from 10.5- or, better, 11- to 12-day-old mouse embryos, we achieve good differentiation in culture, from the blastema stage or early differentiation stages to well-developed and recognizable cartilaginous bone anlagen of the long bones and the paw skeleton (Fig. 41). The reproducibility of the method is excellent if the somite stage at which the limb buds are put into culture is carefully controlled. Using a score system (*Neubert* et al. 1978), it can be shown that the variability of the outcome of the culturing is rather low (Fig. 42).

Using a variety of different compounds with known teratogenic actions, we have been able to produce abnormalities resembling typical malformations as they are seen in in vivo experiments with the in vitro technique (*Neubert* et al. 1974b; *Neubert* et al. 1977). Several experimental setups are possible and the limb buds from treated animals can be cultured or the drug may be added to the culture medium in which normal limbs are developing. A typical abnormality as it can be achieved entirely in vitro is shown in Fig. 41. It should be mentioned that by using different teratogenic compounds it is possible to produce abnormalities which are confined to the paw skeleton or to the "long bones" (*Barrach* et al. 1978).

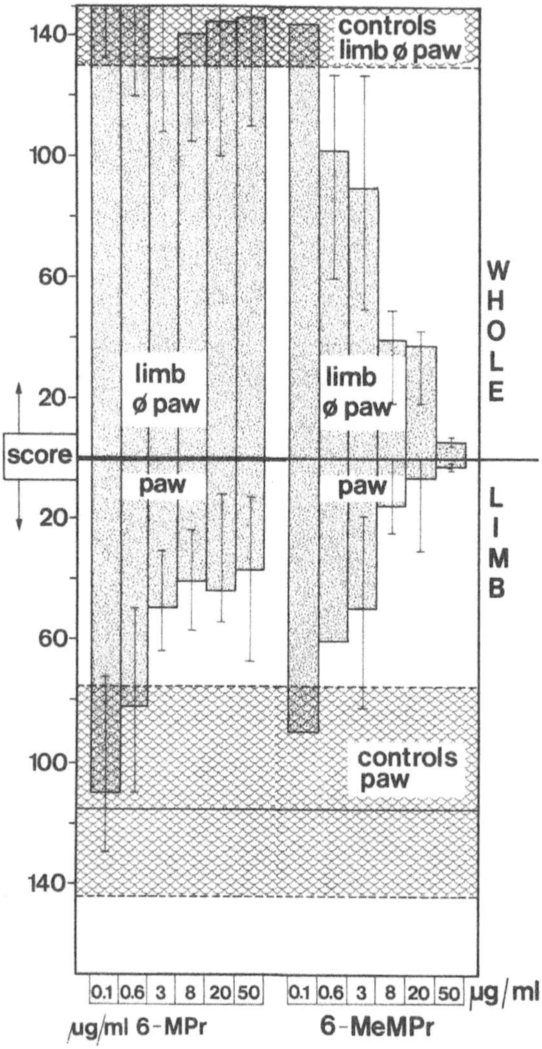

Fig. 43. Quantitative evaluation of an impairment of the differentiation in organ culture produced by 6-mercaptopurine riboside or *6-methyl*mercaptopurine riboside. Quantification was performed with a scoring system developed in our laboratory (*Neubert* et al. 1978). It can be seen that a dose-response relationship can be established and that the patterns of abnormality differ with the two compounds used

With the score system mentioned it has been possible to evaluate drug effects on a semiquantitative basis. An example of such an evaluation is given in Fig. 43. It can be seen that the chemically closely related substances 6-mercaptopurine-riboside and 6-methylmercaptopurine-riboside act on the differentiating limb buds in a dose-dependent manner. But the abnormality induced in vitro by the two substances in quite different: while the effect of 6-mercaptopurine-riboside is confined to the paw skeleton,

Table 13. Some advantages and disadvantages of in vitro methods used in teratologic studies

Advantages	Disadvantages
1) Maternal, nutritional, hormonal, and other factors may be excluded.	1) Complex interactions characteristic for in vivo development cannot be evaluated and the system may only in part resemble in vivo conditions.
2) Drug concentration may be defined more easily. Time of exposure to a drug may be changed systematically. Known metabolites may be tested separately.	2) A possible action of unknown, less characterized, or unstable metabolites may not be recognized.
3) Simpler experimental conditions than in vivo. Biochemical studies, e.g., labeling with radioactive isotopes, are facilitated or rendered possible.	3) Certain embryotoxic effects may not be recognized (growth retardation, embryomortality, prenatally induced defects with postnatal manifestations, etc.).
4) In vitro systems often respond with lower standard deviation than obtained with in vivo studies.	4) Abnormal development may occur in vitro due to certain conditions in culture (false positive) or abnormal reactions found in vivo may not occur in vitro (false negative).

the derivative 6-methylmercaptopurine-riboside equally effects the differentiation of the long bones. This example indicates the specificity of an effect which can be obtained with an in vitro system.

Some of the advantages and disadvantages of the use of in vitro systems in prenatal toxicology are compiled in Table 13. At the moment, we do not feel that the in vitro techniques are capable of replacing in vivo studies, but that they are rather useful additional tools in teratologic research.

VII. Concluding Remarks

Remarkable progress has been made in recent years in research in the field of prenatal toxicology. But prenatal toxicology still has to be regarded as a rather young field of toxicology and much more basic information is needed on almost all levels – biological, biochemical, morphological, toxicologic, and others – before a reliable risk evaluation with respect to the human situation can be attempted, and certainly before human hazards due to prenatally acting agents can be prevented with a high degree of efficiency.

The experience of the last decade has clearly shown that a purely macroscopic, descriptive approach to the field of prenatal toxicology is no longer justified and all the techniques available in modern toxicology must also be applied in teratologic research. Many of the basic problems we are faced with in prenatal toxicology are similar to those in other fields of toxicology. The main problem is still to achieve a quantitative risk assessment for humans from data obtained in animal experiments.

It is still hard to decide whether it is justified to label a chemical as "teratogen." We prefer to state that a compound has a "teratogenic potential" under certain experimental conditions, and it has to be evaluated whether this potential will express itself under defined conditions in humans. At the moment we are still far from being able to satisfactorily make such predictions in the field of teratology, but it should be remembered that the situation is not so different in other fields of toxicology, such as research in mutagenicity or carcinogenicity.

The overlapping of mutagenic, carcinogenic, and teratogenic effects provide an especially challenging field for further research, and many results obtained in one of the three fields will broaden the basis for an understanding of the other toxic actions. This not only applies to the important area of transplacental carcinogenesis, but also to the largely unsolved problems of whether and to what extent a prenatally induced abnormality, which may manifest itself as structural abnormality or even a functional anomaly, may predispose the individual and increase the susceptibility to additional toxic events in adult life, including carcinogenicity.

Acknowledgments: We wish to express our appreciation to *Christiane Duerkop* for her work in producing the figures and *Ulla Schwikowsky* for her work in photography as well as *Susanne Barrach* and *Ruth Kreft* for their help in preparing this manuscript.

Original work mentioned in this paper was supported by grants from Deutsche Forschungsgemeinschaft given to Sfb 29 ("Embryonal-Pharmakologie") at Free University, Berlin.

VIII. Glossary of Terms Used in Prenatal Toxicology

(According to *Neubert* et al. 1978, Role of Pharmacokinetics in Prenatal and Perinatal Toxicology, Georg Thieme Publ. Stuttgart).

Embryo[1]	Developmental stages from the fertilized egg up to the end of organogenesis phase
Fetus	Developmental stages from the end of organogenesis up to birth
Perinatal period	Period around birth, including late fetal and early postnatal life
Embryotoxic or fetotoxic effect, embryotoxicity[1]	All possible types of toxic effects interfering with prenatal development
Abnormality, anomaly	Every structural or functional deviation from normal development
Teratogenic effect teratogenicity[2]	Embryotoxic effect leading to structural abnormalities
Malformation	Structural (gross morphological) abnormality or defect
Embryolethal or fetolethal effect embryo- or fetomortality	Embryotoxic effect incompatible with life
Growth retardation	Embryotoxic effect resulting in a too-small-for-age-fetus; either immature or small but mature
Transplacental carcinogenesis	Fetotoxic (or embryotoxic) effect leading to the development of a tumor in postnatal life caused by an agent applied prenatally
Day 0 of pregnancy[3] (= 1st day of pregnancy) or of gestation[4]	First 24-hour period following conception or mating

1 The term "embryo" is often used to denominate all stages of prenatal development. In this case an "embryotoxic effect" might also be induced late in gestation

2 The term "teratogenic" is often incorrectly used to denominate an "embryotoxic effect"

3 With regard to mother

4 With regard to embryo

References

Adhami H, Noack W (1975) Histological effects of 6-mercaptopurine on the fetal rat central nervous system: A light microscopical study. Teratology 11: 297–312

Asisi A, Merker H-J (1975) Über eine besondere Form der Extremitätenmißbildung bei Ratten nach Gaben von 6-Merkaptopurin am Tag 12 der Schwangerschaft. Drug Res 25: 1924–1926

Babiarz BS, Wee EL, Zimmerman EF (1979) Palate morphogenesis. III. Changes in cell shape and orientation during shelf elevation. Teratology 20: 249–278

Barr M, Brent RL (1970) The relation of the uterine vasculature to fetal growth and the intrauterine position effect in rats. Teratology 3: 251–260

Barrach H-J (1973) Untersuchungen über die Aktivität einiger Fermente des oxidativen Teils des Pentose-Phosphat-Weges im embryonalen Säugetiergewebe und die Beeinflussung durch 6-Aminonicotinamid. Inaugural-Dissertation. Med Fachbereiche, Freie Universität Berlin

Barrach H-J, Baumann I, Neubert D (1978) The applicability of in vitro systems for the evaluation of the significance of pharmacokinetic parameters for the induction of an embryotoxic effect. In: Neubert D, Merker H-J, Nau H, Langman J (eds) Role of pharmacokinetics in prenatal and perinatal toxicology. Georg Thieme Publ, Stuttgart, pp 323–336

Barrach H-J, Grundmann K, Kittel J, Neubert D (1980) Some biochemical and toxicological aspects of mammalian limb development, Conference on Teratology, Carcinogenicity, and Mutagenicity, Sept 17–19, 1979. Hunt Valley Md, USA, in press

Barrach H-J, Neubert D (1980) Significance of organ culture techniques for evaluation of prenatal toxicity. Arch Toxicol 45: 161–187

Barrach H-J, Rautenberg M, Tapken S, Neubert D (1975) Some biochemical characteristics of mouse limb buds differentiating in organ culture. In: Neubert D, Merker H-J (eds) New approaches to the evaluation of abnormal embryonic development. Georg Thieme Publ, Stuttgart, pp 114–132

Bass R (1975) Significance of mitochondrial function for embryonic development: Proposal of a mechanism for the induction of embryolethal effects. In: Neubert D, Merker H-J (eds) New approaches to the evaluation of abnormal embryonic development. Georg Thieme Publ, Stuttgart, pp 524–541

Bass R, Bochert G, Merker H-J, Neubert D (1977) Some aspects of teratogenesis and mutagenesis in mammalian embryos. J Toxicol Environment Health 2: 1353–1374

Bass R, Oerter D (1977) Embryonic development and mitochondrial function. Naunyn-Schmiedeberg's Arch Pharmacol 296: 191–197

Bass R, Schütte I, Nau H (1978) Placental transfer and fetal distribution of thiamphenicol in pregnant rats and humans. In: Neubert D, Merker H-J, Nau H, Langman J (eds) Role of pharmacokinetics in prenatal and perinatal toxicology. Georg Thieme Publ, Stuttgart, pp 507–518

Bass R, Ulbrich B, Welsch F (1978) Thiamphenicol: In vitro accumulation by human placenta and correlation with inhibition of mitochondiral protein synthesis in human and rat placental and fetal mitochondria. In: Neubert D, Merker H-J, Nau H, Langman J (eds) Role of pharmacokinetics in prenatal and perinatal toxicology. Georg Thieme Publ, Stuttgart, pp 519–525

Beck F (1970) Embryonic utilization of histiotroph. In: Bass R, Beck F, Merker H-J, Neubert D, Randhan B (eds) Metabolic pathways in mammalian embryos during organogenesis and its modification by drugs. Free University Press, Berlin, pp 557–574

Beck F (1975) The ferret as a teratological model. In: Neubert D, Merker H-J (eds) New approaches to the evaluation of abnormal embryonic development. Georg Thieme Publ., Stuttgart, pp 8–20

Beck F, Lloyd JB (1966) The teratogenic effects of azo dyes. Adv Teratol 1: 131–193

Beck F, Lloyd JB (1968) Methods for the study of embryotrophic nutrition. Lab Anim 2: 157

Beck F, Lloyd JB, Griffiths A (1967) Lysosomal enzyme inhibition by trypan blue: a theory of teratogenesis. Science (NY) 157: 1180–1182

Becker BA (1974) The statistics of teratology. Teratology 9: 261–262

Bochert G, Rahm U, Schnieders B (1978) Pharmacokinetics of embryotoxic direct acting agents: Comparison of DNA alkylation of various maternal tissues and the embryo during organogenesis. In: Neubert D, Merker H-J, Nau H, Langman J (eds) Role of pharmacokinetics in prenatal and perinatal toxicology. Georg Thieme Publ, Stuttgart, pp 235–251

Bruce NW (1972) Resistance of the rat embryo to ligation of a uterine artery early in gestation. J Reprod Fert 28: 265–267

Brummett ES, Johnson EM (1979) Morphological alterations in the developing fetal rat limb due to maternal injection of chlorambucil. Teratology 20: 279–288

Brunnemann A, Coper H, Neubert D (1964) Biosynthese und Wirkung des 6-Aminonicotinamid-adenindinucleotids (6-ANAD). Naunyn-Schmiedeberg's Arch exp Path Pharmak 246: 437–451

Burki HJ (1974) Mammalian cells: Damage in later replicating DNA as the most efficient cause of reproductive death. Exp Cell Res 87: 277–280

Burton K (1956) A study of the conditions and mechanisms of the reaction for the calometric estimation of deoxyribosenucleic acid. Biochem J 62: 315–323

Caplan AI, Koutroupas S (1973) The control of muscle and cartilage development in the chick limb: The role of differential vascularization. J Embryol Exp Morphol 29: 571–583

Christie GA (1966) Influence of thyroid function on the teratogenic activity of trypan blue in the rat. J Anat 100: 361–368

Coper H, Herken H (1963) Schädigung des Zentralnervensystems durch Antimetaboliten des Nicotinsäureamids. Dtsch med Wschr 41: 1979–1990

Coper H, Lison H, Rommelspacher H, Schulze G, Strauss S (1971) The influence of adrenergic receptor-blocking agents, amphetamine, and 6-aminonicotinamide on thermoregulation. Naunyn-Schmiedebergs Arch Pharmak 270: 378–391

Coper H, Neubert D (1964) Einfluß von NADP-Analogen auf die Reaktionsgeschwindigkeit einiger NADP-bedürftiger Oxydoreduktasen. Biochim Biophys Acta 89: 23–32

Crockroft DL (1977) Post implantation embryo culture. In: Neubert D, Merker H-J, Kwasigroch T.E. (eds) Methods in prenatal toxicology. Georg Thieme Publ, Stuttgart, pp 231–240

Davis HW, Sauter RW (1977) Fluorescence of trypan blue in frozen-dried embryos of the rat. Histochemistry 54: 177–189

Dencker L (1977) Trypan blue accumulation in the embryonic gut of rats and mice during the teratogenic phase. Teratology 15: 179–184

Dietrich LS, Friedland IM, Kaplan LA (1958) Pyridine nucleotide metabolism: Mechanism of action of the niacin antagonist 6-aminonicotinamide. J Biol Chem 233: 964–968

Dixon M, Webb EC (1958) Enzyme techniques. In: Enzymes, 8–34, Academic Press Inc, New York

Edwards MJ, Wanner RA (1977) Cause of maldevelopment; extremes of temperature. In: Wilson JG, Fraser FC (eds) Handbook of teratology, vol I. Plenum Press, New York London, pp 421–444

Epping J (1972) Untersuchungen über das fetale und placentare Wachstum in Abhängigkeit von Implantationsort, Resorptionen, Anzahl der Implantationen und uteriner Blutversorgung. Inaugural Dissertation. Med Fachbereiche, Freie Universität Berlin

Ferguson MWJ (1978) Palatal elevation in the Wistar rat fetus. J Anat 125: 555–577

Franklin JB, Brent RL (1964) The effect of uterine vascular clamping on the development of rat embryos three to fourteen days old. J Morph 115: 273–286

Geber WF (1969) Angiotensin teratogenicity in the fetal hamster. Life Sci 8: 525–531

Gillman J, Gilbert C, Gillman T, Spence I (1948) A preliminary report on hydrocephalus, spina bifida, and other congenital anomalies in the rat produced by trypan blue. S Afr J med Sci 13: 47–90

Goldstein M, Pinsky MF, Fraser FC (1963) Genetically determined organ specific responses to the teratogenic action of 6-aminonicotinamide in the mouse. Genet Res Camb 4: 258–265

Gottschewski GHM (1964) Mammalian blastopathies due to drugs. Nature 201: 1232–1233

Grauwiler J, Schön H (1973) Teratological experiments with ergotamine in mice, rats and rabbits. Teratology 7: 227–236

Greene RM, Kochhar DM (1975) Some aspects of corticosteroid-induced cleft palate. A review. Teratology 11: 47–55

Grünberg H (1963) The pathology of development. Blackwell Scientific Publ, Oxford

Hassel JR, Pratt RM (1977) Elevated levels of c-AMP alters the effect of epidermal growth factor in vitro on programmed cell death in the secondary palatal epithelium. Exp Cell Res 106: 55–62

Healy MJR (1972) Animal litters as experimental units. Appl Stat 21: 155–159

Herbst AL, Poskanzer DC, Robboy SJ, Friedlander L, Scully RE (1975) Prenatal exposure to stilbestrol. A prospective comparison of exposed female offspring with unexposed controls. New Engl J Med 292: 334–339

Herbst AL, Robboy SJ, Scully RE, Poskanzer DC (1974) Clear-cell adenocarcinoma of the vagina and cervix in girls: analysis of 170 registry cases. Amer J Obstet Gynecol 119: 713–724

Herbst AL, Ulfelder H, Poskanzer D (1971) Adenocarcinoma of the vagina, association of maternal stilbestrol therapy with tumor appearance in young women. New Engl J Med 284: 878–881

Herken H, Lange K, Kolbe H (1969) Brain disorders induced by pharmacological blockade of the pentose phosphate pathway. Biochem Biophys Res Communs 36: 93–100

Herken H, Lange K, Kolbe H, Keller K (1974) Antimetabolic action on the pentose phosphate pathway in the central nervous system induced by 6-aminonicotinamide. In: Genazzani E, Herken H (eds) Central nervous system – Studies on metabolic regulation and function. Springer, Berlin Heidelberg New York, pp 41–54

Herken R (1980) Cell cycle phase specificity of hydroxyurea and its effects on the cell kinetics in embryonic spinal cord. Teratology 21: 9–14

Herken R, Schäfer G (1980) Autoradiographic investigation on cell cycle phase specificity of 6-mercaptopurine, in preparation

Herken R, Merker H-J, Krowke R (1978) Investigation of the effect of hydroxyurea on the cell cycle and the development of necrosis in the embryonic CNS of mice. Teratology 18: 103–118

Holmes LB, Trelstad RL (1979) The early limb deformity caused by Acetazolamide. Teratology 20: 289–296

Horakova K, Navarova J, Paterson ARP (1974) The delayed cytotoxic effect of 6-mercaptopurine. Biochim Biophys Acta 366: 333–340

Hurley LS (1977) Nutritional deficiencies and excesses. In: Wilson JG, Fraser FC (eds) Handbook of teratology, vol I. Plenum Press, New York London, pp 261–308

Hurley LS, Cosens G (1970) Teratogenic magnesium deficiency in pregnant rats. Teratology 3: 202 (abstract)

Hurley LS, Everson GJ, Wooten E, Asling CW (1961) Disproportionate growth in offspring of manganese-deficient rats. I. The long bones. J Nutrit 74: 274–282

Hurley LS, Gowan J, Swenerton H (1971) Teratogenic effects of short-term and transitory zinc deficiency in rats. Teratology 4: 199–204

Hurley LS, Mutch PB (1973) Prenatal and postnatal development after transitory gestational zinc deficiency in rats. J Nutrit 103: 649–657

Hurley LS, Swenerton H (1966) Congenital malformation resulting from zinc deficiency in rats. Proc Soc exp Biol Med 123: 692–696

Johnson WJ, McColl JD (1955) 6-aminonicotinamide, a potent nicotinamid antagonist. Science 122: 834

Johnson WJ, McColl JD (1956) Antimetabolite activity of 6-aminonicotinamide. Fed Prod 15: 284

Jusko WJ (1972) Pharmacodynamic principles in chemical teratology: dose effect relationships. J Pharmacol exp Ther 183: 469–480

Kalter H (1974) Choice of the number of sampling units in teratology. Teratology 9: 257–258

Kerr JFR (1972) Shrinkage necrosis of adrenal cartical cells. J Path 107: 217–219

Klingner S (1978) Licht und elektronenmikroskopische Untersuchungen an Mäusefoeten nach Gaben von b-aminoproprionitril. Dissertationsarbeit, Freie Universität Berlin

Kocher W (1977) Action and interaction of chemical and genetic factors in teratogenesis of the limb. In: Bergsma D, Lenz W (eds) Morphogenesis and malformation of the limb, birth defects, original article series vol XIII, 1. Alan Liss Inc, New York, pp 1–18

Kochhar DM (1975) The use of in vitro procedures in teratology. Teratology 11: 273–288

Koehler E, Barrach H-J, Neubert D (1970) Inhibition of NADP dependent oxidoreductases by the 6-aminonicotinamide analogue of NADP. FEBS Letters 6: 225 228

Krowke R, Neubert D (1977) Embryonic intermediary metabolism under normal and pathological conditions. In: Wilson JG, Fraser FC (eds) Handbook of teratology, vol 2, Mechanisms and pathogenesis. Plenum Press, New York London, pp 117–151

Krowke R, Siebert G, Neubert D (1971) Biochemical screening test with ^{14}C-glucose and ^{32}P-phosphate for the evaluation of embryotoxic effects in vivo. Naunyn-Schmiedeberg's Arch Pharmak 271: 274–288

Landauer W (1959) The phenocopy concept: Illusion or reality. Experientia 15: 409–412

Lane JM, Dehm P, Prockop DJ (1971) Effect of a proline analogue azetidin-2-carboxylic acid on collagen synthesis in vivo. I. Arrest of collagen accumulation in growing chick embryos. Biochim Biophys Acta 236: 517–527

Larsson KS (1962) Closure of secondary palate and its relation to sulfomucopolysaccharides. Acta Odontol Scand 20, Suppl 31: 1–35

Leist KH, Grauwiler J (1974) Ergometrine and uteroplacental blood supply in pregnant rats. Teratology 10: 316 (abstract)

Lenz W (1973) Phenocopies. J Med Genet 10: 34–49

Lessmöllmann U, Hinz N, Neubert D (1976) In vitro system for toxicological studies on the development of mammalian limb buds in a chemically defined medium. Arch Toxicol 36: 169–176

Lessmöllmann U, Neubert D, Merker H-J (1975) Mammalian limb buds differentiating in vitro as a test system for the evaluation of embryotoxic effects. In: Neubert D, Merker H-J (eds) New approaches to the evaluation of abnormal embryonic development. Georg Thieme Publ, Stuttgart, pp 99–113

Levene CI, Bates CJ, Baily AJ (1972) Biosynthesis of collagen cross links in cultured 3T6-fibroblasts. Effects of lathyrogens and ascorbic acid. Biochim Biophys Acta 263: 574–582

Lix M (1975) Die Wirkung von Tetrazyklin auf die Skelettentwicklung von Rattenfoetus. Dissertationsarbeit, Freie Universität Berlin

Lloyd JB (1970) Histiotrophic nutrition – a target for "macromolecular" teratogens in rats. In: Bass R, Beck F, Merker H-J, Neubert D, Randhahn B (eds) Metabolic pathways in mammalian embryos during organogenesis and its modification by drugs. Free University Press, Berlin, pp 575–592

Marley PB, Robson JM, Sullivan FM (1967) Embryotoxic and teratogenic action of 5-hydroxytryptamine: Mechanism of action in the rat. Br J Pharmac Chemother 31: 494–505

Merker H-J (1977) Consideration on the problem of critical period. In: Birth defects. Series of the national foundation. Alan Liss Inc, New York, pp 179–202

Merker H-J (1977) Considerations on the problem of critical period during the development of limb skeleton. In: Bergsma D, Lenz W (eds) Morphogenesis and malformation of the limb, birth defects: Original article series, vol XIII, 1. Alan Liss Inc, New York, pp 179–202

Merker H-J, Franke L, Günther Th (1975) The effect of D-penicillamine on the skeletal development of rat foetuses. Naunyn-Schmiedeberg's Arch exp Pharmac 287: 359–376

Merker H-J, Kress K, Kocher W (1980) The relation between hypoplasa, teratogenic risk and pattern of skeleton malformation in rats after application of 6-mercaptopurine. In preparation

Merker H-J, Novak L (1970) Störungen der Zahnentwicklung bei Rattenembryonen nach Gaben von 6-Aminonicotinamid. Experientia 26: 1127

Merker H-J, Novak L, Zimmermann B (1970) Electron microscopic studies on the effect of 6-aminonicotinamid on the mammalian embryos. Naunyn-Schmiedeberg's Arch exp Pharmac 266: 401(A0)

Merker H-J, Pospisil M, Meves P (1975) Cytotoxic effects of 6-mercaptopurine on the limb-bud blastemal cells of rat embryos. Teratology 18: 103–118

Merker H-J, Wedell J, Neubert D (1964) Biochemische und strukturelle Veränderungen an den Zellorganellen der Leber nach vollständiger Kreislauf-Unterbrechung. Naunyn-Schmiedeberg's Arch Pharmac 249: 85–116

Milaire J (1977) Histochemical expression of morphogenetic gradients during limb morphogenesis. In: Bergsma D, Lenz W (eds) Morphogenesis and malformation of the limb, birth defects: Original article series vol XIII, 1. Alan Liss Inc, New York, pp 37–67

Nau H, Neubert D (1978) Development of drug-metabolizing monooxygenase systems in various mammalian species including man. Its significance for transplacental toxicity. In: Neubert D, Merker H-J, Nau H, Langman J (eds) Role of pharmacokinetics in prenatal and perinatal toxicology. Georg Thieme Publ, Stuttgart, pp 13–44

Neubert D (1978) Bedeutung pharmakokinetischer Parameter für die Teratologie. In: Schnieders B, Stille G, Grosdanoff P (eds) Embryotoxikologische Probleme der Arzneimittelforschung, AMI-Berichte 1/78. Dietrich Reimer Verlag, Berlin, pp 83–88

Neubert D (1980) Prospektive in-vitro-Modelle als Ersatz für Langzeituntersuchungen. In: Schnieder B, Grosdanoff P (eds) Zur problematik von chronischen Toxizitätsprüfungen. Dietrich Remmer, Berlin (AMI-Berichte 1/1980, pp 277–287)

Neubert D, Barrach H-J (1977) Significance of in vitro techniques for the evaluation of embryotoxic effects. In: Neubert D, Merker H-J, Kwasigroch TE (eds) Methods in prenatal toxicology, evaluation of embryotoxic effects in experimental animals. Georg Thieme Publ, Stuttgart, pp 202–210

Neubert D, Barrach H-J (1977) Techniques applicable to study morphogenetic differentiation of limb buds in organ culture. In: Neubert D, Merker H-J, Kwasigroch TE (eds) Methods in prenatal toxicology, evaluation of embryotoxic effects in experimental animals. Georg Thieme Publ, Stuttgart, pp 241–251

Neubert D, Barrach H-J (1977) Organotropic effects and dose-response relationship in teratology. In: Neubert D, Merker H-J, Kwasigroch TE (eds) Methods in prenatal toxicology, evaluation of embryotoxic effects in experimental animals. Georg Thieme Publ, Stuttgart, pp 405–412

Neubert D, Barrach H-J (1978) Special aspects of pre- and perinatal toxicology and pharmacology. Advances Pharmacol Therapeut 8: 71–79

Neubert D, Barrach H-J (1980) Effect of environmental agents on embryonic development and the applicability of in vitro techniques for teratological testing, toxicity testing of environmental agents: Current and future requirements. NATO Advanced Study Institute, Monte Carlo, 23–29 Sept 1979. In press
Neubert D, Dillmann I (1972) Embryotoxic effects in mice treated with 2,4,5-trichlorodibenzo-p-dioxin. Naunyn-Schmiedeberg's Arch Pharmacol 272: 243–264
Neubert D, Hinz N, Baumann I, Barrach H-J (1978) Attempt upon a quantitative evaluation of the degree of differentiation of or the degree of interference with development in organ culture. In: Neubert D, Merker H-J, Nau H, Langman J (eds) Role of pharmacokinetics in prenatal and perinatal toxicology. Georg Thieme Publ, Stuttgart, pp 337–349
Neubert D, Lessmöllmann U, Hinz N, Dillmann I, Fuchs G (1977) Interference of 6-mercaptopurine riboside, 6-methylmercaptopurine riboside and azathioprine in the morphogenetic differentiation of mouse extremities in vivo and in organ culture. Naunyn-Schmiedeberg's Arch Pharmacol 298: 93–105
Neubert D, Merker H-J, Barrach H-J, Lessmöllmann U (1976) Biochemical and teratological aspects of mammalian limb bud development in vitro. In: Ebert JD, Marois M (eds) Tests of teratogenicity in vitro. North-Holland Publ Comp, Amsterdam, pp 335–365
Neubert D, Merker H-J, Köhler E, Krowke R, Barrach H-J (1971) Biochemical aspects of teratology. Advances in Biosciences 6: 575–621
Neubert D, Merker H-J, Nau H, LangmanY (eds) (1978) Role of pharmacokinetics in prenatal and perinatal toxicology, 3rd Symposium on prenatal development, Berlin 1978. Georg Thieme Publ, Stuttgart
Neubert D, Merker H-J, Tapken S (1974a) Comparative studies on the prenatal development of mouse extremities in vivo and in organ culture. Naunyn-Schmiedeberg's Arch Pharmacol 286: 251–270
Neubert D, Takpen S, Merker H-J (1974b) Induction of skeletal malformations in organ cultures of mammalian embryonic tissues. Naunyn-Schmiedeberg's Arch Pharmacol 286: 271–282
Neubert D, Zens P, Rothenwallner A, Merker H-J (1973) A survey of the embryotoxic effects of TCDD in mammalian species. Environment Health Perspect 5: 67–79
New DAT (1973) Studies on mammalian fetuses in vitro during the period of organogenesis. In: Austin CR (ed) The mammalian fetus in vitro, Chap 2. Chapman and Hall, London, pp 15–65
Nimni ME, Deshmukh K, Deshmukh A (1970) Mechanism of inhibition of collagen crosslinking and depolymerisation of an incomplete crosslinked form of insoluble collagen caused by D-penicillamin. In: Chemistry and molecular biology of the intercellular matrix, vol 1. Academic Press, New York London, pp 417–430
Oerter D, Bass R (1975) Embryonic development and mitochondrial function. I. Effects of chloramphenicol infusion on the synthesis of cytochrome oxidase and DNA in rat embryos during late organogenesis. Naunyn-Schmiedeberg's Arch Pharmacol 290: 175–189
Pinsky L, Fraser FC (1960) Congenital malformations after a two-hour inactivation of nicotinamide in pregnant mice. Brit med J 2: 195–197
Pratt RM, Goggins JF, Wilk AL, King CTG (1973) Acid mucopolysaccharide synthesis in the secondary palate of the developing rat at the time of rotation and fusion. Devel Biol 32: 230–237
Reddy DV, Adams FH, Baird C (1963) Teratogenic effect of serotonin. J Pediatr 63: 394–397
Röhnelt M (1975) Teratogenicity of diphosphonates in rats. In: Neubert D, Merker H-J (eds) New approaches to the evaluation of abnormal embryonic development. Georg Thieme, Stuttgart, pp 728–745
Ross LM, Walker BE (1967) Movement of palatine shelves in untreated and teratogen-treated mouse embryos. Am J Anat 121: 509–522
Ross RB, Walker BE (1972) Cleft lip and palate. Williams and Wilkins, Baltimore

Rothenwallner A (1974) Die Auslösung von Gaumenspalten durch simultane Applikation zweier Teratogene bei Mäusen. Inaugural-Dissertation. Fachbereich Zahnheilkunde, Freie Universität Berlin

Roussel C, Tuchmann-Duplessis H (1968) Dissociation des actions embryotoxiques et teratogenes du Triton W.R. 1339 chez la souris. CR Acad Sci (Paris) 266: 2171–2174

Ryzlewicz R (1979) Die Wirkung von 6-Mercaptopurin auf die Nierenentwicklung von Rattenembryonen. Dissertationsarbeit an der Freie Universität Berlin

Sadler TW, Cardell RR (1977) Ultrastructural alterations in neuroepithelial cells of mouse embryos exposed to cytotoxic dosis of hydroxyurea. Anat Rec 188: 103–124

Saxen L (1966) Effect of tetracycline on osteogenesis in vitro. J exp Zool 162: 269–294

Schmidt KL (1979) Electron microscope observations of embryos from maternal rats treated with trypan blue. Teratology 19: 285–304

Schultz PW, Reger JF, Schultz RL (1966) Effects of Triton WR-1339 on the rat yolk sac placenta. Amer J Anat 119: 199–234

Schweichel JV, Merker H-J (1973) The morphology of various types of cell death in prenatal tissues. Teratology 7: 253–256

Scott WJ (1978) Cell death and reduced proliferative rate. In: Wilson JG, Fraser FC (eds) Handbook of teratology, vol 2. Plenum Press, New York London, pp 81–98

Spielmann H (1979) Zur Wirkung von Pharmaka in der Präimplantationsphase der Schwangerschaft am Beispiel von Cyclophosphomid. Habilitationsschrift. Freie Universität Berlin

Spielmann H, Eibs HG (1978) Recent progress in teratology: A survey of methods for the study of long actions on the preimplantation embryo. Drug Res 28: 1733–1738

Spielmann H, Eibs HG, Jacob-Müller U (1979) Cyclophosphamide treatment prior to implantation: The effect on embryonic development. In: Persaud TVN (ed) Advances in the study of birth defects, vol 2. MTP Press, Lancaster, pp 95–112

Staples RE, Haseman JK (1974) Selection of appropriate experimental units in teratology. Teratology 9: 259–260

Summerbell D (1974) Interaction between the proximo-distal and antero-posterior coordinates of positional value during the specification of positional information in the early development of chick limb bud. J Embryol Exp Morphol 32: 227–237

Thompson RS, Gautieri RF (1969) Comparison and analysis of the teratogenic effects of serotonin, angiotensin-II, and Bradykinin in mice. J Pharmac Sci 58: 406–412

Tucci SM, Skalko RG (1978) The teratogenic effects of theophylline in mice. Toxicol Letters 1: 337–341

Tuchmann-Duplessis H (1972) Investigations on the mechanism of action of Triton W. R. 1339. In: Bass R, Beck F, Merker H-J, Neubert D, Randhahn B (eds) Metabolic pathways in mammalian embryos during organogenesis and its modification by drugs. Free University Press, Berlin, pp 205–217

Walker BE, Fraser FC (1956) Closure of the secondary palate in three strains of mice. J Embryol Exp Morphol 4: 176–189

Warkany J, Roth CB (1948) Congenital malformations induced in rats by maternal vitamin A deficiency. II. Effect of varying the preparatory diet upon the yield of abnormal young. J Nutrit 35: 1–12

Warkany J, Schraffenberger E (1943) Congenital malformations induced in rats by maternal nutritional deficiency. V. Effects of purified diet lacking riboflavin. Proc Soc exp Biol Med 54: 92–94

Webster DA, Gross J (1970) Studies on the possible mechanisms of programmed cell death in the chick embryo. Develop Biol 22: 157–184

Webster W, Shimada M, Langman J (1973) Effects of fluorodeoxyuridine, colcemid and bromodeoxydeuridine on developing neocortex of the mouse. Am J Anat 137- 67–86

Weil CS (1970) Selection of the valid number of sampling units and a consideration of their combination in toxicological studies involving reproduction, teratogenesis or carcinogenesis. Fd Casmet Toxicol 8: 177–182

Westermann U (1980) Das Wachstumsverhalten des Unterkiefers von Rattenembryonen nach Applikation von 6-MP. Anat Anz Erg Heft. In press

Wieland Th (1977) Modification of actions by phallotoxins. Naturwissenschaften 64: 303–309

Wilkinson GN (1961) Statistical estimations in enzyme kinetics. Biochem 80: 324–332

Williams JR, Little JB, Shipley WV (1974) Association of mammalian cell death with a specific endonucleolytic degradation of DNA. Nature 252: 754–755

Wilson JG (1966) Effects of acute and chronic treatment with actinomycin D on pregnancy and the fetus in the rat. Harper Hosp Bull 24: 109–118

Wilson JG, Shepard TH, Gennaro JF (1963) Studies on the site of teratogenic action of C^{14}-labelled trypan blue. Anat Rec 145: 300

Wolpert L (1969) Positional information and the spatial pattern of cellular differentiation. J Theor Biol 25: 1–47

Wolpert L (1978) Pattern formation in biological development. Scientific Am 239: 154–164

Drug-Induced Cancer

D. SCHMÄHL* and M. HABS

I. Introduction . . . 333
II. Therapeutic Agents Suspected to Induce Cancer . . . 334
1. Arsenic Trioxide . . . 334
2. Sedatives, Anesthetics, Analgesics, and Antihistamines . . . 335
3. Thiouracil, Isonicotinic Acid Hydrazide, Griseofulvin, and Tannin . . . 339
4. Hormones and Miscellaneous Drugs . . . 340
5. Antineoplastic Agents . . . 343
6. Rauwolfia Derivatives and Artificial Sweeteners . . . 352
7. Nitrosatable Agents . . . 355
8. Transplants . . . 356
III. Conclusions . . . 358
References . . . 359

I. Introduction[1]

Today more than ever, drug-induced effects and diseases are gaining in significance. Two factors seem to be largely responsible for this development:

1. The number of drugs and their uses are increasing constantly.

2. More and more drugs are being developed which have far-reaching effects on physiologic and pathologic biochemical reactions.

It has to be stressed that this paper is not intended to disconcert patients or the public. The physician using drugs has been trained to take acute and subacute toxic side effects of drugs into consideration; nowadays he ought to expand this caution to possible chronic toxicity including carcinogenicity.

In addition, it is necessary to undertake a risk-benefit analysis in each individual case, making sure that therapeutic effects are not outweighed by risk. A carcinogenic effect of a drug which may possibly manifest itself many years or even decades after the therapeutic treatment will hardly be of significance if the case has a poor prognosis or there is no alternative to this therapy. If, however, this is not so, then the physician has to consider whether the potentially hazardous drug should be administered or whether alternatives are at hand.

---

* Dedicated to Professor Dr. W. Doerr, Heidelberg, on the occasion of his 65th birthday

1 See also *Clayson* (1972), *Goerttler* (1972), *Schmähl* et al. (1977), *Thomas* (1972), and *Truhaut* (1967). Added in proof: In 1981 an IARC monograph on the evaluation of the carcinogenic risk of chemicals to humans will be published. This monograph will represent the views and expert opinions of an IARC working group on 18 immunosuppressive and cytostatic drugs

From the point of view of overall cancer incidence, drug-induced malignant tumors do not play a very important role. We assume that worldwide, of 10,000 cancer cases one may be induced by drugs. *Jick* and *Smith* (1977) are of the opinion that less than 1% of all cancers can be correlated with known carcinogenic effects of drugs. It is not known how many drugs carrying a carcinogenic risk are being used at present. These rough estimates should not obscure the fact that certain groups of patients who are subjected to a particularly intensive treatment with carcinogenic drugs run a considerably high risk.

The statistical methods of analytic epidemiology have definite limits in detecting slight increases in the frequency of diseases. If a drug increases the risk of developing a relatively frequent tumor type, its detection will consequently be more difficult than the detection of an increased risk of developing a tumor which seldom occurs in the general public.

It is not easy to identify a drug exerting a carcinogenic activity in man. This is primarily due to the fact that a disease is only seldom treated with one drug; usually several are used. Thus it is very difficult to detect the suspect carcinogen in combination therapy, particularly since several drugs may produce mutually modifying effects (*Habs* and *Schmähl* 1979). Furthermore, the often long induction times of iatrogenic tumors are frequently a hindrance to an epidemiologic approach, particularly if the patient no longer knows which drugs or drug combinations he was treated with many years ago. What is true for the patient is of course also applicable to the physician who – at least as far as experiences in the Federal Republic of Germany are concerned – quite frequently is hardly aware of the problems of iatrogenic carcinogenesis. Consequently, the present chapter is also intended to offer information and supplementary medical training. The discussion of radiation as a carcinogen to man is not dealt with in this chapter.

II. Therapeutic Agents Suspected to Induce Cancer

1. Arsenic Trioxide

The earliest reports (more than 160 years ago) on the carcinogenic activity of a drug concern arsenic, which was mainly administered as arsenic trioxide in Fowler's solution in the treatment of psoriasis (*Braun* 1958; *Ehlers* 1968; *Meyhöfer* and *Knoth* 1966; *Neubauer* 1947; *Petzoldt* 1966). Arsenic is said to induce skin carcinomas preceded by melanokeratosis. It has also been suggested, with less evidence, that arsenic causes bronchiogenic carcinomas as well as carcinomas, sarcomas, and hemangioendotheliomas of the liver (*Lee* and *Fraumeni* 1969). According to *Liebegott* (1949), the latent periods of skin carcinomas are 9–17 years, of liver carcinomas, 11–13 years, and of liver sarcomas, 17–21 years. However, much longer latent periods seem probable. Many of these data were obtained from winegrowers who had previously been subjected to arsenic-containing pesticides. Winegrowers from areas such as Kaiserstuhl, Moselle and Rhine districts, and Beaujolais, developed arsenic-induced malignant tumors (*Braun* 1958; *Galy* et al. 1963; *Liebegott* 1949, 1952; *Pein* 1943; *Roth* 1956, 1957; *Thiers* et al. 1967). *Ivankovic* et al. (1979) described lung carcinomas induced in rats after a single intratracheal instillation of an arsenic-containing insecticidal mixture formerly used in vineyards. The carcinogenic effect of arsenic trioxide in man can be regarded as a known and proven cause of occupational diseases and an iatrogenic carcinogen. Accordingly, many physicians have warned against medications containing arsenic (*Ehlers* 1968; *Fierz* 1965; *Gottron* 1954; *Knoth* 1966; *Minkowitz* 1964; *Petzoldt* 1966; *Robson* and *Jelliffe* 1963; *Schuermann* 1957). Since 1959 at the latest, leading German dermatologists have clearly stated that from the dermatologic point of view there is no need for medications containing arsenic. Nevertheless, in 1968 73% of all practicing dermatologists in the Federal Republic of Germany still used arsenic for the treatment of skin diseases (*Ehlers* 1968). This shows that despite numerous warnings, it often takes a long time until findings which demonstrate the hazard of certain medications result in practical implementation. The frequency of arsenic therapy in use today in dermatology is not known. According to personal communications from several dermatologists, arsenic therapy is hardly used any longer by dermatologists.

In spite of the fact that the overall incidence of iatrogenic cancer is small, in a "high-risk group" of patients treated with arsenic trioxide *Fierz* found (1965) that 40% of 262 patients treated with Fowler's solution developed palmar and plantar hyperkeratoses, 8% of which deteriorated into skin carcinomas. This is clearly quite considerable. The same author demonstrated that although increasing doses caused increasing rates of cancer it is difficult to establish a "threshold dose" which would be considered harmless. In some cases he observed tumors already existing after application of approximately only 1 g arsenic trioxide.

Arsenic trioxide has been recorded as an iatrogenic carcinogen to man since 1820 (*Paris* 1820). But it has taken almost 150 years until this knowledge has become well enough known to stop the therapeutic use of arsenic. This has been made easier since there are not many alternatives. In internal medicine, arsenic was also used in a large number of "tonics" of very doubtful therapeutic value. It has to be stressed again that despite the knowledge of its carcinogenic activity, the compound was still used quite frequently in viniculture in the 1930s and 1940s. These inconsistencies hint at a lack of cooperation between different scientific disciplines, for otherwise the approval of arsenic trioxide as a pesticide would not have occurred. A number of occupational carcinomas in winegrowers could have been prevented.

2. Sedatives, Anesthetics, Analgesics, and Antihistamines

Urethan has been used as a sedative in therapy for a long time. It has also served as a solvent in industrial progesterone preparations which were quite frequently administered in the early stage of pregnancy. Its carcinogenic activity was accidentally detected by *Nettleship* (1943). It induces lung tumors (*Guyer* and *Claus* 1947; *Jaffé* 1947; *Shimkin* 1955) in mice and rats (even in germ-free animals), irrespective of the mode of application (*Burstein* and *McIntire* 1968), and, among others, melanotic tumors (*Revière* et al. 1965) in hamsters. According to investigations performed by *Tannenbaum* and *Silverstone* (1958), the compound has to be considered a "multipotential" carcinogen.

$$H_2N{-}\overset{\overset{\displaystyle O}{\|}}{C}{-}O{-}C_2H_5$$

The authors painted a 20% acetone solution of urethan to the skin of mice for 18 months, applying a total dose of up to 1.8 g/animal. At the site of application, no skin tumors occurred, but lung adenomas, carcinomas of the mammary gland, malignant mesenchymal tumors, cystadenomas of the lacrimal glands, and blood cysts of the liver developed, the malignant nature of which was confirmed by their transplantability (*Trainin* 1963). *Toth* et al. (1961) obtained similar results in hamsters. Urethan also has a carcinogenic effect as an aerosol (*Otto* 1966).

The transplacental effects of urethan were demonstrated by *Klein* (1952, 1954) and *Larsen* (1947). *Klein* injected single doses of 15–75 mg/mouse of urethan into the peritoneal cavity of A-strain mice at a late stage of pregnancy (17th to 19th day). The mice were delivered by Caesarean section. About 6 months after birth, lung tumors were observed at a high percentage not only in the mothers, but even in those offspring that were foster-nursed and did not come into contact with urethan again (up to 100% compared with 7.9% in controls). This even applied to fetuses which were exposed to urethan in utero for only 1 h. These results were not only impressive evidence of the irreversibility of this carcinogenic effect, but also showed that the short period of 1 h in which the fetal tissue was exposed to the carcinogenic activity, sufficed to cause irreversible damage to cells, determining that they would result in tumors. Young or unborn individuals appear more sensitive to the carcinogenic activity of urethan than adults (*Klein* 1966; *Vesselinovitch* and *Mihailovich* 1966).

Urethan is also secreted in breast milk. Mice suckled by urethan-treated mothers developed a high percentage of lung tumors (*Fiore-Donati* et al. 1961). With all this evidence it is hard to understand why urethan is still used in therapy today and is still administered to pregnant women as a solvent for hormone preparations. Although complaints have been raised in medical journals, urethan is, to our knowledge, still in use. So far, however, there is no evidence of carcinogenic effects of urethan in man. We are not aware of any adequate epidemiologic studies, however.

The possibility that certain inhalation anesthetics may have a carcinogenic effect in man is of interest because some of these substances have a striking structural similarity to known potent carcinogens to man (*Corbett* 1976) (see Table 1). In this regard it is not only the possible hazard for the patient that is of concern, but even more for the operating-room staff and in particular for the anesthetists. Dentists, too, may run a risk from occupational exposure to anesthetics. The concentrations of these substances reach about 20 ppm in air to which the anesthetists are exposed over several hours per day. These narcotics can still be detected in the exhalation air of anesthetists 7 h to 3 days after a routine occupational exposure. There is an incomplete report that the rate of malformations was higher among progeny of operating-room nurses who had been exposed to these substances during pregnancy. Three neoplasms have been reported in children whose mothers had worked as anethetists during pregnancy (*Corbett* 1976): a neuroblastoma each of the thyroid and the parathyroid glands and a leukemia. In this case, too – analogous to arsenic – certain drugs can involve not only a potential carcinogenic risk for patients, but also an occupational risk.

In 1978, *Waskell* reported mutagenicity tests of anesthetics and their metabolites. Chloral hydrate – a metabolite of trichloroethylene with sedative activity – proved to be a weak mutagen, whereas halothane, isoflurane, methoxyflurane, diazepam, and chlorodiazepoxide showed no mutagenic activity under experimental conditions. For

Table 1. Comparison of the chemical structures of several known human carcinogens with certain inhalation anesthetic agents (according to *Corbett* 1976)

Carcinogens in man	*Inhalation narcotics*
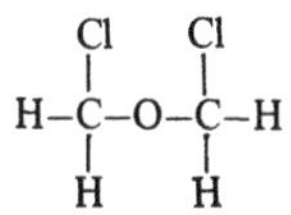 Bis(chloroethyl) ether	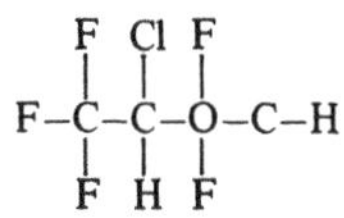 Isoflurane (Forane)
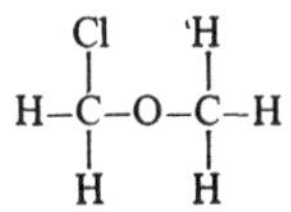 Chloromethyl methyl ether	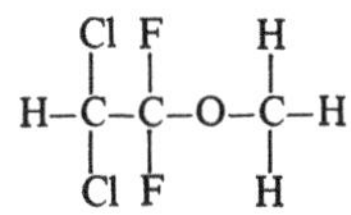 Methoxyflurane (Phenthrane)
	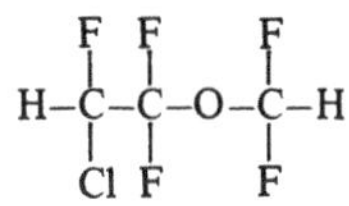 Enflurane (Ethrane)
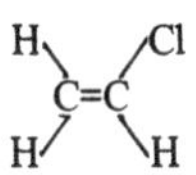 Vinyl chloride	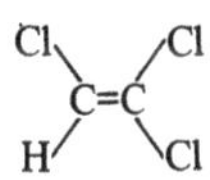 Trichloroethylene

halothane and trilene, a direct interaction with DNA could not be proven. *Baden* et al. (1977) reported that fluroxene (2,2,2-trifluoroethyl vinyl ether) gave a positive reaction after metabolic activation in a mutagenicity test according to Ames. There is an urgent need for studies on the carcinogenicity of inhalation anesthetics in laboratory animals.

Phenobarbital produces liver cell tumors in mice and rats after application of high doses (*Ponomarkov* et al. 1976; *Rossi* et al. 1977), whereas a carcinogenic effect could not be observed after administration of relevant clinical doses (2 mg/kg/week) (*Schmähl* and *Habs* 1976). The liver tumors induced after application of high doses (500 ppm) were similar to those described after application of DDT. Although many authors classified these tumors histologically as definitely malignant, it is still not clear whether this type of tumor may be referred to as a "genuine" neoplasm. Perhaps it is simply a reactive growth induced by a chronic stimulus overstraining the normal metabolic functions of the organ. Epidemiologic investigations on more than 8000 epileptics who had been subjected to phenobarbital medication for years did not demonstrate an increased cancer risk (*Clemmesen* and *Hjalgrim-Jensen* 1978).

In 1965, the suspicion was raised for the first time that after abuse of phenacetin, carcinomas of the renal pelvis may occur (*Hultengren* et al. 1965). Up to 1977, 38 cases of carcinomas of the renal pelvis were reported in the literature, which were possibly caused by phenacetin abuse (*Schmähl* et al. 1977). By 1978, more than 100 cases were known (*Bengtsson* et al. 1978). From 1925 to 1934, before analgesic abuse occurred, *Leistenschneider* and *Ehmann* (1973) observed only one questionable carcinoma of the renal pelvis among 9225 autopsies, whereas in the initial phase of abuse of analgesics (1950–1959) 11 carcinomas of the renal pelvis were observed among 15,635 autopsies, and in the main phase of abuse from 1960 to 1969, 17 cases were found in 21,291 autopsies. These figures suggest that the possible risk of developing a carcinoma of the renal pelvis is low and may be expected only in the case of phenacetin abuse. The experimental findings reported on the carcinogenic activity of phenacetin are contradictory. While *Cuatrecasas* (1978) and *Schmähl* and *Reiter* (1954) did not demonstrate a carcinogenic effect in experimental animals, *Isaka* et al. (1979) and *Johansson* and *Angervall* (1976, 1979) claim to have found one. It is interesting to speculate as to whether this carcinogenic activity is due to genotoxic effects or whether the mechanism is epigenetic resulting from the overt damage caused by large doses and that the existence of a safe dose, i.e., a dose at which no carcinogenic risk can be detected, may be envisaged. It would be imprudent to ban such a drug as important as phenacetin because of the rare cases of carcinomas reported after *abuse* of phenacetin, since the benefit of this drug is doubtless higher than the risk, particularly if the prescribed dosage is observed. Perhaps it would be reasonable to require a doctor's prescription for this substance in order to prevent its abuse.

Hydantoin derivatives, which today are frequently administered as anticonvulsants, have also been suspected to induce occasional malignant lymphomas in man (*Beil* and *Prechtel* 1973; *Hyman* and *Sommers* 1966; *Saltzstein* and *Ackermann* 1959; *Wildhack* 1973). Similarly phenylbutazone has been associated with leukemia (*Bean* 1960; *Chalmers* and *McCarthy* 1964; *Lorenz* and *Gebert* 1968; *Schmähl* et al. 1977).

In particular, those drugs which are prescribed for nonfatal diseases or which are often administered to children should be tested for carcinogenicity *prior* to their use in practice, especially if their chemical structure raises the suspicion of such activity (*Schmähl* 1972). A particularly instructive example is 3-phenyl-5β-diethylamino-ethyl-1,2,4-oxadiazole (*Schmähl* 1972)

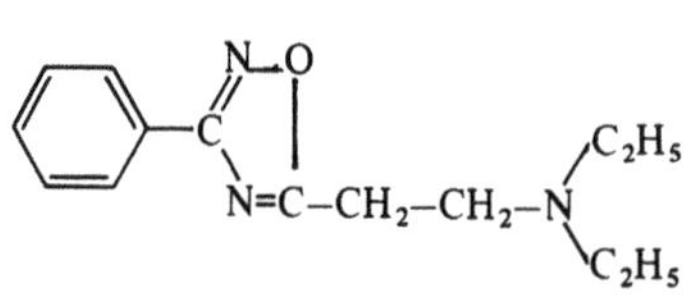

which was intended to be used as a cough medicine. The investigation into carcinogenic effects yielded bladder cancer in rats and dogs (*Barron* 1963), and therefore, the substance was not introduced into therapy.

The antihistaminic drug methapyriline (N,N-dimethyl-N′-(2pyridyl)-N′-(2-thenyl)-ethylenediamine) was recently shown to be carcinogenic in rats. Methapyrilene hydrochloride was mixed with food at a concentration of 0.1% and administered for 64 weeks. The drug induced liver tumors in 92 out of 100 Fischer rats, mainly hepatocellular carcinomas and cholangiocarcinomas. No sex specificity was noted (*Lijinsky* et al. 1980). Methapyrilene and structurally related compounds are presently being investigated in a dose-response study for possible carcinogenic effects in rats at our institute.

3. Thiouracil, Isonicotinic Acid Hydrazide, Griseofulvin and Tannin

Thiouracil, which is used in the therapy of diseases of the thyroid gland, is said to have carcinogenic effects (IARC 1974).

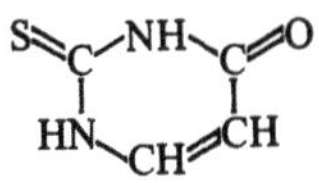

In rats and mice it induces cancer of the thyroid gland and also adenomas of the anterior pituitary lobe. Adenomas of the thyroid gland are also reported to occur in rats after many years' administration of potassium perchlorate (*Kessler* and *Krüskemper* 1966). This finding, however, could not be confirmed by *Osswald* (1968).

A much-discussed problem concerns the experimental findings on the carcinogenic activity of the antitubercular agent isonicotinic acid hydrazide (INH). First observations were reported in 1957 (*Juhasz* et al. 1957). The long-term application of low doses of INH led to an increased occurrence of pulmonary adenomas, lymphosarcomas, and leukemias in mice (*Juhasz* et al. 1963). This effect, however, was not observed in rats (*Peacock* and *Peacock* 1966; *Wolfart* 1960) or hamsters (*Toth* and *Boreisha* 1969). The carcinogenic activity of this substance in mice was repeatedly confirmed (*Biancifiori* and *Severi* 1966; *Mori* et al. 1960; *Toth* and *Rustia* 1967). It induced mainly pulmonary adenomas and occasionally pulmonary carcinomas.

Today INH is used all over the world in the treatment of human tuberculosis, and it has proven to be so effective that ambulatory chemotherapeutic treatment of tuberculosis is sufficient in many cases (*Fox* 1965). So far, no indication or well-founded suspicion relative to a carcinogenic activity of this compound in man has been demonstrated (*Hammond* et al. 1967; *Jung* 1971). However, all these studies suffer from limited duration of observation of INH-treated patients. If the substance were carcinogenic in man, too, we would have to take an induction time of 3 or 4 decades into consideration, as is the case for most known human carcinogens.

INH clearly exemplifies the conflicts which face the clinician who has to decide whether treatment with a possibly carcinogenic drug is justified in man. Benefits and possible hazards have to be weighed in order to arrive at a decision on the use or rejection of the substance. The synthesis of a new substance with the same good antitubercular, but no carcinogenic, activity would doubtless be most desirable.

Griseofulvin, which is occasionally applied in dermatology for the treatment of dermatophytosis, induced hepatomas in mice and tumors of the thyroid gland in rats. In hamsters, however, neoplasms could not be observed (*Epstein* et al. 1967; *Rustia* and *Shubik* 1978).

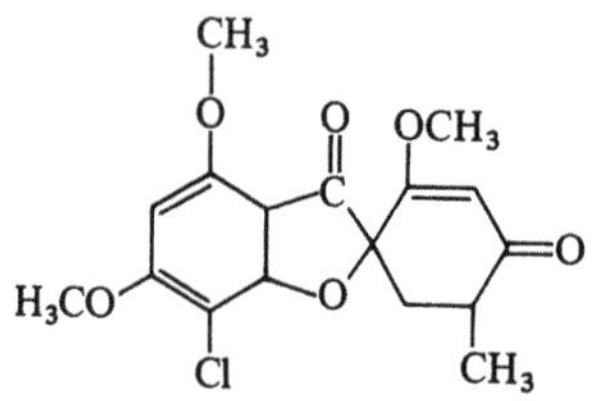

A questionnaire inquiry among 1670 German dermatologists did not establish any evidence of carcinogenic effects in patients treated with griseofulvin (*Götz* and *Reichenberger* 1972).

In this chapter mention should also be made of a naturally occurring substance used in medicine which has a demonstrated carcinogenic effect, namely, tannin (see reference review by *Korpassy* 1961). Its hepatotoxic activity was observed in the wounded of World War II, when extensive burns were treated locally with tannin-containing powders that could be absorbed. These observations initiated closer experimental investigations of the compound with regard to hepatotoxic and carcinogenic effects. In rats tannin induces extensive liver damage with central necroses, hepatic cirrhosis, and cancer after subcutaneous injection of relatively high doses. In mice, however, such alterations could not be observed after application of small doses (*Bichel* and *Bach* 1968). After oral administration liver damage does not occur, because tannin is not, or is only slightly, absorbed through the gastrointestinal tract. Therefore, carcinogenic effects of tannin are not to be expected after oral ingestion, e.g., in tea, wine, or fruits, or for treatment of diarrhea.

In areas with a high tea consumption, such as England and Friesland, no increase in mortality from hepatic cancer has been reported. Attempts to ascribe the local carcinogenicity of plant extracts to their tannin content failed to yield satisfactory results (*Kapadia* et al. 1978).

4. Hormones and Miscellanous Drugs

In 1971, *Herbst* and co-workers demonstrated a strong association between diethylstilbestrol taken during pregnancy and the development of vaginal cancer in female offspring many years later (*Herbst* et al. 1971).

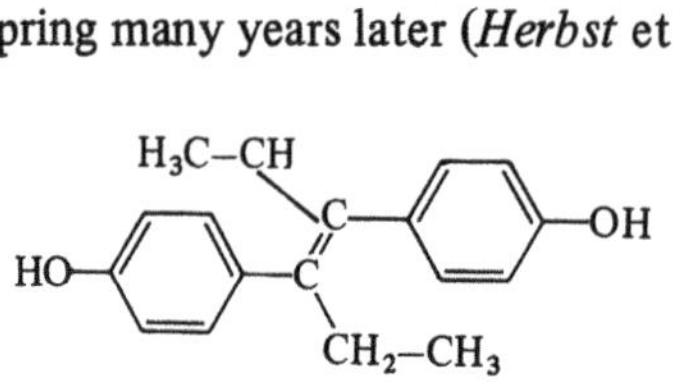

The association between diethylstilbestrol and the clear cell carcinoma of the vagina in young girls whose mothers had been given the compound, in order to prevent a possible abortion, has so far been described in the United States only, but not in German-speaking countries. This may be due to the fact that in these countries natural or synthetic estrogens have not been administered in such high doses for abortion prophylaxis as in the United States (25–100 mg/day), but rather in lower doses in combination with progestogens. *Ulfelder* (1976) described the "syndrome of the stilbestrol-adenosis carcinoma" as one of the few completely new and unexpected medical discoveries of the recent past. Today it is estimated that in the United States about 500,000 to 2 million young women were exposed to diethylstilbestrol in utero, i.e., prenatally. Compared with this large number, the number of clear cell carcinomas of the vagina in exposed offspring observed so far (about 250) is relatively small. Nevertheless, this example of transplacental carcinogenesis induced by diethylstilbestrol shows that we must take transplacental carcinogenic effects of chemical substances into account. It seems, furthermore, that hormonal imbalances in pregnant women may basically condition the development of neonates toward malignant growth of certain organs or organ systems. Comparative and similar results were obtained experimentally in hamsters (*Rustia* and *Shubik* 1976).

The possible "carcinogenic or promoting effect of hormones" has recently received worldwide notice with respect to the widespread administration of contraceptives and anabolic steroids. Remarkably, it has been known since 1941 that estrogens can have a tumor-inducing effect in various animal species (*Gardner* 1941). In man the localization of tumors which can develop due to such hormonal disturbances is essentially restricted to two organs, namely the liver and the endometrium.

In 1970, *Baum* tried to publish the first observations on liver tumors in women who had taken oral contraceptives over a long period of time. However, the editors of the journal to which the paper was submitted rejected the data and the author's conclusions as "ridiculous" (for references see *Klatskin* 1977). Furthermore, the statistical significance of the observations described was doubted. In the early 1970s, the time seemed ripe to communicate such data, and corresponding case reports were published (*Baum* et al. 1973). In 1977, world literature recorded 237 well-documented cases of association between the occurrence of liver tumors and the administration of oral contraceptives. The number of cases reported since then has surely increased considerably, although it seems to be small in comparison with the several million women taking oral contraceptives. The liver tumors observed included histologically benign hepatocellular adenomas up to hepatocellular carcinomas (*Klatskin* 1977; *Scheuer* and *Lehmann* 1977; *Pike* et al. 1977). Since adenomas tend to rupture, patients with adenomas often die from acute hemorrhage into the peritoneal cavity. *Scheuer* and *Lehmann* (1977) published a review of all relevant data in the German literature. Although the causal association between administration of oral contraceptives and the rare occurrence of liver tumors has not yet been accepted generally, it is recommended that young women especially should not take these drugs over a long period without interruption, but should instead take them intermittently (see also Table 2). However, it cannot be guaranteed that longer drug-free intervals in the administration of oral contraceptives will definitely inhibit the risk of tumor induction in predisposed women. It is unknown whether existing alterations in the liver cells will regress during these pauses. Since a dose-time-response relationship seems to exist for the induction of hepatogenic tumors associated with the administration of hormonal contraceptives, a reduction of the tumor risk is likely if the organism is exposed less to these preparations.

Table 2. Duration of the administration of oral contraceptives in 34 case-control pairs (according to *Edmondson* et al. 1976)

Duration (months)	Cases	Controls	Risk
⩽ 12	6	15	1.0
13– 36	4	8	1.3
37– 60	8	7	2.9
61– 84	4	2	5.0
85–108	4	1	10.0
⩾ 109	8	1	20.0

Obviously the risk of inducing liver tumors during treatment with anabolic steroids seems to be less clear. Until 1977, 18 cases had been reported (for references see *Scheuer* and *Lehmann* 1977). It is remarkable, though, that all these patients suffered from a basic disease which possibly predisposed them to develop liver tumors. These diseases were mainly Fanconi anemia, idiopathic aplastic anemia, as well as hormonal disturbances, such as hypopituitarism or kryptorchism.

Anabolic steroids are doubtless valuable drugs which show very beneficial effects against certain diseases and today are considered indispensable. Doubts have to be raised, however, from the medical as well as the toxicologic viewpoint, as to whether they should be given to competitive sportsmen who are actually healthy and do not need any drug treatment. Although to our knowledge liver tumors induced by anabolic steroids have not yet been described for this group, the principle should be adopted here, too, that drugs should be used for the treatment of diseases only.

Since the early 1970s, a constant increase in endometrial carcinomas has been registered in the United States (*Weiss* et al. 1976). This disease is said to be enhanced by a high estrogen level which occurs in women who have estrogen-secreting ovarial tumors or cysts or take estrogen-containing drugs (*Antunes* et al. 1979; *Mack* et al. 1976; *Weiss* et al. 1976; *Jick* et al. 1979). In a case-control study comprising 451 carcinoma cases and 888 controls, it was demonstrated in the United States that women who took estrogens postmenopausally ran a sixfold higher risk of developing cancer of the endometrium. A dose dependency could be shown: women who had been administered conjugated estrogens for more than 5 years showed a 15-fold higher risk than controls (*Antunes* et al. 1979). In the United States the results of this investigation led to demands for a more strict indication of use prior to estrogen treatment. In the Federal Republic of Germany, the discussion about a possible risk of developing estrogen-induced tumors has not yet been concluded (*Herold* et al. 1979; *Lingemann* 1979).

Schindler (1976) demonstrated that in adipose tissue of patients with endometrial carcinomas, a significantly increased aromatization of androstendione to estrogen takes place. An association between endometrial carcinomas and the extraglandular production of estrogen seems to exist. In experiments with rabbits, it was possible to produce endometrial carcinomas after intramuscular injection of high doses of the synthetic estrogen diethylstilbestrol (*Meissner* et al. 1957). It has been observed that after treatment with high doses of estrogen in cases of breast cancer, endometrial carcinomas occurred (*Khandekar* et al. 1978). The administration of estrogen postmenopausally is supposed to increase the risk of developing breast cancer slightly. Dose-response relationships seem to be conceivable (*Hoover* et al. 1976). The publications cited above are often based on single observations only. When estrogens are administered over long periods of time and in high doses, the target organs are subjected to a constant proliferative stimulus, which in individual cases may induce a cancerous growth, probably via an epigenetic mechanism.

Before turning to three further, and practically very important, groups of substances, we have to mention that, on the basis of experimental observations and a few rare cases, some other drugs have been discussed as potential carcinogens in man (literature review by *Schmähl* et al. 1977), including tar-containing ointments (*Hirohata* et al. 1973); β-phenylethylhydrazine sulfate, used in the treatment of depressions (*Toth* 1976); ethylmethanesulfonate, which was to be used as a contraceptive for men (*Hrushesky* et al. 1972); and, last but not least, niridazole (1-(5-nitro-2-thiazolyl)-2-imidazolidinone, Ambilhar), which is widely used for the treatment of schistosomiasis and amebiasis, particularly in tropical regions (*Urman* et al. 1975).

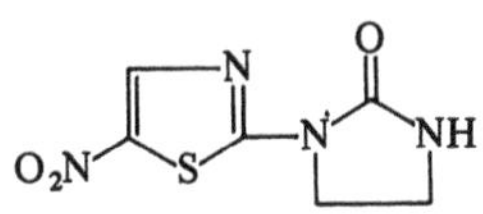

It should be mentioned that there are many nitrofuran drugs. A number of nitrofuran derivatives have been identified as strong carcinogens in experiments (*Cohen* et al. 1973). However, there seems to exist a strict structure-response relationship according to which the presently used therapeutic drugs having a nitrofuran base have so far proven not to be "risky."

A preliminary study by *Reddy* and *Qureshi* (1979) and yet unpublished results of studies carried out in the United States indicate a carcinogenic activity of the lipid-reducing drugs clofibrate and fenofibrate after chronic application to rats and mice. Malignant tumors of the liver, lung and pancreas were induced. These investigation results still need to be confirmed. Since, however, lipid-reducing drugs are frequently used, doctors should be aware of the possible risk involved in long-term administration.

In an ongoing lifetime study carried out in our laboratory an alkaloid extract from Senecio Fuchsii that mostly contains fuchsisenecionin proved to be hepatocarcinogenic in rats, affecting females more than males. The mechanism of the observed carcinogenic action is still unknown. In Germany Senecio Fuchsii extracts are used as teas for diabetics and are applied systemically against uterine bleedings.

5. Antineoplastic Agents

Antineoplastic agents, particularly those of the alkylating type, have proven to be carcinogenic in experimental studies, as well as according to numerous case reports in man. The relevant references comprising the corresponding experimental data have recently been compiled (*Schmähl* et al. 1977; *Schmähl* and *Habs* 1978). We will therefore not repeat the experimental data in this chapter.

Seen historically, the carcinogenic activity of cancer chemotherapeutic agents, including most of the alkylating agents and ethylene imine compounds, has been known from experimental investigations for 3 decades. In the later 1960s, Japanese investigators indicated that following exposure to mustard gas, neoplasms may occur in the respiratory tract of man (*Sato* et al. 1967; *Wada* et al. 1968). Thus it was found that among workers who had been employed in the production of mustard gas in the years between 1929 and 1945 the rate of malignant tumors of the respiratory tract was 33-fold higher than in the general population. German authors (*Weiß* and *Weiß* 1975, 1976) confirmed the results of these Japanese investigators. Besides a statistically proven increased occurrence of bronchus carcinomas in former mustard gas-exposed workers, carcinomas of the urinary bladder and leukemias were observed to a threefold higher extent than expected. Also, the occurrence of glioblastomas and neurofibromas in association with exposure to N-mustard has been discussed. Already in 1970, *Lindenfelser* referred to the occurrence of cancer of the urinary bladder as a later effect of exposure to chemical warfare agents.

These observations in occupational medicine, as well as the large amount of experimental data on carcinogenic effects of such drugs, caused us to test alkylating agents in particular, and, in addition, antimetabolites, antineoplastic natural substances, and antibiotics in comparative and quantitative dose-response investigations (*Schmähl* 1967; *Schmähl* 1972; *Schmähl* and *Habs* 1979). Our earlier studies can be summarized as follows: at a dose corresponding to that administered clinically to patients, alkylating compounds induced significant carcinogenic effects in rats which are approximately equivalent to those of whole-body X-ray radiation. Compared with untreated controls, we observed a four- to sixfold increase in tumor yield. The antimetabolites investigated by us (methotrexate, 6-mercaptopurine, 5-fluorouracil) as well as vinblastine and demecolcine (Colcemid) (desacetyl-methylcolchicine), did not prove to be carcinogenic. Regarding tumor localization, no predilection for certain organ sites could be seen in our experiments; however, an increase in leukemias and hemangiosarcomas was recorded (*Weisburger* 1977).

Using cyclophosphamide as a model, since it is one of the most frequently used chemotherapeutic alkylating agents, we undertook some quantitative experiments. Our primary

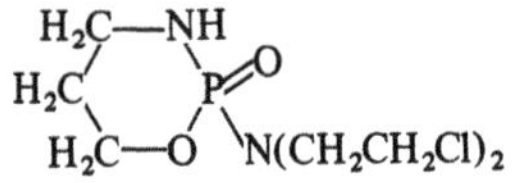

objective was to determine whether small doses, lower than those presently used in clinical chemotherapy, are carcinogenic or not. Rats were given various doses orally, the lowest dose being only 25% of the dose used in man in "maintenance therapy." Tables 3 and 4 show the carcinogenic effect of these small doses. In our experiments we found the same types of malignant tumors as those described following treatment with cyclophosphamide and other alkylating agents used in the therapy of human cancer diseases, namely, carcinomas of the urinary bladder (*Lenzin* et al. 1978; *Niederle* and *Müller* 1978; *Pearson* and *Soloway* 1978; *Petri* and *Altwein* 1978; *Rupprecht* and

Table 3. Carcinogenic action of low-dose cyclophosphamide given orally to Sprague-Dawley rats in a lifetime experiment. Survival times and tumor incidences

Group	No. of animals[a]		Individual[b] dose (mg/kg)	Median survival[c] time (days)		Animals with malignant tumors[d] Males			Females			Median tumor induction time (days)	
	m	f		m	f	Abs.	%	%stand.	Abs.	%	%stand.	m	f
I	31	27	2.5	638	642	13	42	76	9	33	87	610	650
II	35	33	1.25	646	720	15	43	50	11	33	65	620	620
III	36	37	0.63	808	889	14	39	23	13	35	43	699	789
IV	34	37	0.31	906	934	11	32	6	11	30	27	861	792
V	38	34	0	759	985	4	11	11	5	15	15	654	896

[a] Number of evaluable animals alive when the first animal died with a malignant tumor (m, day 357, f, day 404); at the start of the experiment each group comprised 40 males and 40 females

[b] Applied in drinking water 5 times/week

[c] Based on total number of animals minus animals not examined because of autolysis or cannibalism

[d] Based on number of evaluable animals

Table 4. Carcinogenic action of low-dose cyclophosphamide given orally to Sprague-Dawley rats in a lifetime experiment. Tumor localization

Group	Urinary bladder					Lymphoid and hemato-poietic tissue		Nervous system		Vascular system		Uterus		Adrenal	Liver	Mammary gland	Testis	Others
	No_m [a]	No_f [b]	No_t [c]	MIT [d]	N_1 [e]	No_t	MIT	No_t	MIT	No_t	MIT	No_t	MIT	No_t	No_t	No_t	No_t	No_t
I	7	1	8	619	4	4	–	1	–	3	–	1	–	3	1	–	–	3
II	5	–	5	697	7	6	755	6	646	7	532	–	–	3	–	1	1	5
III	2	–	2	–	11	6	807	5	710	2	–	6	798	3	1	1	1	4
IV	2	–	2	–	6	3	–	7	767	4	–	2	–	2	–	1	–	5
V	–	–	–	–	1	–	–	1	–	1	–	4	–	1	–	1	–	1

[a] Number of male rats with tumor

[b] Number of female rats with tumor

[c] Total number of rats with tumors (if animals had more than one tumor, the latter was counted separately)

[d] Median induction time (days given if ⩾ 5 animals were diagnosed with malignant tumors of the same organotropism)

[e] Number of additional animals with benign tumors of the urinary bladder

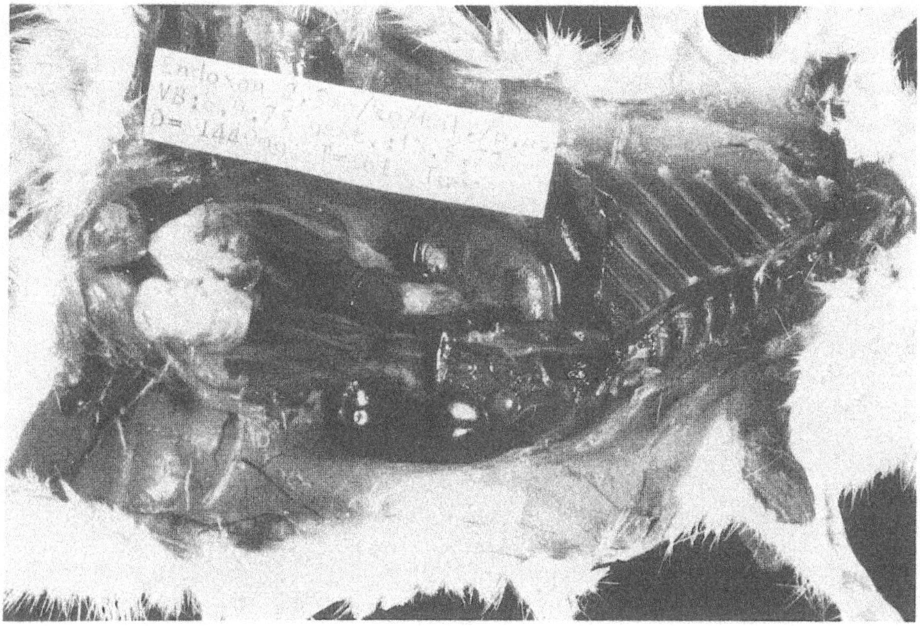

Fig. 1. Macroscopic view of a cyclophosphamide-induced carcinoma of the urinary bladder

Blessing 1973; *Dale* and *Smith* 1974; *Wall* and *Clausen* 1975; *Worth* 1971; *Beyer-Boon* et al. 1978; *Richtmeier* 1975) and leukemias (*Gutjahr* and *Spranger* 1975; *Karchmer* et al. 1974; *Petersen* 1973; *Khandekar* et al. 1977; *Labedzki* et al. 1976; *Reimer* et al. 1977; *Rowley* et al. 1977; *Smit* and *Meyler* 1970; *Sotrel* et al. 1976; *Schmalzl* et al. 1975; *Puri* and *Campbell* 1977) (Figs. 1–4).

In 1968 *Chaves* had already shown that after a single intraperitoneal application of cyclophosphamide, rats developed hyperplasia in the mucosa of the urinary bladder.

In the case of carcinogenesis induced by alkylating cytostatic agents, the animal experiments predicted results seen several years later in man. It is hard to understand why, despite these data, cytostatic agents with structural formulae suggesting a carcinogenic activity have been put on the market. A typical example is chlornaphazine.

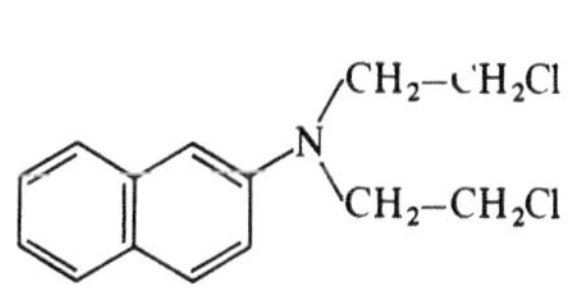

It contains a mustard group at the basic molecule of β-naphthylamine. During metabolism the chloroethyl function is probably cleaved off so that β-naphthylamine is formed, the carcinogenic effect of which has been known for many decades. Chlornaphazine has been used in the treatment of polycythemia, predominantly in Scandinavian countries, and has led to carcinomas of the urinary bladder (Table 5), in many

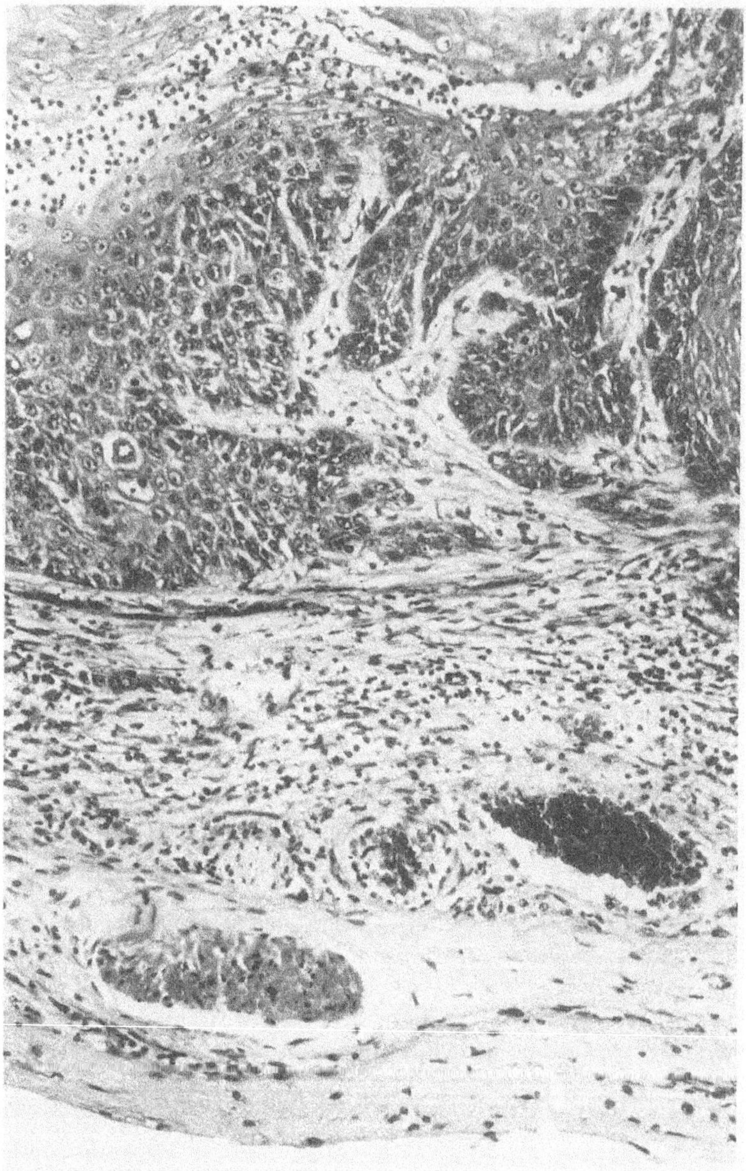

Fig. 2. Microscopic view of a cyclophosphamide-induced carcinoma of the urinary bladder

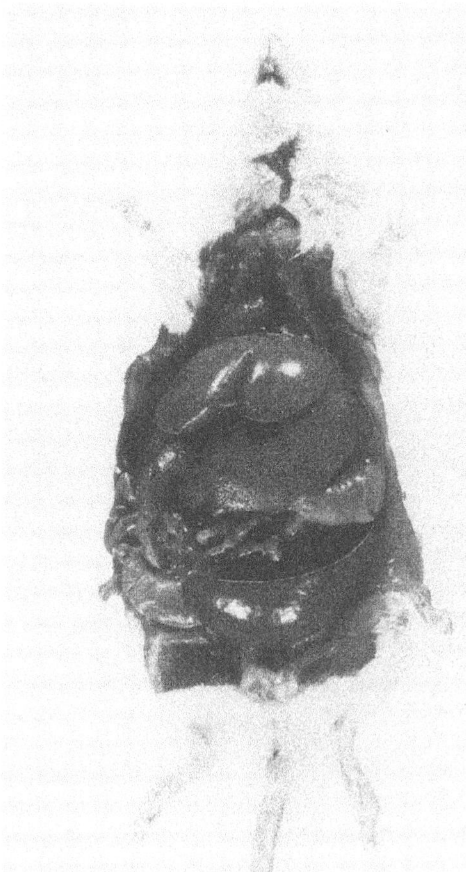

Fig. 3. Macroscopic view of a cyclophosphamide-induced leukemia with marked splenomegaly

cases after surprisingly short induction times (2–10 years) (*Thiede* and *Christensen* 1969; *Videbaek* 1964). The carcinomas of the urinary bladder induced by chlornaphazine in man could obviously have been avoided, if the physicians employing this agent had had better knowledge about the association between chemical structure and carcinogenic activity, for, as stated above, the carcinogenic activity of this compound was predictable.

The existence of much experimental and clinical data has resulted in the reporting of the induction of secondary tumors by cytostatic agents more and more often by clinicians (*Harris* 1976; *Hartwich* and *Butzler* 1971; *Hunstein* and *Rehn* 1975). This

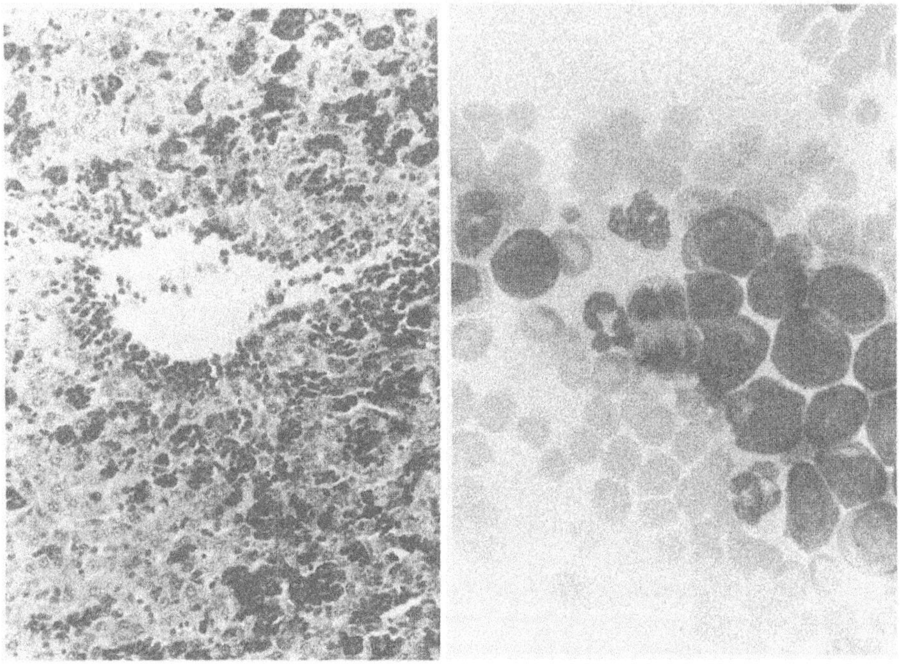

Fig. 4. Microscopic view of a cyclophosphamide-induced leukemia in the liver and peripheral blood

even includes attempts to quantify the risk of developing secondary tumors in patients subjected to radiologic and chemotherapeutic treatment. Thus, *Delbrück* and collaborators (1978) stated that the risk of inducing an acute leukemia in patients subjected to intensive radiology and chemotherapy of malignant lymphomas was 50- to 100-fold higher than in the general population. Similar conclusions were reached by *DeVita* et al. (1973), who consider the risk of inducing long-term complications after chemotherapy of Hodgkin's disease, i.e., induction of secondary tumors, to be 3.5–30 times higher than in the general population. The latency period up to the occurrence of a therapy-induced leukemia is the shorter the more intensively the chemo- or radiotherapy was carried out (*Cadman* et al. 1977), suggesting a dose-response relationship. *Chabner* (1977) calculated that patients with ovarian carcinomas who had been subjected to intensive chemotherapy with alkylating agents ran a 21- to 26-fold higher risk of developing an acute leukemia within 2 years after the beginning of therapy than those in the general population of the same age. For patients who survived the first 2 years after treatment, the risk was calculated to be 66–170 times higher. When looking at these figures, it should be kept in mind that definitely not all cases of secondary tumors induced by chemotherapy are detected and published. We know of a number of unpublished cases in which a secondary tumor (bladder cancer) was most probably induced by chemotherapeutic treatment.

The drugs used in cancer chemotherapy – alkylating agents as well as antimetabolites or antibiotics of the adriamycin type – represent highly reactive substances which should be employed only in cases with a correspondingly poor prognosis. For many years we have again and again stressed this (*Schmähl* 1967; *Schmähl* and *Osswald* 1970; *Schmähl* et al. 1977); we consider it all the more necessary if these antineoplastic substances are recommended for use in diseases without a fatal prognosis, such as Dupuytren's contracture (*Aron* 1968), multiple sclerosis (*Danielczyk* 1970), or lupus erythematosus (*Brook* 1969). Today, even psoriasis – though only in its most serious form – is treated with cytostatic agents, although dermatologists are fully aware of the possible risk of inducing a secondary tumor and should exercise a more restrictive prescription policy (*Bailin* et al. 1975; *Kelleter* et al. 1972; *Rassner* 1973).

The mechanism of action in carcinogenesis induced by cytostatic agents has been a topic of numerous discussions. Some authors (*Arseneau* et al. 1977; *Penn* 1974) believe that the immunosuppressive activities of cytostatic agents are primarily responsible for their carcinogenic effect. Our own investigations, however, do not confirm this supposition (*Schmähl* and *Osswald* 1970; *Schmähl* 1977). On the contrary, we found that chemical carcinogenesis is not related to the immune status of the host.

An increasing number of nitrosoureas have recently been introduced into cytostatic therapy (*Carter* et al. 1972; *Douglass* et al. 1976; *Schabel* 1976). Among the nitrosoureas there are many substances which exert a strong carcinogenic effect in animal experiments (*Druckrey* et al. 1967; *Habs* and *Schmähl* 1976). In 1978, *Schmähl* and *Habs* reported on the carcinogenic activity of some analogues of bis-chloroethylnitrosourea after repeated intraperitoneal administration to rats.

$$ClCH_2CH_2\underset{}{\overset{NO}{\overset{|}{N}}}CONHCH_2CH_2Cl \qquad \text{1,3–bis(2–chloroethyl)–1– nitrosourea}$$

Chlorozotocin has been shown to be a strong carcinogen (*Habs* et al. 1979). *Eisenbrand* (1979) reported that the carcinogenicity and the cytostatic activity of nitrosourea derivatives are not necessarily linked to each other. There have also been first reports on the carcinogenic activities of N-nitrosoureas in man (*Cohen* et al. 1976; *Jochimsen* et al. 1976). In an experimental study on inoculated leukemia, *Zeller* and *Schmähl* (1979) reported that after curative treatment with BCNU, secondary tumors occur in 11% of the treated animals which were caused by the BCNU treatment. Further animal experiments are needed to show whether or not it will be possible to reduce the carcinogenic activity of these highly potent cytostatics without decreasing their cytostatic activity. If various drugs with the same cytostatic effect on tumors of a certain organ are available, those compounds should preferably be selected for clinical trials which exhibited no or only a weak carcinogenic potency in animal experiments.

The existing experimental and clinical data on carcinogenesis induced by cytostatic substances permit us to draw the following conclusions, which were already published in a similar form in 1967 (*Schmähl* 1967):

1. Cytostatic agents should be used only in cases with a poor prognosis; this includes all those cancers which occur systemically or can no longer be treated by "classical" therapy. It is important, however, to know whether the tumor in question is chemosensitive as far as one can tell with existing knowledge.

2. Nonmalignant diseases should be treated with cytostatic agents only if no alternative is available.

3. Particular restraint should be exercised in using carcinogenic cytostatic agents in experimental "adjuvant" chemotherapy, because by randomizing the patients, potentially healthy people who have already been cured by a classical treatment might be subjected to potential hazards. Special caution is required if young patients are affected. This warning seems to be particularly justified, since some cases of leukemia in man have been described after adjuvant chemotherapy of breast cancer (*Lerner* 1977). If the adjuvant chemotherapy with carcinogenic alkylating compounds is applied indiscriminately, it is to be expected that a large number of patients who have been subjected to this treatment will later on develop a secondary tumor induced by the adjuvant chemotherapy.

In ongoing animal experiments with rats, we have tested the CMF scheme (cyclophosphamide – methotrexate – 5-fluorouracil) recommended by *Bonadonna* (1976) for the adjuvant chemotherapy of breast cancer, and we have so far detected marked carcinogenic effects with this combination. In accordance with our former investigations, it seems likely that a major part of this carcinogenic effect has to be attributed to cyclophosphamide. We are therefore now investigating whether cyclophosphamide may be substituted by another noncarcinogenic cytostatic agent while maintaining the same therapeutic effectiveness in the new cimbination. The results of our investigations will be published in due time.

4. The implementation of cytostatic therapy should be carried out by clinicians who have special experience in this field of chemotherapy. Inexperienced physicians should never employ this form of treatment in cancer patients.

The development of our knowledge of carcinogenesis induced by cytostatic agents in experimental animals and in man during the last 2 decades has precisely predicted the "late effects" observed in man. The detection of these late effects has initiated more restrictive practices in chemotherapy. These more restrictive practices will hopefully protect patients against possible late effect in the future. In the case of otherwise incurable diseases, such as Hodgkin's disease and plasmocytomas, these late effects will have to be endured in order to prevent acute danger to life.

6. Rauwolfia Derivatives and Artificial Sweeteners

Finally we want to report on two examples of potentially carcinogenic drugs, which may demonstrate how this topic should not be dealt with – especially in public. In 1974, two epidemiologic studies were published, suggesting that Rauwolfia derivatives may induce breast cancer in women (*Armstrong* et al. 1974; *Heinonen* et al. 1974). Taking the global use of these drugs into consideration, the public was quickly upset. Furthermore, "critical" comments appeared in newspapers and on the radio in which the medical profession was accused of irresponsibility because doctors had treated many patients with an allegedly carcinogenic drug over long periods. The methodical setup which led to the assumption of a correlation between the use of Rauwolfia preparations and the development of breast cancer was subjected to a critical examination by *Immich* (1974). He concluded that the described results of epidemiologic studies were "methodical artefacts." Additional investigations in different countries (*Aromaa* et al. 1976; *Laska* et al. 1975; *O'Fallon* et al. 1975) showed that there is no association between application of Rauwolfia preparations and the development of breast cancer. A commission established in 1976 by the German Federal Health Agency (Bundesgesundheitsamt) came to the conclusion that "the suspicion that reserpine might induce or promote breast cancer could not be confirmed by the existing data" (*Gross* 1976). Today no one seriously considers the possibility of a cancer-inducing effect of Rauwolfia preparations in man.

A second example of a questionable procedure leading to considerable concern among parts of the population involves the alleged cancer-inducing effects of artificial sweeteners (cyclamate, saccharin). This discussion has been continuing in public for many years. Artificial sweeteners are used medically in the treatment of diabetes or adiposity in a large number of people, and as such, they belong to the category of drugs in a broader sense. In the United States and Canada (for literature review see *Schmähl* 1978a), both compounds were found to cause cancer of the urinary bladder in rats if they were fed chronically and over several generations in daily doses of more than 5 g/kg body weight. In Germany diabetics ingest an average of 1–5 mg/kg of saccharin per day, the maximum being already an exteme value. Comparison of the dose relationship shows that in the animal experiment the dose administered was 1000-fold higher than the dose administered to man. Assuming that a man consumed about 1 kg of food per day, this would mean that, when extrapolating the animal experiment to man, the food would have to contain 50 g saccharin to induce a demonstrable carcinogenic effect. This example demonstrates the unreality of the experimental setup. Animal experiments in several species in which the saccharin dose administered was lower, e.g., 500, 200, or 50 mg/kg body weight, did not produce any carcinogenic effect. Similar results were obtained in experiments carried out at our institute (*Schmähl* 1973).

The large number of negative findings obtained in various laboratories all over the world seems to indicate that even in cases of 100- to 200-fold overdoses, a cancer-inducing effect is not to be expected, not even in sensitive animal species such as rats. As far as is known, pure saccharin does not act genotoxically (*Pool* 1978). In usual mutagenicity tests the results proved to be negative (overview by *Guggenheim* 1979). *Hicks* and *Chowaniec* (1977) carried out animal experiments on carcinogenicity in which, after application of a locally active carcinogen into the urinary bladder, an artificial sweetener was orally administered in high doses over long periods of time. Considerably increased tumor incidences were diagnosed in those animals which had been subjected to the combination treatment. This experimental setup, however, does not prove a carcinogenic effect of saccharin. The acute toxic effect of the carcinogen induces a profound inflammation of the mucosa of the urinary bladder. It seems likely that this inflammation is chronically maintained by the saccharin excreted in the urine. The fact, however, that carcinomas can develop on the basis of chronic inflammations was already demonstrated by *Narat* in 1925. By dropping hydrochloric acid or potassium hydroxide solution, respectively, on mouse skin he induced chronic ulcers, which in the course of time were modified into carcinomas. We have reproduced and confirmed these experiments (*Schmähl* and *Habs* unpublished). This epigenetic process

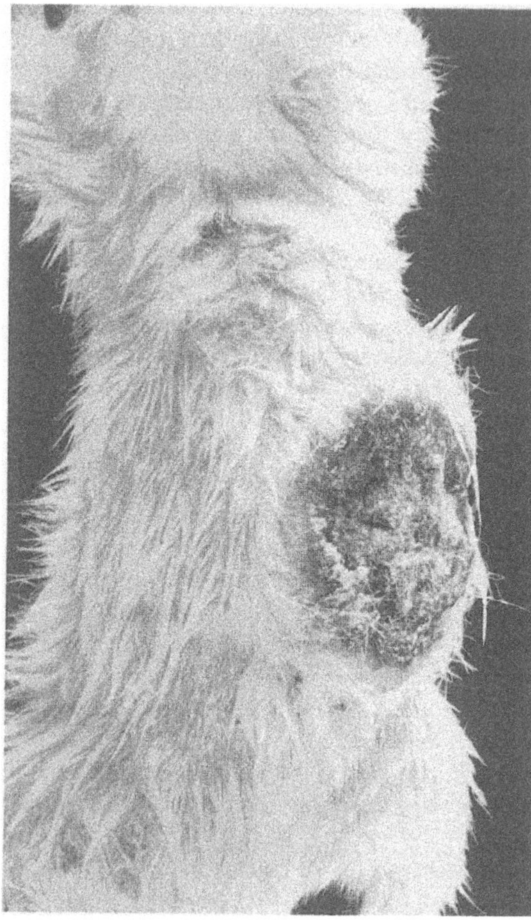

Fig. 5. Squamous cell carcinoma induced by chronic dropping of hydrochloric acid to mouse skin

of carcinogenesis should, of course not be interpreted to the effect that hydrochloric acid and KOH are to be regarded as "genuine" carcinogens (Fig. 5).

Our own ongoing experiments, in which the transplacental application of saccharin and cyclamate in pregnant rats is under investigation, has not caused any transplacental carcinogenesis so far (1.5 years since the onset of the experiments). Thus, there is no reason to ascribe a carcinogenic effect in man to cyclamate or saccharin, particularly since further epidemiologic studies did not demonstrate this either (*Armstrong* and *Doll* 1974; *Armstrong* et al. 1976; *Guggenheim* 1979). In our experiments we did not observe any promoting effect of simultaneously administered artificial sweeteners on the carcinogenesis induced by N-nitroso compounds in the urinary bladder. Despite all the excitement and concern among the public, the discussion about the possible carcinogenicity of cyclamate or saccharin has brought about a positive result. Commercially available saccharin often used to contain considerable amounts of contominants, predominantly o-toluenesulfonamide (a possibly weak carcinogen which in animal experiments induced tumors of the urinary bladder (*Schmähl* 1978b); the saccharin sold today in Germany includes less than 10 ppm of this contaminant, i.e., saccharine is now less contaminated.

7. Nitrosatable Agents

An important problem still remains to be discussed. Many drugs are or contain nitrosatable agents which, when they react with nitrite, especially in the acid medium of gastric juice, can be converted to N-nitroso compounds or release carcinogenic nitrosamines (see Table 5).

Table 5. Reaction of some drugs with nitrite to nitrosamines under "stomachlike" conditions (pH 1–2, 37°C)

Drug	Nitrosamine formed	Carcinogenicity	Reaction yield
Amidopyrene (Pyramidon)	Dimethylnitrosamine	+++	High
Oxytetracyclin	Dimethylnitrosamine	+++	Medium
Chlorpromazine	Dimethlynitrosamine	+++	Low
Dextropropoxyphene	Dimethylnitrosamine	+++	Low
Methadone	Dimethylnitrosamine	+++	Low
Methapyrilene	Dimethylnitrosamine	+++	Low
Lucanthone	Diethylnitrosamine	+++	Medium
Quinacrine	Diethylnitrosamine	+++	Medium
Disulfiram	Diethylnitrosamine	+++	Low
Nicethamide	Diethylnitrosamine	+++	Low
Tolazamide	N-nitrosohexamethylene imine	++	Low
Cyclizine	Nitrosopiperazine and	++	Low
	Dinitrosopiperazine	++	Low
Ephedrine	N-nitrosoephedrine	++	Medium
Phenmetrazine	N-nitrosophenmetrazine	–	Medium
Methylphenidate	N-nitrosomethylphenidate	–	Medium
Phenacetin	N-nitroso-2-nitro-4-ethoxy-acetanilide	?	Medium

This process can be crucial if the yield is very high and the nitrosamine formed has a strong carcinogenic activity, as is the case with aminopyrine for example (*Lijinsky* and *Taylor* 1977; *Taylor* and *Lijinsky* 1975).

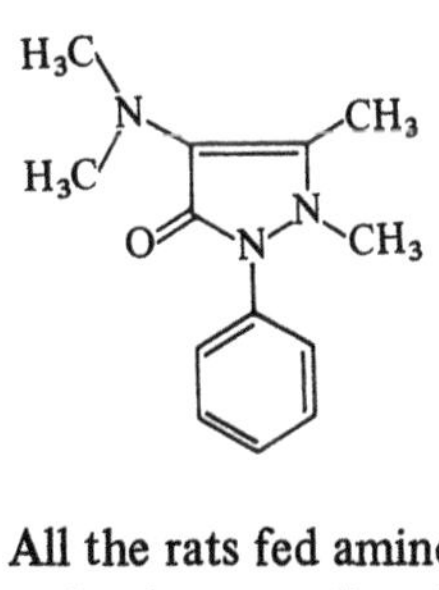

All the rats fed aminopyrine together with nitrite developed liver cancer after only 7 months, because dimethylnitrosamine was formed in the stomach. When treating the animals with only pyramidon or nitrite, respectively, a carcinogenic effect could not be observed. Thus, drugs which are not carcinogenic as such, but have an appropriate chemical structure, may serve as precursors for the formation of carcinogenic nitrosamines if they are brought into contract with nitrite (see also *Walker* et al. 1976). Such a danger arises particularly if (1) the nitrosamine formed has a strong carcinogenic effect, (2) the yield is very high, and (3) the respective drug is administered frequently and possibly over long periods of time. Case reports show a possible risk of inducing gastric cancer in patients who have taken cimetidine (*Lancet* 1979), a drug that can be nitrosated. The nitrosated chemical shows mutagenic activity in the Ames assay system (*Pool* 1979). Long-term bioassays are under way in our laboratory, in which possible carcinogenic potentials are to be assessed.

If, however, the rate of conversion is low and the drug is not applied too frequently, then the possible hazard seems to be negligible (*Eisenbrand* et al. 1978). For practical purposes it can be recommended to measure first in short-term in vitro systems whether the respective nitrosatable drug forms or releases an N-nitroso compound at a considerable rate due to reaction with nitrite. If this is the case, the corresponding compound should be tested for possible mutagenic and carcinogenic effects, including the testing of the drug as such or in combination with nitrite. This procedure seems unnecessary in the case of substances which are used only for extremely serious diseases.

8. Transplants

The literature of the early 1960s shows an increasing number of reports on the occurrence of malignant tumors after organ transplantation (*Enderlin* and *Guisan* 1973; *Guisan* et al. 1973; *Penn* and *Starzl* 1972; *McCann* 1969). The frequency of such tumors is about 5% in recipients of transplants 12–36 months after the operation, thus being many times higher than that of age-matched comparative groups. It is particularly striking that predominantly tumors of the lymphatic system, but also malignant epithelial tumors, are found. Often these are multiple tumors (*Mendelsohn* 1976).

The induction time of these tumors is comparatively short; mostly they occur within 1–5 years after the transplantation of an organ.

In order to make successful organ transplantation possible, immunosuppressive therapy has to be used to prevent graft rejection. Originally this was done using X-ray irradiation or alkylating agents or corticosteroids; nowadays, antimetabolites and corticosteroids are used more often. The question arises whether the malignant tumors occurring after organ transplantation are caused by chemical agents which had to be administered to prevent graft rejection, or whether different mechanisms are involved. It may be that the induced immunosuppression can modify the chemical carcinogenesis in some way or other.

The short induction time of only a few years speaks against the hypothesis that this type of tumor involves the same mechanism of action as classical carcinogenesis (*Schmähl* 1977). Furthermore, the frequent occurrence of lymphoreticular malignant tumors is noticed and cannot be explained by effects of known chemical carcinogens. An interesting parallel between tumors occurring after organ transplantation and experience in pediatrics is to be observed. Children who were born with an immunodeficiency (Wiscott-Aldrich syndrome, agammaglobulinemia, ataxia teleangiectatica, etc.) have an extremely high tendency to develop cancer. Until the 16th year of age, they run about a 10,000-fold higher risk of developing cancer than normal children (*Waldmann* et al. 1972; *Swift* et al. 1976; *Hamoudi* et al. 1974; *Gatti* and *Good* 1971). From these observations it may be assumed that immunosuppression as such – be it chemically induced or congenital – may have a "carcinogenic" effect.

Against this assumption, however, weighty objections have been raised (*Gleichmann* and *Gleichmann* 1973). The most important of these is the fact that experimentally immunosuppressive measures have not been found to induce cancer or promote the activity of chemical carcinogens (*Andrew* 1974; *Waynforth* and *Magee* 1974; *Kroes* et al. 1975; *Anderson* et al. 1978). In extensive investigations using various models, we were not able to demonstrate a promoting (or inhibiting) effect of immunosuppressive (or immune-stimulating) actions on chemical carcinogenesis (*Schmähl* and *Osswald* 1970; *Schmähl* et al. 1971; *Schmähl* 1971; *Schmähl* et al. 1974; *Scherf* and *Schmähl* 1975; *Schmähl* et al. 1976a, b; *Scherf* et al. 1969, 1970; *Scherf* 1972, 1976; *Schmähl* 1975). The necessary association between the carcinogenic and the immunotoxic effect of chemical carcinogens could not be established.

It appears that the immunologic status of the total organism does not determine the effectiveness of chemical carcinogens. It is therefore conceivable that in "immunocarcinogenesis," oncogenic viruses may have a causal significance (*Schmähl* 1977). This is just as hypothetical as the view that the chemical substances applied to induce immunosuppression might cause this type of carcinogenesis. These observations provide a very important research stimulus which might contribute to detecting a mechanism of carcinogenesis in man.

Finally, we would like to hint at the possibility that iatrogenic tumors may also be caused by surgical interventions, putting special emphasis on sarcomas from foreign bodies and scars. Occasionally, the occurrence of sarcomas is associated with foreign body implants. In experiments, various plastic materials, but also metals and other materials such as ivory, were shown to induce sarcomas at the site of implantation in the animal (reference review by *Ott* et al. 1963). There are several case reports in which the occurrence of sarcomas in postoperative scars is described. For sarcomas induced by foreign bodies as well as in scars, a common pathology can be assumed (*Ott* 1970). Considering the large number of surgical interventions during recent years, the risk of developing a scar sarcoma seems to be extremely low. Also, we assume that a number of cases have not been reported. An increased frequency of malignant tumors is reported in the gastric stump after Billroth's operation and in the intestinal tract after cholecystectomy (*Capron* et al. 1978). There is current discussion as to whether tumors may increasingly occur at the stoma after implantation of a preternatural anus (reference review by *Schmähl* et al. 1977). Among others, *Dahm, Werner* and coworkers as well as *Ivankovic* investigated experimentally the possible increased effects of chemical carcinogens in resected organs of the gastrointestinal tract (*Dahm* and *Werner* 1973, 1975; *Dahm* and *de Heer* 1976; *Werner* et al. 1977; *de Heer* and *Werner* 1978; *Junghans* et al. 1977; *Rumpf* et al. 1978). In carcinogenesis experiments, the effect of locally active carcinogens was increased in animals with gastric stumps in comparison to normal animals. Thus, the administration of 1,2-dimethylhydrazine – a substance which preferably induces interstinal tumors – led to tumors at the preternatural anus in rats after a short induction time (*Ivankovic* 1979) (Fig. 6).

Resections in the gastrointestinal tract with end-to-end anastomosis, however, did

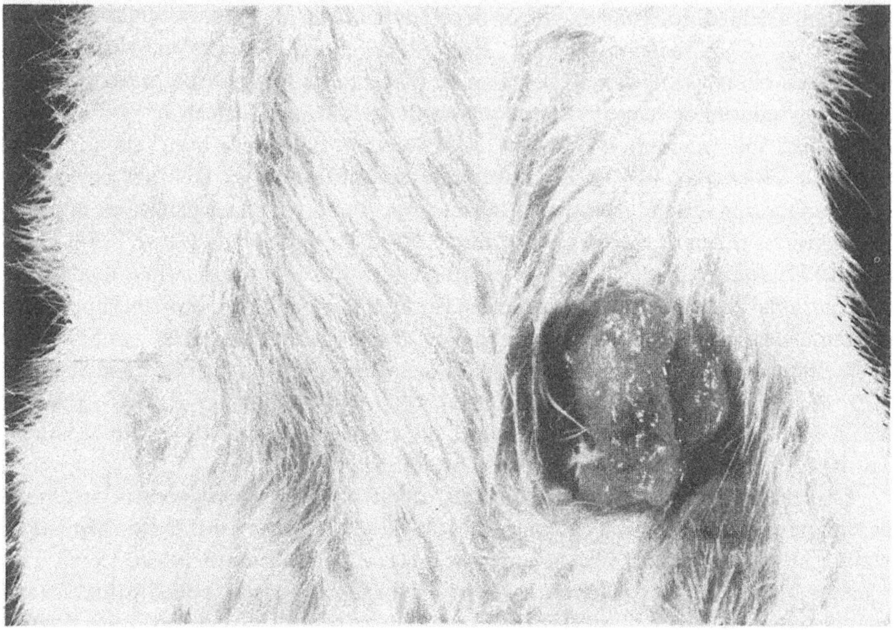

Fig. 6. Adenocarcinoma induced by 1,2-dimethylhydrazine at the site of operation in an animal with preternatural anus

not affect the carcinogenesis in the remaining intestinal sections of animals (*de Heer* and *Werner* 1978). Contrary to this result, *Williamson* and collaborators (1978) found a promotion of acetoxymethane-induced colonic neoplasia after resection of the proximal small bowel.

If there is an operation-dependent increased cancer risk for man in the gastrointestinal tract, it may be considered negligible. At present, restraint from performing operations on the basis of possible cancer risks cannot be recommended, since the existing data are not yet sufficient to justify such a decision.

III. Conclusions

There are a number of drugs for different therapeutic uses which show cancer-inducing properties. Besides drug-induced iatrogenic tumors, there is also experimental and clinical evidence indicating an increased cancer risk after certain operative interventions, e.g., foreign-body and scar sarcomas and colon cancer after resection in the gastrointestinal tract. The number of iatrogenic cancers among the overall cancer incidence in man is very low, but carcinogenic drugs are often used in the treatment of certain diseases. The decision on the implementation of a therapy with carcinogenic drugs should therefore be taken critically in each individual case. Since the so-called postoperative adjuvant chemotherapy, which is meant to be a metastasis-inhibiting preventive measure, is at present still in the stage of experimental clinical trials, it should be implemented only within the scope of clinical studies in cooperation with skilled oncologists. During selection of drugs and drug combinations for clinical test-

Table 6. Drugs which have to be considered as potential carcinogens for man on the basis of experimental investitations or casuistic reports.
Carcinogenic action of drugs in man

Definite/likely	Possible	Unlikely/not assessable
Alkylating agents	Adriamycin	Ethylmethane sulfonate
(lost derivatives,	Anabolics	Cantharidin
ethylene imines)	Antimetabolites	Cyclamate
Arsenic trioxide	Chloramphenicol	Fuchsin
Diethylstilbestrol	Contraceptives	Hexamethylene tetramine
(transplacental)	Furium	Iron dextran
Procarbazine	Griseofulvin	Isonicotinic acid hydrazide
Nitrosoureas	Halogenated paraffins	Lactams
Streptozotocin	Hydantoin derivatives	Metronidazol
	Lysergides	Paraffin oils
	Niridazoles	Phenobarbital
	Nitrofuran derivatives	Phenylethylene hydrazine
	Oestrogens	Polyvinyl pyrrolidone and similar plasma-expanding agents
	Phenacetin	Potassium perchlorate
	Phenylbutazone	Pronethalol
	Quinolin derivatives	Reserpine
	Tannin (epicutaneous)	Saccharin
	Tar ointments	Safrole
	Thiouracil	Tannin (oral)
	Urethan	

ing, the possible risk of inducing iatrogenic secondary tumors should always be kept in mind.

In Table 6, we compiled those drugs which to our knowledge have been suspected or are still suspected to be possible carcinogens, attempting to make a qualitative assessment of the carcinogenic risk arising from their therapeutic use for man. Included are some substances, e.g., contraceptives or phenacetin, the carcinogenic effect of which to man could be made most likely in individual cases. We classified these drugs as "possible" carcinogens only because the risk arising from their application is obviously very low.

Since the pathologist is often the one who at autopsy sets up an exact epicrisis, he might find associations between administered drugs and the formation of a tumor. From the viewpoint of the etiology of malignant tumors, it would be desirable if findings concerning the topic of this chapter were reported, because they might then influence toxicologic research.

References

Anderson LM, Budinger JM, Maronpot RR, Good RA (1978) Transplacental lung tumorigenesis in the athymic mouse. Cancer Res 38: 137–141

Andrew EJ (1974) Failure of immunosurveillance against chemically induced in situ tumors in mice. J Natl Cancer Inst 52: 729–732

Antunes CMF, Stolley PD, Rosenshein NB, Davies JL, Tonascia JA, Brown C, Burnett L, Rutledge A, Pokempner M, Garcia R (1979) Endometrial cancer and estrogen use. Report of a large case-control study. New Engl J Med 300: 9–13

Armstrong B, Doll R (1974) Bladder cancer mortality in England and Wales in relation to cigarette smoking and saccharin consumption. Brit J Prev Med 28: 233–240

Armstrong B, Stevens N, Doll R (1974) Retrospective study of the association between use of rauwolfia derivatives and breast cancer in English women. Lancet II: 672–675

Armstrong B, Lea AJ, Adelstein AM, Donovan JW, White GC, Ruttle S (1976) Cancer mortality and saccharin consumption in diabetics. Brit J Prev Soc Med 30: 151–157

Aromaa A, Hakama M, Hakulinen T, Saxen E, Teppo L, Idänpään-Heikkilä J (1976) Breast cancer and use of rauwolfia and other antihypertensive agents in hypertensive patients: A nationwide case-control study in Finland. Int J Cancer 18: 727–738

Aron E (1968) Le traitement médical de la maladie de Dupuytren par un agent cytostatique (méthyl-hydrazine). La Presse Medicale 76 (41): 1956

Arseneau JC, Canellos GP, Johnson R, DeVita VT (1977) Risk of new cancers in patients with Hodgkin's disease. Cancer 40: 1912–1916

Baden JM, Kelley M, Wharton RS, Hitt BA, Simmon VF, Mazze RI (1977) Mutagenicity of halogenated ether anesthetics. Anesthesiology 46: 346–350

Bailin PL, Tindall JP, Roenigk HH, Hogan MD (1975) Is methotrexate therapy for psoriasis carcinogenic? A modified retrospective-prospective analysis. JAMA 232: 359–362

Barron CN (1963) Observations on the chronic toxicity of 3-phenyl-5β-diethylaminoethyl-1,2,4-oxadiazole in the rat and dog. Exp Molec Path (Suppl) 2: 1–27

Baum JK, Holtz F, Bockstein JJ, Klein EW (1973) Possible association between benign hepatomas and oral contraceptives. Lancet II: 926–929

Bean RHD (1960) Phenylbutazone and leukaemia: A possible association. Brit Med J II: 1552

Beil E, Prechtel K (1973) Malignes Lymphom oder Hydantoin-Lymphadenopathie? Münch Med Wschr 115 (45): 2033–2039

Bengtsson U, Johansson S, Angervall L (1978) Malignancies of the urinary tract and their relation to analgesic abuse. Kidney International 13: 107–113

Beyer-Boon ME, DeVoogt HJ, Schaberg A (1978) The effects of cyclophosphamide treatment on the epithelium and stroma of the urinary bladder. Europ J Cancer 14: 1029–1035

Biancifiori C, Severi L (1966) The relation of isoniazid (INH) and allied compounds to carcinogenesis in some species of small laboratory animals: A review. Brit J Cancer 20: 528–538

Bichel J, Bach A (1968) Investigation on the toxicity of small chronic doses of tannic acid with special reference to possible carcinogenicity. Acta Pharmacol Toxicol 26: 41–45

Bonadonna G, Brusamolino E, Valagussa P, Rossi A, Brugnatelli L, Brambilla C, DeLena M, Tancini L, Bajetta E, Musumeci R, Veronesi U (1976) Combination chemotherapy as an adjuvant treatment in operable breast cancer. New Eng J Med 294: 405–410

Braun W (1958) Krebs an Haut und inneren Organen, hervorgerufen durch Arsen. Dtsch Med Wschr 83: 870–872

Brook CGD (1969) Psychosis in systemic lupus erythematosus (SLE) and the response to cyclophosphamide. Proc Roy Soc Med Vol 62: 28

Burstein N, McIntire KR (1968) Urethan-induced pulmonary tumors in germ-free mice. Proc Amer Assoc Cancer Res 9: 11

Cadman EC, Capizzi RL, Bertino JR (1977) Acute nonlymphocytic leukemia. A delayed complication of Hodgkin's disease therapy: Analysis of 109 cases. Cancer 40: 1280–1296

Capron JP, Delamarre J, Canarelli JP, Brousse N, Dupas JL (1978) La cholecystectomie favorise-t-elle l'apparition du cancer rectocolique? Gastroenterol Clin Biol 2 (4): 383–389
Carter SK, Schabel FM Jr, Broder JE (1972) 1,3-Bis-(2-chloroethyl)-1-nitrosourea (BCNU) and other nitrosoureas in cancer treatment. Adv Cancer Res 16: 237–332
Chabner BA (1977) Second neoplasm – a complication of cancer chemotherapy. New Engl J Med 297: 213–214
Chalmers TM, MacCarthy DD (1964) Phenylbutazone therapy associated with leukaemia. Brit Med J I: 747
Chaves E (1968) Induction of bladder hyperplasia in rats after a single dose of cyclophosphamide. Rev Franç Études Clin Biol 13: 51–61
Clayson DB (1972) Carcinogenic hazards due to drugs. In: Meyler L, Peck HM (eds) Drug-induced diseases vol 4. Excerpta Medica Monograph, Amsterdam, pp 91–109
Clemmesen J, Hjalgrim-Jensen S (1978) Is phenobarbital carcinogenic? A follow-up of 8078 epileptics. Ecotox Environm Safety 1: 457–470
Cohen SM, Lower GM, Ertürk E, Bryan GT (1973) Comparative carcinogenicity in Swiss mice of N-[4-(5-nitro-2-furyl)-2-thiazolyl] acetamide and structurally related 5-nitrofurans and 4-nitrobenzenes. Cancer Res 33: 1593–1597
Cohen RJ, Wiernik PH, Walker MD (1976) Acute nonlymphocytic leukemia associated with nitrosourea chemotherapy: Report of two cases. Cancer Treatment Rep 60: 1257–1261
Corbett TH (1976) Cancer and congenital anomalies associated with anesthetics. Ann New York Acad Sci 271: 58–66
Cuatrecasas P (1978) Phenacetin studies. Science 203: 6–7
Dahm K, DeHeer K (1976) Cancer risk of the stomach resected for ulcer: The role of duodenogastric reflux. Z Krebsforsch 87: 343–344
Dahm K, Werner B (1973) Anastomosenkarzinom im resezierten Magen der Ratte nach Gabe von N-Methyl-N'-nitro-N-nitrosoguanidin. Dtsch Med Wschr 98: 2486–2487
Dahm K, Werner B (1975) Das Karzinom im operierten Magen. Dtsch Med Wschr 100: 1073–1078
Dale GA, Smith RB (1974) Transitional cell carcinoma of the bladder associated with cyclophosphamide. J Urology 112: 603–604
Danielszyk W (1970) Erfahrungen mit Zytostatika bei der multiplen Sklerose. Wien Klin Wschr 82(40): 697–699
DeHeer K, Werner B (1978) Colonic carcinogenesis in the rat after resection. In: Gerard A (ed) Gastrointestinal tumors. A clinical and experimental approach. Pergamon Press, Oxford New York Toronto Sydney Paris Frankfurt, pp 83–88
Delbrück H, Teillet F, Andrieu JM, Schmitt G, Bayle O, Wetter O (1978) Langzeitkomplikationen bei Patienten mit malignen Lymphomen nach Chemo- und (oder) Strahlentherapie. Dtsch Med Wschr 103: 789–793
DeVita VT, Arseneau JC, Sherins RJ, Canellos GP, Young RC (1973) Intensive chemotherapy for Hodgkin's disease: Long-term complications. In: Natl Cancer Inst Monograph 36, pp 447–454
Douglass D, Levin PT, Moertel CG (1976) Nitrosoureas: Useful agents for the treatment of advances gastrointestinal cancer. Cancer Treatment Rep 60: 757–759
Druckrey H, Preussmann R, Ivankovic S, Schmähl D (1967) Organotrope carcinogene Wirkung bei 65 verschiedenen N-Nitroso-Verbindungen an BD-Ratten. Z Krebsforsch 69: 103–201
Edmondson HA, Henderson B, Benton B (1976) Liver cell adenomas associated with use of oral contraceptives. New Engl J Med 294: 470–472
Ehlers G (1968) Klinische und histologische Untersuchungen zur Frage arzneimittelbedingter Arsen-Tumoren. Z Haut-Geschl-Krkh 43: 763–774

Eisenbrand G, Preussmann R, Schmähl D (1978) Carcinogenicity of N-nitrosoephedrine in rats. Cancer Letters 5: 103–106

Eisenbrand G (1979) Carcinogenic action of BCNU analogs after repeated intraperitoneal application to Sprague-Dawley (SD) rats. Proc Amer Assoc Cancer Res 20: 46

Enderlin F, Guisan Y (1973) Maligne Tumoren unter Immunosuppression, ein neues Problem beim Transplantatempfänger. Helv Chir Acta 40: 773–776

Epstein SS, Andrea J, Joshi S, Mantel N (1967) Hepatocarcinogenicity of griseofulvin following parenteral administration to infant mice. Cancer Res 27: 1900–1906

Fierz U (1965) Katamnestische Untersuchungen über die Nebenwirkungen der Therapie mit anorganischem Arsen bei Hautkrankheiten. Dermatologica 131: 41–58

Fiore-Donati L, De Benedictis G, Maiorano G, Chieco-Bianchi L (1961) Development of pulmonary adenomas in mice suckled by mothers receiving urethan. Naturwiss 48: 409–410

Fox WW (1965) Recent advances in the chemotherapy of tuberculosis. Adv Chemother 2: 197–267

Galy O, Touraine R, Brune J, Roudier P, Gallois P (1963) Le cancer poulmonaire d'origine arsénical des vignerons de Beaujolais. J Franç Med Chir Thor 17(3): 303–311

Gardner WU (1941) The effect of estrogen on the incidence of mammary and pituitary tumors in hybrid mice. Cancer Res 11: 345–358

Gatti RA, Good RA (1971) Occurrence of malignancy in immunodeficiency diseases. A literature review. Cancer 28: 89–98

Gleichmann H, Gleichmann E (1973) Immunosuppression and neoplasia I. A critical review of experimental carcinogenesis and the immunesurveillance theory. Klin Wschr 51: 255–259

Goerttler K (1972) Models and facts in iatrogenic cancerogenesis (report). Verh Dtsch Ges Path 56: 138–164

Götz H, Reichenberger M (1972) Ergebnisse einer Fragebogenaktion bei 1670 Dermatologen der Bundesrepublik Deutschland über Nebenwirkungen bei der Griseofulvintherapie. Hautarzt 23: 485–492

Gottron HA (1954) Gegenwartsfragen beim Hautcarcinom. Med Klin 49: 1553–1560

Gross F (1976) Abschließende Stellungnahme zur Frage eines erhöhten Brustkrebsrisikos durch Rauwolfia-Präparate. Dtsch Ärzteblatt 73: 2370

Guggenheim B (ed) (1979) Health and sugar substitutes. S Karger, Basel München New York Sydney

Guisan Y, Enderlin F, Harder F, Brunner F, Thiel G, Bernhardt JP, Schädeli J, Mihatsch M (1973) Malignomas après transplantation. Schweiz Med Wschr 103: 577–585

Gutjahr P, Spranger J (1975) Acute leukemia following anticancer treatment. J Pediatrics 87: 1004

Guyer MF, Claus PE (1947) Tumor of the lung in rats following injections of urethane (ethyl carbamate). Cancer Res 7: 342–345

Habs M, Schmähl D (1976) Influence of five different postnatal lifelong treatments on the transplacental carcinogenicity of ethylnitrosourea in Sprague Dawley rats. Cancer Letters 2: 93–100

Habs M, Eisenbrand G, Schmähl D (1979) Carcinogenic activity in Sprague-Dawley rats of 2-[3-(2-chloroethyl)-3-nitrosoureido]-D-glucopyranose (chlorozotocin). Cancer Letters 8: 133–137

Habs M, Schmähl D (1979) Carcinogenic action od CMF treatment in rats. In: Current chemotherapy. Proc 11th Int Congr Chemother II, pp 1711–1713

Hammond EC, Selikoff IJ, Robitzek EH (1967) Isoniazid therapy in relation to later occurrence of cancer in adults and in infants. Brit Med J II: 792–795

Hamoudi AB, Ertel I, Newton WA, Reiner CB, Clatworthy HW (1974) Multiple neoplasms in an adolescent child associated with IgA deficiency. Cancer 33: 1134–1144

Harris CC (1976) The carcinogenicity of anticancer drugs: A hazard in man. Cancer 37(2): 1014–1023

Hartwich G, Butzler W (1971) Zweittumoren bei Hämoblastosen unter zytostatischer Therapie. Med Klin 66(43): 1445–1450

Heinonen OP, Shapiro S, Tuominen L, Turunen MI (1974) Reserpine use in relation to breast cancer. Lancet II: 675–677

Herbst AL, Ulfelder H, Poskanzer DC (1971) Adenocarcinoma of the vagina: Association of maternal stilboestrol therapy with tumour appearance in young women. New Eng J Med 284: 878–881

Herold G, Krause D, Taubert H-D, Baumann R (1979) Das klimakterische Syndrom: Substitutionstherapie mit Östrogenen. Dtsch Ärzteblatt 27: 1814–1815

Hicks RM, Chowaniec J (1977) The importance of synergy between weak carcinogens in the induction of bladder cancer in experimental animals and humans. Cancer Res 37: 2943–3949

Hirohata T, Masuda Y, Horie A, Kuratsune M (1973) Carcinogenicity of tar-containing skin drugs: Animal experiment and chemical analysis. Gann 64: 323–330

Hoover R, Gray LA, Cole P, MacMahon B (1976) Menopausal estrogens and breast cancer. New Engl J Med 295(8): 401–405

Hrushesky W, Sampson D, Murphy GP (1972) Carcinogenicity of ethylmethanesulfonate. J Natl Cancer Inst 49: 1077–1083

Hultengren N, Lagergren C, Ljungrist A (1965) Carcinoma of the renal pelvis in renal papillary necrosis. Acta Chir Scand 130: 314–320

Hunstein W, Rehn K (1975) Tumorinduktion durch Zytostatika beim Menschen. Dtsch Med Wschr 100: 155–158

Hyman GA, Sommers SC (1966) The development of Hodgkin's disease and lymphoma during anticonvulsant therapy. Blood 28: 416–427

IARC Monographs on the evaluation of carcinogenic risk of chemicals to man. Some anti-thyroid and related substances, nitrofurans and industrial chemicals. Vol 7, IARC Lyon, pp 85–94 (1974)

Immich H (1974) Assoziation zwischen Reserpin-Medikation und Brustkrebs? Dtsch Ärzteblatt 71(42): 2997–2999

Isaka H, Yoshii H, Otsuji A, Koike K, Nagai Y, Koura M, Sugiyashu K, Kanabayashi T (1979) Tumors of Sprague-Dawley rats induced by long-term feeding of phenacetin. Gann 70(1): 29–36

Ivankovic S, Eisenbrand G, Preussmann R (1979) Lung carcinoma induction in BD rats after single intratracheal instillation of an arsenic-containing pesticide mixture formerly used in vineyards. Int J Cancer 24: 786–788

Ivankovic S (1979) Personal communication

Jaffé WG (1947) Carcinogenic action of ethyl urethane on rats. Cancer Res 7: 107–112

Jick H, Smith PG (1977) Regularly used drugs and cancer. In: Hiatt HH, Watson JG, Winsten JA (eds) Origins of human cancer. Cold Spring Harbor. A: 389–398

Jick H, Watkins RN, Hunter JR, Dinan BJ, Madsen S, Rothman KJ, Walker AM (1979) Replacement estrogens and endometrial cancer. New Engl J Med 300(5): 218–222

Jochimsen PR, Pearlman NW, Lawton RL (1976) Pancreatic carcinoma as a sequel to therapy of lymphoma. J Surg Oncol 8: 461–464

Johansson S, Angervall L (1976) Urothelial changes of the renal papillae in Sprague-Dawley rats induced by long-term feeding of phenacetin. Acta Path Microbiol, Scand A 84: 375–383

Johansson S, Angervall L (1979) Carcinogenicity of phenacetin. Science 204 (4389): 130

Juhasz J, Baló J, Kendrey G (1957) Über die geschwulsterzeugende Wirkung des Isonicotinsäurehydrazid (INH). Z Krebsforsch 62: 188–196

Juhasz J, Baló J, Szende B (1963) Neue experimentelle Angaben zur geschwulsterzeugenden Wirkung des Isonicotinsäurehydrazid (INH). Z Krebsforsch 65: 434–439

Jung HD (1971) Zur fraglichen Induzierung von Bronchial- und Hautkarzinom durch INH (Isoniazid) am Beispiel der Tuberculosis luposa. Z Erkrank Atmungsorg 135: 31–38

Junghans K, Seufert R, v Gerstenberg L, Ivankovic S (1977) Chemically induced carcinogenesis in the stomach of the rat after vagotomy and resection. Proc Int Congr Surg Kyoto, Japan

Kapadia GJ, Chung EB, Ghosh B, Shukla YN, Basak SP, Morton JF, Pradhan SN (1978) Carcinogenicity of some folk medicinal herbs in rats. J Natl Cancer Inst 60: 683–686

Karchmer RK, Amare M, Larsen WE, Mallouk AG, Caldwell GG (1974) Alkylating agents as leukemogens in multiple myeloma. Cancer 33: 1103–1107

Kelleter R, Kuhn D, Schnyder UW, Schröter R (1972) Lymphoretikuläre Hyperplasie nach dreijähriger Methotrexatbehandlung einer Psoriasis. Dtsch Med Wschr 97(13): 514–516

Kessler FJ, Krüskemper HL (1966) Experimentelle Schilddrüsentumoren durch mehrjährige Zufuhr von Kaliumperchlorat. Klin Wschr 44(19): 1154–1156

Khandekar JD, Kurtides ES, Stalzer RC (1977) Acute erythroleukemia complicating prolonged chemotherapy for ovarian carcinoma. Arch Intern Med 137: 355–356

Khandekar JD, Victor TA, Mukhopadhyaya P (1978) Endometrial carcinoma following estrogen therapy for breast cancer. Arch Intern Med 138: 539–541

Klatskin G (1977) Hepatic tumors: Possible relationship to use of oral contraceptives. Gastroenterology 73: 386–394

Klein M (1952) The transplacental effect of urethan on lung tumorigenesis in mice. J Natl Cancer Inst 13: 1003–1010

Klein M (1954) Induction of lung adenomas following exposure of pregnant newborn, and immature male mice to urethan. Cancer Res 14: 438–440

Klein M (1966) Influence of age on induction with urethan of hepatomas and other tumors in infant mice. J Natl Cancer Inst 36: 1111–1120

Knoth W (1966) Arsenbehandlung. Arch Klin Exp Dermatol 227: 228–234

Korpassy B (1961) Tannins as hepatic carcinogens. Progr Exp Tumor Res 2: 245–290

Kroes R, Berkvens JM, Weisburger JH (1975) Immunosuppression in primary liver and colon tumor induction with N-hydroxy-N-2-fluorenylacetamide and azoxymethane. Cancer Res 35: 2651–2656

Labedzki L, Fuchs HJ, Grips KH (1976) Plasmozytom und finale unreifzellige Leukose. Dtsch Med Wschr 101(4): 108–111

Lancet I (1979) Gastric cancer in patients who have taken cimetidine. Lancet I: 1234–1236

Larsen CD (1947) Pulmonary-tumor induction by transplacental exposure to urethane. J Natl Cancer Inst 8: 63–70

Laska EM, Siegel C, Meisner M, Fischer S, Wanderling J (1975) Matched-pairs study of reserpine use and breast cancer. Lancet II: 296–300

Lee AM, Fraumeni JF (1969) Arsenic and respiratory cancer in man: An occupational study. J Natl Cancer Inst 42: 1045–1052

Leistenschneider W, Ehmann R (1973) Nierenbeckenkarzinom nach Phenazetinabusus. Schweiz Med Wschr 103: 433–439

Lenzin A, Cavalli F, Sonntag R, Zimmermann A (1978) Blasenkarzinom bei langjähriger Behandlung mit Cyclophosphamid wegen multiplem Myelom. Urologie A17: 105–108

Lerner H (1977) Second malignancies diagnosed in breast cancer patients while receiving adjuvant chemotherapy at the Pennsylvania Hospital. Proc Amer Assoc Cancer Res 18: 340

Liebegott G (1949) Pathologische Anatomie der chronischen Arsenvergiftung. Dtsch Med Wschr 27/28: 855–856

Liebegott G (1952) Über die Beziehungen zwischen chronischer Arsenvergiftung und malignen Neubildungen. Zbl Arbeitsmed Arbeitsschutz 2: 15–16

Lijinsky W, Taylor HW (1977) Feeding tests in rats on mixtures of nitrite with secondary and tertiary amines of environmental importance. Fd Cosmet Toxicol 15: 269–274

Lijinsky W, Reuber MD, Blackwell BN (1980) Liver tumors in rats by chronic oral administration of the antihistaminic methapyrilene hydrochloride. Science 209: 817–819

Lindenfelser R (1970) Harnblasenkrebs als Spätfolge chemischer Kampfstoffe. Z Urol 63: 175–177

Lingemann CH (ed) (1979) Recent results in cancer research. Vol 66 Carcinogenic hormones. Springer, Berlin Heidelberg New York

Lorenz K, Gebert P (1968) Maligne Retikulose nach Phenylbutazon-Therapie. Münch Med Wschr 110(40): 2283–2287

Mack TM, Pike MC, Henderson BE, Pfeffer RI, Gerkins VR, Arthur M, Brown SE (1976) Estrogens and endometrial cancer in a retirement community. New Engl J Med 294: 1262–1267

McCann CF (1969) Primary malignancy in patients undergoing immunosuppression for renal transplantation. Transplantation 8: 209–212

Meissner WA, Sommers SC, Sherman G (1957) Endometrial hyperplasia, endometrial carcinoma, and endometriosis produced experimentally by estrogen. Cancer 10: 500–509

Mendelsohn G (1976) Multiple tumors in a renal transplant recipient. John Hopkins' Med J 139: 253–256

Meyhöfer W, Knoth W (1966) Über die Auswirkung einer langjährigen antipsoriatischen Arsentherapie auf mehrere Organe unter besonderer Berücksichtigung andrologischer Befunde. Hautarzt 17(7): 309–313

Minkowitz S (1964) Multiple carcinomata following ingestion of medicinal arsenic. Ann Intern Med 61: 296–299

Mori K, Yasuno A, Matsumoto K (1960) Induction of pulmonary tumors in mice with isonicotinic acid hydrazid. Gann 51: 83–89

Narat JK (1925) Experimental production of malignant growth by simple chemicals. J Cancer Res 9: 135–147

Nettleship A, Henshaw PS, Meyer HL (1943) Induction of pulmonary tumors in mice with ethyl carbamate (urethane). J Natl Cancer Inst 4: 309–319

Neubauer O (1947) Arsenical cancer: A review. Brit J Cancer 1: 192–251

Niederle N, Müller H (1978) Harnblasenkarzinom im Verlauf einer chronischen myeloischen Leukämie. Dtsch Med Wschr 103(34): 1346

O'Fallon WM, Labarthe DR, Kurland LT (1975) Rauwolfia derivatives and breast cancer. Lancer II: 292–296

Osswald H (1968) Prüfung von Kaliumchlorat auf cancerogene Wirkung. Arzneimittel-Forsch 18: 121–122

Ott G (1970) Fremdkörpersarkome. In: Leuthardt F, Schoen R, Schwiegk H, Studer A, Zollinger HU (eds) Exp Med Path Klin. Springer, Berlin Heidelberg New York

Ott G, Vollmar J, Hieronymi G (1963) Krebsgefährdung nach Implantation von Kunststoffen. Langenbecks Arch Klin Chir 302: 608–628

Otto H, Plötz D (1966) Experimentelle Tumorinduktion mit Urethanaerosolen. Z Krebsforsch 68: 284–292

Paris JA (1820) Pharmacologica. 3 Edition. Philips, London, pp 132–134

Peacock A, Peacock PR (1966) The results of prolonged administration of isoniazid to mice, rats, and hamsters. Brit J Cancer 20: 307–325

Pearson RM, Soloway MS (1978) Does cyclophosphamide induce bladder cancer? Urology XI(5): 437–447

Pein H (1943) Über die Krebsentstehung bei der chronischen Arsenvergiftung. Dtsch Arch Klin Med 190: 429–443

Penn I (1974) Chemical immunosuppression and human cancer. Cancer 34: 1474–1480

Penn I, Starzl TE (1972) Malignant tumors arising de novo in immunosuppressed organ transplant recipients. Transplantation 14: 407–417
Petersen HS (1973) Erythroleukaemia in a melphalan-treated patient with primary macroglobulinaemia. Scand J Hämatol 10: 5–11
Petri E, Altwein JE (1978) Cyclophosphamid und Harnblasenkarzinom. Dtsch Med Wschr 103(1): 30–32
Petzoldt D (1966) Stellung und Wert der Arsen-Behandlung aus dermatologischer Sicht. Dtsch Med Wschr 91(19): 909–910
Pike MC, Edmondson HA, Brenton B, Henderson BE (1977) Liver adenomas and oral contraceptives. In: Hiatt HH, Watson JD, Winsten JA (eds) Origins of human cancer. A Cold Spring Harbor 423–427
Ponomarkov V, Tomatis L, Turusov V (1976) The effect of long-term administration of phenobarbitone in CF-1 mice. Cancer Letters 1: 165–172
Pool BL (1978) Non-mutagenicity of saccharin. Toxicology 11: 95–97
Pool BL (1979) Personal communication
Puri HC, Campbell RA (1977) Cyclophosphamide and malignancy. Lancet I: 1306
Rassner G (1973) Psoriasis – ihre zytostatische Behandlung und Amethopterin (Methotrexat). Fortschr Med 91(9): 381–390
Reddy JK, Qureshi SA (1979) Tumorigenicity of the hypolipidemic peroxisome proliferator ethyl α-p-chlorophenoxy isobutyrate (clofibrate) in rats. Br J Cancer 40: 476–482
Reimer RR, Hoover R, Fraumeni JF, Young RC (1977) Acute leukemia after alkylating-agent therapy of ovarian cancer. New Engl J Med 297(4): 177–181
Richtmeier AJ (1975) Urinary-bladder tumors after cyclophosphamide. New Engl J Med 293: 1045–1046
Rivière MR, Oberman B, Arnold J, Guérin M (1965) Tumeurs mélaniques et mélanomes induit chez le Hamster doré par application cutanée de carbamate d'ethyle (urethane). Bull Cancer 52: 127–144
Robson AO, Jelliffe AM (1963) Medicinal arsenic poisoning and lung cancer. Brit Med J II: 207
Rossi L, Ravera M, Repetti G, Santi L (1977) Long-term administeration of DDT or phenobarbital-Na in Wistar rats. Int J Cancer 19: 179–185
Roth F (1956) Über die chronische Arsenvergiftung der Moselwinzer unter besonderer Berücksichtigung des Arsenkrebses. Z Krebsforsch 61: 287–319
Roth F (1957) Arsen – Leber – Tumoren (Haemangioendotheliom). Z Krebsforsch 61: 468–503
Rowley JD, Golomb HM, Vardiman J (1977) Acute leukemia after treatment of lymphoma. New Engl J Med 297(18): 1013
Rumpf P, Schacht U, Palomba P, Kremer K, Schmitz H, Borchard F (1978) Chemisch induzierte Karzinogenese des Rattenmagens nach Vagotomie und Resektion. Z Gastroenterol 16: 85–94
Rupprecht L, Blessing MH (1973) Fibrosarkom der Harnblase nach siebenjähriger Chemotherapie einer Lymphogranulomatose im Kindesalter. Dtsch Med Wschr 98 (36): 1663–1665
Rustia M, Shubik P (1976) Transplacental effects of diethylstilbestrol on the genital tract of hamster offspring. Cancer Letters 1: 139–146
Rustia M, Shubik P (1978) Thyroid tumours in rats and hepatomas in mice after griseofulvin treatment. Brit J Cancer 38: 237–249
Saltzstein SL, Ackermann LV (1959) Lymphoadenopathy induced by anticonvulsant drugs and mimicking clinically and pathologically malignant lymphomas. Cancer 12: 164–182
Sato T, Utsumi S, Kajikawa K, Ikeda H (1967) A case of cancer of the larynx found in mustard gas poisoning. Jap J Otol 70(11): 1773–1778
Schabel FM (1976) Nitrosoureas: A review of experimental antitumor activity. Cancer Treatment Rep 60: 665–698

Scherf HR (1972) Untersuchungen an männlichen Sprague-Dawley-Ratten über Zusammenhänge zwischen der immundepressiven und der carcinogenen Wirkung bei vier N-Nitroso-Verbindungen. Z Krebsforsch 77: 189–193

Scherf HR (1976) The effect of 4-dimethylaminoazobenzene and azobenzene on the immune reaction of male Sprague-Dawley rats. Z Krebsforsch 87: 327–332

Scherf HR, Schmähl D (1975) Experimental investigation on immunodepressive properties of carcinogenic substances in male Sprague-Dawley rats. In: Recent results in cancer research, vol 52: 76–87

Scherf HR, Karsten C, Krüger C (1969) Tierexperimentelle Untersuchungen über immunsuppressive Wirkungen von Cytostatica. Langenbeck's Arch Chir 325: 1028–1033

Scherf HR, Krüger C, Karsten C (1970) Untersuchungen an Ratten über immunosuppressive Eigenschaften von Cytostatica unter besonderer Berücksichtigung der carcinogenen Wirkung. Arzneimittel-Forsch 20: 1467–1470

Scheuer A, Lehmann FG (1977) Lebertumoren bei Therapie mit Kontrazeptiva und Anabolika. Internist 18: 208–214

Schindler AE (1976) Estrogens and endometrial cancer: Aspects of etiology and survival rate. Arch Geschwulstforsch 46(5): 345–349

Schmähl D (1967) Karzinogene Wirkung von Cyclophosphamid und Triazichon bei Ratten. Dtsch Med Wschr 92(25): 1150–1152

Schmähl D (1971) Karzinogenese und Immundepression. Dtsch Med Wschr 96(45): 1771–1772

Schmähl D (1972) Toxikologische Probleme der iatrogenen Carcinogenese. Verh Dtsch Ges Path 56: 133–138

Schmähl D (1973) Fehlen einer kanzerogenen Wirkung von Cyclamat, Cyclohexylamin und Saccharin bei Ratten. Arzneimittel-Forsch 23: 1466–1470

Schmähl D (1975) Experimental investigations with anti-cancer drugs for carcinogenicity with special reference to immune depression. In: Recent results in cancer research, vol 52. Springer, Berlin Heidelberg New York, pp 18–28

Schmähl D (1977) Carcinogenic action of anticancer drugs with special reference to immunosuppression. Cancer 40: 1927–1929

Schmähl D (1978a) Saccharin und Blasenkrebs. Dtsch Med Wschr 103(3): 91–92

Schmähl D (1978b) Experiments on the carcinogenic effect of orthotoluol-sulfonamide (OTS). Z Krebsforsch 91: 19–22

Schmähl D, Habs M (1976) Life-span investigations for carcinogenicity of some immune-stimulating, immunodepressive and neurotropic substances in Sprague-Dawley rats. Z Krebsforsch 86: 77–84

Schmähl D, Habs M (1978) Experimental carcinogenesis of antitumour drugs. Cancer Treatment Rev 5: 175–184

Schmähl D, Habs M (1979) Carcinogenic action of low-dose cyclophosphamide given orally to Sprague-Dawley rats in a life-time experiment. Int J Cancer 23: 706–712

Schmähl D, Osswald H (1970) Experimentelle Untersuchungen über carcinogene Wirkungen von Krebschemotherapeutica und Immunosuppressiva. Arzneimittel-Forsch 20: 1461–1467

Schmähl D, Reiter A (1954) Fehlen einer cancerogenen Wirkung beim Phenacetin. Arzneimittel-Forsch 4: 404–405

Schmähl D, Wagner R, Scherf HR (1971) Der Einfluß von Immunosuppressiva auf die Cancerisierung der Rattenleber durch Diäthylnitrosamin und die Fibrosarkomentstehung durch 3,4-Benzpyren. Arzneimittel-Forsch 21: 403–404

Schmähl D, Mundt D, Schmidt KG (1974) Experimental investigations on the influence upon the chemical carcinogenesis. 1st communication: studies with ethylnitrosourea. Z Krebsforsch 82: 91–100

Schmähl D, Habs M, Diehl B (1976a) Experimental investigations on the influence upon the chemical carcinogenesis. IInd communication: studies with 3,4-benzopyrene. Z Krebsforsch 86: 85–88

Schmähl D, Danisman A, Habs M, Diehl B (1976b) Experimental investigations on the influence upon the chemical carcinogenesis. IIIrd communication: studies with 1,2-dimethylhydrazine. Z Krebsforsch 86: 89–94

Schmalzl F, Keiser G, Kresbach E, Fritz H, Asamer H, Braunsteiner H (1975) Plasmozytom, Alkylantien und akute myelogene Leukämien. Dtsch Med Wschr 100(39): 1961–1967

Schuermann H (1957) Neuere Therapie der Psoriasis vulgaris universalia. Med Klin 52: 1686

Shimkin MB (1955) Pulmonary tumors in experimental animals. Adv Cancer Res 3: 223–267

Smit CG, Meyler L (1970) Acute myeloid leukaemia after treatment with cytostatic agents. Lancer II: 671–672

Sotrel G, Jafari K, Lash AF, Stepto RC (1976) Acute leukemia in advanced ovarian carcinoma after treatment with alkylating agents. Obstet Gyn 47: 67s–71s

Swift M, Sholman L, Perry M, Chase C (1976) Malignant neoplasms in the families of patients with ataxia telangiectasia. Cancer Res 36: 209–215

Tannenbaum A, Silverstone H (1958) Urethan (ethyl carbamate) as a multipotential carcinogen. Cancer Res 18: 1225–1231

Taylor HW, Lijinsky W (1975) Tumor induction in rats by feeding aminopyrine or oxytetracycline with nitrite. Int J Cancer 16: 211–215

Thiede T, Christensen BC (1969) Bladder tumours induced by chlornaphazine. Acta Med Scand 185: 133–137

Thiers H, Colomb D, Moulin G, Colin I (1967) Le cancer cutane arsenical des viticulteurs du Beaujolais. Ann Dermatol Syphil 94: 133–158

Thomas C (1972) Systematic of iatrogenic carcinogenesis (report). Verh Dtsch Ges Path 56: 126–132

Toth B (1976) Tumorigenicity of β-phenylethylhydrazine sulfate in mice. Cancer Res 36: 917–921

Toth B, Boreisha I (1969) Tumorigenesis with isonicotinic acid hydrazide and urethan in the Syrian golden hamster. Europ J Cancer 5: 165–171

Toth B, Rustia M (1967) The effect of isonicotinic acid hydrazide on the development of tumors. Int J Cancer 2: 413–420

Toth B, Tomatis L, Shubik P (1961) Multipotential carcinogenesis with urethan in the Syrian golden hamster. Cancer Res 21: 1537–1541

Trainin N (1963) Neoplastic nature of liver "blood cysts" induced by urethan in mice. J Natl Cancer Inst 31: 1489–1499

Truhaut R (ed) Potential carcinogenic hazards from drugs. Evaluation of risks. UICC Monograph series vol 7. Springer, Berlin Heidelberg New York

Ulfelder H (1976) The stilbestrol-adenosis-carcinoma syndrome. Cancer 38: 426–431

Urman HK, Bulay O, Clayson DB, Shubik P (1975) Carcinogenic effects of niridazole. Cancer Letters 1: 69–74

Vesselinovitch SD, Mihailovich N (1966) Significance of newborn age and dose of urethan in leukemogenesis. Cancer Res 26: 1633–1637

Videbaek A (1964) Chlornaphazine (Erysan) may induce cancer of the urinary bladder. Acta Med Scand 176: 45–50

Wada S, Miyanishi M, Nishimoto K, Kambe S, Miller RW (1968) Mustard gas as a cause of respiratory neoplasia in man. Lancet I: 1161–1163

Waldmann TA, Strober W, Blaese RM (1972) Immunodeficiency diseases and malignancy. Various immunologic deficiencies of man and the role of immune processes in the control of malignant disease. Ann Intern Med 77: 605–628

Walker EA, Bogovski P, Griciute L (eds) Environmental N-nitroso compounds. Analysis and formation. IARC Sci Publ No 14, Lyon, France

Wall RL, Clausen KP (1975) Carcinoma of the urinary bladder in patients receiving cyclophosphamide. New Engl J Med 293: 271–273

Waskell L (1978) Study of the mutagenicity of anesthetics and their metabolites. Mutation Res 57: 141–153

Waynforth HB, Magee PN (1974) The effect of N-nitroso-N-methylurea and N-dimethylnitrosamine on cell mediated and humoral immune responses in rats and mice. Brit J Cancer 30: 512–523

Weisburger EK (1977) Bioassay program for carcinogenic hazards of cancer chemotherapeutic agents. Cancer 40: 1935–1949

Weiß A, Weiß B (1975) Karzinogenese durch Lost-Exposition beim Menschen, ein wichtiger Hinweis für die Alkylantien-Therapie. Dtsch Med Wschr 100(17): 923

Weiß A, Weiß B (1976) Glioblastom und Neurofibrom nach Lost-Einwirkung. Münch Med Wschr 118(27): 875–878

Weiss NS, Szekely DR, Austin DF (1976) Increasing incidence of endometrial cancer in the United States. New Engl J Med 294: 1259–1262

Werner B, DeHeer K, Mitschke H (1977) Cholecystectomy and carcinoma of the colon. Z. Krebsforsch 88: 223–230

Wildhack R (1973) Leukämie nach Hydantoin-Behandlung. Münch Med Wschr 115 (28): 1275–1279

Williamson RCN, Bauer FLR, Oscarson JEA, Ross JS, Malt RA (1978) Promotion of azoxymethane-induced colonic neoplasia by resection of the proximal small bowel. Cancer Res 38: 3212–3217

Wolfart W (1960) Ruft Isonikotinsäurehydrazid Tumoren hervor? Dtsch Med Wschr 85(37): 1655–1657

Worth PHL (1971) Cyclophosphamide and the bladder. Brit Med J II: 182

Zeller WJ, Schmähl D (1979) Development of second malignancies in rats after cure of acute leukemia L5222 by single doses of 2-chloroethylnitrosoureas. J Cancer Res Clin Oncol 95: 83–86

Subject Index

The numbers set in *italics* refer to those pages on which the respective catch-word is discussed in detail

absorption *24*
acetaminophen 78, 196, 203
acetanilide 31
acetazolamide 268
acetic acid 28
acetophenitidin 203
acetosalicylic acid 75, 78, 196, 203
acetoxymethane 358
acetylate 28
acetylcholine 44
– receptors 44
acetyl-hydrazide 28
acetylhydrazine 83
acetyl transferase activity 83
acidosis 201
aciduria, paradoxical 232
achlorhydria 24
acute easinophilic cholangiohepatitis 108
– glomerulonephritis 191, 202
– interstitial nephritis *185*
– liver dystrophy 77, 83, 86, 91
– – failure 76, 86
– – injury *76*
– tubular necrosis 145, 151, 162, 187, 192, 193, 194, 219
Addison's disease 226
additive effect 279
adenoma, hepatocellular 112
–, mononodular 110, 116
–, multinodular 110, 111, 115, 116, 117, 119, 121
–, uninodular 115, 116, 118, 121
adrenaline 21, 35, 46
adriamycin 350, 359
agammaglobulinemia 356
agranular endoplasmic reticulum 70, 71, 78, 83
– – reticulum, hypertrophy 70, *71*, 96, 97
agranulocytosis 18, 19, 55, 154
ajmaline 85, 86, 87, 97, 104
alcohol-induced fatty changes 85
alcoholic centrolobular sclerosis 107
– cholestasis 94
– hepatitis 109
alcoholism, chronic 85, 102
aldehyde-fuchsin staining 71
aldophosphamide 37
aldosterone 232, 233
alkaline phosphatase 93
alkalosis, metabolic 231
alkylating agents 358
allergen triggers 56
allergic drug reactions, classification *56*
– vasculitis 189
allergy *51, 53*
allopurinol 35, 37, 40, 102, 104, 186, 189, 190
aloe 219
alprenolol 29
alveolitis, extrinsic allergic 59
amanitine 78
Ambilhar 343
amebiasis 343
amelia 273
amidopyrene (Pyramidon) 355
aminoglycoside antibiotics 39
δ-aminolaevulinic acid-synthetase 51
6-amino nicotinamide 251, 271, 272, 275, 278, 281, 282, 305, 306, 307, 308, 309, 311, 312, 313, 314, 315, 316
– – -analogue of NADP 309, 310, 312
aminonucleoside 146, *147*, 149, 150
– nephrosis *147*, 150, 158, 159, 171, 173
aminophenazone 75
2-aminopropionitrile 287
aminopyrine 18, 33, 355
amitriptyline 37
amphetamine 36, 45
amphotericin B 193, 219
ampicillin 39, 185, 187
amylobarbitone 31

amyloidosis 203
anabolic steroids 71, 94, 95, 96, 110, 121, 341, *342*, 359
anaemia 48, 49, 56, 190, 196, 201, 202
–, aplastic 2, 4, 121, 154
–, haemolytic 56, 58
–, idiopathic auto-immune 58
–, megaloblastic 34
anaesthesia, general 50
analgesic nephropathy 184, *196*
analgesics 49, 71, 75, 104, 194, 195, *335*
anaphylactic shock, acute 52, 53, 55, 56
anaphylactoid reactions 57
anaphylaxis 2, 19, 53, 55, 56, *57*
androstendione 342
anemia, idiopathic aplastic 342
anesthetics 335, *336*
angiitis 194
angina pectoris 8
angiotensine 255
anorexia nervosa 218, 220, 222, 230, 234
anthraquinone 219
anthracycline 149
antiarrhythmic drugs 85, 97
anti-basement-membrane glomerulonephritis 153, 163, 173, 174
antibiotics 185, 192, 194, 218, 344, 350
antibodies, IgE 56, 57, 59
–, IgG 56, 57, 58, 156, 158, 165, 172, 189
–, IgM 56, 57, 58, 165, 170, 171, 189
anticholinergic drugs 19, 43
anticoagulants 43
anticonvulsants 338
antidepressants 85
–, tricyclic 27, 36, 46
antiepileptic drugs 22, 34, 71, 90, 168
antifungal agents *193*
antihistamines 22, *335*
antihypertensives 166
antimalarials 48, 49
antimetabolites 97, 344, 350, 356, 359
antineoplastic agents *343*
antineoplastic drugs 19, 37
antipyrin 29, 30, 31, 33, 186
antirheumatic drugs 97
antituberculous drugs 79, 83, 84, 85, 86, 107, 185, 194, *195*
anti-tubular basement membrane nephritis 189
antigen-antibody complexes, circulating 146, 152, 173
– –, in situ formation 146, 152, 156, 173
antigenic determinant 52
antigenic effect 82
antinuclear factor antibodies 29
aplastic anaemia 2, 4, 121, 154
– –, idopathic 342
apnea 46
arrhythmia, cardiac 2
arsenic 109
arsenic trioxide *334*, 359
arthritis, chronic 10
–, rheumatoid *51*, 54, 153, 159
Arthus phenomenon 152
Arthus-type skin reaction 59
artificial sweeteners 353
ascites 31
aseptic papillary necrosis 196, 199, 200, 201, 202, 203, 204
aspirin 10, 18, 21, 24, 43, 48, 52, 55, 57, 59, 78, 85, 104, 107, 204
asthma 43, 54, 55, 57, 59
ataxia 32
ataxia teleangiectatica 356
atophan 80
atopic disease 54
– eczema 55
atopy *54*
Auriothan 159
Auro-Detoxin 159
aurothioglucose 159
aurothiopolypeptide 159
auto-immune cytotoxic reaction *58*
azathioprine 37, 97, 110, 114, 146, 150, 186

background, genetic 285
β-adrenergic blocking drugs 43
Billroth's operation 357
Bis(chloroethyl) ether 337
B-lymphocytes 54, 55
bacitracin 46
barbiturates 22, 33, 42, 51, 71, 166
Bartter's syndrome 218, 226, 227, 228, 229, 230
basophils 55, 56
beclomethasone 21
Benzerazide 35
benzodiazepine 22, 27
benzpyrene 33
benzylpenicilloyl 189
beromycin 189
bile acids 85, 93, 94

bile excretion, delay 80
biliary cirrhosis, primary 100, 153
bilirubin 93
bioactivation *37*, 39
bioavailability 22, 23, 24, 25, 29, 31
bioinactivation 50
biotransformation *28*, 34, 70, 104, 108
bisacodyl 219
bladder carcinoma 338, 344, 347, 348, 350, 353, 354
bradykinin 255
bland cholestasis 95
breast cancer 342, 352, 353
blocking antibodies 53, 56
blood-brain barrier 27
blood eosinophilia 186, 190, 195
Boeck granulomes 102
bone marrow aplasia 37
– –, suppression 149
boric acid 21
breast disease 10
broad spectrum antibiotics 21
5-bromodeoxyuridine 272
bromosulphthalein 57
brondius carcinoma 344
brucellosis 191
Budd-Chiari disease 112, 114

caffeine 203
calcium 50
canalicular cholestasis 95
cancer, vaginal 4, 5, 340
canrenone 24, 37
cantharidin 359
Captopril *165*
carbamazepine 21, 33, 35, 37, 55, 72, 73, 166
– epoxides 37
carbenicillin 31, 39, 185, 218
carbenoxolone 218
carbimazol 186
carbon tetrachloride 78, 107
carcinogenesis 266
–, transplacental 244, 264, 322, 323, 341
carcinogenic effect 322
carcinogenicity 242, 322
cardiac arrhythmia 2
– dysrhythmias 19, 43
cardiotoxicity 149
cardiovascular disease 6, 8
– mortality, tolbutamide-induced 3
cascara 219
cataract 7
catecholamines 44, 46
cathartic drugs *218*
causal genesis 292
cell-ballooning 85
cell-mediated immune reaction 152
cell-mediated reactions *59*
cell proliferation, regenerative 76
cellular hydrops 85, 93
centrolobular liver necrosis 77, 78, 81, 84, 86, 91, 107, 114
– sclerosis, alcoholic 107
cephalosporin 55, 57, 58, 185, 193
cephalotin 192, 193
cephazolin 39
cerebrospinal fluid 27
ceroid pigment 90, 104
Chagas' disease 147
chenodesoxycholic acid 110
chinoline derivatives 49
chloralhydrate 26, 336
chloramphenicol 2, 3, 4, 19, 23, 30, 31, 35, 48, 185, 261, 273, 359
chloramphenicol-induced aplastic anemia 3, 4
chlornaphazine *347*
chlorinated hydrocarbons 33
chlormethiazole 23, 30, 31
p-chloro-acetanilide 47
chlorodiazepoxide 336
chloroform 78
chloromethyl methyl ether 337
chlorophenoxybutyric acid 40
chlorozotocin 351
chlorpromazine 58, 80, 95, 97, 98, 100, 104, 166, 355
chlorthalidone 185, 219
cholangiohepatitis, acute eosinophilic 108
cholangiolitic cholestasis 95
cholangitis 100
–, destructive nonsuppurative 100
–, eosinophilic 94, 104
cholecalciterol 34
cholecystectomy 357
cholecystographic dyes 59
cholestatic effect, obligatory 80
– hepatitis 100
– –, drug-induced 95
– hepatopathy 76
– jaundice 51
– lesions 70, 77, 84, *91*
– reactions 76, 77, 78, 80, 93
"cholestatic hepatosis" 76, 97
cholestasis 76, 77, 80, 83, 85, 86, 87, *91*, 104, 108, 110, 119

cholestasis, alcoholic 94
–, bland 95
–, canalicular 95
–, cholangiolitic 95
–, cytotoxic 85
– during pregnancy 95
–, hepatocanalicular 95
–, primary intralobular 100, 102
–, prolonged 104
–, uncomplicated 95
"cholestais with hepatitis" 77
chronic active hepatitis 104, 153
– arthritis 10
– hepatitis 69
– –, drug induced 106
– viral hepatitis 108
chrysotherapy 159
cimetidine 356
Cinchophen 18, 97
cirrhosis 30, 31, 43, 106, 107, 109
–, postdystrophic 86, 107
–, postnecrotic 86, 107
–, primary biliary 100, 153
clearing up 94
clear cell carcinoma of the vagina 340
cleft palate 259, 262, 267, 268, 269, 272, 275, 276, 280, 281, 283, 315
clindomycin 31, 46
clofibrate 40, 343
clonidine 46
clotting factors 43
CMF scheme (cyclophosphamide-methotrexate-5-fluorouracil) 352
cobalt-chloride 38
codeine 57
cohort study 2, 3, 6
Colcemid 344
colic, renal 193, 196
colistin 46, 185, 193
colitis, pseudomembranous 4
–, ulcerative 229
combined cytotoxic-cholestatic drug injury 91
complement 56, 58
concentric lamellar bodies 73
congenital functional anomalies 244
Conn's syndrome 218, 222
contact cathartics 219
– dermatitis 56, 59, 152
contraceptives 4, 7, 8, 9, 10, 13, 33, 51, 71, 81, 83, 86, 92, 93, 94, *95*, 96, 97, 100, 110, 111, 112, 114, 115, 116, 117, 119, 120, 121, 166, *341*, 359
– for men 343
contraindication 8, 10
controlled hypothermia 312
Coomb's test, indirect 58
copper sulphate 21
coralgil 109
coronary death 6
– heart disease 6, 8
corticosteroids 33, 42, 43, 356
creatinine phosphokinase 50
crescent formation 148, 154, 172
cross-allergy *53*
curare-like action 46
cutaneous erythema 55
cyclamate *353*, 359
cyclizine 355
cyclopenthiazide 219
cyclophosphamide (Endoxan) 37, 38, 146, 150, 151, 251, 275, 281, 282, 286, 298, 344, 345, 346, 347, 348, 349, 350
cylindruria 192, 193
cytochrome P_{450}-type system *251*
cytosine arabinoside 271, 272
cytostatic drugs 80, 85, 86, 87, 97, 114, 146, 149, *150*
cysteamine 38
cysteine 38
cystinuria 153
cytotoxic cholestasis 85
– effect 81, 82, 248
– hepatopathy 77, 80
– hepatosis 77, 80
– injuries, direct 81
– –, indirect 81
– lesions *85*, 107
– liver dystrophy 77
– – injury 77
– necrotizing hepatopathy 77
– reaction 293, 299, 301, 304
– reactions 56, *57*, 76, 77, 78, 80

dapsone 29
daunomycin 146, *149*
– nephrosis *149*
daunorubicin 146, *149*
deafness, ethacrynic-acid-induced 1
DDT 73, 337
delayed type of hypersensitivity 59
demecolcine 344
demethylchlortetracycline 57
DPH syndrome 244
dermatitis, exfoliative 190
desacetylrifampicin 37
desipramine 46
N-desmethyldiazepam 37
destructive interstitial nephritis 222

destructive nonsuppurative cholangitis 100
de Vita schedule 80, 86
dexamethason 267, 275, 281, 282
dexamethasone 42
dextran 52, 57
dextrapropoxyphene 35
dextropropoxyphene 355
diabetes 256, 353
diabetes insipidus 21
– mellitus 43, 202
diarrhea, chronic 222
diazepam 26, 27, 30, 31, 37, 71, 102, 336
diacetylmorphine *170*
diazoxide 25, 26
dichloralphenazone 33
dicoumarol 33, 35
diethyleneglykol 47
diethylmaleate 38
diethylstilbestrol 4, 5, 244, *340*, 342, 359
digitalis 19, 43, 46
– toxicity 43, 46
digitoxin 22
digoxin 22, 23, 24, 25, 39
dimethylhydrazine 357, 358
diphenylhydantoin 287
dimethylnitrosamine 355
dimethocyphenyl-penicilloyl 189
diphenyldramine 33
diphenylhydantoin 72, 73, 83, 166, 186
diphenylhydrazine 86, 87
diphenylmethane 219
diphtheria 186
diplopia 32
disulfiram 35, 355
Distraneurine *164*
diuretic drugs 172, 173, 185, *218*
L-dopa 24, 35, 45, 46
– -induced dyskinesias 45
dopamine 35, 45
dose specifity 266, *273*
drug allergy *51*, *53*
– hepatitis, "fulminating" 76
– –, unspecific 91
– – with cholestasis 95
– -induced cholestatic hepatitis 95
– – chronic hepatitis 106
– – hepatitis 70, 76
– – hepatitis with cholestasis 91
– – hepatopathy 70, 77
– – injury 70
– – jaundice 95
– -metabolizing system 78
– reactions, type A *19*
– –, type B 19, *47*
– specifity 266, *271*
– toxicity 5, 14, *17*, 44
ductal proliferation 109
Dupuytren's contracture 351
dysentery 221
dysrhythmias, cardiac 19

EDTA intoxication 222
eczema 54, 55
–, atopic 55
electrolyte imbalance 172
embryolethal effect 243, 244, 285, 323
embryomortality 244, *259*, 321, 323
embryotoxic effect 243, 244, 245, 246, 250, 251, 255, 256, 271, 321, 323
embryotoxicity 286, 323
emodin 219
encephalopathy 43
–, hepatic 31
endometrial cancer, estrogen-induced 3, 7
endometrial carcinoma 342
endophlebitis 110
– hepatica obliterans 112, 114
endoplasmic reticulum, agranular 70, 71, 78, 83
– –, agranular (smooth), hypertrophy 70, *71*, 96, 97
Endoxan (cyclophosphamide) 146, 150, 275, 281, 282, 286, 298, 344, 345, 346, 347, 348, 349, 350
enflurane 337
enzyme-inhibition 29, *34*
enzyme-induction 29, *33*, 70, 71
eosinophilic cholangiohepatitis, acute 108
– cholangitis 94, 104
– granulocytes 78, 84, 86, 90, 91, 94, 100, 101, 102, 104, 108
– infiltration 78, 81, 83, 84, 94, 95
– pericholangitis 94
ephedrine 36, 355
epithelioid cell granulomas 78, 100, 101, 102, 115, 119
– – reaction, minifocal 102
ergotamine 255
erythema, cutaneous 55
erythromycin 23, 39, 55
– estolate 23
– propionate 23
erythropoietin deficiency 202
estrogen 3, 7, 80, 81, 83, 95, 110, 114, 119, *341*, 359

estrogen-induced endometrial cancer 3, 7
ethacrinic acid 1, 26, 40, 219
– – -induced deafness 1
ethanol 33
ether cyclopropane 50
ethosuximide 55, 166
Ethrane 337
ethylene imine 359
ethylmethane sulfonate 343, 359
exanthema 186, 190
exfoliative dermatitis 190
extoplasma 94
extrinsic allergic alveolitis 59

facultative hepatotoxicity 76, *80*
Fanconi anaemia 121, 342
– syndrome 47, 193, 218, 219
"fast acetylators" 83
fatty acids 33
– changes, alcohol-induced 85
– infiltration 78, 79, 82, 83, 85, 86, 87, 109
– liver of pregnancy 80, 85
fava beans 48
"feathery degeneration" 85, 92, 93, 94
fenofibrate 343
ferment induction 83
fetomortality 244, 323
fetotoxic effect 243, 244, 246, 250, 251, 323
fibrosis, portal 106, 109
fluorescein 57
5-fluoro-uracil 37, 344
fluroxene 337
focal multinodular hyperplasia 115, 116, 117, 118, 119
– necroses 86, 90, 112
– sclerosing glomerulonephritis 170, 171
– sclerosis 148, 170
folic acid 22, 33, 34
– – antagonists 108
– – deficiency 22, 34, 286
formal genesis 292
Fowler solution 109, 334, 335
frusemide 38, 40, 43
Fuchsin 359
fuchsisenecionin 343
"fulminating drug hepatitis" 76
– viral hepatitis 86
functional anomalies, congenital 244
furazolidone 54
Furium 359
Furosemide 185, 219, 220

gallamine 46
gallbladder disease 7
gastric cancer 356
– hemorrhage 18, 43
– ulcer 202
gastrointestinal bleeding 21, 43
gene defect, inheritable 245, 246
general anaesthesia 50
genesis, causal 292
–, formal 292
genetic background 285
gentamicin 22, 39, 46, 185, 191, 192
giant cells 92, 93, 94, 100, 101, 102, 190
– mitochondria 96, 151
glafenin 185, 193
"glatte Nebenkerne" 73
glaucoma 42, 43
glioblastoma 344
glomerulonephritis 59, 148, 170, 172, 194, 229
–, acute 191, 202
–, anti-basement-membrane 153, 163, 173, 174
–, chronic proliferating 148
–, focal sclerosing 170, 171
–, gold-induced *159*
–, immune-complex 145, 148, 152, 153, 154, 158, 161, 163, 164, 165, 168, 169, 170, 171, 173
–, membrane-proliferative 170
–, mesangioproliferative 148, 154, 168, 169
–, perimembranous 154, 155, 156, 157, 158, 159, 160, 162, 163, 164, 165
–, proliferating intercapillary 151, 171
glomerulosclerosis 148
–, focal 229
glucocorticoids 272, 286
glucocorticoid therapy 85, 110
glucose-6-phosphate dehydrogenase 48, 49
– – deficiency *48*, 49
glucosuria 190
glucuronic acid 28
glutamine 28
glutethimide 33, 51
gluthathione 38, 78
–, reduced 48
– -reductase 48, 49
– – deficiency *49*
glycine 28
glycogen 71, 85, 86, 99
– storage 85, 86, 87
gold-induced glomerulonephritis *159*

gold nephropathy *159*, 162, 163
– preparations *159*, 173
Goodpasture syndrome 146, 153, 171, *172*
Goormaghtigh cells 224, 225, 226, 234
gout 43
granular endoplasmic membranes 71
granulomatous reaction 78, 80, 81, 82, 84, 100, 101, *102*, 104
grey baby syndrome 30
griseofulvin 51, 166, *339*, 359
"ground-glass hepatocytes" 71
grouped necroses 77
growth retardation 244, 256, 257, 259, 260, 261, 264, 274, 278, 313, 321, 323
guanethidine 23, 24, 27
N-guanine 285
O-guanine
guanoxan 166

Hb_{Zurich} 49
HbH disease 49
HB_s antigen 71
HB_s-bearing cells 72, 73
haematuria 154, 170, 186, 190, 192, 193, 196, 201
haemoglobin 48, 49
–, inactive 201
haemoglobins, drug-sensitive 49
haemolysis 48, 49, 56, 58, 194
haemolytic accidents 58
– crises 48, 49
– reactions 57, 58
haemoptysis 172
HLA alloantigens 51
– allogens 54
– serotype 54
halogenated paraffins 359
halothane 50, 80, 81, 82, 83, 84, 85, 86, 102, 104, 336, 337
hay-fever 54
heart failure 43
Heinz bodies 49
hemangioendothelioma 334
hemangiosarcoma 344
hemorrhage, gastric 18
hemosiderin 90
heparin 57
hepatic coma 30
– disease 50
– encephalopathy 31
– precoma 43, 44
hepatitis 2, 23, 28, 58, 69, 190
–, acute viral 30
–, alcoholic 109
–, cholestatic forms 100
–, chronic 69
–, – active 104, 153
–, –, drug-induced 106
–, – viral 108
–, "drug induced" 70, 76
–, lupoid 106
–, viral 77, 91
hepatoblastoma, mixed 121
hepatocanalicular cholestasis 95
hepatocellular carcinoma *120*
hepatocyte turnover 76
hepatoma 339
hepatopathy 70
–, cholestatic 76
–, cytotoxic 77, 80
–, – necrotizing 77
–, toxic 77, 80
hepatoportal sclerosis 109
hepatosis, cholestatic 76
–, cytotoxic 77, 80
hepatotoxic properties 23
hepatotoxity 38
–, facultative 76, *80*
–, intrinsic 76
–, obligatory 76, 78, 80, 85
hepatovascular lesions *109*
heroin 57, *170*
herpetic eruptions 43
hexamethalentetramine 359
hexobarbitone 31
Heymann nephritis 146, 153, 161, 164
histamine 56
– releasers 57
histiotrophic nutrition 252
Hodgkin's disease 55, 350, 352
hydantoin 102, 166, *167*, 338, 359
hydralazine 24, 29, 33, 102, 166, 167, 168, 169
hydrocarbons, volatile *171*
hydrochlorthiazide 24, 219
hydronephrosis 203
hydropic changes 82, 83, 85, 86, 87, 94, 99, 100, 109
hydrops, cellular 85, 93
5-hydroxytryptamine 35, 255
hydroxyurea 298, 299, 301
hyperaldosteronism 220
–, secondary 232
hyperbilirubinaemia 31
hypercholesterinaemia 100
hypercholesterolaemia 34
hyperglycaemia 43
hyperkalaemia 2, 50
hyperplasia, focal multinodular 115, 116, 117, 118, 119

hyperplasia, numerical, of liver cells 73
hypersensitivity 81
– icterus 95
–, delayed type 59
– reactions 81
hypertension 196, 198, 201
hyperthermia, malignant *50*
hypertriglyceridaemia 34
hypoalbuminemia 26, 31
hypokalaemic nephropathy 146, 173, 217
hypopituitarism 342
hypoprothrombinemia 42
hyposensitisation 56
hyposensitivity 44
hypothermia, controlled 312

IgE antibodies 56, 57, 59
– mediated rhinitis 54
IgG antibodies 56, 57, 58, 156, 158, 165, 172, 189
IgM antibodies 56, 57, 58, 165, 170, 171, 189
idiosyncrasy 81
"idiosyncratic liver lesions" 76
immune complex reactions *58*
– – formtion, in situ 146, 152, 156, 173
– – glomerulonephritis 145, 148, 152, 153, 154, 158, 161, 163, 164, 165, 168, 169, 170, 171, 173
– complexes, circulating 146, 152, 173
– reaction, cell-mediated 152
– type cytotoxic reaction 58
"immunocarcinogenesis" 357
immunodeficiency 356
– syndromes 55
immunosuppressive therapy 356
Imurek 146, 150
incomplete karyokinesis 76
indirect cytotoxic injuries 81
indomethacin 43
infarction, myocardial 3, 6, 8, 10, 13
INH = isonicotinic acid hydrazide *339*
inheritable gene defect 245, 246
insufficiency, renal 147, 149, 162, 172, 184, 196, 201, 202
insulin 36
interference 245
interstitial lung fibrosis 153
– nephritis 162
– –, acute *185*
– –, destructive 222
intrinsic hepatotoxicity 76
iodinated contrast media 57
ionizing irradiation 114
iproniazid 84
irradiation, ionizing 114
isoflurane 336, 337
isoniazid 24, 28, 29, 31, 35, 39, 79, 80, 83, 84, 104, 107, 166, 167
isonicotinic acid hydrazide (INH) *339*, 359

jaundice 18, 50, 80, 93, 95, 97, 100
–, cholestatic 51
– of pregnancy 83, 95
juxtaglomerular apparatus 224, *225*, 234

kaliopenic nephropathy 221
kanamycin 39, 46, 185, 192, 193
karyokinesis, incomplete 76
karyokinetic process 91
kidney disease 39
kryptorchism 342
Kupffer cells 75, 90, 91, 92, 93, 100, 104, 109

labetalol 31
Lactams 359
LE cells 58
lamellar bodies, concentric 73
laryngeal edema, acute 52, 56, 59
lathyrogenic substances 287, 291, 300
laxatives 84, 90, 94, 97, 98, 104, 108, 109, 172, 173, *218*
laurylsylphate 23
leptospirosis 191
lethality 257
leukemia 38, 339, 344, 347, 350, 351, 352
leukaemias 55, 203
leukocyturia 196, 201
leukopenia 56
levamisole 51
Liddle's syndrome 218
lignocaine 29, 31, 37
lincomycin 4, 39, 46
lipid metabolism 34
– peroxidation 75, 78
lipofuscin 71, 74, 75, 104, 226
– -like substances 198, 199, 202
lipofuscinosis 71, 74, 75
lipophagic granulomas 102
lithium 205
litter effect *257*
liver adenoma 110, 111, 112, *115*
– carcinoma 337, 338, 341, 343, 355
– cell necrosis 78, 80, 83, 86, 95, 97, 107, 108, 109

liver cell necroses, single 72, 73, 75, 77, 78, 82, 85, 86, 87, 90, 91, 92, 93, 94, 95, 96, 98, 100, 101, 102, 104, 108, 109
– cirrhosis 30, 31, 43, 106, 107, 109, 340
– –, postdystrophic 86, 107
– –, postnecrotic 86, 107
– –, primary biliary 100, 153
– damage 340
– disease 30, 31
– dystrophy 78, 83
– –, acute 77, 83, 86, 91
– –, cytotoxic 77
– –, subacute 82, 83, 86
– failure, acute 76, 86
– fibrosis 107, 108
– injury, acute *76*
– –, chronic *104*
– –, cytotoxic 77
– necrosis, centrolobular 77, 78, 81, 84, 86, 91, 107, 114
– tumors *115*, 341, 342, 343
– –, benign 4, 9
– –, steroid-induced 112, *115*
local anaesthetics 57
Lopirin *165*
lost-derivatives 359
lucanthone 355
lung fibrosis, interstitial 153
lung tumors 339, 343
lupoid hepatitis 106
lupus erythematosus 351
lupus erythematosus, systemic 29, 54, 153, 154, 158, *166*
lymphoma 107, 108, 203
lymphoma, malignant 338, 350, 356
lymphosarcoma 110
lysergides 359
lysine hydroxylase 287
lysosome-induced necrosis *293*

macrophages 75, 90, 91
macula densa 224, 225, 226
magnesium deficiency 252
malformations 255, 257, 259, 261, 267, 268, 285, 292, 314, 316, 323
Maliasin 168
malignant hyperthermia *50*
malignant lymphoma 338, 350, 356
Mallory bodies 109
MAO = monoamine oxidase 35
– -inhibitors 35, 36, 37
mast-cells 55, 56, 198
M. Banti 109
medroxyprogesterone 33
medullary sponge kidney 203
megaloblastic anaemia 34
meganuclei 76, 104
melanokeratosis 334
membrane-proliferative glomerulonephritis 170
miningitis 27
meningocele 255
meningo-encephalitis 59
mephenytoin 166
meprobamate 31
mercaptobenzothiazole 59
6-mercaptopurine 35, 37, 80, 97, 114, 251, 272, 278, 290, 294, 295, 296, 297, 298, 299, 302, 304, 344
– riboside 277, 286, 320, 321
mercuric salts 145, 162
mercury nephropathy *162*
merthiolate 47
mesangio-proliferative glomerulonephritis 148, 154, 168, 169
mesenchymal reactions 81
metabolic alkalosis 231
metabolites, reactive 81
Metalcaptase 146
methadone 171, 355
metapyrilene 338, 355
– hydrochloride 338
methagualone 33
methemoglobin 48, 201
methicillin 185, 187, 189, 190, 195
methotrexate 80, 102, 107, 109, 110, 344
methoxyflurane 50, 336, 337
3-methylcholanthrene 38
α-methyl-dopa 36, 58, 80, 86, 102, 104, 107, 109, 166, 167
6-methylmercaptopurine riboside 320
methylphenidate 355
methylsergit 166
methyltestosterone 94, 100
methylthiouracil 97, 166
metoclopramide 25
metoprolol 24
metronidazol 359
microangiopathy 198
micrognathia 255
minifocal epithelioid cell reaction 102
minipill 95, 96, 119
mitomycin 80
mithramycin 80
monilial infection 21
monoamine oxidase 35
– – inhibitors 35, 36, 37
mononucleosis 191
morphine 22, 43, 57

multinodular adenoma 110, 111, 115, 116, 117, 119, 121
– hyperplasia 115, 116, 117, 118, 119
multiple sclerosis 351
multivesicular bodies 227, 234
muscular rigidity 50
mushroom poisoning 107
mustard gas 344
N-mustard 344
mutagenic effect *245*, 322
mutagenicity 242, 322
mutation 244
myasthenia gravis 46
myelin bodies 109
myelocele 255
myelooptic neuropathy, subacute 8
myelosuppression 19
myocardial infarction 3, 6, 8, 10, 13
myocarditis 58, 59

NADPH 48
nafcillin 185
nalidixic acid 26
naloxone 46
"Nebenkerne, glatte" 73
necrosis, centrolobular 77, 78, 81, 84, 86, 91, 107, 114
–, tubular 145, 151, 162, 187, 192, 193, 194, 219
Neo-Citrollamin 168
neomycin 46, 193
neonatal alcohol syndrome 244
nephritis, acute interstitial *185*
–, anti-tubular basement membrane 189
–, interstitial 162
–, –, destructive 222
–, potassium-losing 233
–, primarily chronic interstitial *205*
nephrocalcinosis 194
nephrolithiasis 201
nephropathy 18
–, hypokalaemic 146, 173, *217*
nephrosclerosis 230
nephrotic syndrome 145, 147, 149, 151, 152, 154, 157, 158, 159, 162, 164, 165, 168, 170, 173, 191
nephrotoxicity 47
neuroblastoma 336
neurofibroma 344
neurohypophyseal system 231
neuropathy, peripheral 28
nicetamide 355
nickel sulphate 59
nicotinamide 309
– -adenine dinucleotide phosphate (NADP) 309, 310, 312
nicotinic acid 261
niridazole 343, 359
nitrite *355*
nitroazepam 29, 43
nitrofuran 343, 359
nitrofurantoin 24, 40, 48, 53, 57
nitrosamine 73, 355
nitrosatable agents *355*
nitrosoureas 351, 359
N-nitrosurea 251
nitrous oxide 50
nonsensitive icterus 95
noradrenaline 27, 35, 44, 46
norethrandolone 110
norpethidine 37, 38, 40
nortryptyline 37
Novacyl 263
"nuclear unrest" 76

obligatory cholestatic effect 80
– hepatotoxicity 76, 78, 80, 85
oculo-muco-cutaneous syndrome 18
omphalocele 255
oncogenic viruses 357
opiates 46
orcein staining 71
organotropic effects *266*
osteomalacia 18, 34
ototoxicity 39
ovarial tumors, estrogen-secreting 342
ovarian carcinoma 350
ovarian cyst 10
over-additive effect 279
ovulation inhibitors see contraceptives
oxacillin 185
oxidized glutathione 242
h-oxy-nicotinic acid 263
oxyphenbutazone 37
oxyphenisatin 84, 90, 94, 97, 98, 104, 106, 108
oxypurinol 37
oxytetracycline 287, 355

pancreas tumors 343
papillary necrosis, aseptic 196, 199, 200, 201, 202, 203, 204
para-aminosalicylic acid (PAS) 25, 48, 59, 166, 194
paracetamol 24, 29, 30, 31, 37, 38, 78, 85, 86, 97, 107, 196
paradoxical aciduria 232
paraffin oils 359
paraimalintartrate 85, 97, 106
paraldehyde 21
paraphenylendiamine 59
parkinsonism 2, 41, 45

PAS = para-aminosalicylic acid 25, 48, 59, 166, 194
peliosis hepatis 110, 111, 112, 114, 118, 120
–, major form 112
–, minor form 112
D-penicillamine 287, 288, 289, 290
penicillamine 51, 146, *151*, *153*, 166, 168, 169, 173
– nephropathy *153*, 159, 160, 161, 162, 163, 169
– polylysine 159
penicillin 19, 22, 27, 40, 52, 53, 55, 57, 58, 59, 84, 100, 101, 102, 104, 152, 153, 166, 185, 187, 189, 194, 195, 218
– -induced anaphylaxis 1
penicilloic acid 158, 159
– aldehyde 158, 159
penicilloyl determinant 53
– group derivatives 52
pentobarbitone 29, 31
pentose phosphate pathway 313
peptic ulcer 7, 10, 43, 44
peptides 52
perchlorate 146, 152
perhexiline maleate 109
perimembranous glomerulonephritis 154, 155, 156, 157, 158, 159, 160, 162, 163, 164, 165
peritonitis, sclerosing 4
pethidine 31, 36, 37, 38, 40, 57
petrol intoxication 172
phase specifity *266*
phenacetin 18, 23, 37, 47, 48, 74, 75, 78, 194, *196*, 203, 205, 337, 338, 355, 359
– kidney 196
phenelzine 29
pheneturide 33, 35, 166
phenindione 186, 187, 190, 191
phenmetrazine 355
phenobarbital 78, 186, 337, 359
phenobarbitone 24, 29, 31, 33, 37, 38, 40
phenocopia 246, 247
phenolisatin 106, 108
phenolphthalein 219
phenothiazine 27, 36, 41, 45, 46, 312
phenoxybenzamine 46
Phenthrane 337
phenylbutazon 26, 31, 35, 37, 43, 85, 97, 102, 166, 186, 195, 338, 359
β-phenylethylhydrazine sulfane 343, 359
phenyramidole 35
phenytoin 18, 19, 22, 25, 26, 29, 32, 33, 35, 36, 51, 55, 59, 90, 166
– acid 22
– intoxication 22, 35
phocomelia 4
–, thalidomide-induced 3, 4
phospholipidosis, drug-induced 109
photosensitivity 47
photosensitization 53
piecemeal necrosis 109
pigment granules (deposits) 74, 75
pigmentation 199, 202
pill cholestasis 95
piperonylbutoxide 38
pivampicillin 24
placenta 28
plant-like cells 85
plasma cells 55
plasmacytoma 203, 352
– -protein binding 25, 26, 27, 42
– renin 233, 234
pneumonitis 59
polydactyly 267, 273, 301, 302
polyarteriitis nodosa 59
polycyclic hydrocarbons 33
polymyxin B 57, 185, 193, 195
polyneuritis 59
polyvinyl pyrrolidone 359
porphyria *51*
–, acute intermittent 51
portal fibrosis 106, 109
postdystrophic cirrhosis 86, 107
postnecrotic cirrhosis 86, 107
potassium 44
– bichromate 59
– chlorazepate 37
– depletion 43
– -losing nephritis 233
– perchlorate 339
potentiation 279
practolol 4, 18, 22, 24, 166, 167
prednisolone 26
prednisone 26, 31, 47
pregnancy 29, 33
– jaundice 83, 95
prenatal toxicology 243, 245
prepiliosis 112
prick-in skin tests 54
primaquine 48, 49
primary biliary cirrhosis 100
primarily chronic interstitial nephritis *205*
primidone 37, 166
probenicid 146, 151
procainamide 24, 29, 37, 39, 166, 167, 168, 169

procaine 59
procarbazine 359
prochlorperazine 41
progesterone 95, 261, 263, 335
progestogens 341
proliferating glomerulonephritis, chronic 148
– intercapillary glomerulonephritis 151, 171
proline hydroxylase 287
pronethalol 359
propanolol 21, 24, 31, 46
propantheline 25
propylthiouracile 97, 166, 168
probenecid 27, 40
procarbazine 37
prostaglandins 227, 231
prostaglandin synthesis 204, 227, 231
proteinuria 145, 147, 148, 150, 154, 156, 157, 158, 159, 162, 168, 170, 173, 190, 192, 193
pseudo-Bartter's syndrome 226, 229
pseudocholinesterase 50
pseudomembranous colitis 4
pseudoxanthoma 100
psoriasis 107, 109, 334, 351
psychopharmacological agents 71, 72, 73, 86, 87, 97, 104
pulmonary bleeding 172
pulmonary tumors 339, 343
puromycin 147
pyelonephritis 196
–, chronic 203, 223
Pyramidon 355
pyridine nucleotide analogues 310
pyuria 193
–, sterile 201

quinacrine 355
quinidine 24, 40, 46, 48, 58, 102
quinine 41, 48, 58
quinolin 359

Rauwolfia derivatives *352*
reactive metabolites 81
reagin antibodies 56
– -mediated allergy 54
regenerative cell proliferation 76
renal artery stenosis 203
– colic 193, 196
– disease 50
– excretion 39
– failure 21, 29, 225
– –, acute 184, 190, 191, 192, 193, 194, 195
– insufficiency 80, 147, 149, 162, 172, 184, 196, 201, 202
– –, acute 186
– –, chronic 145, 184, 190, 197
– tuberculosis 203
– vein thrombosis 203
renin concentrations 233, 234
renomedullary interstitial cell tumors 227
replication 284
reserpine 36, 116, 353, 359
respiratory disease 22
responsiveness *48*
retinoic acid 269, 270
rhesus factor 58
rheumatoid arthritis *51*, 54, 153, 159
rhinitis 55
–, IgE mediated 54
rickets 18, 34
rifampicin 25, 31, 33, 37, 58, 79, 80, 84, 185, 195
rigidity, muscular 50
ring tests 159
risk pregnancy 256

saccharin *353*, 359
safrole 359
salicylates 24, 40, 43, 202
salicylic acids 27, 33
salvarsan 100
sarcoid-like lesions 102
Saridon nephritis 196
scarlet fever 186
schistosomiasis 343
scleroderma 153
sclerosing peritonitis 4
sclerosis, hepatoportal 109
sedatives *335*
Senecio alkaloids 114
Senecio Fuchsii 343
senna 219
sensitization 53, 57
sepsis 186
serotonin 44, 255
serum sickness syndrome 56, 58, 59, 152
sex hormone metabolism 34
shock 187
– necroses 91
shrinkage necrosis *292*, 295, 296, 297
Shy-Drager syndrome 44
sickle cell anemia 202
single cell necroses 72, 73, 75, 77, 78, 82, 85, 86, 87, 90, 91, 92, 93, 94, 95, 96, 98, 100, 101, 102, 104, 108, 109

skin reactions, allergic 154
– test 57
sklerosis, focal 148
SLE = systemic lupus erythematosus 153, 154, 158, *166*
"slow acetylator" 83
small-for-date-baby 244, 264, 323
smooth endoplasmic reticulum, hypertrophy 70
sodium aurothiomalate 51, 159
– dehydrocholate 57
– valproate 55
sonne dysentery 221
species specifity *273*
spironolactone 24, 37
steroid aerosols 21
– hormones 33, 42, 43, 80, 112, 118, 190
– icterus 95
– -induced cholestasis 95
– – liver tumors, benign 112, *115*
steroids, anabolic 71, 94, 96, 110, 121, 341, *342*
stibophen 58
streptomyces peucetius 149
streptomycin 46, 57, 59, 166, 193
streptozotocin 359
subacute liver dystrophy 82, 83, 86
– myelooptic neuropathy (SMON) 8
succcinamide 166
succinylcholine 46
sulfahemoglobin 201
sulphadiazine-silver *165*
sulphadimethoxine 49
sulphamilamide 47
sulphate ions 28
sulphonamides 29, 48, 49, 51, 52, 54, 58, 97, 102, 166, 185, 187, 189, 193
sulphonylureas 36, 54, 58
sulthiame 35, 36
supersensitivity *44*
suxamethonium 50
– hypersensitivity *50*
sweeteners, artificial 353
swelling necrosis *293*
systemic lupus erythematosus 29, 47, 153, 154, 158, *166*
steady state concentration 22, 27, 32

tannic acid 78
tannin 340, 359
tardive dyskinesia 45
tar ointments 343, 359
Tauredon 159
teratogenesis 18
teratogenic action 243
– effect 242, 243, 244, *245*, 249, 255, 277, 278, 279, 283, *284*, 322, 323
teratogenicity 242, *259*, 323
testosterone 121
tetrachlorodibenzo-p-dioxin 262, 267, 275, 276, 281, 282, 286
tetracycline 24, 39, 46, 47, 80, 85, 166, 187, 193, 219
thalidomide 2, 3, 4, 18, 247, 273, 286
– -induced phocomelia 3, 4
thalassaemia 49
T-helper cells 55
theophylline 31, 314
thiamazol 97
thiamine 57
thiamphenicol 261, 273
thiazide 36, 40, 43, 185, 189, 219
thioacetamide 73
thioquanine 114
thiourazil 59, *339*, 359
thiourea 41
thorotrast 114
thrombocytopenia 154, 159
thrombembolism 8, 9, 10, *51*
thyroid gland cancer 339
thyrostatic drugs 93, 97, 166, 168
T-lymphocytes 54, 55, 59
tobramycin 39, 191, 192
tolazamide 355
tolbutamide 3, 5, 6, 23, 31, 35, 51, 146, 152
– -induced cardiovascular mortality 3, 5
tolerance *44*
o-toluene sulfonamide 354
toxic hepatopathy 77, 80
– liver injuries 81
toxicity 5, 14
toxicology, prenatal 243
tracheo-oesophageal fistula 269
transcription 284
transfusion of incompatible blood 57
translation 284
transplacental carcinogenesis 244, 264, 322, 323, 341
– effect 336
transplants *356*
Trenimon 146, 150
trichloroacetic acid 26
trichloroethylene 336, 337
trichlorophenoxyacetic acid 267, 281, 282
tricyclic antidepressants 27
triethylenebenzoquinidine 146, 150

tridione *164*, 168
trilene 337
trimethadione *164*, 166
– nephropathy *164*
trioxydone 166
Triton WR 1339 252, 261, 263
Trolovol 146
trypan blue 252, 286
Trypanosoma cruzi 147
tuberculosis 112
–, renal 203
tuberculostatic drugs 79, 83, 84, 85, 86, 107, 185, 194, 195
tubocurarine 46, 50, 57
tubular atrophy 222, 224, 225, 231, 233
– necrosis 145, 151, 162, 187, 192, 193, 194, 219
turpentine oil 59
tyramine 35, 36

ulcer, peptic 7, 10
ulcerative colitis 229
uncomplicated cholestasis 95
universal teratogenic action 285
unspecific drug hepatitis 91
– – hepatitis with cholestasis 95
uraemia 26, 40, 172, 193
uretero sigmoidostomy 218, 222
urethan 114, *335*, 359
uricosurics 97
urinary tract infections 199, 201, 202, 225
urticaria 52, 55, 56, 59
urothelium, carcinoma 202
uterine vessels 256
uveitis 190

vaccines 52, 57, 59
vacuolar degeneration 217, 221, 222, 234, 293
vaginal cancer 4, 5, 340
vasculitis 58
–, allergic 189
vinblastin 344
vinylchloride 337
viral hepatitis 91
– –, active chronic 91
– –, chronic 108
– –, fulminating 86
viruses, oncogenic 357
vitamin A 286
– deficiency 252
vitamin D 22, 33, 34
– – deficiency 22
– K 42, 48
voncomycin 39
virus-induced hepatitis 77

warfarin 23, 26, 33, 42
– -resistance 42
whole-body X-ray radiation 344
Wilson's disease 153
Wiscott-Aldrich syndrome 356

Zentropil 168
zinc deficiency 252, 286

Index to Volumes 62–68 Current Topics in Pathology

Volume 62

C.R. Austin, Developmental Anomalies Arising from Errors of Fertilization and Cleavage . . . 3
D. Szöllösi, Oocyte Maturation and Paternal Contribution to the Embryo in Mammals . . . 9
W. Engel, W. Franke, Maternal Storage in the Mammalian Oocyte . . . 29
Ch. Epstein, The Genetic Activity of the Early Mammalian Embryo . . . 53
H.W. Denker, Formation of the Blastocyst: Determination of Trophoblast and Embryonic Knot . . . 59
C. Lutwak-Mann, The Response of the Preimplantation Embryo to Exogenous Factors . . . 83
H. Spielmann, Embryo Transfer Technique and Action of Drugs on the Preimplantation Embryo . . . 87
H.M. Beier, Uterine Secretion Protein Patterns Under Hormonal Influences . . . 105
L. Saxén, M. Karkinen-Jääskeläinen, I. Saxén, Organ Culture in Teratology . . . 123
V.H. Ferm, Teratogenic Effects and Placental Permeability of Heavy Metals . . . 145
O. Bomsel-Helmreich, Experimental Heteroploidy in Mammals . . . 155
A. Gropp, B. Putz, U. Zimmermann, Autosomal Monosomy and Trisomy Causing Developmental Failure . . . 177
J.G. Boué, A. Boué, Chromosomal Anomalies in Early Spontaneous Abortion . 193

Volume 63

Aa, Johansen, Early Gastric Cancer . . . 1
H. Thompson, Pathology of Coeliac Disease . . . 49
K. Elster, Histologic Classification of Gastric Polyps . . . 77
H.T. Enterline, Polys and Cancer of the Large Bowel . . . 95
M.I. Filipe, A.C. Branfoot, Mucin Histochemistry of the Colon . . . 143
R.H. Riddel, The Precarcinomatous Phase of Ulcerative Colitis . . . 179
I.M.P. Dawson, The Endocrine Cells of the Gastro-Intestinal Tract and the Neoplasms which Arise from Them . . . 221
J.M. Skinner, R. Whitehead, Immunological Aspects of Gastro-Intestinal Pathology . . . 259
D.M. Goldenberg, Oncofetal and Other Tumor Associated Antigens of the Human Digestive System . . . 289

Volume 64

S. Widgren, Pulmonary Hypertension Related to Aminorex Intake (Histologic, Ultrastructural, and Morphometric Studies of 37 Cases in Switzerland) . . . 1
J.L. van Lancker, DNA Injuries, Their Repair, and Carcinogenesis . . . 65
C. Thomas, H.J. Steinhardt, K. Küchemann, D. Maas, U.N. Riede, Soft Tissue Tumors in the Rat (Pathogenesis and Histopathology) . . . 129
K. Salfelder, K. Ueda, E.L. Quiroga, J. Schwarz, Visceral Candidosis (Anatomic Study of 34 Cases) . . . 177

Volume 65

H.-V. Gärtner, T. Watanabe, V. Ott, A. Adam, A. Bohle, H.H. Edel, R. Kluthe, E. Renner, F. Scheler, R.M. Schmülling, H.G. Sieberth, Correlations Between Morphologic and Clinical Features in Idiopathic Perimembranous Glomerulonephritis 1
J. Thiele, Human Parathyroid Gland: A Freeze Fracture and Thin Section Study 31
A. Bohle, U. Helmchen, K.E. Grund, H.-V. Gärtner, D. Meyer, K.D. Bock, M. Bulla, P. Bünger, L. Diekmann, U. Frotscher, K. Hayduk, W. Köster, M. Strauch, F. Scheler, H. Christ, Malignant Nephrosclerosis in Patients with Hemolytic Uremic Syndrome. 81
A.M. Novi, Liver Carcinogenesis in Rats After Aflatoxin B_1 Administration . . . 115
J. Schwarz, K. Salfelder, Blastomycosis 165

Volume 66

B. Sandstedt, The Placenta and Low Birth Weight 1
W.-W. Höpker, B. Ohlendorf, Placental Insufficiency 57
L. Olding, Interactions Between Maternal and Fetal/Neonatal Lymphocytes. . . 83
J.P. Kraehenbuhl, C. Bron, B. Sordat, Transfer of Humoral Secretory and Cellular Immunity from Mother to Offspring 105
H. Soma, Single Umbilical Artery with Congenital Malformations. 159
S. Panem, C-Type Virus Expression in the Placenta 175
M. Bibbo, Transplacental Effects of Diethylstilbestrol 191

Volume 67

W. Schlake, K. Nomura, Histogenesis of Carcinoma in the Glandular Stomach of the Rat After B I Resection 1
P. Höhn, Morphology and Morphogenesis of Experimentally Induced Small Intestinal Tumors 69
E. Kunze, Development of Urinary Bladder Cancer in the Rat 145
Ch. Witting, B-Lymphocytes in Carcinogenesis 233

Volume 68

G.T. Simon, Ultrastructure of Acute Inflammation 1
J.B. Hay, H.Z. Movat, Hyperemia, Stasis, and Increase in Vascular Permeability: New Methods for Their Quantitation. 33
P.C. Wilkinson, J.M. Lackie, The Adhesion, Migration and Chemotaxis of Leucocytes in Inflammation 47
J.B. Hay, Kinetics of the Inflammatory Response in Regional Lymph 89
H.Z. Movat, The Kinin System and its Relation to Other Systems. 111
J.O. Minta, H.Z. Movat, The Complement System and Inflammation. 135
R. van Furth, R. Willemze, Phagocytic Cells During an Acute Inflammatory Reaction 179
S. Wasi, H.Z. Movat, Phlogistic Substances in Neutrophil Leukocyte Lysosomes: Their Possible Role in Vivo and Their in Vitro Properties 213
M.C. Cohen, S. Cohen, Cellular Hypersensitivity and Inflammation. 239
M.G. Johnston, J.B. Hay, M.Z. Movat, The Role of Prostaglandins in Inflammation 259

www.ingramcontent.com/pod-product-compliance
Ingram Content Group UK Ltd.
Pitfield, Milton Keynes, MK11 3LW, UK
UKHW052339030826
474029UK00003B/149

* 9 7 8 3 6 4 2 6 7 8 6 3 9 *